New Frontiers in Malaria Research

New Frontiers in Malaria Research

Editor: Gianna Watson

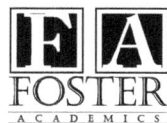

FA
FOSTER
ACADEMICS

www.fosteracademics.com

www.fosteracademics.com

FA FOSTER
ACADEMICS

Cataloging-in-Publication Data

New frontiers in malaria research / edited by Gianna Watson.
      p. cm.
Includes bibliographical references and index.
ISBN 978-1-63242-849-3
1. Malaria. 2. Malaria--Research. 3. Malaria--Prevention. 4. Communicable diseases.
5. Infection. I. Watson, Gianna.
RC156 .N49 2019
616.936 2--dc23

© Foster Academics, 2019

Foster Academics,
118-35 Queens Blvd., Suite 400,
Forest Hills, NY 11375, USA

ISBN 978-1-63242-849-3 (Hardback)

Contents

Permissions

List of Contributors

Index

Preface

Malaria is a chronic infectious disease caused by single-celled microorganisms belonging to the Plasmodium group. It can be caused by five species of Plasmodium, namely, P. falciparum, P. vivax, P. malariae, P. ovale, and P. knowlesi. However, it is most commonly caused by P. falciparum. Its common symptoms include headache, tiredness, vomiting and fever. The microscopic examination of blood by using blood films is the most common diagnostic method. Other diagnostic tests include malaria antigen detection tests and microscopy. Treatment methods include the intake of artemisinin, lumefantrine, mefloquine and sulfadoxine/pyrimethamine. This book will also provide interesting topics for research, which interested readers can take up. It strives to provide a fair idea about malaria and to help develop a better understanding of the latest advances within the field of malaria research. This book includes contributions of experts and researchers, which will provide innovative insights into this disease.

The researches compiled throughout the book are authentic and of high quality, combining several disciplines and from very diverse regions from around the world. Drawing on the contributions of many researchers from diverse countries, the book's objective is to provide the readers with the latest achievements in the area of research. This book will surely be a source of knowledge to all interested and researching the field.

In the end, I would like to express my deep sense of gratitude to all the authors for meeting the set deadlines in completing and submitting their research chapters. I would also like to thank the publisher for the support offered to us throughout the course of the book. Finally, I extend my sincere thanks to my family for being a constant source of inspiration and encouragement.

Editor

Whole genome sequencing and microsatellite analysis of the *Plasmodium falciparum* E5 NF54 strain show that the *var*, *rifin* and *stevor* gene families follow Mendelian inheritance

Ellen Bruske[1], Thomas D. Otto[2,3]* and Matthias Frank[1]*

Abstract

Background: *Plasmodium falciparum* exhibits a high degree of inter-isolate genetic diversity in its variant surface antigen (VSA) families: *P. falciparum* erythrocyte membrane protein 1, repetitive interspersed family (RIFIN) and subtelomeric variable open reading frame (STEVOR). The role of recombination for the generation of this diversity is a subject of ongoing research. Here the genome of E5, a sibling of the 3D7 genome strain is presented. Short and long read whole genome sequencing (WGS) techniques (Ilumina, Pacific Bioscience) and a set of 84 microsatellites (MS) were employed to characterize the 3D7 and non-3D7 parts of the E5 genome. This is the first time that VSA genes in sibling parasites were analysed with long read sequencing technology.

Results: Of the 5733 E5 genes only 278 genes, mostly *var* and *rifin/stevor* genes, had no orthologues in the 3D7 genome. WGS and MS analysis revealed that chromosomal crossovers occurred at a rate of 0–3 per chromosome. *var, stevor* and *rifin* genes were inherited within the respective non-3D7 or 3D7 chromosomal context. 54 of the 84 MS PCR fragments correctly identified the respective MS as 3D7- or non-3D7 and this correlated with *var* and *rifin/stevor* gene inheritance in the adjacent chromosomal regions. E5 had 61 *var* and 189 *rifin/stevor* genes. One large non-chromosomal recombination event resulted in a new *var* gene on chromosome 14. The remainder of the E5 3D7-type subtelomeric and central regions were identical to 3D7.

Conclusions: The data show that the *rifin/stevor* and *var* gene families represent the most diverse compartments of the *P. falciparum* genome but that the majority of *var* genes are inherited without alterations within their respective parental chromosomal context. Furthermore, MS genotyping with 54 MS can successfully distinguish between two sibling progeny of a natural *P. falciparum* cross and thus can be used to investigate identity by descent in field isolates.

Keywords: *var* genes, Recombination, E5, 3D7, NF54, Variant surface antigens, Antigenic variation, Epigenetic, PfEMP1, RIFIN, STEVOR, Microsatellites, Whole genome sequencing, Cross over recombination, Non cross over recombination

*Correspondence: ThomasDan.Otto@glasgow.ac.uk; matthias.
frank@praxis-frank-tuebingen.de
[1] Institute of Tropical Medicine, University of Tuebingen, Wilhelmstr. 27,
72074 Tuebingen, Germany[3] Present Address: Centre of Immunobiology,
Institute of Infection, Immunity & Inflammation, College of Medical,
Veterinary and Life Sciences, University of Glasgow, Glasgow, UK
Full list of author information is available at the end of the article

Background

The malaria parasite *Plasmodium falciparum* is the most prevalent malaria species found on the African continent [1] and is responsible for 90% of deaths from malaria [2]. The NF54 isolate derives from an infection obtained near Schiphol Airport in the Netherlands [3]. Two sibling parasites, 3D7 and E5, were independently isolated by limiting dilution from the original NF54 culture [3, 4]. The 3D7 clone has been used in the malaria genome sequencing project [5], revealing that the *P. falciparum* genome consists of a 23 Mb nuclear genome with 14 chromosomes and around 5500 genes [6]. E5 was incidentally indentified during transfection experiments of the original NF54 culture [4] and has previously been characterized by PCR cloning and gene specific PCR [7]. Whole genome sequencing of *P. falciparum* is complicated by the special properties of the *P. falciparum* genome: it is very AT-rich and contains many repetitive regions and homopolymer runs, especially in its intergenic regions, complicating the assembly of genome data [8–10]. It has recently been shown that the genome can be divided into a core genome (95%) hypervariable regions (5%) [10, 11]. Unambiguous alignments of sequence data of different strains are only possible in the core regions and not in the hypervariable regions that harbour the majority of the variant surface antigen (VSA) gene families [12–14].

To date, five multicopy gene families that encode VSAs have been described in *P. falciparum*: *stevor* (subtelomeric variable open reading frame) [15], *rif* (repetitive interspersed family) [16], *pfmc-2tm* (*P. falciparum* Maurer's clefts two transmembrane) [17], *surfin* (surface associated interspersed genes) [18] and *var* [19]. The best investigated VSA is *P. falciparum* erythrocyte membrane protein 1 (PfEMP1) [6, 20, 21]. PfEMP1 is encoded by the multicopy *var* gene family that consists of about 60 *var* (variability) genes per *P. falciparum* genome [19]. Antigenic variation is primarily mediated by mutually exclusive expression of 1 of the 60 *var* genes per infected red blood cell. The subtelomeric position of most *var* genes [14] predisposes them to recombination contributing to the diversity of PfEMP1 [22]. PfEMP1 is transported to the surface of infected red blood cells and acts as a receptor for the surface receptors on endothelial host cells. This cytoadhesion prevents clearance of the red blood cells by the spleen. Different forms of PfEMP1 possess different binding specificities and individual PfEMP1 variants have been associated with distinct malaria syndromes such as malaria in pregnancy or cerebral malaria [23–28].

In endemic regions, antibodies to PfEMP1 develop early in life have and have been shown to correlate with the development of protective immunity [29]. To escape the human immune response, *P. falciparum* can switch the PfEMP1-variant expressed on the surface of infected red blood cells. Recent investigations also support a role for the non-PfEMP1 VSA proteins in cytoadhesion, antigenic variation and as targets of the human immune response [30–32]. The non-PfEMP1 VSA families are located in close proximity to the *var* genes within the hypervariable regions of the *P. falciparum* chromosomes. The chromosomal position of the VSA gene families thus complicates their genetic analysis. Because of this position the VSA gene families were excluded from a recent extensive analysis of progenies of experimental *P. falciparum* crosses [10].

The aim of this work was to characterize VSA-gene family inheritance in a NF54 clone with WGS technology. To provide a framework to investigate identity by descent (IBD) in field isolates a set of 84 microsatellites was evaluated for its ability to distinguish between the 3D7 and non-3D7 parts of the E5 genome. Microsatellites are variable numbers of tandem repeats in DNA [33]. They have the advantage that they are locus-specific and highly polymorphic. Because most microsatellites are located in non-coding regions they are not subject to purifying selection. The original work by Walliker, Wellems and Su has generated a large repository of MS primers that were originally used to determine the genetic basis of chloroquine resistance [34] and erythrocyte invasion in progeny of experimental genetic crosses [35] as well as multiple other fundamental aspects of *P. falciparum* biology (summarized in Figan et al. [36]). MS flanking drug resistance loci have also been employed to determine the size of genetic sweeps in population based studies [37, 38]. A 12-locus primer set developed by Anderson et al. [39] has been used by many investigators to assess the genetic diversity of field isolates [40, 41]. Recently, Figan et al. [36] identified 12 MS markers that can reliably differentiate progeny from experimental crosses. However, the small number of MS precludes an analysis of chromosomal inheritance. Therefore, here we evaluate a set of 84 microsatellite alleles distributed over the 14 *P. falciparum* chromosomes to type chromosomal regions as 3D7- or non-3D7.

Genome changes in progeny of a *P. falciparum* cross are a consequence of crossover or non-crossover recombination [10, 42]. Crossover recombination represent, a reciprocal exchange between homologous chromosomes during meiosis, whereas non-cross over recombination results in the duplication of a sequence from a donor sites that replaces a sequence at an acceptor site (also referred to as a gene conversion).

The analysis of E5 offered the opportunity to investigate crossover and non-crossover recombination in a natural sibling of the 3D7 genome clone. Zero to three cross- overs per chromosome were identified. VSA gene families were inherited in their respective parental chromosomal background. The chromosomal distribution of VSA genes in E5 was virtually identical to 3D7. The *var* and *rifin/stevor* gene families represented the most genetically distinct parts of the E5 genome. However, only one definite non-crossover recombination event among non-3D7 and 3D7 *var* genes was detected.

Methods

Parasites, cell culture and generation of DNA

The NF54-C2 clone (isogenic with 3D7) [43, 44] and the NF 54 E5 [4] clone were used for in vivo microsatellite typing. Parasites were cultivated in RPMI 1640 medium completed with 10% Albumax concentrate (Gibco), 2 mM Glutamine, 0.05 mg/ml Gentamicin and 25 mM Hepes buffer (Sigma) at 2.5% haematocrit of 0+ erythrocytes from a local blood bank. Culture flasks were kept at 37 °C under standard parasite cell culture conditions (5% O_2, 5% CO_2, 90% N_2). At a parasitaemia of ca. 4%, the erythrocytes were spun down and parasite DNA was extracted from the pellet using the QiAmp DNA Blood Midi Kit according to the manufacturer's manual.

var gene PCR and Sanger sequencing

PCR using *var*-specific primers from Salanti et al. [26] with modifications [44] was carried out using the following conditions: 94 °C 3 min, 94 °C 30 s, 48 °C 45 s for 30× cycles, then 70 °C 30 s, 70 °C 3 min. PCR products were run on a 1% agarose gel, bands were cut out and purified with NucleoSpin® Extract Kit (Macherey–Nagel) according to the manufacturer's protocol. Preparation of the DNA for sequencing was as follows: the reaction mix containing 1× sequencing buffer, 10% Big Dye Terminator v1.1 (Applied Biosystems), sequencing buffer (Applied Biosystems), 125 μM primer, 60% dH$_2$O, 1–5 ng DNA were run with the following conditions: 94 °C 10 s, 50 °C 5 s, 25 cycles, 60 °C 4 min. All samples were purified using a 6.7% Sephadex (w/v) column. Sequences were aligned and a consensus sequence was generated with the help of BioEdit sequence alignment editor (http://www.mbio.ncsu.edu/BioEdit/bioedit.html).

Microsatellite primer selection

For each of the 14 chromosomes microsatellites (MS) were selected with the help of the NCBI map viewer database (http://www.ncbi.nlm.nih.gov/mapview/maps.cgi). The initial selection of MS was based on the unpublished analysis of the 3D7xHB3 cross (kindly provided by Akhil Vaidya, Department of Microbiology and Immunology, Drexel University College of Medicine, Philadelphia, Pennsylvania, USA). A total of 84 MS were evaluated. In order to allow cross reference to MS alleles employed in other MS genotyping investigations 4 microsatellites

evaluated by Anderson et al. [39] were also included. Subsequently, 4 MS per chromosome were selected for the genotyping of E5 and NF54C2. In general, 3 MS were located in subtelomeric regions and 1 in a central chromosomal region. For chromosome 7, 5 MS were chosen. The MS 9B12, located 1.4 Kb downstream the chloroquine (CQ) resistance gene *pfcrt* [38] and MS B5M77, which is located 18.1 Kb upstream of the *pfcrt* locus were also included. 9B12 is highly conserved in chloroquine resistant strains. B5M77 is positioned at the 3' end of the "chloroquine resistance genetic sweep" area and thus exhibits low allele diversity in resistant strains but high allele diversity even in chloroquine sensitive strains [38, 45].

Microsatellite PCR

Microsatellite PCR was performed using the following conditions: 5 μl DNA were used in a 50 μl reaction containing 1× PCR buffer, 1.5 mM MgCl$_2$, 0.08 μM dNTPs and 0.25 μM primer. For fragment analysis, the forward primer was labelled at its 5' end (Eurofins Genomics). Four different dyes were used per chromosome (Table 1). The program was as follows: 94 °C 5 min, 94 °C 20 s, 45 °C 10 s, 40 °C 10 s, 60 °C 30 s, 40×, 65 °C 2 min. PCR products were checked on a 1.5–2% agarose gel.

MS sequence analysis

To verify the MS position, all MS were amplified from NF54 C2 DNA and the reaction products were sequenced. The obtained sequences were manually aligned with the 3D7 MS sequence in the database. Only MS PCR primers pairs that amplified the 3D7 reference sequence were used for the fragment analysis.

Fragment analysis

PCR products were all diluted 1:200 with water. A master mix was prepared with 5 μl H$_2$O and 5 μl Formamide (Hi-Di Life Technologies) and − 0.1 μl Standard (LIZ 500 Life Technologies). Per singleplex reaction 10 μl master mix and 1 μl diluted PCR product were used. For multiplex fragment analysis 10 μl master mix and 1 μl diluted PCR product of each PCR reaction were used. The mix was heated at 95 °C for 3 min and immediately chilled on ice for a few minutes before fragment analysis. Analysis was done in 96-well plates (Biozym Scientific GmbH) with the Applied Biosystems ABI Prism 3130xl Genetic Analyzer and data were evaluated using GeneMapper v 4.1.

Chimera breakpoint PCR

PCR across the breakpoint of the chimeric *var* gene in E5 containing an E5-like half downstream and a part (approx. 3 kb) of the 3D7 *var* gene Pf3D7_083350

Table 1 Microsatellite coordinates on the respective chromosomes, primer sequences and the dyes used are depicted

Chromosome	Microsatellite	Position on chromosome (3D7/NCBI-Map viewer)[centiMorgan]	Fwd rimer (5´-3´)	Rev primer (5´-3´)	Fluorophore
1	C1M38	124812 .. 124973	GCCATATCATCGGTAATAAT	CTGGTTGAATGATCTAAGAA	ATTO 565
	C1M39	182870 .. 183017	GTAAATCGTTAACATATTCAC	CATGTATGATCTATGTCCAAA	ATTO 550
	B7M97	216,927 .. 217,120	TATCTTCAAACGATTTGGAA	ATGGAAGTCTTCTTCATCATG	YY
	C1M13	551434 .. 551570	GGGATATAATATTATGTTATTG	AATCACCTACACGATACAAC	FAM
2	KPG	105,531 .. 105,694	TCTAATAACGTAAGTTCA	TGGAGTAAATATTGTTCA	ATTO 565
	C2M20	147593 .. 147729	CAGGGTTCATGTTATATTGA	AGGAGAACCTCACAGTAAT	ATTO 550
	C2M11	457780 .. 457922	CATTCAAGTGTATTATCATTA	TGCATTTGGAGTGAGCTT	YY
	BM41	772378 .. 772535	CATGTTTATTATGATTGGGAA	TAATGATCCATGTACCTTTCC	FAM
3	C3M29	148906 ..149074	GAGAGCAAAAATGGCAGAAG	TCATTAATCCTCTTAACTACA	ATTO 550
	C3M27	222118 .. 222274	AGTATCATATTTGGTTAGATC	TTTGGTTAACAAATTTCCTAC	PET
	C3M33	502303 .. 502453	CTTATAAAAGAATTACCTGG	TTGTTACATTTTAAATGGTAC	YY
	C3M45	937398 .. 937557	CGAAAAGATAACTTACACATT	AATCATATCATATATGCAAGC	FAM
4	C4M62	108839 .. 109123	GAATTCACTTAAATGTATTTATTTG	GACACAAGTTATTTTGTGAAT	ATTO 565
	C3M35	796589 .. 796807	GGAAATATATATCATACTTGG	TTTTTGGTGTCGGTTATTTT	YY
	B5M109	1011330 .. 1011466	AAAAAAATAAATAATAATAATAAC	TGTGGGGAAATATTTGTCG	ATTO 550
	B5M51	1057107 .. 1057335	AACACAACATATGAATTCTCC	TCTTTCCATCTTTATCGTTC	FAM
5	B5M58	140933 .. 141164	AAATGTTATATCATTTGGGGA	AGTGGATCATATATTTAATGC	NED
	B5M96	232350 .. 232518	ATATCAGGAGTATGGTTTTG	AAAAAAGGCTAGGTAAAATTC	ATTO 565
	C5M12	683546 .. 683730	TCAAAGTATAAATATAACCAC	CTAATAAGGTTGATGTTACTTCC	YY
	B5M94	1212784 .. 1212947	GGGTTCTTAATATTTTTTACC	CATATCAAAATTCATCATTTCT	FAM
6	BM70	258517 .. 258701	GGAAAATATCCCAGAAAAGG	GGAACAAAAAAAAAAAGGAAA	FAM
	Ta109	800986 .. 801159	GGTTAAATCAGGACAACAT	CCTATACCAAACATGCTAAA	YY
	TA1	899,844 .. 900,029	CCGTCATAAGTGCAGAGC	TTTTATCTTCATCCCCACA	ATTO 550
	Ta24	1101542 .. 1101734	CATAGATACATCAAACATAA	TAAATAAAAATTTATTCCTG	ATTO 565
7	B5M77	290289 .. 290433	TAAAGTCTTTCAATACATATG	GAAATAATTTCATATACACAC	ATTO 565
	9B12	313,056 .. 313,217	ATATATTCCAGTATGTTCGC	AATGATACAATGGGATTTAC	
	C13M30	599702 .. 599908	CCTTTTGGGGTTTAAATGTA	TGGAGATGGAACATGGAAAA	YY
	BM51	1030760 .. 1030899	TAATAATATTAATGGTGGTGA	TAATTGTATGACTTCGAGAAT	NED
	ebp	1271522 .. 1271662	TTCACAAGCCAAATATCA	ATTCATAACTCCTTCAGA	FAM
8	hrp2	98739 .. 98901	CGTAAGCATTTTAATTGCA	TAAATGCGGAATTATTCTA	ATTO 550
	BM5	123670 .. 123810	GAAAGTAGATTGTAGTATTTA	TACACATGAATGATTTAATCA	FAM
	BM16	575427 .. 575586	GCTCCTCAATAAATTGTTAT	TCTGTTGCCTCTCAGACAAT	YY
	BM62	1201795 .. 1201968	TCTGATGGTATAACCAGATAC	GATATAGCGAATTCTTAAGAG	ATTO 565
9	B7M57	125063 .. 125286	GTAAGAATAGATTTAACAAATG	AAGAGAAAGAGAGAAAAAATG	FAM
	C9M103	743822 .. 743972	ATTAGATATTTATAATGAACGG	ATGTGTACGTGTCGAATACT	ATTO 550
	BM54	817042 .. 817208	GATGAATATTATGAGGAAAAC	TCATCATAATTAACAATATGG	YY
	C9M43	1430410 .. 1430541	GACACACATATAGTAATAGA	GATATACATATATGGACATAT	ATTO 565
10	C4M3	57991 .. 58168	GTTGTTTCGGCAATTTACCT	TTAATGCAATTTATTATCAC	ATTO 565
	B7M101	194437 .. 194637	TATATGGAAGTTTTCTTCAGG	CTATGTTTATGTTAATTATTGC	ATTO 550
	B7M46	763306 .. 763479	AGCCATTCGTAAACTGCCT	CACTATCAATATAAGTATCC	YY
	ta40	1322577 .. 1322793	AAGGGATTGCTGCAAGGT	CATCAATAAAATCACTACTA	FAM
11	Ta119	627614 .. 627856	TCCTCGATTATATTATTGCA	TAATACATTCCCATTAGATG	ATTO 565
	C12M110	1515255 .. 1515393	GATGATAAATATGCACCCATC	TTCATGTATATGCATATATAC	YY
	ta117	1790958 .. 1791137	ATCTCTACCTCAACCACCA	TGTGTTACCACCATTGTTA	ATTO 550
	Resa2	1990946 ..1991063	CTATTTGTTTATAGTTATGTA	TTTAATGTAGTGTCATGAA	FAM
12	C12M30	0	CTTCAATAAGGGAAAATCCA	TAATAGTAAGTAAAGTCACA	ATTO 550
	TA121	168703 .. 168863	ACTTGTCAAGTGCTCATCA	TTTGTAATTTTCACTAGGAT	FAM
	Ta34	1144887 .. 1145007	AACATAGCCAAATCGCAC	CCATTTGATGTGTCATCAC	YY
	Ta48	2032882 .. 2033158	TTTTGATATCTCTCAATCAT	CTTCACGACAGAGGTGTC	ATTO 565
13	B8M6	703669 .. 703794	ATGATGCAGAAAAGAATAAAT	GTGATGGTTTCTCAAATTTGG	FAM
	C1M70	1457131 .. 1457306	ATATCGAAAGGTGAATAGAAA	ATAATTAATATGGTCATATGG	YY
	ta60	2584963 .. 2585166	CTCAAAGAGAAATAATTCA	AAAAAGGAGGATAAATACAT	ATTO 565
	C14M35	2664073 .. 2664255	ATCCCTACATGAATAAAATG	TCCCTTATGTATACTTCCAC	ATTO 550
14	C14M59	125828 .. 126006	AGTACAAAGAAGTATATCCAT	CTTATAATAGATAAATGTGTC	ATTO 565
	RHO1	419854 .. 420048	TGTAAAAAATAGACATTTCA	AAAAACGAAAATACAACCAA	FAM
	Ta88	1610557 .. 1610781	CTGGTAACGATGGAAAAGC	TACGCTTATTGTTATTACTCA	YY
	Pf9607	2315888 .. 2315994	TTTAAAGACCGATCATCA	AGTAGCACAACAATAACA	ATTO 550

upstream was done using the primers PFE5_F1 (5'-CGC CATAGTATCACCAATGC-3') and PF3D7083350_R2 (5'-CCCGACGTGGTACACCTG-3') with the following conditions: 3 min 94 °C, 10 s 94 °C, 30 s 56 °C, 30 s 72 °C, 3 min 72 °C, 40 cycles, using 5 μl DNA template (concentration up to 5 ng), 2.5 μM primer, 0.2 mM MgCl₂, 0.2 mM dNTPs. PCR products were checked on an 1% agarose gel.

Whole genome sequencing

Illumina
Genomic DNA of E5 was sheared into 250–350 bp fragments by focused ultrasonication [Covaris Adaptive Focused Acoustics technology (AFA Inc., Woburn, USA)]. An amplification-free Illumina library [46] was prepared and sequenced on a Illumina GAII (150 bp) platform according to the manufacturer's standard sequencing protocol. Reads were mapped with smalt (ftp://ftp.sanger.ac.uk/pub/resources/software/smalt/,parameter–x–a 1000). Variants were called with gatk against the *P. falciparum* version 3 assembly from geneDB [47, 48].

Pacific bioscience reads
From the same DNA, SMRTbell template library using the Pacific Biosciences issued protocol (20 kb Template Preparation Using BluePippin Size-Selection System) were generated. Five SMRT cells were sequenced on the PacBio RS II platform using P5 polymerase and chemistry version 3. Raw sequence data were deposited in the European Nucleotide Archive under accession number ERS500965.

Sequence processing
Sequence data from the SMRT cells were assembled with HGAP. As expected genome size 23.5 Mb was used. Next, the contigs were further improved with IPA (https://github.com/ThomasDOtto/IPA). The script performs following steps: delete small contigs, identify overlapping contigs with low Illumina coverage, order contigs against the *P. falciparum* 3D7 reference using ABACAS2 [49], corrects errors with Illumina reads using iCORN2 [50], circularizes the two plastid genomes with circulator [51] and renames the chromosomes and contigs. The draft genome was annotated with companion [52], using *P. falciparum* 3D7 version 3 from October 2015 as reference.

Bioinformatic sequence analysis
Using Artemis [53] and bamview [54], a free genome browser and annotation tool, and the Artemis Comparison Tool (ACT) [54, 55], a pairwise comparison tool of DNA sequences from the Wellcome Trust Sanger Institute (Hinxton, UK) to visualize similarities and differences between genomes, the genome of 3D7 (serving as reference) was compared with E5. By laying one sequence over the other, coverage and single nucleotide polymorphism (SNP) maps of the E5 reads over the 3D7 genome can be loaded into the program. The SNP map served as a tool to detect differences between 3D7 and E5. Areas with low SNP frequency and even Illumina read coverage were defined as 3D7 chromosomal areas. To find shared proteins between PfE5 and Pf3D7, they were compared (ignoring alternative splicing) with a BLASTp (E-value cutoff 1e−6) and then clustered with orthomcl version 1.4, default parameter [56].

Results

Analysis of chromosomal inheritance in E5
To characterize chromosomal regions of E5 as 3D7 or non-3D7 a set 84 MS primer pairs was evaluated for multiplex PCR with fluorescent probes. First, all MS were amplified under the same set of PCR conditions from 3D7 DNA. Most of the reactions resulted in a clear product after gel electrophoresis. Sanger sequencing and manual alignment of the sequences to the 3D7 reference genome showed that 57 of the 84 MS PCR fragments could be unambiguously aligned to the target MS sequence, whereas 27 MS resulted in sequences that either did not amplify or could not be aligned with the target sequence (Additional file 1).

57 MS were, therefore, employed for genotyping (Table 1). All MS were amplified from E5 and 3D7 DNA and MS length was determined by capillary fragment analysis. Each chromosome was characterized at 4–5 MS loci. An MS allele was designated as 3D7-type, if the fragment length difference was ≤3 bp between E5 and 3D7. E5 had 37 3D7-type and 20 non-3D7 MS alleles (Table 2). On chromosomes 1, 3, 6 and 9 all MS alleles were 3D7-type. The remaining 10 E5 chromosomes were composed of 3D7 and non-3D7 MS alleles. The pattern of MS allele distribution suggested that large chromosomal haplotypes were inherited together, however the distant spacing of the MS markers precluded fine scale mapping. The latter was only achieved for the area of chromosome 7 that harbours the chloroquine resistance gene *pfcrt*. The microsatellites 9B12, located 1.4 Kb downstream of *pfcrt* [34, 45] and B5M77, located 18.1 Kb upstream of this locus, had 3D7-type alleles in E5. Thus, MS in the "genetic sweep" area were the same in E5 and 3D7, suggesting that in both clones this chromosomal fragment was inherited as a 3D7-type haplotype.

To further evaluate chromosomal inheritance we next characterized E5 and 3D7 with a 3D7 specific *var* gene primer set. This revealed overall good correlation between the presence of 3D7 *var* genes and 3D7 MS alleles in the respective chromosomal areas (Table 2).

Table 2 Genotyping based on microsatellite fragment length and 3D7 specific *var* gene PCR

Chromosome	MS	*Var* gene	Expected length (NCBI)	Length 3D7	Length E5
1		PF3D7_0100100			
		PF3D7_0100300			
	C1M38		160	165	165
	C1M39		150	151	151
	B7M97		194	190	190
	C1M13		137	136	136
		PF3D7_0115700			
2		PF3D7_0200100			
	KPG		161	167	163
	C2M20		127	139	123
	C2M11		143	139	139
	BM41		158	159	159
		PF3D7_0223500			
3		PF3D7_0300100			
	C3M29		169	ich	174
	C3M27		157	160	160
	C3M33		151	150	150
	C3M45		210	160	160
		PF3D7_0324900			
4		PF3D7_0400100			
		PF3D7_0400400			
	C4M62		285	291	221
		PF3D7_0412900			
		PF3D7_0413100			
		PF3D7_0412400			
		PF3D7_0412700			
	C3M35		219	216	174
		PF3D7_0420900			
		PF3D7_0420700			
		PF3D7_0421100			
		PF3D7_0421300			
	B5M109		137	140	158
	B5M51		229	227	214
		PF3D7_0425800			
		PF3D7_0426000			
5		PF3D7_0500100			
	B5M58		232	236	215
	B5M96		169	173	173
	C5M12		185	183	183
	B5M94		164	163	131
6		PF3D7_0600200			
		PF3D7_0600400			
	BM70		185	185	185
		PF3D7_0617400			
	Ta109		174	173	174
	Ta1		168	188	188
	Ta24		193	194	194
		PF3D7_0632500			
		PF3D7_0632800			
7		PF3D7_0700100			
	B5M77		145	148	148
	9B12		165	160	160
		PF3D7_0711700			
		PF3D7_0712300			
		PF3D7_0712400			
		PF3D7_0712600			
		PF3D7_0712800			
		PF3D7_0712900			
	C13M30		207	205	205
	BM51		140	144	140
	ebp		141	138	138
		PF3D7_0733000			
8		PF3D7_0800100			
		PF3D7_0800200			
		PF3D7_0800300			
	hrp2		163	163	164
	BM5		141	140	140
		PF3D7_0808600			
		PF3D7_0808700			
		PF3D7_0809100			
	BM16		160	159	159
	BM62		174	176	164
		PF3D7_0833500			
9		PF3D7_0900100			
	B7M57		224	225	225
	C9M103		151	154	154
	BM54		167	167	167
	C9M43		132	134	134
		PF3D7_0937600			
		PF3D7_0937800			
10		PF3D7_1000100			
	C4M3		178	179	174
	B7M101		201	204	185
	B7M46		174	170	151
	Ta40		217	215	212
		PF3D7_1041300			
11		PF3D7_1100100			
		PF3D7_1100200			
	Ta119		243	247	247
	C12M110		139	160	134
	Ta117		180	181	180
	Resa2		118	115	115
		PF3D7_1150400			
12	C12M30		158	114	114
		PF3D7_1200100			
		PF3D7_1200400			
		PF3D7_1200600/ var2csa			
	Ta121		161	158	164
		PF3D7_1219300			
	Ta34		121	116	117
		PF3D7_1240300			
		PF3D7_1240400			
		PF3D7_1240600			
		PF3D7_1240900			
	Ta48		277	276	270
		PF3D7_1255200			
13		PF3D7_1300100			
		PF3D7_1300300			
	B8M6		126	122	125
	C1M70		176	174	174
	ta60		204	206	199
	C14M35		183	181	151
		PF3D7_1373500			
14	C14M59		179	181	158
	RHO1		195	195	195
	Ta88		225	223	223
	Pf9607		107	111	111

Table 2 (continued)

The MS individual fragment lengths are shown for 3D7 and E5 as well as for the in silico 3D7 microsatellite lengths in the NCBI database. MS alleles with > 3 bp size difference between 3D7 and E5 are typed as non-3D7 (grey). 3D7 alleles are white, non-3D7 alleles are grey. 3D7 *var* gene amplification on E5 DNA was verified by targeted Sanger sequencing of PCR fragments. Note that the table differs from Table 1 in Frank et al. [7] at the 5′ end of Chromosome 7 (reannotation of PF3D7_0700100 previously Mal8P1.220) and at the 3′ end of Chromosome 13: PF3D7_1373500 (previously MAL13P1.356)

However, in a few telomeric areas MS and *var* gene typing did not correlate. This was most noticeable on chromosome 7 (*ebp*), 8 (*hrpII*) and 12 (C12M30) where the MS genotyping suggested a 3D7 chromosomal haplotype but the adjacent 3D7 *var* genes were not amplified from E5.

Comparison of the PCR fragment lengths of the 57 MS after amplification on 3D7 DNA with the "in silico" length of the respective MS in the 3D7 genome (version 3) revealed, that 21 MS exhibited a size difference of > 3 bp thus raising the question of the validity of some of the MS typing results.

To validate the MS and *var* gene haplotyping results E5 was characterized by whole genome Illumina sequencing resulting in a E5 genome with > 100× coverage. Mapping of E5 onto the 3D7 reference sequence revealed areas with many SNPs and low coverage, which were defined as non-3D7 (E5-type) and areas with only few SNPs and even median coverage which were regarded as 3D7-type (Fig. 1a). Fragment analysis as well as WGS both showed the same pattern of cross overs in chromosomes 1–14 in clone E5 (compared to 3D7 reference) (Fig. 1b) and confirmed that chromosomes 1, 3, 6 and 9 of E5 were identical with 3D7 and thus appeared to have been inherited without cross overs. In the remaining 10 chromosomes between one to three cross overs per chromosome were detected by Illumina WGS. WGS haplotyping of the telomeric areas of chromosome 7, 8 and 12 typed these areas as non-3D7, confirming the *var* PCR genotype. In contrast MS genotyping of the same areas (*ebp*, *hrp2* and C12M30) showed identical alleles between E5 and 3D7 suggesting a 3D7-haplotype. Together the data suggested that these 3 MS were not sufficiently diverse to allow haplotyping of sibling parasites and they were, therefore, excluded from further analysis. In summary, 54 MS allele typing results were confirmed by WGS as being 3D7 or non-3D7. Overall, the MS and WGS data showed that genetic exchange in the progeny of a natural genetic cross occurred at a rate of 0–3 crossover per chromosome. Allthough *var* gene fragment haplotyping correlated well with microsatellite and WGS haplotyping the Illumina read length precluded a exact anaylsis of VSA gene family inheritance in E5.

Anaylsis of VSA gene family inheritance in E5

Short read assemblies do not permit the accurate assembly of non-reference subtelomeric regions, therefore VSA family inheritance in E5 was assessed by long read Pacific Bioscience sequencing technology. This resulted in an assembly of 58 contigs. Using IPA, the number of contigs was reduced to 29, including the apicoplast and mitochondrial genomes, resulting in a total assembly length of 23.3 Mb.

Annotation of the assembly generated 5733 genes (Table 3). Overall the E5 genome showed a highly conserved structure compared to the 3D7 reference genome. Of the 5733 E5 genes all except 278 had orthologues in the 3D7 genome. These 278 genes were, therefore, designated as singletons (Fig. 2). The *rifin/stevor* and *var* families had 58 singletons and 11 singletons respectively and together represented the largest group of genes with known function among the singletons (Additional file 2).

The Pacific Bioscience genome assembly confirmed the Illumina haplotyping and furthermore enabled a detailed analysis of the chromosomal areas harbouring VSA gene families. VSA family genes consisted of: 62 full length *var* genes (61 LARSFADIG motifs), 32 *var* pseudo-genes, 189 *rifin/stevor* genes, 20 *rifin/stevor* pseudo-genes, 8 *sur-fins*, 6 *Pfmc-2TM* genes and 2 *Pfmc-2TM* pseudo-genes. Comparison of the Pacific Bioscience E5 genome with the 3D7 genome showed that the VSA antigen families have virtually the same size (Table 4). Both clones share the same distribution of VSA genes into subtelomeric and central regions as 3D7 (genome sequence vs.3) (Fig. 3). One miss-assembly in the first *var* gene cluster of chromosome 4 was detected (Additional file 3).

3D7 VSA genes were surrounded by 3D7-type chromosomal areas. Similarly, the non-3D7 (E5 specific) VSA sequences mapped to non-3D7 chromosomal areas. Interestingly for the E5 part that is identical to 3D7 the majority was co-linear with the respective areas in 3D7. Only one large scale recombination event was detected in the 3D7-type subtelomeric regions of E5 (see below).

Based on the Pacific Bioscience assembly the correlation of telomeric MS genotype and *var* gene genotyping was reevaluated (Fig. 3). Of the 54 MS, 27 were located in vicinity of telomeric regions (distance range 50–1,000,000 kb from the telomeres). 11 MS carried 3D7 alleles and 16 non-3D7 alleles. In 26 of the corresponding 27 telomeric areas the *var* gene alleles correlated with the MS alleles. The only exception was the 5′ end of

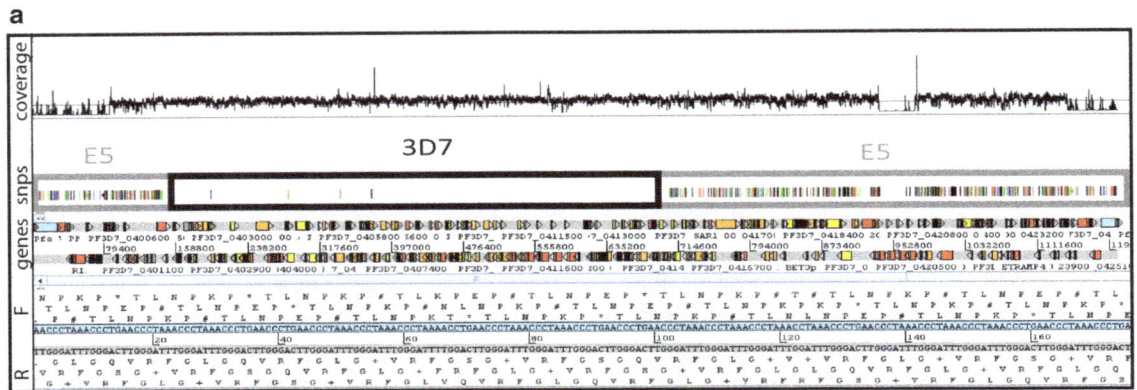

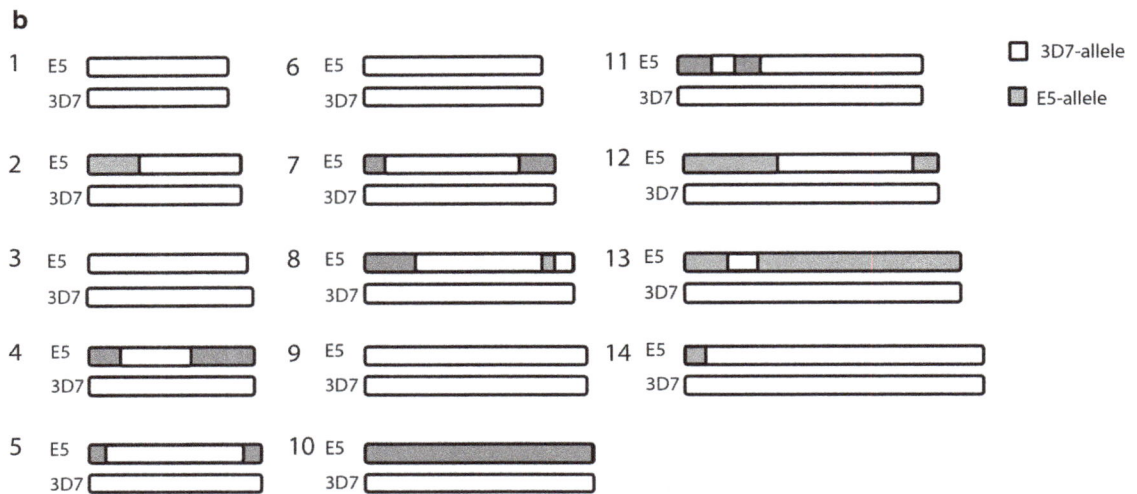

Fig. 1 a 3D7 Artemis view of chromosome 4 showing snp plots and coverage in comparison to E5. Areas with many SNPs and low coverage were defined as non-3D7 (E5-type), those with only few SNPs and a high coverage were regarded as 3D7-type. **b** Chromosome map deriving from illumina whole genome sequencing data showing putative crossovers in the individual chromosomes of 3D7 compared to E5. 3D7-alleles are depicted in white, parts distinct from 3D7 ("E5-alleles") in grey

Table 3 *Plasmodium falciparum* NF54 E5 genome characteristics

Number of annotated regions/sequences	29
Number of genes	5733
Gene density (genes/megabase)	240.97
Number of coding genes	5607
Number of pseudogenes	126
tRNA	105
Overall GC%	19.28
Coding GC%	23.9

chromosome 11 that carried non-3D7 *var* genes but the next MS TA119 located at approximately 600 kb had a 3D7 allele. WGS showed that a chromosomal crossover had occurred 5′ to TA119. WGS and MS data thus clearly

showed that *var* gene inheritance followed a Mendelian pattern.

To estimate the contribution of non-crossover recombination to VSA diversity the *var* gene family of E5 was evaluated. E5 specific *var* genes that shared sequences between 50 and 500 bp with 3D7 were identified and then manually verified using the ACT program. This identified one previously described *var* gene in E5 (PfE5_120005800) that shares 105 bp with Pf3D7_0937800 that is present in E5 and 3D7 on chromosome 9.

A new chimera (preliminary nomenclature: PfE5_232200) was located on chromosome 14. It shares one half of exon 1 of the *var* gene Pf3D7_0833500 (MAL7P1.212, approx. 3 kb) and the remainder of the subtelomeric area with 3D7. The rest of the *var* gene is E5-specific (Additional file 4). The same but complete

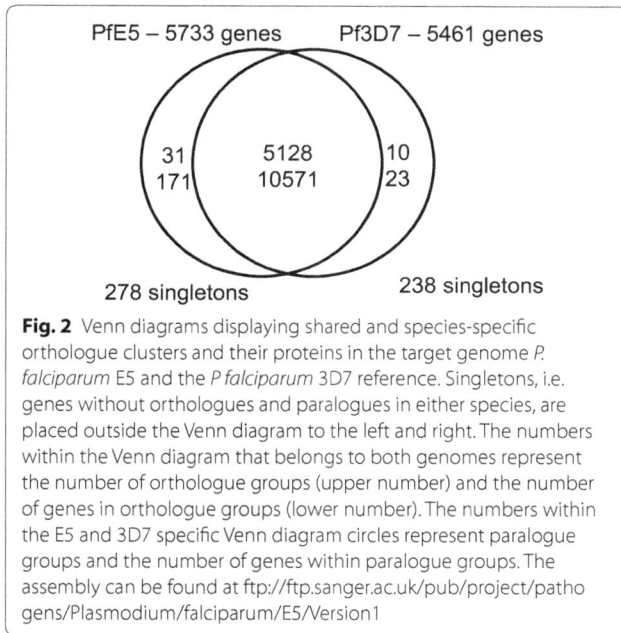

Fig. 2 Venn diagrams displaying shared and species-specific orthologue clusters and their proteins in the target genome *P. falciparum* E5 and the *P falciparum* 3D7 reference. Singletons, i.e. genes without orthologues and paralogues in either species, are placed outside the Venn diagram to the left and right. The numbers within the Venn diagram that belongs to both genomes represent the number of orthologue groups (upper number) and the number of genes in orthologue groups (lower number). The numbers within the E5 and 3D7 specific Venn diagram circles represent paralogue groups and the number of genes within paralogue groups. The assembly can be found at ftp://ftp.sanger.ac.uk/pub/project/pathogens/Plasmodium/falciparum/E5/Version1

Table 4 3D7 and E5 VSA-gene families

VSA-gene family	Genes in 3D7	Genes in E5
var (≥ 4 kb)	61	62
rifin + stevors	190	189
pfmc-2tm	12	6
Surfin	7	8

3D7 data was retrieved from GeneDB [47]

var gene Pf3D7_0833500 is also found on chromosome 8 of 3D7 and E5. PCR analysis across the breakpoint in E5, coming from the E5-specific part of the *var* gene and going into the 3D7-type *var* gene, yielded a product and thus verified the result in vivo (Fig. 4). Together the data suggest that the telomeric end of chromosomes 14 up to the middle of the *var* gene is duplicated. Both chimeric genes thus appear to have resulted from a partial duplication of a 3D7 *var* gene.

Discussion

3D7 and E5 were both cloned from the original NF54 isolate [3, 4] and thus represent progeny of a natural genetic cross. Although the parents of this cross are not known, a previous analysis of 32 progeny of the 7G8XGB4 experimental cross [57] has shown that the two parental genomes are inherited on average at a ratio of 1:1 per progeny. Given that approximately 50% of the E5 genome is identical to 3D7 this suggests that 3D7 is isogenic with one parent of this cross. Thus, analysis of E5 allowed an

assessment of chromosomal crossovers as well as non-crossover recombination in a progeny clone of a natural genetic cross.

In this work, the E5 genome was characterized with MS genotyping as well as short and long read WGS techniques. All genotyping approaches suggested a chromosomal recombination rate of 0–3 crossovers per chromosome, consistent with previously reported crossover rates in progeny of experimental genetic crosses [10, 57]. Similarly, all methods indicated that inheritance of VSA gene families occurred within the context of the respective parental haplotypes. A comprehensive analysis of VSA inheritance was however only possible with long read Pacific Biosciene WGS, because the readlength of > 8000 base pairs enabled an accurate assembly of the highly variable telomeric and central chromosomal parts that harbour the VSA gene families. This analysis showed that the VSA gene families have almost the same number of genes in E5 and 3D7.

Annotation of the E5 genome revealed a total of 5733 genes. This number is slightly higher than the 5500 genes in the 3D7 reference genome and is explained by the fact that companion annotation tool overpredicts open reading frames [52]. Genome wide comparison by orthomcl-analysis revealed that the E5 and 3D7 genomes consisted of > 95% genes that had orthologues in both genomes. Only approximately 4% of the E5 and 3D7 genes were singletons and the *rifin/stevor* and *var* genes represented the largest group of genes with known functions among the singletons. Despite this, the total number of identified singleton *var* genes was lower in the orthomcl-analysis than the number of unique E5 *var* genes identified by direct sequence alignment. The underestimation of *var* gene diversity by the orthomcl-analysis is likely due to highly conserved exon II sequences. Overall the data are clearly consistent with the previously reported high genetic diversity of VSA gene families compared to the highly conserved *P. falciparum* core genome.

The *var* gene family has long been shown to be prone to recombination during meiosis [7, 42, 58–60] and mitosis [9, 61, 62]. Furthermore, several investigations have recently quantified mitotic *var* gene recombination rates [9, 62] in different strains. Analysis of the 3D7 and E5 genomes revealed that E5 had a total of 62 *var* genes (compared to 61 *var* genes in the 3D7 reference genome). The "additional" new *var* gene was generated by recombination between a 3D7 *var* gene on chromosome 8 and an E5 specific *var* gene on chromosome 14. 3D7 has no full *var* gene on chromosome 14, but recently Otto et al. showed that 8 of 10 field isolates carry a *var* gene in this subtelomere of chromosome 14 [11]. This shows that non-chromosomal recombination can expand the *var* gene repertoire of individual strains but that the sites of

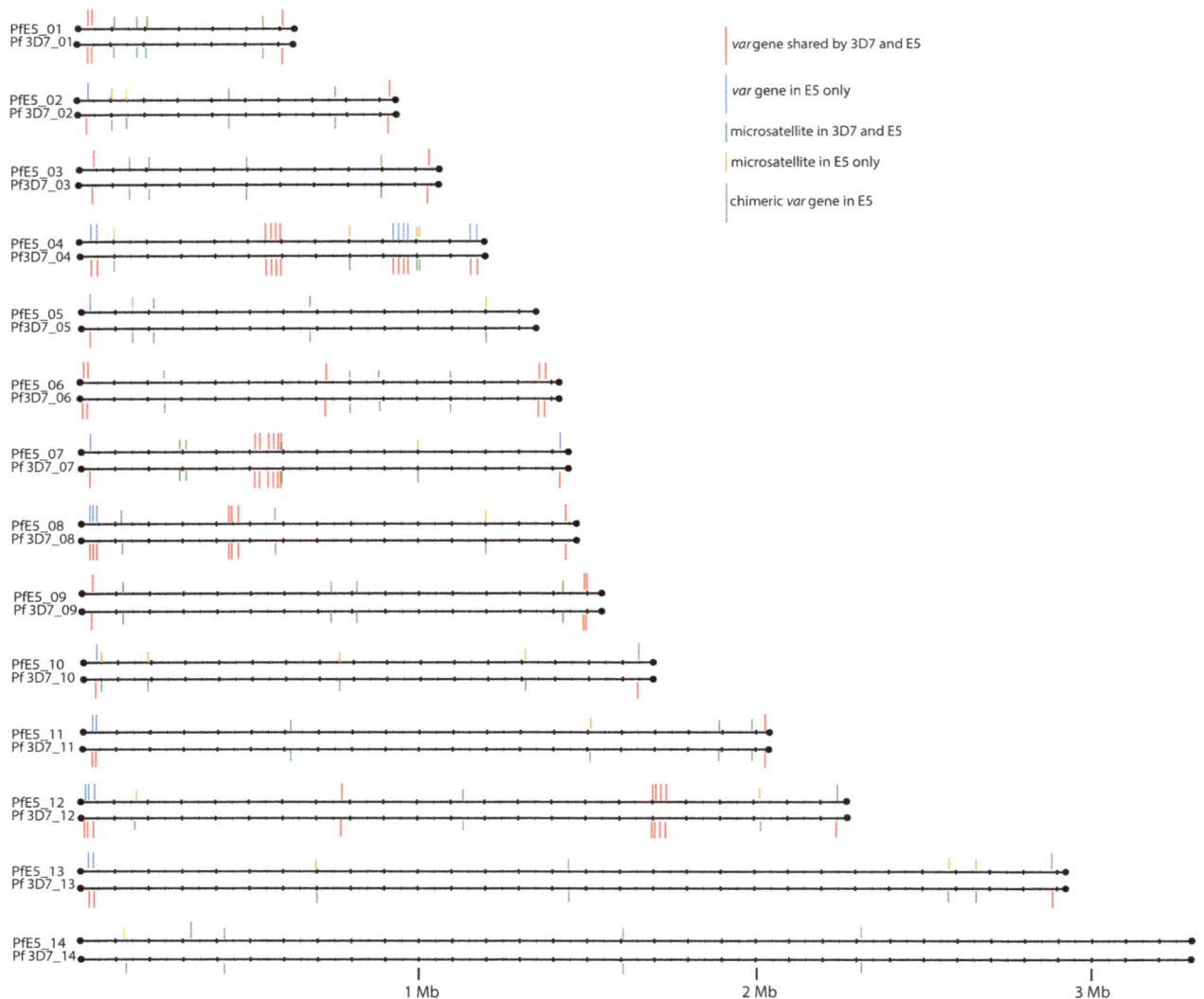

Fig. 3 E5 and 3D7 have the same *var* gene distribution into telomeric repeats and central clusters. *var* genes that are identical between E5 and 3D7 are coloured in red. *var* genes only found in E5 are blue. MS that are identical between E5 and 3D7 are coloured in green. MS that are only found in E5 are coloured in orange. The E5 chimeric *var* gene on chromosome 14 is depicted in grey. Note that for clarity reasons only the *var* genes are depicted. The exact chromosomal location of the *rifin/stevor* gene positions can be found at ftp://ftp.sanger.ac.uk/pub/project/pathogens/Plasm odium/falciparum/E5/Version1

these changes appear to be conserved across different isolates. The presence of an intact "3D7 donor" sequence suggests that the chimeric *var* gene is the result of a gene conversion event as it has been reported previously for the *var* gene family [42, 61]. Recently Calhoun et al. [63] showed that experimentaly induced double stranded breaks are repaired by the "telomerase healing" pathway. Indeed their work showed a similar non-crossover recombination event resulting in the replacement of a chromosome 13 telomere by a chromosome 9 telomere, thereby creating a new chimeric *var* gene on chromosome 13. The data presented here thus support a role

for telomere healing in the generation of VSA gene family genetic diversity. A previously described chimeric *var* gene sequence [7] that carries a 105 bp 3D7 fragment within the DBL of the E5 *var* gene was reidentified in the current analysis and the corresponding "3D7 donor" *var* gene was localized to chromosome 9. This chimeric sequence is located within a hypervariable DBL block that has been shown to exhibit high sequence variability in field isolates [64]. Larger population based studies with long read WGS are necessary to determine if this type short chimeric sequence represent

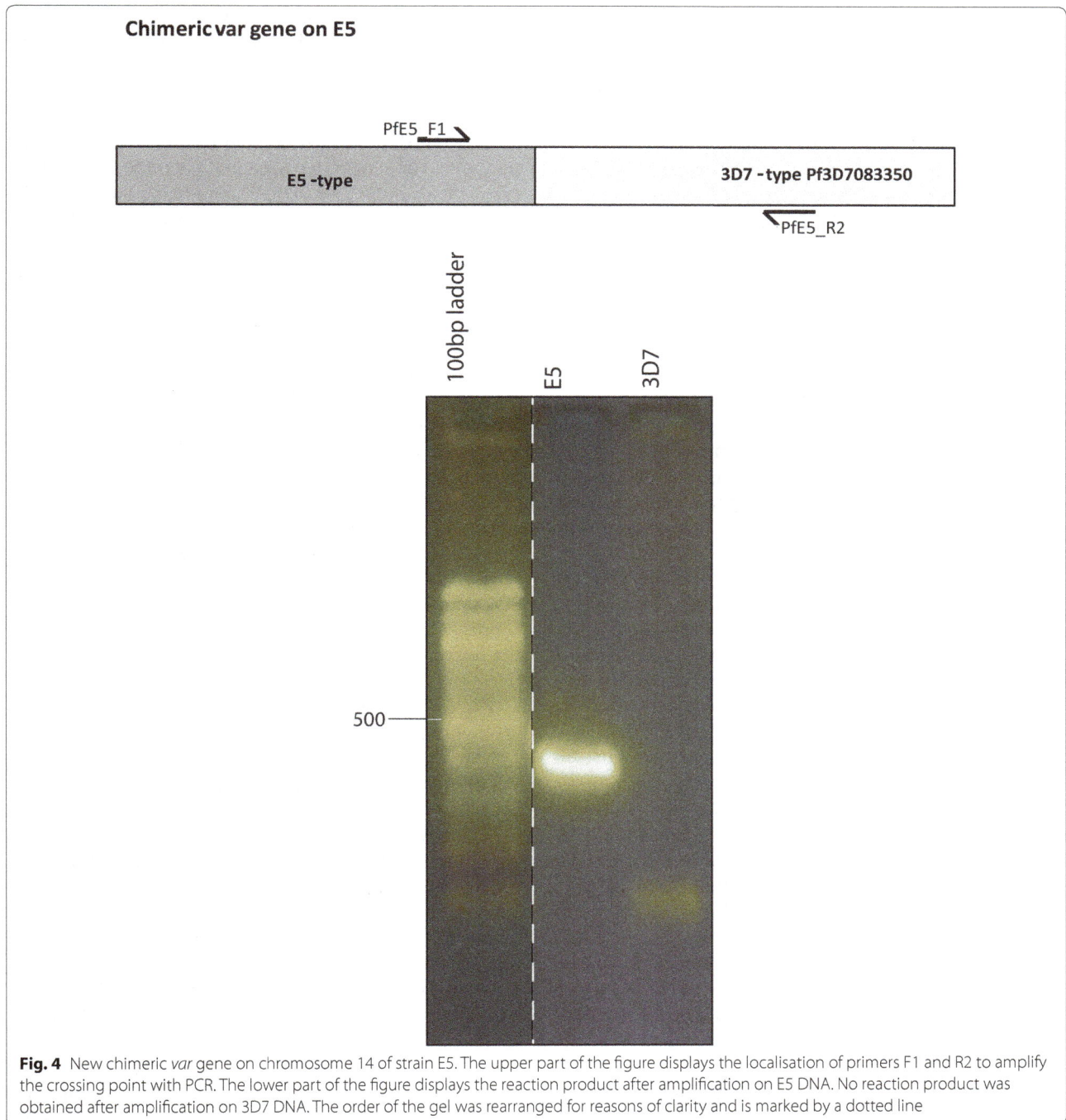

Fig. 4 New chimeric *var* gene on chromosome 14 of strain E5. The upper part of the figure displays the localisation of primers F1 and R2 to amplify the crossing point with PCR. The lower part of the figure displays the reaction product after amplification on E5 DNA. No reaction product was obtained after amplification on 3D7 DNA. The order of the gel was rearranged for reasons of clarity and is marked by a dotted line

true non-chromosomal recombination or simply random sharing of sequences among the global *var* gene population.

The VSA gene families of *P. falciparum* are located in subtelomeric regions and internal clusters. The boundaries between the VSA containing areas and the stable core genome have recently been newly defined by Otto et al. [11], through the analysis of 10 newly cultured field isolates from different geographic regions, by long read Pacific Bioscience sequencing technology. The beginning of the subtelomeric region was defined as the point were newly assembled genomes stop aligning with the 3D7 reference genome, however recombination within the subtelomeric regions was not able to be assessed because the analysed strains were not genetically related. In contrast in this work the analysis of the 3D7-type subtelomeric and central areas of the E5 genome with short and long read WGS enabled an assessment of recombination in the VSA harbouring parts of the E5 genome. Analysis of the 3D7-like subtelomeres and internal clusters by short read WGS exhibited moderate SNP frequency and low coverage and thus suggested relatively frequent sequence alterations compared to the 3D7 refrence sequence. This likely reflects the difficulty of short read sequencing technology in the characterization of DNA sequences with high AT content and an abundance of repetitive DNA elements. In contrast long read WGS data of the subtelomeres and central clusters only identified one large scale recombination event showing that most of the 3D7-type subtelomeric sequences were indeed co-linear with the original 3D7 sequences. Together these data indicate that the majority of subtelomeres of *P. falciparum* are highly conserved across progeny from genetic crosses and that long read sequencing technology is more appropriate for the characterization of the genome areas harbouring VSA gene families.

3D7 and E5 both originate from the same NF54 culture and, therefore, have been in tissue culture for approximately the same time. The highly conserved nature of the E5 genome parts harbouring the 3D7-VSA gene families suggests that mitotic non-chromosomal recombination alone is insufficient to explain the global genetic diversity of the *var* gene family [65]. This suggests that the selective pressure of the host immune system is essential for the expansion of parasite populations with new chimeric *var* genes and thus for the generation of the seemingly endless diversity of the global *var* gene repertoire. Furthermore, the high degree of genetic diversity in the *rifin/stevor* gene families indicates that these non-PfEMP1 VSAs may be under similar diversifying selection as the *var* gene family [29–32].

Larger studies of progeny from natural genetic crosses with long read sequencing technology are necessary to examine the possible role of acquired immunity in the generation the *var* gene and *rifin/stevor* genetic diversity at the population level.

While there has been a long standing interest in the analysis of VSA families from different laboratory strains, recently field isolate VSA gene families have moved into the focus. In this context it has become clear that progeny of natural genetic crosses that show IBD are far more prevalent than previously thought [66].

In order to establish a method that can reliably differentiate between different progeny of a natural genetic cross, a set of 84 MS primers from the NIH database was evaluated for its ability to identify the 3D7 and non-3D7 parts of the E5 genome. 27 MS primers resulted in

erroneous genotyping with the PCR conditions applied in this work. This is likely due to the fact that one standardized set of PCR conditions was applied for all primers and no attempts to optimize individual reaction conditions were made. However, even with these standard PCR conditions, 54 of 57 MS genotyping results were confirmed by WGS. 3 MS loci (*ebp, hrp2* and C12M30) showed the same alleles in E5 and 3D7, despite being located in the non-3D7 part of E5. Two of these MS were located within the open reading frames of *ebp* and *hrp2* indicating that these genes are not sufficiently diverse to distinguish between sibling parasites.

Comparative genotyping of E5 and 3D7 with 54 MS genotyping was accomplished within a few days and the use of different fluorophores for different MS on each chromosome enabled "head to head" genotyping of individual E5 and 3D7 chromosomes by multiplex PCR-reactions. This is the first time that MS genotyping has been directly compared to WGS. MS length differences of < 3 bp diffrences between E5 and 3D7 correctly identified the 3D7-type parts of the E5 genome. In some of these 3D7-type MS alleles the PCR fragment length differed from the in silico length of the respective MS in the 3D7 genome (version 3). This is most likely due to DNA slippage during PCR DNA replication. However, given the fact the PCR fragment length of these MS were identical after amplification of E5 and 3D7 this phenomenon appears to be higly reproducible and does not lead to erroneous genotyping.

Recently, Figan et al. [36] identified a set of 12 different microsatellite markers that reliably distinguish between progeny of 4 different experimental genetic crosses. The PCR conditions employed by Figan et al. and the PCR conditions in this work were almost identical suggesting that the two primer sets could be combined for rapid genotyping of field isolates.

SNP barcoding has recently emerged as a genome wide typing technique and has been used to investigate *Plasmodium* and the origin of its genotypes [67, 68]. The barcoding genotyping technique, which is based on a 23 single nucleotide polymorphisms (SNPs) and on high-quality raw sequence data [69], detects differences in the organelle genomes of *P. falciparum* and thus is not suitable for characterization of chromosomal inheritance. Similarly, another SNP assay developed some years earlier, is based on 24 SNP loci that are distributed unevenly across the genome, i.e. some chromosomes do not have SNP markers and others only 1 marker, thus tracking chromosomal cross over events is not possible [70].

SNP and WGS analysis are expensive and depend on the availability of high quality sequence data as well as extensive bioinformatic expertise. Therefore SNP and WGS can only be applied to subsets of *P. falciparum* lines and are usually carried out in specialized centres with extensive resources. In contrast MS genotyping and data analysis can be carried out in smaller centres, potentially enabling investigator driven analysis and identification of *P. falciparum* strains most suitable for subsequent WGS analyses in specialized centres.

The vast majority of the confirmed 54 MS are located in the non-coding parts of the *P. falciparum* genome. Consequently, they are not under purifying selection and may reflect the underlying genetic plasticity of the *P. falciparum* genome more accurately than methods that are based on the detection of SNPs of coding regions.

Future analysis of natural *P. falciparum* cross progeny from semi-immune and non-immune individuals may allow insights into the factors that drive crossover and and non-crossover recombination in *P. falciparum*. In this context MS genotyping may be used to determine IBD in field isolate progeny and to identify parasites clones most suitable for WGS analysis.

Conclusion

The data presented in this work show that the *var* and *rifin/stevor* gene families represent the most diverse parts of the *P. falciparum* genome, but that the majority of the VSA genes are inherited without alteration in a Mendelian fashion. Furthermore, MS genotyping data correlate well with WGS data suggesting that MS genotyping can be employed to define IBD in progeny of natural *P. falciparum* crosses.

Additional files

Additional file 1. MS Primers that generated PCR products that could not be aligned to the 3D7 MS refrence sequence.

Additional file 2. Singelton genes within the E5 genome.

Additional file 3. ACT view showing a miss-assembly between E5 and 3D7 in the first *var* gene cluster of chromosome 4. The blue bars at the top represent the E5 bin contig, matching to an area on E5.

Additional file 4. ACT screenshot of *var* chimera, box. The top sequence (chromosome 8 of PfE5) is identical to Pf3D7 (middle track, chromosome 8), but does not finish with a telomer. The sequence left hand site of the *var* gene in 3D7 up to the chromosome end (telomer repeat marked with T) is shared to chromosome 14 of PfE5 (lowest track). The black blast hits between the identity of 95–100%. *For visualisation reasons, the chromosome 14 of PfE5 was complemented. So the *var* chimera in PfE5 is on the left hand site of chr14 and on the forward strand.

Authors' contributions

MF conceived the project and integrated the different datasets. EB conducted the MS genotyping experiments and analyzed the MS and the short read WGS data. TO assembled the E5 genome with short and long WGS data and performed the de novo annotation of the E5 genome based on long read sequencing data. All authors wrote the manuscript. All authors read and approved the final manuscript.

Author details

[1] Institute of Tropical Medicine, University of Tuebingen, Wilhelmstr. 27, 72074 Tuebingen, Germany. [2] Malaria Programme, Wellcome Trust Sanger Institute, Hinxton CB10 1SA, UK. [3] Present Address: Centre of Immunobiology, Institute of Infection, Immunity & Inflammation, College of Medical, Veterinary and Life Sciences, University of Glasgow, Glasgow, UK.

Acknowledgements

We are indebted to Chris Newbold without whom this paper would never have been possible. Chris facilitated the sequencing of E5 and brought us (EB, MF and TO) together as scientists. We thank Kathrin Vrankovijc, Johanna Volk, Sandra Dimonte and Andrea Weierich and all trainees for the their assistance in evaluating the microsatellite analysis by targeted Sanger sequencing and establishing the multiplex PCR assay and Matt Berriman and Mandy Sanders for the help with the Illumina and Pacific Bioscience sequencing. We thank Akhil Vaidya for providing us with the MS set that was utilized for the analysis of the 3D7xHB3 cross.

Competing interests

The authors declare that they have no competing interests.

Funding

MF and EB were funded by the BMBF-Grant 01KA110 of the German ministry for education and research (BMBF). TO was supported by the Wellcome Trust (098051).

References

1. WHO | Malaria. WHO. http://www.who.int/mediacentre/factsheets/fs094/en/. Accessed 16 July 2017.
2. WHO | World Malaria Report 2016. WHO. http://www.who.int/malaria/publications/world_malaria_report_2016/en/. Accessed 1 Dec 2017.
3. Ponnudurai T, Leeuwenberg AD, Meuwissen JH. Chloroquine sensitivity of isolates of Plasmodium falciparum adapted to in vitro culture. Trop Geogr Med. 1981;33:50–4.
4. Frank M, Dzikowski R, Costantini D, Amulic B, Berdougo E, Deitsch K. Strict pairing of var promoters and introns is required for var gene silencing in the malaria parasite Plasmodium falciparum. J Biol Chem. 2006;281:9942–52.
5. Hall N, Pain A, Berriman M, Churcher C, Harris B, Harris D, et al. Sequence of Plasmodium falciparum chromosomes 1, 3–9 and 13. Nature. 2002;419:527–31.
6. Gardner MJ, Hall N, Fung E, White O, Berriman M, Hyman RW, et al. Genome sequence of the human malaria parasite Plasmodium falciparum. Nature. 2002;419:498–511.
7. Frank M, Kirkman L, Costantini D, Sanyal S, Lavazec C, Templeton TJ, et al. Frequent recombination events generate diversity within the multi-copy variant antigen gene families of Plasmodium falciparum. Int J Parasitol. 2008;38:1099–109.
8. Vembar SS, Seetin M, Lambert C, Nattestad M, Schatz MC, Baybayan P, et al. Complete telomere-to-telomere de novo assembly of the

   Plasmodium falciparum genome through long-read (>11 kb), single molecule, real-time sequencing. DNA Res Int J Rapid Publ Rep Genes Genomes. 2016;23:339–51.

9. Hamilton WL, Claessens A, Otto TD, Kekre M, Fairhurst RM, Rayner JC, et al. Extreme mutation bias and high AT content in *Plasmodium falciparum*. Nucleic Acids Res. 2017;45:1889–901.

10. Miles A, Iqbal Z, Vauterin P, Pearson R, Campino S, Theron M, et al. Indels, structural variation, and recombination drive genomic diversity in *Plasmodium falciparum*. Genome Res. 2016;26:1288–99.

11. Otto TD, Böhme U, Sanders M, Reid A, Bruske EI, Duffy CW, et al. Long read assemblies of geographically dispersed *Plasmodium falciparum* isolates reveal highly structured subtelomeres. Wellcome Open Res. 2018;3:52.

12. Rubio JP, Thompson JK, Cowman AF. The var genes of *Plasmodium falciparum* are located in the subtelomeric region of most chromosomes. EMBO J. 1996;15:4069–77.

13. Hernandez-Rivas R, Mattei D, Sterkers Y, Peterson DS, Wellems TE, Scherf A. Expressed var genes are found in *Plasmodium falciparum* subtelomeric regions. Mol Cell Biol. 1997;17:604–11.

14. Fischer K, Horrocks P, Preuss M, Wiesner J, Wünsch S, Camargo AA, et al. Expression of var genes located within polymorphic subtelomeric domains of *Plasmodium falciparum* chromosomes. Mol Cell Biol. 1997;17:3679–86.

15. Cheng Q, Cloonan N, Fischer K, Thompson J, Waine G, Lanzer M, et al. stevor and rif are *Plasmodium falciparum* multicopy gene families which potentially encode variant antigens. Mol Biochem Parasitol. 1998;97(1–2):161–76.

16. Fernandez V, Hommel M, Chen Q, Hagblom P, Wahlgren M. Small, clonally variant antigens expressed on the surface of the *Plasmodium falciparum*–infected erythrocyte are encoded by the rif gene family and are the target of human immune responses. J Exp Med. 1999;190:1393–404.

17. Sam-Yellowe TY, Florens L, Johnson JR, Wang T, Drazba JA, Le Roch KG, et al. A Plasmodium gene family encoding maurer's cleft membrane proteins: structural properties and expression profiling. Genome Res. 2004;14:1052–9.

18. Winter G, Kawai S, Haeggström M, Kaneko O, von Euler A, Kawazu S, et al. SURFIN is a polymorphic antigen expressed on *Plasmodium falciparum* merozoites and infected erythrocytes. J Exp Med. 2005;201:1853–63.

19. Su X, Heatwole VM, Wertheimer SP, Guinet F, Herrfeldt JA, Peterson DS, et al. The large diverse gene family var encodes proteins involved in cytoadherence and antigenic variation of *Plasmodium falciparum*-infected erythrocytes. Cell. 1995;82:89–100.

20. Baruch DI, Pasloske BL, Singh HB, Bi X, Ma XC, Feldman M, et al. Cloning the *P. falciparum* gene encoding PfEMP1, a malarial variant antigen and adherence receptor on the surface of parasitized human erythrocytes. Cell. 1995;82:77–87.

21. Smith JD, Rowe JA, Higgins MK, Lavstsen T. Malaria's deadly grip: cytoadhesion of *Plasmodium falciparum* infected erythrocytes. Cell Microbiol. 2013;15:1976–83.

22. Kyes S, Horrocks P, Newbold C. Antigenic variation at the infected red cell surface in malaria. Annu Rev Microbiol. 2001;55:673–707.

23. Bernabeu M, Danziger SA, Avril M, Vaz M, Babar PH, Brazier AJ, et al. Severe adult malaria is associated with specific PfEMP1 adhesion types and high parasite biomass. Proc Natl Acad Sci USA. 2016;113:E3270–9.

24. Nunes-Silva S, Dechavanne S, Moussiliou A, Pstrąg N, Semblat J-P, Gangnard S, et al. Beninese children with cerebral malaria do not develop humoral immunity against the IT4-VAR19-DC8 PfEMP1 variant linked to EPCR and brain endothelial binding. Malar J. 2015;14:493.

25. Avril M, Bernabeu M, Benjamin M, Brazier AJ, Smith JD. Interaction between endothelial protein C receptor and intercellular adhesion molecule 1 to mediate binding of *Plasmodium falciparum*-infected erythrocytes to endothelial cells. mBio. 2016;7:e00615–6.

26. Salanti A, Staalsoe T, Lavstsen T, Jensen ATR, Sowa MPK, Arnot DE, et al. Selective upregulation of a single distinctly structured var gene in chondroitin sulphate A-adhering *Plasmodium falciparum* involved in pregnancy-associated malaria. Mol Microbiol. 2003;49:179–91.

27. Lau CKY, Turner L, Jespersen JS, Lowe ED, Petersen B, Wang CW, et al. Structural conservation despite huge sequence diversity allows EPCR

binding by the PfEMP1 family implicated in severe childhood malaria. Cell Host Microbe. 2015;17:118–29.

28. Turner L, Lavstsen T, Berger SS, Wang CW, Petersen JEV, Avril M, et al. Severe malaria is associated with parasite binding to endothelial protein C receptor. Nature. 2013;498:502–5.

29. Chan J-A, Howell KB, Reiling L, Ataide R, Mackintosh CL, Fowkes FJI, et al. Targets of antibodies against *Plasmodium falciparum*–infected erythrocytes in malaria immunity. J Clin Invest. 2012;122:3227–38.

30. Bruske EI, Dimonte S, Enderes C, Tschan S, Flötenmeyer M, Koch I, et al. In Vitro variant surface antigen expression in *Plasmodium falciparum* parasites from a semi-immune individual is not correlated with var gene transcription. PLoS ONE. 2016;11:e0166135.

31. Tan J, Pieper K, Piccoli L, Abdi A, Perez MF, Geiger R, et al. A LAIR1 insertion generates broadly reactive antibodies against malaria variant antigens. Nature. 2016;529:105–9.

32. Niang M, Yan Yam X, Preiser PR. The *Plasmodium falciparum* STEVOR multigene family mediates antigenic variation of the infected erythrocyte. PLoS Pathog. 2009;5:e1000307.

33. Ellegren H. Microsatellites: simple sequences with complex evolution. Nat Rev Genet. 2004;5:435–45.

34. Wellems TE, Walker-Jonah A, Panton LJ. Genetic mapping of the chloroquine-resistance locus on *Plasmodium falciparum* chromosome 7. Proc Natl Acad Sci U S A. 1991;88:3382–6.

35. Hayton K, Gaur D, Liu A, Takahashi J, Henschen B, Singh S, et al. Erythrocyte binding protein PfRH5 polymorphisms determine species-specific pathways of *Plasmodium falciparum* invasion. Cell Host Microbe. 2008;4:40–51.

36. Figan CE, Sá JM, Mu J, Melendez-Muniz VA, Liu CH, Wellems TE. A set of microsatellite markers to differentiate *Plasmodium falciparum* progeny of four genetic crosses. Malar J. 2018;17:60.

37. Roper C, Pearce R, Nair S, Sharp B, Nosten F, Anderson T. Intercontinental spread of pyrimethamine-resistant malaria. Science. 2004;305:1124.

38. Wootton JC, Feng X, Ferdig MT, Cooper RA, Mu J, Baruch DI, et al. Genetic diversity and chloroquine selective sweeps in *Plasmodium falciparum*. Nature. 2002;418:320–3.

39. Anderson TJC, Su X-Z, Bockarie M, Lagog M, Day KP. Twelve microsatellite markers for characterization of *Plasmodium falciparum* from finger-prick blood samples. Parasitology. 1999;119:113–25.

40. Nabet C, Doumbo S, Jeddi F, Konaté S, Manciulli T, Fofana B, et al. Genetic diversity of *Plasmodium falciparum* in human malaria cases in Mali. Malar J. 2016;15:353.

41. Hong NV, Delgado-Ratto C, Thanh PV, Van den Eede P, Guetens P, Binh NTH, et al. Population genetics of *Plasmodium vivax* in four rural communities in Central Vietnam. PLoS Negl Trop Dis. 2016;10:e0004434.

42. Freitas-Junior LH, Bottius E, Pirrit LA, Deitsch KW, Scheidig C, Guinet F, et al. Frequent ectopic recombination of virulence factor genes in telomeric chromosome clusters of *P. falciparum*. Nature. 2000;407:1018–22.

43. Frank M, Dzikowski R, Amulic B, Deitsch K. Variable switching rates of malaria virulence genes are associated with chromosomal position and gene subclass. Mol Microbiol. 2007;64:1486–98.

44. Enderes C, Kombila D, Dal-Bianco M, Dzikowski R, Kremsner P, Frank M. Var Gene promoter activation in clonal *Plasmodium falciparum* isolates follows a hierarchy and suggests a conserved switching program that is independent of genetic background. J Infect Dis. 2011;204:1620–31.

45. Frank M, Lehners N, Mayengue PI, Gabor J, Dal-Bianco M, Kombila DU, et al. A 13-year analysis of *Plasmodium falciparum* populations reveals high conservation of the mutant pfcrt haplotype despite the withdrawal of chloroquine from national treatment guidelines in Gabon. Malar J. 2011;10:304.

46. Kozarewa I, Ning Z, Quail MA, Sanders MJ, Berriman M, Turner DJ. Amplification-free Illumina sequencing-library preparation facilitates improved mapping and assembly of (G+C)-biased genomes. Nat Methods. 2009;6:291–5.

47. Logan-Klumpler FJ, De Silva N, Boehme U, Rogers MB, Velarde G, McQuillan JA, et al. GeneDB—an annotation database for pathogens. Nucleic Acids Res. 2012;40(Database issue):D98–108.

48. DePristo MA, Banks E, Poplin RE, Garimella KV, Maguire JR, Hartl C, et al. A framework for variation discovery and genotyping using next-generation DNA sequencing data. Nat Genet. 2011;43:491–8.

49. Assefa S, Keane TM, Otto TD, Newbold C, Berriman M. ABACAS: algorithm-based automatic contiguation of assembled sequences. Bioinformatics. 2009;25:1968–9.

50. Otto TD, Sanders M, Berriman M, Newbold C. Iterative correction of reference nucleotides (iCORN) using second generation sequencing technology. Bioinformatics. 2010;26:1704–7.

51. Hunt M, Silva ND, Otto TD, Parkhill J, Keane JA, Harris SR. Circlator: automated circularization of genome assemblies using long sequencing reads. Genome Biol. 2015;16:294.

52. Steinbiss S, Silva-Franco F, Brunk B, Foth B, Hertz-Fowler C, Berriman M, et al. Companion: a web server for annotation and analysis of parasite genomes. Nucleic Acids Res. 2016;44(Web Server issue):W29–34.

53. Rutherford K, Parkhill J, Crook J, Horsnell T, Rice P, Rajandream MA, Barrell B. Artemis: sequence visualization and annotation. Bioinformatics. 2000;16:944–5.

54. Carver T, Harris SR, Otto TD, Berriman M, Parkhill J, McQuillan JA. BamView: visualizing and interpretation of next-generation sequencing read alignments. Brief Bioinf. 2013;14:203–12.

55. Carver TJ, Rutherford KM, Berriman M, Rajandream MA, Barrell BG, Parkhill J. ACT: the artemis comparison tool. Bioinformatics. 2005;21:3422–3.

56. Li L, Stoeckert CJ, Roos DS. OrthoMCL: identification of ortholog groups for eukaryotic genomes. Genome Res. 2003;13:2178–89.

57. Jiang H, Li N, Gopalan V, Zilversmit MM, Varma S, Nagarajan V, et al. High recombination rates and hotspots in a Plasmodium falciparum genetic cross. Genome Biol. 2011;12:R33.

58. Deitsch KW, del Pinal A, Wellems TE. Intra-cluster recombination and var transcription switches in the antigenic variation of Plasmodium falciparum. Mol Biochem Parasitol. 1999;101:107–16.

59. Rask TS, Hansen DA, Theander TG, Gorm Pedersen A, Lavstsen T. Plasmodium falciparum erythrocyte membrane protein 1 diversity in seven genomes—divide and conquer. PLoS Comput Biol. 2010;6:e1000933.

60. Sander AF, Lavstsen T, Rask TS, Lisby M, Salanti A, Fordyce SL, et al. DNA secondary structures are associated with recombination in major Plasmodium falciparum variable surface antigen gene families. Nucleic Acids Res. 2014;42:2270–81.

61. Bopp SER, Manary MJ, Bright AT, Johnston GL, Dharia NV, Luna FL, et al. Mitotic evolution of Plasmodium falciparum shows a stable core genome but recombination in antigen families. PLoS Genet. 2013;9:e1003293.

62. Claessens A, Hamilton WL, Kekre M, Otto TD, Faizullabhoy A, Rayner JC, et al. Generation of antigenic diversity in Plasmodium falciparum by structured rearrangement of var genes during mitosis. PLoS Genet. 2014;10:e1004812.

63. Calhoun SF, Reed J, Alexander N, Mason CE, Deitsch KW, Kirkman LA. Chromosome end repair and genome stability in Plasmodium falciparum. mBio. 2017;8:e00547–617.

64. Bull PC, Buckee CO, Kyes S, Kortok MM, Thathy V, Guyah B, et al. Plasmodium falciparum antigenic variation. Mapping mosaic var gene sequences onto a network of shared, highly polymorphic sequence blocks. Mol Microbiol. 2008;68:1519–34.

65. Barry AE, Leliwa-Sytek A, Tavul L, Imrie H, Migot-Nabias F, Brown SM, et al. Population genomics of the immune evasion (var) genes of Plasmodium falciparum. PLoS Pathog. 2007;3:e34.

66. Taylor AR, Schaffner SF, Cerqueira GC, Nkhoma SC, Anderson TJC, Sriprawat K, et al. Quantifying connectivity between local Plasmodium falciparum malaria parasite populations using identity by descent. PLoS Genet. 2017;13:e1007065.

67. Su X. Tracing the geographic origins of Plasmodium falciparum malaria parasites. Pathog Glob Health. 2014;108:261–2.

68. Manske M, Miotto O, Campino S, Auburn S, Almagro-Garcia J, Maslen G, et al. Analysis of Plasmodium falciparum diversity in natural infections by deep sequencing. Nature. 2012;487:375–9.

69. Preston MD, Campino S, Assefa SA, Echeverry DF, Ocholla H, Amambua-Ngwa A, et al. A barcode of organellar genome polymorphisms identifies the geographic origin of Plasmodium falciparum strains. Nat Commun. 2014;5:4052.

70. Daniels R, Volkman SK, Milner DA, Mahesh N, Neafsey DE, Park DJ, et al. A general SNP-based molecular barcode for Plasmodium falciparum identification and tracking. Malar J. 2008;7:223.

2

Towards a re-emergence of chloroquine sensitivity in Côte d'Ivoire?

Oléfongo Dagnogo[1,2], Aristide Berenger Ako[2], Lacinan Ouattara[3], Noel Dougba Dago[4], David N'golo Coulibaly[2], André Offianan Touré[2] and Joseph Allico Djaman[1,2]*

Abstract

Background: Resistance of *Plasmodium falciparum* to anti-malarial drugs has hampered efforts to eradicate malaria. Recent reports of a decline in the prevalence of chloroquine-resistant *P. falciparum* in several countries, including Malawi and Zambia, is raising the hope of reintroducing chloroquine in the near future, ideally in combination with another anti-malarial drug for the treatment of uncomplicated malaria. In Côte d'Ivoire, the decrease in the clinical efficacy of chloroquine, in addition to a high proportion of clinical isolates carrying the Thr-76 mutant allele of the *pfcrt* gene, had led to the discontinuation of the use of chloroquine in 2004. Previous studies have indicated the persistence of a high prevalence of the Thr-76 mutant allele despite the withdrawal of chloroquine as first-line anti-malarial drug. This present study is conducted to determine the prevalence of the Thr-76T mutant allele of the Pfcrt gene after a decade of the ban on the sale and use of chloroquine in Côte d'Ivoire.

Results: Analysis of the 64 sequences from all three study sites indicated a prevalence of 15% (10/64) of the Thr-76 mutant allele against 62% (40/64) of the Lys-76 wild-type allele. No mutation of the allele Thr-76 was observed at Anonkoua Kouté while this mutant allele was in 31% (5/16) and 25% (5/20) of isolate sequences from Port-Bouët and Ayamé respectively.

Conclusion: More than a decade after the discontinuation of the use of chloroquine in Côte d'Ivoire, the proportion of parasites sensitive to this anti-malarial seems to increase in Anonkoua-kouté, Port-bouët and Ayamé.

Keywords: Pfcrt, Thr-76, Chloroquine sensitivity, Côte d'Ivoire, Antimalarial drug resistance

Background

Malaria remains a major public health problem in the world. According to the World Health Organization (WHO), 212 million cases of malaria were recorded in 2015, of which 429,000 led to death, of which 92% occurred in Africa with 70% of children under 5 years of age [1]. Up to 1990, chloroquine (CQ) was the main malaria treatment therapy thanks to its efficacy, safety, low cost and antipyretic properties. In the late 1950s, resistance to CQ emerged in different parts of the world, first in South-East Asia and South America (Colombia and Venezuela) [2–5]. The resistance to CQ spread rapidly and was detected in West Africa in the 80s and 90s [6, 7].

In Côte d'Ivoire, the prevalence of CQ-resistant parasites that used to be very low in 1987 with only three confirmed cases of chloroquine resistance (CQR) appeared to have increased [8, 9]. Indeed, high prevalence of the K76T mutation, a key mutation associated with *Plasmodium falciparum* resistance to CQ, have been reported in Yopougon in Abidjan (65%), Bonoua (100%), Samo (95%) and Adzopé (62%) [10]. Recent reports of a decline in the prevalence of chloroquine-resistant *P. falciparum* in several countries, including Malawi and Zambia, raise the hope of reintroducing chloroquine in the near future ideally in combination with another anti-malarial drug for the treatment of uncomplicated malaria [11, 12]. It could possibly be given to non-vulnerable groups, but it requires close monitoring of possible reemergence of CQ

*Correspondence: djamanj@yahoo.fr; josephdjaman@pasteur.ci
[2] Institut Pasteur de Côte d'Ivoire, 01 BP 490, Abidjan 01, Côte d'Ivoire
Full list of author information is available at the end of the article

resistance development. Indeed, it has been suggested that effective and sustained withdrawal of CQ could lead to the reappearance of CQ-sensitive *P. falciparum*. It is the case in East Africa, particularly in Malawi and Kenya where a re-emergence of this sensitivity to CQ was reported after the discontinuation of its uses in 1993 and 1999, respectively [11, 12]. Some studies in Cameroon (Central Africa) and in Senegal (West Africa) [13–15], have reported the same trend for susceptibility to CQ after withdrawal as first-line malaria treatment.

In Côte d'Ivoire, the decreasing clinical efficacy of chloroquine, in addition to a high proportion of resistant isolates, led the Ivorian health authorities to call for withdrawal and discontinuation of the use of chloroquine in 2004 in favor of artemisinin-based combination therapy (ACT) as a first-line treatment for uncomplicated malaria. This study aimed to investigate the prevalence of the K76T mutation a little more than a decade after the official withdrawal of CQ in uncomplicated malaria treatment management in Côte d'Ivoire.

Methods
Study site
This was a prospective study that took place in three different health centers, Anonkoua Kouté, Port-Bouët general hospital and Ayamé from February to August 2015. All these sites are located in the southern region of Côte d'Ivoire where the climate is equatorial with annual rainfall exceeding 1700 mm of rain and the temperature varies between 27 and 33 °C. Malaria is seasonal, more frequent during the rainy season from June to September with peaks prevalence rate and incidence in October–November. *Plasmodium falciparum* is the dominant species with more than 90% of malaria parasites identified. The main vectors of malaria in this study area (the southern forest zone of Côte d'Ivoire) are the members of the complexes *Anopheles gambiae* sensu lato (s.l.) and *Anopheles funestus* s.l. [16].

Anonkoua-kouté Health Centre and Ayamé General Hospital were selected based on the high annual incidences of malaria cases records. In addition, these health centers are chosen for several years as the main sites for performing multicenter clinical efficacy tests by the Malaria Unit of Institut Pasteur of Côte d'Ivoire. Port Bouët general hospital was selected for this study not only because of the constantly high annual incidences of malaria cases, but also and especially because of its swampy environment often used for market garden produces.

Study population and sample collection
All patients clinically suspected to have malaria at Anonkoua Kouté Health Center, Port-Bouët general hospitals and Ayamé during the study period were eligible. However, after informed consent, blood samples were collected from patients who are over 2 years of age with an axillary temperature greater than 37.5 °C and suffering from uncomplicated *P. falciparum* malaria confirmed by microscopic examination.

Blood sample
In each patient who have been confirmed of having malaria by microscopic examination, approximately 2–5 mL of venous blood was collected in an EDTA tube. Approximately 50 µL of whole blood was dropped on Whatman 3 MM filter paper discs [dried blood spots (DBS)] using a micropipette with filter cones. The papers containing the blood spots were dried for about 60–120 min at room temperature away from dust. Unused blood contained in the EDTA tube was stored in microtubes at − 20 °C for possible subsequent utilization.

Extraction of *Plasmodium falciparum* genomic DNA
Plasmodial DNA was extracted with methanol from DBS cut into small pieces were immersed in 1 mL of washing buffer (950 µL of 1× PBS plus 50 µL of 10% saponin) and incubated overnight at 4 °C [17]. The wash buffer was removed and 150 µL of methanol were added. After a 20 min incubation, the methanol was gently removed and the samples were dried at room temperature for 2 h before adding 300 µL of sterilized water. The samples were then heated at 99 °C in a thermo-mixer for 30 min to elute the DNA. After removing the confetti debris, the DNA extracts were aliquoted into a 1.5 mL Eppendorf tube and stored at − 20 °C.

Amplification of the *pfcrt* gene
The pfcrt gene was amplified by nested PCR using a specific pair of primers and a commercial DNA polymerase kit called 5× FIREPol Blend Master Mix with mM $MgCl_2$. This kit is a pre-mix (for the reaction mixture) ready to use composed of DNA polymerase (FIREPol® DNA polymerase), buffer (5× Blend Master Mix Buffer), $MgCl_2$ (7.5 mM $MgCl_2$) and dNTPs (2 mM dNTPs of each). For primary PCR, the primer pairs used for amplification of the *pfcrt* gene were 72_97EF (5′GACCTTAACAGGTGG CTCAC)/72_97ER (5′TTTATTGGTAGGTGGAATAG). The primary PCR of this gene was carried out in a reaction volume of 25 µL containing: 0.625 µL of each primer, 3 µL of plasmodial DNA, 5 µL of Taq DNA polymerase and 15.75 µL of milliQ water. The mixture was then put into a PTC-100TM thermocycler (Eppendorf Mastercycler, PTC-100 Peltier Thermal Cycler), programmed as follows: Initial denaturation at 95 °C for 15 min followed by 30 denaturation cycles at 95 °C for 30 s, hybridization

at 58 °C for 2 min and extension at 72 °C for 2 min. Finally, a terminal extension at 72 °C for 10 min.

The second PCR was carried out on the amplification products of the primary PCR in a reaction volume of 50 µL containing: 1.25 µL of each primer, 5 µL of amplification product (amplicon) of the first PCR, of 5 µL of Taq DNA polymerase and 37.5 µL of milliQ water. The primer pairs used for the secondary PCR were SecIF (5′ GGTAAATGTGCTCATGTGTTTAAACTTATT)/SecIR (5′ TTACTTTTGAATTTCCCTTTTTATTTCCA). The secondary PCR was performed with the same thermocycler used for the primary PCR with the following program: Initial denaturation at 95 °C for 15 min followed by 30 denaturation cycles at 95 °C for 30 s, hybridization at 60 °C for one minute and extension at 72 °C for 1 min. Finally, a terminal extension at 72 °C for 10 min.

Detection and analysis of PCR products

The amplification products were migrated on a 1.5% agarose gel containing ethidium bromide (EtBr). After migration, the gel was recovered and then observed under a UV lamp using the UV transilluminator (Gel DocTM EZ Imager). The presence or absence of bands made it possible to judge the effectiveness of the PCR.

Sequencing amplification

The amplified DNA fragments (*pfcrt* gene) of *P. falciparum* were sequenced according to the Sanger method by the company Eurofins MWG operon (Cochin sequencing platform). Samples were dropped to the platform in a microplate (Greiner Bio-one-652270B) along with a deposit slip that was sent to the platform's email address. A reaction medium was prepared for the PCR-nested sense primer (sequencing primer) from the amplification products. In each well of the microplate, a volume of 13 µL of amplification product was added to 2 µL of sequencing primer at 10 µM. Wells containing the sequencing reaction medium were sealed with cap strips (4titude-044737) before covering the entire surface of the microplate with an adhesive film (AmpliSeal, Greiner Bio-one-676040). This microplate containing the samples was sent to the platform for sequencing.

After the sequencing reaction, the received DNA sequences were recovered as fasta. In this study, it is the sequences corresponding to the *pfcrt* gene of the isolates collected. The use of the software BioEdit made it possible to analyse the sequences to search for possible mutations. Indeed, the loci of interest, namely the codons at position 74, 75, 76 of the *PfCRT* polypeptide or the nucleotides at position 222, 225, 228 of the *pfcrt* gene were identified and analysed after a parallel alignment of two or more DNA sequences, including the reference sequence *pfcrt* gene, by maximizing the number of identical nucleotides or residues, while minimizing the number of mismatches and voids.

Statistical analysis of data

Data were collected on a standard questionnaire tested and validated. They were then entered and analysed on the statistical software R; version 3.2.2 [18]. The χ^2 comparison test of three averages was used to compare the prevalence of the molecular marker of CQ resistance (*pfcrt* K76T). The χ^2 test was used to determine whether the molecular marker prevalence can be considered to be all equal (null hypothesis H0) or if two or more prevalence are different (alternative hypothesis Ha). A difference and/or statistical association was considered significant if p of the test $\chi^2 < 0.05$.

Results

A total of 64 persons infected with *P. falciparum* were selected for this study, including 41 (64%) women and 23 (36%) men. The average age of the patients was 17 years (age ranging from 2 to 62 years) (Table 1). In addition, the parasite densities varied from 1200 to 200,000 parasites/µL with average parasite densities of 22,900; 9193 and 42,327 parasites/µL at Anonkoua Kouté, Port-Bouët and Ayamé, respectively (Table 1 and Fig. 1). A significant difference (p = 0.002) was observed between the parasite densities at Port-Bouët and Ayamé. The mean parasite density in all three sites was 24,806 parasites/µL.

Table 1 Samples used for molecular analysis of chloroquine chemoresistance

Sites	Period of collection in 2015	Age group (years)	DBS collected	Average Parasite density (µL/mm³)
Anonkoua-kouté	February–March	2–53	28	22,900
Port-Bouët	April–May–July	2–62	16	9193
Ayamé	June–July–August	2–55	20	42,327
Total			64	24,806

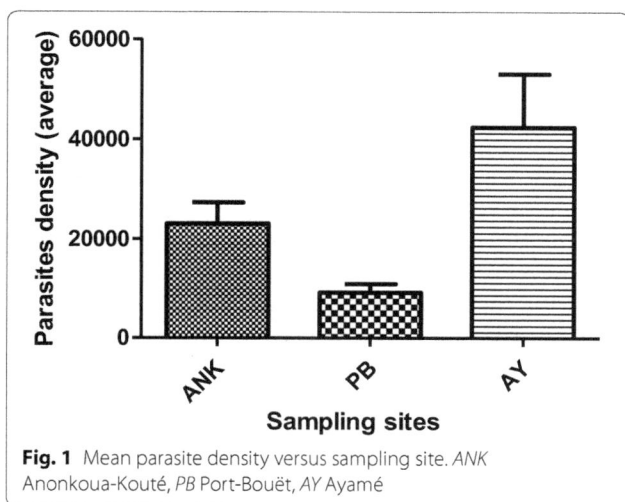

Fig. 1 Mean parasite density versus sampling site. *ANK* Anonkoua-Kouté, *PB* Port-Bouët, *AY* Ayamé

Table 2 Prevalence of the individual alleles of the *pfcrt* gene in the study sites

Codons	Alleles	Sample size (N = 64)	
		n = 59	%
Crt_74	Wild		
	Met-74	47	73
	Ile-74	5	7
	Mutants		
	Lys-74	1	1
	Leu-74	5	7
	Trp-74	1	1
Crt_75		n = 64	%
	Wild		
	Asn-75	48	75
	Glu-75	5	7
	Mutants		
	Lys-75	6	9
	Tyr-75	5	7
Crt_76		n = 64	%
	Wild		
	Lys-76	40	62
	Thr-76	10	15
	Mutants		
	Gly-76	1	1
	Ile-76	1	1
	Gln-76	16	25

"N" represents the total number of isolates sequenced at the three sites. "n" represents the number of isolates sequenced successfully by codon

Prevalence of the individual alleles of the *pfcrt* gene and molecular analysis of the corresponding genotypes

Across all the three study sites, the results indicated that the prevalence of wild-type isolates Met-74 (73%), Asn-75 (75%), Lys-76 (62%) is higher than those isolates carrying mutations of the *pfcrt* gene Ile-74 (7%), Glu-75 (7%) and Thr-76 (15%) (Table 2). Molecular analysis of the genotypes corresponding to the *pfcrt* gene shows that the MNK genotype (wild type) was predominant with a prevalence of 62% (Table 3). In contrast, single genotypes mutant, double mutant and triple mutant were observed with respective prevalence of 12%, 6% and 18%.

Among the triple mutant genotypes, there was a predominance of isolates carrying IET and LKQ with respective prevalence of 6% and 9%. The analysis also found single mutant MNT (9%) and double mutant MYQ (6%) genotypes (Table 3).

Prevalence of wild-type Lys-76 and Thr-76 mutants of the *pfcrt* gene at Anonkoua-Kouté, Port-Bouët and Ayamé

No Thr-76 mutation was observed in Anonkoua-Kouté while this mutant allele was found in 31% and 25% of the sequences of the isolates from Port-Bouët and Ayamé, respectively, as indicated in Table 4. The highest prevalence of the Thr-76 allele were found in Port-Bouët (31%) and Ayamé (25%) (Table 4). Moreover, in all the study sites no significant difference (P = 0.955) was observed in the prevalence of the wild-type Lys-76 allele, Anonkoua-Kouté (60%), Port-Bouët (62%) and Ayamé (65%).

Discussion

Previous studies carried out in West Africa and particularly in Côte d'Ivoire showed a strong correlation between the Thr-76 mutation of the *pfcrt* gene and the therapeutic failures on one hand, and between the Thr-76 mutation of the *pfcrt* gene and in vitro chemoresistance of *P. falciparum* isolates to chloroquine [19–22] on the other hand.

Results indicate that in all three study sites, the mutant allele Thr-76 (15%) was associated with mutant Ile-74 (7%) and Glu-75 (7%) in isolates at very low proportion compared to wild-type alleles Lys-76 (62%), Met-74 (73%) and Asn-75 (75%). In addition, the wild allele Lys-76 was observed in Anonkoua-Kouté, Port-Bouët and Ayamé 60%, 62% and 65%, respectively.

These results contrasted those obtained (for the Thr-76 mutation) in 2006 (65%) in Yopougon, Abidjan [8], in 2005 (100% and 95%) in Bonoua and Samo respectively [10] and in 2010 (62%) in Adzopé [9]. However, the data are in accordance with Gharbi et al. [23] who, after modelling chloroquine resistance in Côte d'Ivoire from the Thr-76 allele with samples from travelers

Table 3 Prevalence of genotypes corresponding to *pfcrt*

pfcrt key codons	Genotypes			Sample size (N = 64)
	M74I	**N75E**	**K76T**	**n (%)**
Wild type	M	N	K	*40 (62)*
Single mutations				8 (12)
	M	N	*T*	6 (9)
	Others			2 (3)
Double mutations	M	*Y*	*Q*	*4 (6)*
Triple mutations				*12 (18)*
	L	*K*	*Q*	6 (9)
	I	*E*	*T*	4 (6)
	K	*E*	*G*	1 (1)
	I	*Y*	*I*	1 (1)

A capital letter in the "genotype" column represents the one-letter code of amino acids. The amino acids resulting from the mutation of *pfcrt* are underlined and in italic. The determined prevalences correspond to the number of observations on the number of successes per gene

Table 4 Prevalence of the wild-type Lys-76 and the mutant Thr-76 of the *pfcrt* gene in Anonkoua-Kouté, Port-Bouët and Ayamé

Codon	Alleles	Anonkoua-Kouté: N = 28 n (%)	Port-Bouët: N = 16 n (%)	Ayamé: N = 20 n (%)	p-value (χ^2 test)
Lys-76-Thr	Lys-76	17 (60)	10 (62)	13 (65)	0.955
	Thr-76	*0 (0)*	*5 (31)*	*5 (25)*	–

The mutated amino acids are italic. "N" represents the total number of isolates sequenced successfully per study site. "n" represents the number of isolates sequenced successfully at the codon Crt_76

The list of other mutants is in Table 2

The χ^2 test could not be performed for the mutants because of the value less than 5 in a cell

returning to Côte d'Ivoire reported a decrease in prevalence from 63 to 37% of Thr-76 allele.

Normally, the prevalence of the Thr-76 mutation should be reduced because parasites that carry the Lys-76 wild-type allele have a survival advantage in the absence of drug pressure [24]. Indeed, when drug pressure is low, drug resistance is accompanied by a reduction in the genetic performance of resistant parasites compared to susceptible parasites [25, 26]. Thus, when the drug pressure decreases, the proportion of sensitive parasites increases and that of the resistant parasites decreases [11].

The low prevalence observed for Thr-76 isolates may be due to a number of factors, the main one being the effective withdrawal of CQ in Côte d'Ivoire. Indeed, CQ

has always been prescribed and/or delivered in Côte d'Ivoire for the treatment of uncomplicated malaria [27] until 2007, when it was withdrawn in favor of amodiaquine (AQ) [28]. However, the substitution of amodiaquine would have delayed the decline since AQ also selects for the Thr-76 allele of *pfcrt* [29] in contrary to the countries where the decline has been most precipitous thanks to an intensive deployment of lumefantrine as part of Coartem. The data generated are in line with these observations, since artemether-lumefantrine (AL) was officially used as first-line treatment in Côte d'Ivoire by year 2013. It was, therefore, necessary to wait a few years to observe a possible significant decrease in chloroquine-resistant *P. falciparum* isolates. Thus, the public authorities have had to intensify awareness campaigns to inform the population and the medical staff, to take action to fight against the illegal sale of anti-malarial drug on parallel markets (street drugs). All these actions eventually made effective the removal of the CQ and that would be the basis of the increase in the prevalence of chloroquine-sensitive parasites. In addition, government control over pharmaceutical distribution channels and drug supply chains in the public and private sectors has reduced the use of non-recommended drugs such as CQ [30, 31]. For example, in Malawi, the successful implementation of national information campaigns and the effective control of drug delivery patterns has led, 10 years later, to the re-emergence of sensitivity to CQ [32]. The context in Côte d'Ivoire is also different from what was reported in French Guyana where, despite the fixation of the IET genotype, the return to sensitivity was observed thanks to the acquisition of the C350R mutation in parasites carrying the Lys-76 allele [33]. No mutation of the Thr-76 allele was observed in Anonkoua Kouté while this mutant allele was carried by 31% and 25% of isolates from Port-Bouët and Ayamé, respectively.

These prevalence of the Thr-76 mutation in Port-Bouët and Ayamé could be related to the effects of migratory movements of the populations towards these areas. Indeed, these two communities are characterized by a strong agroeconomic activity (livestock, farming, and fishing) with many rivers, large farms that attract many indigenes and non-indigenes from the subregion. These populations mainly occupy the villages (Ayamé) and the many precarious neighbourhoods (Port-Bouët) where most households often do not have access to national information thus depriving them of awareness campaigns for the withdrawal and abandon of the CQ. Thus, these households opt for anti-malarial treatments without consultation (self-medication), thus maintaining drug pressure [34]. The populations migrating from neighbouring West African countries to these localities may also be potential carriers of resistant parasites, which could explain the prevalence of the Thr-76 mutation observed in these areas.

Therefore, the withdrawal of chloroquine and the introduction of ACT seem to promote the re-emergence of CQ-sensitive isolates. It would be desirable to carry out another study that could be extended to several localities with a larger number of samples to confirm this decrease of CQ-resistant parasites in Côte d'Ivoire. Thus, if the proportion of chloroquine-resistant parasites decreases at the national level to an undetectable level of *pfcrt* mutants, a reintroduction of chloroquine in combination with other anti-malarial drug for malaria treatment and prophylaxis may be considered, as Malawi has done [11].

Conclusion

The present study showed that the CQ resistance has decreased in Côte d'Ivoire in Anonkoua-Kouté, Port-Bouët and Ayamé communities since its withdrawal in 2004. This decrease in CQ resistance seems to be related to the efficiency and the success of the policy of abandoning the use of CQ in Côte d'Ivoire. Therefore, the withdrawal of chloroquine (CQ) and the introduction of ACT for the treatment of uncomplicated malaria in Côte d'Ivoire appear to favour the re-emergence of isolates sensitive to CQ. However, even if the proportion of chloroquine-sensitive parasites seems to increase in Anonkoua-Kouté, Port-Bouët and Ayamé, a reintroduction of chloroquine in malaria treatment cannot be recommended currently in Côte d'Ivoire.

Abbreviations
ACT: artemisinin-based combination therapy; AQ: amodiaquine; CQ: chloroquine; CQR: chloroquine resistance; DNA: deoxyribonucleic acid; EDTA: ethylene diamine tetraacetic; PBS: phosphate buffered saline; PCR: polymerase chain reaction; NCER: National Committee on Ethics and Research; WHO: World Health Organization.

Authors' contributions
DO: blood collection, designed and realized the technical manipulations, CND directed technical manipulations, AAB and DDN realized the statistical treatment, OL contributed to the drafting of the manuscript, TOA followed the realization of the project, DAJ conceived the project. Each author participated sufficiently in the work to take public responsibility for appropriate portions of the content. All authors read and approved the final manuscript.

Author details
¹ UFR Biosciences, Félix Houphouët-Boigny University, BP V 34, Abidjan 01, Côte d'Ivoire. ² Institut Pasteur de Côte d'Ivoire, 01 BP 490, Abidjan 01, Côte d'Ivoire. ³ Department of Food Science and Technology, Nangui Abrogoua University, 02 BP 801, Abidjan 02, Côte d'Ivoire. ⁴ UFR Sciences Biologiques, Péléforo Gon Coulibaly University, BP1328 Korhogo, Côte d'Ivoire.

Acknowledgements
The authors express their profound gratitude to the Pasteur Institute of Côte d'Ivoire who allowed us to use the facilities of the molecular biology platform of the Institut Pasteur of Côte d'Ivoire to perform the PCR tests.

Competing interests
The authors declare that they have no competing interests.

Funding
The study was carried out on own funds.

References
1. WHO. World malaria report. Geneva: World Health Organization; 2016.
2. Harinasuta T, Suntharasamai P, Viravan C, Ravel P, Ma L, Tichit M, et al. Chloroquine-resistant falciparum malaria in Thailand. Lancet. 1965;286:657–60.
3. Young MD, Moore DV. Chloroquine resistance in *Plasmodium falciparum*. Am J Trop Med Hyg. 1961;10:317–20.
4. Payne D. Did medicated salt hasten the spread of chloroquine resistance in *Plasmodium falciparum*? Parasitol Today. 1988;4:112–5.
5. Peters W. Chemotherapy and drug resistance in malaria. New York: Academic Press Ltd; 1987. p. 542.
6. Hellgren U, Ardal OK, Lebbad M, Rombo L. Is chloroquine-resistant *Plasmodium falciparum* malaria emerging in Senegal or The Gambia? Trans R Soc Trop Med Hyg. 1987;81:728.
7. Kyrönseppä H, Lumio J, Ukkonen R, Pettersson T. Chloroquine-resistant malaria from Angola. Lancet. 1984;1:1244.
8. Djaman J, Ahibo H, Yapi HF, Bla KB, Ouattara L, Yavo W, et al. Molecular monitoring of *Plasmodium falciparum* malaria isolates in Côte d'Ivoire: genetic markers (dhfr-ts, dhps, pfcrt, pfmdr-1) for antimalarial-drugs resistance. Eur J Sci Res. 2010;40:461–70.
9. Ouattara L, Bla KB, Assi SB, Yavo W, Djaman AJ. pfcrt and dhfr-ts sequences for monitoring drug resistance in Adzopé Area of Côte d'Ivoire after the withdrawal of chloroquine and pyrimethamine. Trop J Pharm Res. 2010;9:568.
10. Johansson M, Penali LK, Assanvo SP, Ako BA, Offianan AT, Johansson M, et al. Molecular analysis of markers associated with chloroquine and sulfadoxine/pyrimethamine resistance in *Plasmodium falciparum* malaria parasites from southeastern Côte-d'Ivoire by the time of artemisinin-based combination therapy adoption in 2005. Infect Drug Resist. 2012;5:113–20.
11. Kublin JG, Cortese JF, Njunju EM, Mukadam RA, Wirima JJ, Kazembe PN, et al. Reemergence of chloroquine-sensitive Plasmodium falciparum malaria after cessation of chloroquine use in Malawi. J Infect Dis. 2003;187:1870–5.
12. Mwai L, Ochong E, Abdirahman A, Kiara SM, Ward S, Kokwaro G, et al. Chloroquine resistance before and after its withdrawal in Kenya. Malar J. 2009;8:106.
13. Ndam NT, Basco LK, Ngane VF, Ayouba A, Ngolle EM, Deloron P, et al. Reemergence of chloroquine-sensitive pfcrt K76 *Plasmodium falciparum* genotype in southeastern Cameroon. Malar J. 2017;16:130.
14. Dieng Y, Gaye O, Faye B, Tine R, Ndiaye M, Ndiaye JL, et al. Assessment of the molecular marker of *Plasmodium falciparum* chloroquine resistance (Pfcrt) in Senegal after several years of chloroquine withdrawal. Am J Trop Med Hyg. 2012;87:640–5.
15. Wurtz N, Fall B, Pascual A, Diawara S, Sow K, Baret E, et al. Prevalence of

molecular markers of *Plasmodium falciparum* drug resistance in Dakar, Senegal. Malar J. 2012;11:197.

16. Adja AM, N'goran EK, Koudou BG, Dia I, Kengne P, Fontenille D, et al. Contribution of *Anopheles funestus, An. gambiae* and *An. nili* (Diptera: Culicidae) to the perennial malaria transmission in the southern and western forest areas of Côte d'Ivoire. Ann Trop Med Parasitol. 2011;105:13–24.

17. Miguel RB, Coura JR, Samudio F, Suárez-Mutis MC. Evaluation of three different DNA extraction methods from blood samples collected in dried filter paper in Plasmodium subpatent infections from the Amazon region in Brazil. Rev Inst Med Trop Sao Paulo. 2013;55:205–8.

18. Team RC. R: A language and environment for statistical computing. R Found Stat Comput 2008.

19. Djimdé A, Doumbo OK, Cortese JF, Kayentao K, Doumbo S, Diourté Y, et al. A molecular marker for chloroquine-resistant falciparum malaria. N Engl J Med. 2001;344:257–63.

20. Djaman JA, Bla BK, Yavo W, Yapi HF, Mazabraud A, Basco LK. Polymorphism of PFCRT and PFMDR-1 genes of *Plasmodium falciparum* and chloroquine susceptibility in Côte d'Ivoire. Acta Protozool. 2007;46:361–5.

21. Figueiredo P, Benchimol C, Lopes D, Bernardino L, do Rosario VE, Varandas L, et al. Prevalence of *pfmdr1, pfcrt, pfdhfr* and *pfdhps* mutations associated with drug resistance, in Luanda, Angola. Malar J. 2008;7:236.

22. Bridges DJ, Molyneux M, Nkhoma S. Low level genotypic chloroquine resistance near Malawi's northern border with Tanzania. Trop Med Int Health. 2009;14:1093–6.

23. Gharbi M, Flegg J, Pradines B, Berenger A, Ndiaye M, Djimde AA, et al. Surveillance of travellers: an additional tool for tracking antimalarial drug resistance in endemic countries. PLoS One. 2013;8:e77775.

24. Laufer MK, Plowe CV. Withdrawing antimalarial drugs: impact on parasite resistance and implications for malaria treatment policies. Drug Resist Updat. 2004;7:279–88.

25. Gadalla NB, Elzaki SE, Mukhtar E, Warhurst DC, El-Sayed B, Sutherland CJ. Dynamics of pfcrt alleles CVMNK and CVIET in chloroquine-treated Sudanese patients infected with *Plasmodium falciparum*. Malar J. 2010;9:74.

26. Ord R, Alexander N, Dunyo S, Hallett R, Jawara M, Targett G, et al. Seasonal carriage of pfcrt and pfmdr1 alleles in Gambian Plasmodium falciparum imply reduced fitness of chloroquine-resistant parasites. J Infect Dis. 2007;196:1613–9.

27. Kiki-Barro CP, Konan FN, Yavo W, Kassi R, Menan EIH, Djohan V, et al. [Antimalaria drug delivery in pharmacies in non-severe malaria treatment. A survey on the quality of the treatment: the case of Bouake (Côte d'Ivoire)] (in French). Sante. 2004;14:75–9.

28. MSHP: Arrêté No 24/CAB/MSHP Du 12 Janvier 2007 Portant Institution d'un Schéma Thérapeutique pour Traitement du Paludisme en Côte d'Ivoire. Abidjan; 2007.

29. Sisowath C, Petersen I, Veiga MI, Mårtensson A, Premji Z, Björkman A, et al. *In vivo* selection of *Plasmodium falciparum* parasites carrying the chloroquine-susceptible pfcrt K76 allele after treatment with artemether–lumefantrine in Africa. J Infect Dis. 2009;199:750–7.

30. Talisuna AO, Adibaku S, Amojah CN, Amofah GK, Aubyn V, Dodoo A, et al. The affordable medicines facility-malaria—a success in peril. Malar J. 2012;11:370.

31. Tougher S, Ye Y, Amuasi JH, Kourgueni IA, Thomson R, Goodman C, et al. Effect of the Affordable Medicines Facility-Malaria (AMFm) on the availability, price, and market share of quality-assured artemisinin-based combination therapies in seven countries: a before-and-after analysis of outlet survey data. Lancet. 2012;380:1916–26.

32. Laufer MK, Thesing PC, Eddington ND, Masonga R, Dzinjalamala FK, Takala SL, et al. Return of chloroquine antimalarial efficacy in Malawi. N Engl J Med. 2006;355:1959–66.

33. Pelleau S, Moss EL, Dhingra SK, Volney B, Casteras J, Gabryszewski SJ, et al. Adaptive evolution of malaria parasites in French Guiana: reversal of chloroquine resistance by acquisition of a mutation in pfcrt. Proc Natl Acad Sci USA. 2015;112:11672–7.

34. Kouadio AS, Ciss, G, Obrist B, Wyss K, Zinsstag J, Yao YJ, et al. Fardeau économique du paludisme sur les ménages démunis des quartiers défavorisés d'Abidjan, Cote d'Ivoire. VertigO. 2006, Hors Serie 3.

3

'For the poor, sleep is leisure': understanding perceptions, barriers and motivators to mosquito net care and repair

Zawadi M. Mboma[1,2]*, Angel Dillip[1], Karen Kramer[3,4,5], Hannah Koenker[6], George Greer[7] and Lena M. Lorenz[1,2]

Abstract

Background: The rate of physical deterioration of long-lasting insecticidal nets (LLINs) varies by household practices, net brand and environment. One way to sustain the protection provided by LLINs against malaria is through day-to-day care, and repairing holes as and when they occur. To ensure LLIN coverage is high between mass campaigns and, as international donor funds decrease, personal responsibility to maintain nets in good condition is becoming more important. This study aimed to understand local barriers and motivators to net care and repair in southern Tanzania in a community that receives free LLINs through a school-based distribution mechanism.

Methods: Qualitative research methods were applied in a rural and peri-urban village in Ruangwa district. Focus group discussions (FGDs) were conducted for five groups of 8–12 participants; (1) key informants, (2) young men (18–24 years old), (3) women (> 18 years) with children under the age of five, (4) older men (> 25 years), and (5) older women with or without children (> 25 years). In each village, five men, five women with or without children, and five women with children under the age of five were recruited for in-depth interviews (IDIs). After each IDI and FGD with women with young children, participants were guided through a participatory activity. The study also counted the number and size of holes in nets currently used by IDI participants to determine their physical degradation status.

Results: A general willingness to care and repair mosquito nets was observed in Ruangwa district for the love of a good night's sleep free of mosquito bites or noises. Net care was preferred over repair, especially among women who were the primary caretakers. The main motivation to look after nets was protection against mosquito bites and malaria. Washing nets occurred as frequently as every other week in some households to ensure cleanliness, which prevented other dirt-related problems such as sneezing and headaches. Barriers to net care included care not being a priority in the day-to-day activities and lack of net retreatment kits. Net repair was reported to be a temporary measure and necessary as soon as a hole was identified. However, during the net assessment and participatory activity, it became clear that people did not actually repair smaller holes. Protection against mosquitoes, malaria and cost saving from replacing nets were identified as motivators for net repair. Barriers to net repair included it not being a priority to repair holes that could be tucked under the mattress and lack of knowledge on when to repair nets.

Conclusion: In Ruangwa, net care was defined as overall net maintenance, such as cleanliness, and not directly associated with the prevention of damage as reported in other studies. Net repair was reported as a temporary measure before the acquisition of a new net, hence not a priority in a busy household. Inconsistencies were observed between

*Correspondence: zmageni@ihi.or.tz
[1] Ifakara Health Institute, Dar-es-Salaam, Tanzania
Full list of author information is available at the end of the article

reported intentions to repair mosquito nets and current net condition. Targeted education through health facilities and community change agents are potential means to overcome barriers to net care and repair.

Keywords: Long-lasting insecticidal nets (LLINs), Mosquito net, Net care, Net repair, Malaria Tanzania, Health Belief Model

Background

The Government of Tanzania has made considerable effort in achieving universal coverage for its population with Long-Lasting Insecticidal Nets (LLINs) through a number of continuous and keep-up distribution mechanisms [1–3]. The physical deterioration of the net, while inevitable with time, varies by product type, household practices (e.g. use, washing) and environment (e.g. type of sleeping space) [4–8]. One of the ways to sustain the protection provided by LLINs is through personal responsibility of households to care for LLINs day-by-day [9]. Extending the lifespan of LLINs is important to reduce the frequency of net replacements and maintain high access to LLINs between distributions, to ensure continuing health gains from the use of nets [5].

The World Health Organization Pesticide Evaluation Scheme (WHOPES), now replaced by the Prequalification Team (PQT), recommends that LLINs remain effective after 20 standard washes and last 3 years under field conditions [10]. Manufacturers instruct specific care practices to prolong the useful life of the LLIN, such as hanging the net low enough to touch the ground or tucking underneath the mattress, washing gently with soap and water but not bleach, drying nets in the shade and avoiding direct sunlight, keeping net away from direct flames and repairing holes as soon as possible [11]. However, it is unclear how many households receive their nets with the packaging or if those who receive the instructions on the packaging understand and practice them.

Net care (i.e. hanging of net, daily storage/tying up net over sleeping space, washing, drying, seasonal storage) and repair (i.e. sewing, knotting, patching) practices are similar across communities, but vary in priority between households [12–14]. In Senegal [13], Nigeria [14] and Mali [12], net care was preferred and more common than repair. In Uganda [5], nets perceived too torn were most likely to be repurposed for alternative uses around the house rather than repaired. In urban Dar-es-Salaam, requesting users to reduce washing frequency to maintain enough insecticide on nets was deemed impractical [15]. This variation in priority of performing net care and repair practices emphasizes the need to integrate local and culturally-fitting messaging with ongoing malaria interventions rather than promoting blanket universal recommendations across all endemic countries [16].

This study was conducted in southern Tanzania (Ruangwa district, Lindi region; Fig. 1) in 2016 after the third round of continuous LLIN distribution through the School Net Programme (SNP) conducted in 2015. Malaria prevalence in children under five in the Lindi Region remains high at 17.4% as per the 2015–2016 national health survey [17]. Starting in 2013, the SNP was introduced as a pilot "keep-up" strategy to supplement mass distribution campaigns as a means to maintain universal coverage of LLINs prior to its national roll-out [18, 19]. The programme distributes LLINs each year to school-going children in alternating classes (primary classes 1, 2, 3, 4, 5 and 7, secondary classes/forms 2 and 4) [18, 20, 21]. Ninety-eight percent of all registered students and teachers in Ruangwa district received LLINs through the SNP programme [20]. Generally in Lindi region, ownership of at least one LLIN was 70% while ownership of at least one LLIN for every two people who slept in the household the night prior to the survey was 47% according to the 2015–2016 National Health Survey [17]. Specifically, monitoring of SNP rounds 1 and 2 recorded ownership of at least one LLIN in all the SNP participating regions (Ruvuma, Lindi and Mtwara) to be 76% and 79%, respectively [21]. The analysis of the third mosquito net distribution is still ongoing. The SNP also promoted sharing of surplus nets with neighbours who did not own mosquito nets. Long-lasting insecticidal nets were to remain available to pregnant women and infants during antenatal and immunization visits at their attending health facility through the Tanzania National Voucher Scheme (TNVS) [18, 19]. Unfortunately, the TNVS was discontinued in 2014 and a replacement system (free nets during antenatal and immunization visits (ANC/EPI)) was not implemented until June 2016 (pers. Comm. Ikupa Akim, National Malaria Control Programme) [21, 22]. Alternative sources of mosquito nets (treated and untreated) are through the commercial sector (local market, kiosks) for those without school-going children.

The objective of this study was to explore local perceptions and practices of net care and repair in a community that continuously receives LLINs. Specifically, actions associated with different levels of net damage, motivators and barriers associated with net care and repair, and perceptions on how to overcome those reported barriers were assessed. The study approach was based on the Health Belief Model (HBM) [23], which has been useful

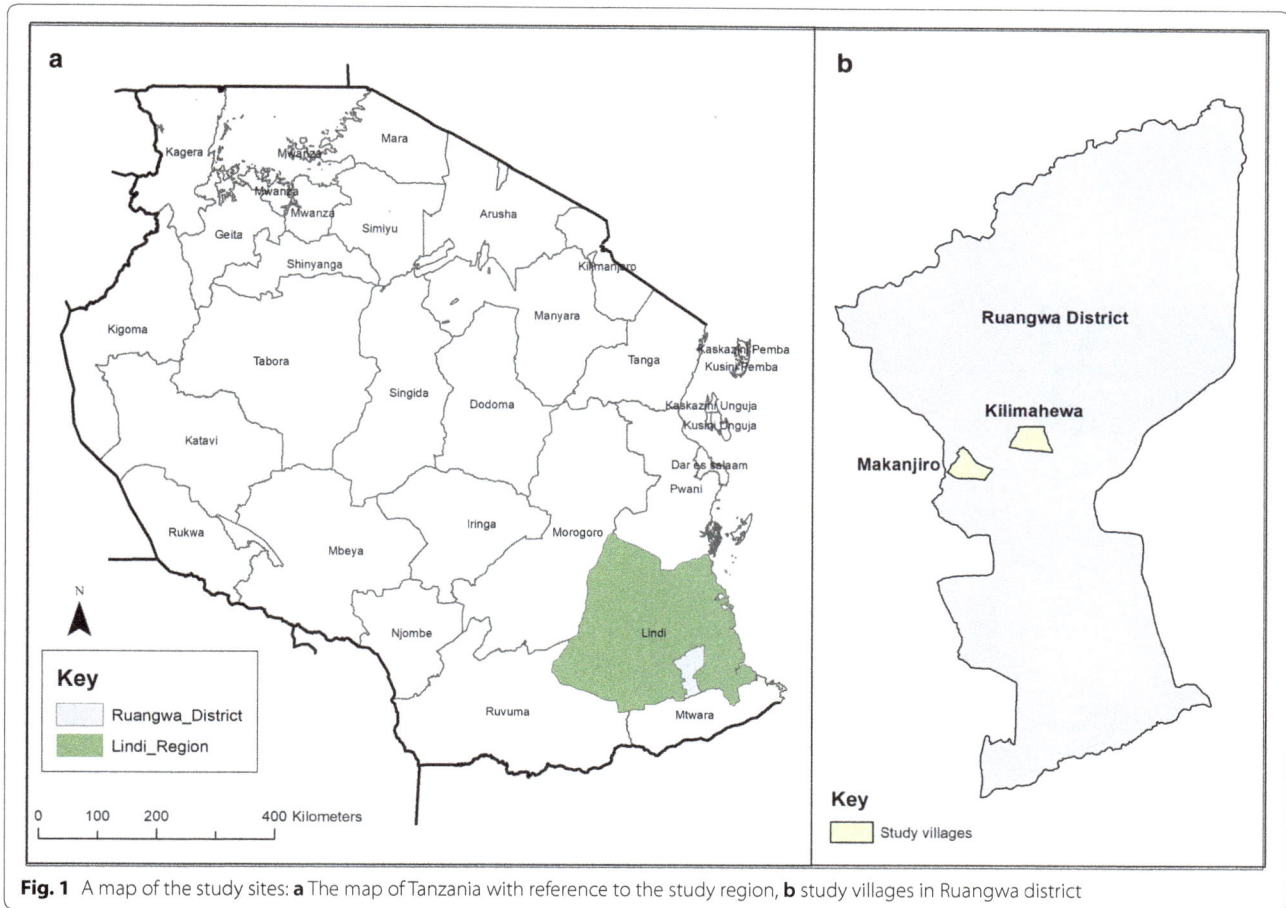

Fig. 1 A map of the study sites: **a** The map of Tanzania with reference to the study region, **b** study villages in Ruangwa district

to explain and predict human-disease interactions in previous studies [13, 24]. The model assumes that individuals will (a) opt to care for and repair their LLINs because of their perception that malaria is a major threat to their health (perceived severity and susceptibility), (b) identify themselves as capable to perform day-to-day care and repair activities (self-efficacy) based on modifying factors such as personal and net characteristics and external and internal cues to action, and (c) maintain nets as a means to protect themselves against malaria (perceived benefits increasing likelihood of action) (Fig. 2).

Understanding variations in local perceptions, motivators and barriers to net care and repair is key for the National Malaria Control Programme (NMCP) to optimize cost-effectiveness with fewer net replacements through suitable Behaviour-Change Communication (BCC). Exposure to effective BCC about net care and repair has been observed to improve overall net condition [25, 26]. However, repairs alone were not found sufficient to improve physical condition [25, 26], leading to the U.S President's Malaria Initiative (PMI) to change their policy to support only net care initiatives promoting

BCC that protects nets from damage and improve net use [27]. Reinforcing Tanzania's BCC strategy to include relatable positive messages could inspire appropriate net care actions. The study expected participants to put high value on net care and repair to maintain intact nets as a valuable commodity that protects them against malaria, which they see as a major threat to their health (Fig. 2).

Methods
Study site
The study was conducted in Makanjiro (rural) and Kilimahewa (peri-urban) villages in Ruangwa District, Lindi Region (Fig. 1). Ruangwa District was one of two districts in Southern Zone enrolled in the population arm of the Sentinel Panel of Districts (SPD), Sample Vital registration with Verbal Autopsy (SAVVY) project based at the Ifakara Health Institute (IHI) [28]. Makanjiro and Kilimahewa villages were randomly selected from a pool of 15 villages enrolled in the SAVVY project. The primary malaria vectors in Tanzania are *Anopheles gambiae* sensu stricto, *Anopheles funestus* (both vectors indoor resting) and *Anopheles arabiensis* (outdoor resting) [19,

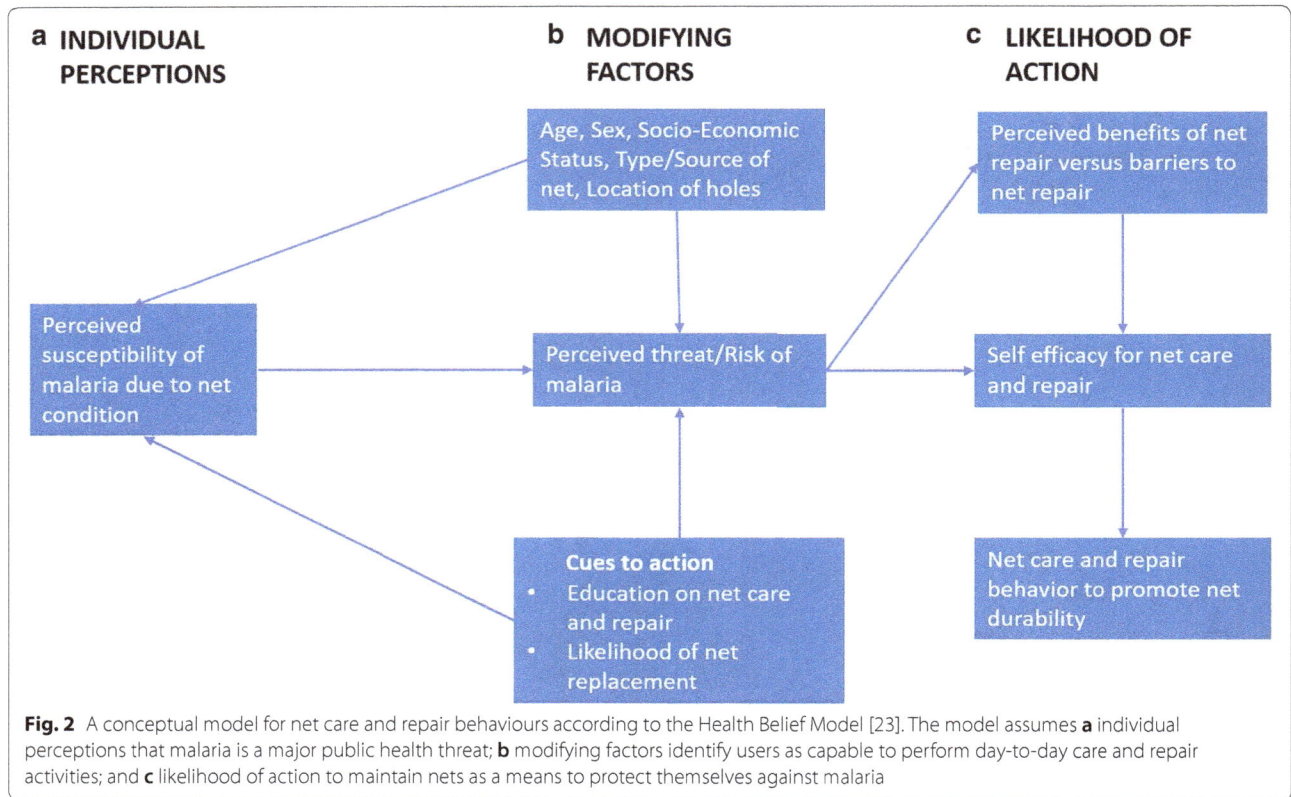

Fig. 2 A conceptual model for net care and repair behaviours according to the Health Belief Model [23]. The model assumes **a** individual perceptions that malaria is a major public health threat; **b** modifying factors identify users as capable to perform day-to-day care and repair activities; and **c** likelihood of action to maintain nets as a means to protect themselves against malaria

29–32]. Lindi region has one major rainy season per year (March–May) at the end of which peak malaria transmission occurs [19].

Ethical approval and consent to participate
Ethical approval was obtained from the Ifakara Health Institute (Ref: IHI/IRB/No: 015-2016), and the National Institute of Medical Research, Tanzania (Ref: NIMR/HQ/R.8a/Vol. IX/2193). The study was only administered to participants above 18 years of age upon written informed consent.

Data collection
Data was collected through a mix of qualitative research methods, namely Focus Group Discussions (FGDs), In-Depth Interviews (IDIs) and a Participatory Activity (PA). Study participants were selected purposively with the assistance of village leaders. Participants were eligible if they were above 18 years of age, had lived in the village for a minimum of 12 months, and owned at least one LLIN in their household.

In 2016, a pilot study was conducted in Pemba Mnazi (rural Dar-es-Salaam) to ensure research tools were locally appropriate. All FGDs and IDIs were conducted in Kiswahili language and audio-recorded with hand-held digital devices. In addition, notes were taken during each

interview. Interviews were guided by a topic guide containing a priori themes identified through literature and based on the theoretical framework of the HBM model (Fig. 2). Participants were encouraged to narrate their day-to-day activities regarding care and repair of LLINs. The topic guide was used to probe where necessary. The sample size of 30 IDIs and 10 FGDs were determined by reviewing similar studies [5, 13, 14] to capture variation of responses from different participant groups. Response saturation [33] was reached after three FGDs and five IDIs, but sampling was continued to ensure emerging themes were not missed.

Structured participant questionnaire
Prior to the start of any FGD or IDI, researchers administered a simple structured questionnaire to collect non-identifying socio-demographic information about each participant, including sex, age, education, number of children, participation in the SNP and exposure to BCC messaging in the past 6 months.

Focus group discussions
Five FGDs were conducted in each village. Four FGDs were conducted with community members and one with key village informants (i.e. religious, traditional/village leaders, and influential people). The community

members were split into four groups of 8–12 participants each. Focus Group Discussions were conducted separately for young men (18–24 years old), women (> 18 years) with children under the age of five, older men (> 25 years), and older women with or without children (> 25 years old).

In-depth interviews

In each of the two villages, five men, five women with or without children, and five women with children under the age of five were recruited for IDIs. In-Depth Interviews were conducted primarily at the study participant's home or space of comfort with minimal distraction from children and neighbours to provide a confidential environment for them to discuss in detail their attitudes and actions towards net care and repair.

Participatory activity and mosquito net assessment

After each IDI and the FGD with women with children under the age of five, participants were guided through a participatory activity (PA). Study participants were shown individually labelled nets with different levels of damage and repair (Table 1) and were asked to decide between four actions for each net: (1) do nothing and continue to use; (2) repair and continue to use; (3) no longer use net but use it for something else in the household; or (4) no longer use it and discard the net. The level of damage and evidence of repair presented during the PA was to mimic observations from other field studies [34, 35]. Study participants were asked to make

two choices for each net to explore current actions and understanding of net care and repair with social norms and discuss the reasons for their choices; (1) what they *would* do; and (2) what they think they *should* do.

To compare reported intentions during the PA with actual behaviour, the net used by the person being interviewed was assessed onsite at the end of each IDI. The number, size and location of holes and evidence of repair were recorded, and participants were asked to reflect on the status of their nets and their reported attitudes to care and repair. The holes were assessed using the World Health Organization (WHO) hole size descriptions and categorized as either "good" (<79 cm^2 hole surface area), "damaged" (80–789 cm^2) or "too torn" (> 790 cm^2) [10].

Data management and analysis

All audio-recorded data from the FGDs and IDIs were transcribed and spot-checked by both the interviewer and note-taker involved in the interview. Following approval of transcripts, interview summaries were written for each FGD and IDI. Data analysis was conducted following thematic framework analysis procedures [36] to specifically explore study objectives. The thematic framework analysis included familiarization of data, identification of the thematic framework, indexing, charting, mapping and interpretation [37–40]. An initial coding framework was created using the topic guide. All four researchers who participated in the data collection then independently conducted an inductive thematic analysis of the interview summaries and a preliminary

Table 1 Responses for action on nets with different damage and repair attributes presented in the participatory activity

Net ID	Number of holes	Hole sizes[a]	Hole location[b]	Repair[c]	Category[d]	Common "would do" response	Common "should do" response
1	1	"Size 2"	Bottom	No	Good	Repair and continue to use	Repair and continue to use
2	1	"Size 2"	Roof	No	Good	Repair and continue to use	Repair and continue to use
3	18	15 × "Size 1", 3 × "Size 2"	Mix	No	Damaged	Discard; or use it for alternative purposes	Repair and
4	9	8 × "Size 1", 1 × "Size 3"	"Size 1" top, "Size 3" bottom	No	Damaged	Repair and continue to use	Repair and continue to use
5	2	1 × "Size 2", 1 × "Size 4"	"Size 4" roof, "Size 2" bottom	No	Damaged	Repair and continue to use	Repair and continue to use
6	2	1 × "Size 2", 1 × "Size 4"	"Size 4" roof, "Size 2" bottom	Partial (Size 4)	Damaged	Repair and continue to use	Repair and continue to use
7	25	22 × "Size 1", 1 × "Size 2", 2 × "Size 3"	Mix	No	Damaged	Repair and continue to use; Discard; or use it for alternative purposes	Repair and continue to use

[a] Hole size categories based on the WHO guidelines [10]: "Size 1": smaller than a thumb (0.5–2 cm), "Size 2": larger than a thumb but smaller than a fist (2–10 cm), "Size 3": larger than a fist but smaller than a head (10–25 cm) and "Size 4": larger than a head (> 25 cm)

[b] Each side panel split into top half and bottom half

[c] Type of repair: Sewing with needle and thread (as per SNP BCC messaging)

[d] Physical damage categories based on total hole surface area [10]: good: <79 cm^2, Damaged: 80–789 cm^2 and Too Torn: > 790 cm^2

coding framework was established including sub-themes relevant to study objectives. Names and all individual identifiers were removed from transcripts.

The transcripts were then entered into NVivo 11 Pro software (QSR International Pty Ltd, Australia) for final data management, indexing, and identification of associated narratives to the study objectives. Data collected were organised by coding responses under each theme identified in the final codes to allow within and between participant group analysis. Data from the structured questionnaires was summarized. Triangulation was done to compare (a) responses given during the PA, (b) observations made in the mosquito net assessment, and (c) participant reflections of their current net status to provide in-depth context and to validate findings.

Results

A total of 118 individuals from the two villages were interviewed (male: n=56; female: n=62). Fifty-eight people were from the village of Makanjiro (rural) and 60 from the village of Kilimahewa (peri-urban). The highest level of education attained by the majority of the study participants (n=87) was completion of primary school. Ninety-one participants reported to have received their LLIN from the SNP while 27 nets were purchased from local stores. There are no data on whether shop-bought nets were treated or untreated. Eighty-six of the 263 children of the study participants were attending primary school and therefore eligible for a mosquito net through the SNP. On average, the study participants received 0.5 SNP nets per year. Of the 118 interviewed participants, 87 had been exposed to BCC about malaria in the past 6 months. The most recalled BCC messages were to hang the net, sleep underneath the net and use the net all year round.

Perceived threat

Malaria was unanimously perceived to be a major public health threat in Ruangwa. The disease was mainly associated with death, miscarriage and poverty. Illness forced individuals to be away from the workforce while malaria treatment increased household costs. The disease was reported to weaken the bodies of those who suffered from it, and the repercussions would be worse if the head of household fell ill as reiterated by a woman in Kilimahewa.

"Yes, I am unable to perform any of my tasks because I am sick. I am unable to care for my children or work. If the father, who is the head of household, falls sick, it is even worse as there is no-one to provide." (IDI participant, Woman with child under the age of

five, Kilimahewa)

Generally, the importance of mosquito nets for protection against malaria mosquitoes was reported as the main driver of motivation to care and repair nets by the majority of the study participants.

"The net protects me so that a mosquito who would bite and infect me with malaria cannot reach me." (IDI participant, Man, Kilimahewa)

Participants reported a high risk of being bitten by mosquitoes and valued the protection of the nets from mosquitoes which aided better sleep.

"For the poor, sleep is leisure. If you hear noises from such insects, you will not sleep." (FGD Participant, Makanjiro, Older man)

Mosquito nets used by children, especially those under the age of five, were most likely to be repaired first. This was because young children were reported to be most vulnerable to the disease and not able to care for or repair their own nets. Male key informants and older men reported their own personal nets to be of top priority for repair as they were the breadwinners of the family. Older women specifically reported to repair damaged household items, including nets and clothes, in one sitting rather than repairing each item soon after each hole was identified.

Nails on bed frame edges were reported as the primary cause of damage because of the daily tucking and untucking from underneath the mattress. Other causes of damage included children playing with the net, pulling the net too much to fit a bed that is bigger than the net, edges of the wooden frame "besela" used to hang the net, and household pests and rodents.

Net care

Net care was primarily defined as washing, tying up the net over the sleeping space in the morning and lowering it in the evening for use, and seasonal storage. Upon probing, hanging nets after washing and drying nets inside or outside the household were acknowledged as other practices associated with care.

Nets were usually washed within the household compound in a basin or bucket with soap and water as soon as the net was perceived to be dirty. Most participants reported washing their nets every other week. Washing the net ensured cleanliness, which also prevented other dirt-related problems such as sneezing and headaches. Tying up nets over the sleeping space in the morning and lowering it in the evening for use was done to avoid mosquitoes and other insects from hiding inside the net during the day. Seasonal storage, a result of seasonal net use, differed between the two villages. Kilimahewa (peri-urban) residents reported using mosquito nets throughout the year whereas Makanjiro (rural) residents only used their nets during the rainy season when mosquito prevalence increased, except for households with children under the age of 5.

> *"We use mosquito nets during rainy season, because there are a lot of swamps and mosquitoes, but during the dry season, there are no mosquitoes. We store the nets." (FGD participant, Older Woman. Makanjiro)*

When describing barriers to net care or repair, study participants were quick to separate themselves from the subject and started speaking in the third person. Reported barriers to net care included care not being a priority in the day-to-day activities, "negligence" and lack of net "Ngao" (net retreatment kits that used to be sold over the counter but were discontinued in 2009 after the introduction of LLINs). Women attributed being pre-occupied by other household activities such as sweeping and cooking, which left them too exhausted by the end of the day to then take particular care of the net. It was also reported difficult to keep up with small children who would play and tug on the nets if tied above the sleeping space.

> *"Other people do not have time to relax at home because they are so preoccupied by other household activities that they even forget to tie up nets in the morning." (IDI Participant, Woman, Kilimahewa).*

The majority of participants reported that other community members were negligent as they did not clean or care for their personal items. These community members were not expected to make time to wash or care for the nets provided to them. There were concerns that nets needed to be re-treated with insecticides after each wash to activate the insecticide for continued protection as was previously recommended with *"Ngao"* net retreatment kits. The lack of net retreatment kits at the markets left many heads of households in dilemma of how frequently to wash their nets.

> *"For most residents here, our households are of dirt floors, so when you sweep the house, in no time your net is dirty." (FGD Participant, Older Men, Kilimahewa).*

Key informants reported poverty as the underlying barrier to net care. The general household environment such as mud floors and grass/thatch roofs makes it difficult to care for one's net every day. Resources such as a wooden frame "besela" required to hang up the net during the day were also not available for all.

> *"For many it is about their general standard of living. It is not only difficult to care for their nets but also for other household items such as clothes." (FGD Participant, Young Man, Kilimahewa)*

Net repair

Net repair was reported necessary as soon a hole was identified and defined as either sewing and/or tying knots (Fig. 3). Upon probing, adding patches to holes was dismissed as an option for net repair. Though patches of old clothes were easy to find, sewing them on the net reduced the airflow inside the net, and was hence not seen as a practical solution for repair.

Blocking the entry of mosquitoes into the net was crucial, because,

> *"if mosquitoes enter the net because I do not repair it, the children will get malaria and I will have to stop doing everything else to take care of them and maybe even get malaria myself." (IDI participant, Woman with child under the age of five, Makanjiro)*

Study participants generally echoed their huge dependence on freely-distributed nets as the primary source and means of protection against malaria. While nets were available at the local shops, the costs were perceived too high even for untreated nets (approximately TZS 10,000, USD\$4.50). Replacement schedules of the free SNP nets were largely unclear to residents in the study villages so extending the life of a net until a replacement net arrives, free or bought, was reported crucial to ensure household members remain protected for as long as possible.

Net repair was perceived a social responsibility for all LLIN recipients. Through net repair, community members, who are the workforce to build the Tanzanian nation, would be protected from the deadly disease of malaria.

> *"When we join forces and work together, we create a workforce that a village such as ours depends on for development. But when community members fall sick with malaria, we lose the workforce in the village, and also as a nation." (FGD participant, Key Informant, Makanjiro)*

Net repair was largely reported as a temporary measure before the acquisition of a new net, hence not a matter of priority. Some participants reported sewing a net as too much work, while others reported not knowing how to sew a net given the varying material type and mesh size of the net itself. The lack of educational sessions on when to repair nets was also reported as a barrier. When holes were not repaired, the number and size of holes

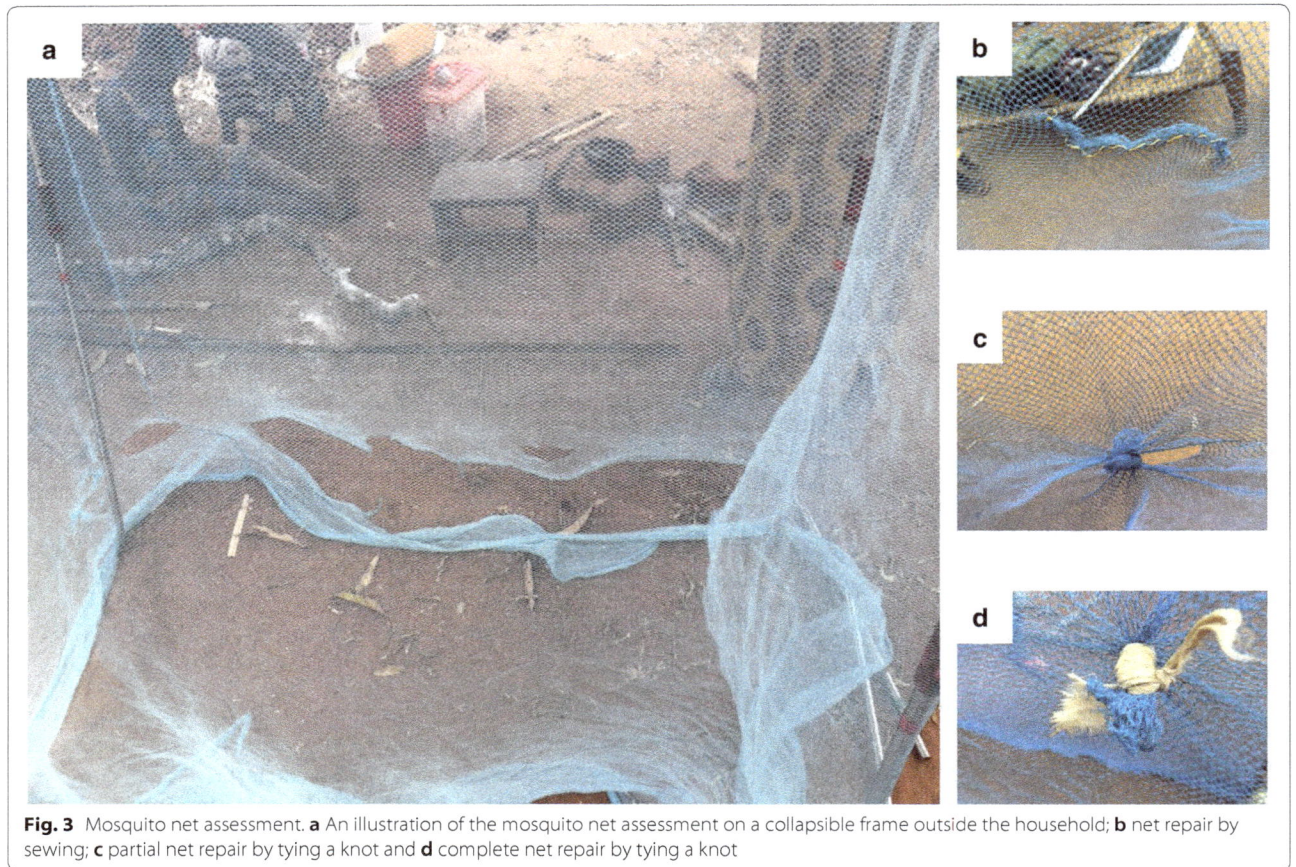

Fig. 3 Mosquito net assessment. **a** An illustration of the mosquito net assessment on a collapsible frame outside the household; **b** net repair by sewing; **c** partial net repair by tying a knot and **d** complete net repair by tying a knot

increased until nets were perceived to be "too torn" to be worth repairing.

> *"Some do not know what to do when they identify a hole on the net. Some do not even recognize that the hole should be repaired to adequately protect themselves from malaria." (IDI participant, Woman, Kilimahewa)*

Mechanistic problems reported included regular needles being too small to grip properly and close the hole whereas tying a knot was only feasible for some types of holes (Fig. 3). Lack of self-initiative to explore and find alternative solutions, for example using bigger needle and thicker thread to repair the net, was reported as a potential barrier for others to repair their nets. Some participants also reported lack of sewing kits (needle and thread) for net repair readily available in their households. Key informants highlighted that some tailors refused to mend nets as nets were perceived as too personal to be repaired by them.

Self-efficacy to care for and repair nets

Both men and women reported their capabilities to perform all the basic care and repair practices such as washing, hanging, tying up the net above sleeping space, storing it away and knotting. However, the wife or woman was seen as the one solely responsible for net care and repair in households irrespective of her economic role (i.e. whether she was head of household or also worked). The man's main contributions were to act as the catalyst (proposing when care actions such as washing should be performed) and the financial decision-maker (net repair and/or replacement decisions). In the absence of a woman (unmarried, widowed or travelling wife), men reported to care for and repair their own nets but in the confines of their household in seclusion from the public. Children aged 13 and above, irrespective of their gender, could take responsibility of their own nets. Parental check-up became less common due to cultural norms that refrain mothers from entering their sons' room and the father a daughter's room once the children reached puberty.

Mosquito net assessment

Of the nets presented during the Participatory Activity (PA), the following five net IDs from the PA; 1, 3, 4, 5 and 7 (Table 1), were most comparable to those from participating households in terms of level of damage and lack of repair (Table 2). All participants reported they *would* repair the single hole identified at the bottom of net ID 1. The horizontal tear was perceived easy to sew together if sewing materials were readily available in their households. Alternatively, participants suggested that the hole located at the bottom could be tucked under the mattress. Most study participants reported they would discard Net ID 3 (18 holes) or use it for alternative purposes around the household such as an additional cushion under the mattress or fencing the flower garden. The holes were perceived to be too many and too scattered to repair. As with Net ID 1, the hole located at the bottom of Net ID 4 (9 holes) was reported to be either repaired or tucked underneath because *"it [the single hole] is located*

at the bottom. After tucking the net under the mattress, mosquitoes cannot get through." (IDI participant, Older Man, Kilimahewa).

Very few of the small holes located at the top were noticed by participants, and those that did identify them, did not mention any action to repair them. Participants responded they would either repair and continue to use net ID 5 (2 holes) or use it for alternative purposes around the house depending on their financial status when the holes were identified. A few reported they would seek out the local tailor to repair the large hole at the top. Reponses for net ID 7 (25 holes) were mixed with some ready to use it for alternative purposes while others would repair and continue to use it. However, it was unanimously echoed that all the nets presented in the PA were still usable and *should* be repaired as the holes were not overwhelming in number or size. Study participants did not perceive any of the nets presented to be too torn; therefore, they *should* all be repaired for continued use of

Table 2 Mosquito net assessment findings by In-Depth Interview participant groups and village

Village/participant group	Net type	Number of holes	Hole sizes[a]	Hole location[b]	Repair[c]	Category[d]
Kilimahewa (peri-urban)						
Man	LLIN	3	3 × "Size 1"	Bottom	0	Good
Man	LLIN	3	3 × "Size 1"	Bottom	0	Good
Man	LLIN	36	17 × "Size 1", 19 × "Size 2"	Top, bottom, roof	5	Damaged
Man	Unknown	31	16 × "Size 1", 14 × "Size 2", 1 × "Size 3"	Top, bottom	1	Damaged
Man	Untreated	3	3 × "Size 1"	Bottom	0	Good
Woman	LLIN	9	8 × "Size 1", 1 × "Size 2"	Top, bottom	0	Good
Woman	LLIN	1	1 × "Size 2"	Bottom	0	Good
Woman	LLIN	1	1 × "Size 1"	Top	0	Good
Woman	LLIN	7	6 × "Size 1", 1 × "Size 2"	Bottom	2	Good
Woman	LLIN	21	19 × "Size 1", 2 × "Size 2"	Top, bottom	0	Damaged
Woman with under 5	Unknown	106	98 × "Size 1", 8 × "Size 2"	Top, bottom, roof	2	Damaged
Woman with under 5	Untreated	4	2 × "Size 1", 2 × "Size 2"	Bottom	0	Good
Woman with under 5	LLIN	2	2 × "Size 1"	Top, bottom	0	Good
Woman with under 5	LLIN	13	2 × "Size 1", 10 × "Size 2", 1 × "Size 3"	Bottom	0	Damaged
Woman with under 5	LLIN	4	1 × "Size 1", 3 × "Size 2"	Top, bottom	2	Damaged
Makanjiro (rural)						
Man	LLIN	4	2 × "Size 2", 1 × "Size 3", 1 × "Size 4"	Top, bottom	0	Too torn
Man	LLIN	12	12 × "Size 1"	Bottom	0	Good
Man	LLIN	21	8 × "Size 1", 13 × "Size 2"	Bottom	5	Damaged
Man	LLIN	2	2 × "Size 1"	Bottom	1	Good
Man	LLIN	4	1 × "Size 1", 1 × "Size 2", 2 × "Size 3"	Top, bottom	0	Damaged
Woman	LLIN	0	–		0	Good
Woman	LLIN	0	–		0	Good

[a] Hole size categories based on the WHO guidelines [10]: "Size 1": smaller than a thumb (0.5–2 cm), "Size 2": larger than a thumb but smaller than a fist (2–10 cm), "Size 3": larger than a fist but smaller than a head (10–25 cm) and "Size 4": larger than a head (> 25 cm)

[b] Each side panel split into top half and bottom half

[c] Number of holes repaired on the net. Type of repair varied as per Fig. 3 including sewing and knotting

[d] Physical damage categories based on total hole surface area [10]: Good: < 79 cm^2, Damaged: 80–789 cm^2 and Too Torn: > 790 cm^2

protection against malaria, particularly when left with no money to acquire a new net (Table 1).

Generally, mosquito nets assessed in peri-urban Kilimahewa were in "good" condition (n = 10) while the remaining handful of nets (n = 5) were "damaged" as per WHO hole sizes categories [10] (Table 2). The condition of nets assessed in Makanjiro varied much more: Two nets were in as good as new condition (no holes), four nets had some holes but were still in "good" condition, five nets were "damaged", and four nets were "too torn" (Table 2). Of the 30 nets assessed across the two villages, only five nets in Kilimahewa and three nets in Makanjiro showed any evidence of repair by sewing or knotting.

The most common response during the PA was to repair and continue to use nets, and everyone reported they should repair and continue to use. However, actual evidence of repair in nets from households was scarce (Table 2). When asked, the main reasons given for not repairing nets were; (1) not being able to identify most of the holes while inside the households due to poor lighting, and (2) tucking holes located at the bottom underneath the mattress. Study participants did indicate that the net assessment exercise encouraged them to repair the holes in their nets and that they would assess all other nets present in their households for damage following the end of the interview.

Cues to action

Given that the SNP was the primary source of nets in the study villages, it was suggested that parents should be invited to the schools for educational sessions on net care and repair so that they could engage better daily in the maintenance of LLINs to prevent malaria.

It was proposed that Community Health Workers and other experts from the district headquarters should train people on the importance of nets, how to care for nets and when to repair them. However, there were some participants that cautioned:

"Mosquito nets are private items that one has to have self-initiative to take care of. Educational sessions on such sensitive matters can be deemed offensive by the recipient of the net" (FGD participant, Older Man, Makanjiro).

The women generally echoed that men were equally as capable to perform both care and repair duties within households, hence should also participate in day-to-day activities. Net manufacturing companies were requested to produce stronger nets. It was also requested that net retreatment kits *"Ngao"* should be restocked in the commercial markets as it was reassuring to retreat a net after each wash to ensure it would repel or kill mosquitoes upon contact.

Upon probing, mass washing sessions, inclusion of leaflets and sewing kits in the packaging, and road shows were perceived as other measures to encourage net maintenance and general cleanliness. However, it was emphasized that the leader of the mass washing initiative should be someone not associated with the village to avoid passing judgement and spreading gossip of the status of nets within the village.

Information on leaflets attached on the packaging of nets was received with mixed reviews. While those in Kilimahewa received it well, study participants in Makanjiro worried for the illiterate who were perceived to be the majority in the village despite previous distributions including leaflets with pictorial demonstrations. Interactive educational sessions by community health workers and experts during road shows were proposed to be more informational.

Discussion

Though not unanimously actioned, there was a general readiness to care for and repair mosquito nets in southern Tanzania for the love of a good night's sleep free of mosquito bites or noises, as observed in other studies across sub-Sahara Africa [5, 12–14]. Response saturation was reached quickly in our study among participant groups and between villages, and responses of motivators and perceived challenges were similar to those of other studies in sub-Saharan Africa. This implies that general motivators and barriers to net care and repair are comparable across a range of cultural settings. These results are discussed using the theoretical framework presented in Fig. 1 and based on the HBM [23]. This study found that malaria was perceived to be a major threat and that mosquito nets were considered a useful tool against mosquito bites and to reduce health expenses associated with disease (individual perceptions; Fig. 2). Most people felt they were able to take good care of their nets and repair them when necessary (self-efficacy), although net repair was most commonly seen as a temporary measure and net care was performed mainly to keep nets clean and free of insects rather than to specifically prolong the lifespan of the net (potential barriers). A discrepancy was found between what people reported they did or knew they should do and actual condition of the nets. This highlights potential gaps in knowledge and uncovers the lack of an important motivator to care and repair: the better the net condition, the better the protection against malaria (likelihood of action).

Study participants much preferred net care over repair, which was similar to studies in West and East Africa [5, 12–14]. In southern Tanzania, the motivation for net care was generally associated with overall net maintenance such as cleanliness and preventing mosquitoes and other insects from hiding inside the net, and not directly associated with the prevention of damage as in other studies. Similarly to other studies, however, dirty nets were perceived harmful to one's health and shameful to society [5, 13–15]. Clean nets were seen as aesthetically pleasing and a show of a responsible woman. Some net owners reported to wash their nets almost every other week (approximately 26 washes a year) as was also observed in Uganda [5] and Peru [41]. Tanzania's School Net Programme BCC messaging currently lacks a recommendation for washing frequency and only states to "*wash your net when it gets dirty and dry it in the shade to preserve the effectiveness of the insecticide of the net*" (Pamela Kweka [John Hopkins Centre for Communications Programs in Tanzania] *pers. comm.*). The existing BCC also does not address the fact that LLINs do not require the "Ngao" net retreatment kits. Households were left in a dilemma as they wanted clean nets, yet also wanted to maintain the active chemical content. If they did not wash the nets, they got negative reactions from family members. If they did wash their nets frequently, the nets were deemed ineffective to sleep under after about a year. In Kenya, increased washing frequency was associated with decreased physical condition of nets [8]. In Tanzania, 45% of nets were in bad condition after washing them four to seven times a year and insecticidal content was also observed to be low [42].

Behavioural Change Communication should be updated to include a realistic recommendation regarding washing frequency as was done in Peru [41], keeping in mind that expecting people to refrain from washing their subjectively dirty nets is unrealistic [15]. Behaviour Change Communication should also highlight the importance of preventing damage on nets while promoting preventative net maintenance behaviours, such as tying up the net over the sleeping space or storing nets safely away from children or rodents when not in use [23].

Although participants stated that nets were important to protect against malaria, net repair was only seen as a temporary measure before acquisition of a new net as was also found in Senegal [13, 43]. People much preferred receiving brand-new nets for free and only uncertainty around distribution schedules motivated net repair. Although people reported that net repair was necessary as soon as a small hole was identified, inconsistencies were observed between such reported intentions and the physical condition of nets observed inside households [5, 14]. The lack of priority to repair nets led to the accumulation of holes with time. Nets observed to be "too torn" showed no more evidence of repair and were from households of women (self-reported primary caretakers) (Table 2). Households with poor lighting, which were the majority in the study villages, have more difficulty in identifying holes for repair. Using a frame, which stretched the material as was done in this study, allowed participants to easily identify the smallest of holes. This, however, is an unlikely method for household members to regularly assess their own nets so they can determine the appropriate action. When the net is removed from its hanging place, it is normally crumpled together in a ball of fabric, making it difficult to identify small holes. Many larger holes were observed at the bottom of the nets and respondents most often said they would tuck those holes underneath the mattress. The convenience of tucking holes underneath the mattress fostered neglect for other holes. Thus, holes that could not be tucked underneath the mattress were stretched and became larger over time.

Mechanistic challenges may have contributed to the low occurrence of repairs. Net repairs by sewing was largely dependent on other household items requiring sewing, was time consuming and needed financial investment of a bigger needle and thicker thread (Fig. 3b). Alternatively, knotting was either partial or pulled a lot of net material together depending on the size of the hole, potentially creating other mosquito entry points (Fig. 3c, d). In Nigeria, net repairs were not sufficient to improve overall status, i.e. shift nets from the "damaged" to the "good" WHO category [25], irrespective of the increase in proportion of repairs on torn nets [44].

Lack of knowledge or misconceptions (e.g. Ngao) were identified as key barriers to effective care and repair practices. Existing SNP BCC primarily targeted primary and secondary school children through posters and a weekly radio programme called "Pata Pata" jingle. Children were advised to inform their parents or caretakers of care and repair practices. Subsequently this may have created a knowledge gap where some parents and caretakers received limited or diluted information from their children. Workshops engaging parents, who have primary responsibility of taking care of the nets, were requested. Behavioural Change Communication for SNP should build on existing practices around the villages to share public health information of the developments of malaria control interventions such as the transition from use of untreated nets, retreatments kits and now LLINs [45] to ensure appropriate continued community-wide engagement in net maintenance. Women of Makanjiro village reported increased motivation to care for their LLINs following a Community Change Agent's educational session in their small group "Vikoba" meetings. Community-wide engagements in Ghana [46], Cambodia [47] and Madagascar [48] have had positive effects on promoting interactions with malaria control interventions and should become a more regular feature as part of continuous net distribution mechanisms in Tanzania.

The BCC messages that were recalled by household members emphasize the proper use of LLINs. It is therefore important to evolve the BCC strategy to include positive social norms, e.g. the personal responsibility to maintain nets in good condition [5, 13], especially as the SNP is now embedded into the NMCP LLIN strategy and has expanded its distribution to the Lake Zone [27]. Messages should incorporate net care as part of a daily routine and not as an additional burden to ensure that the luxury from a good night's sleep and health gains are maintained.

Study limitations

Though sampling was continued even after response saturation was reached, these findings only reflect the attitudes and actions of those interviewed and not the entire Lindi region or other zones in Tanzania where residents with school-going children continuously receive nets from the SNP. Although the researchers explained they were not health workers or involved in the SNP distribution process, there remains a possibility that study participants missed the distinctions, potentially biasing responses to be favourable towards mosquito nets and reported care and repair behaviours. The mosquito net assessment and PA were done outside the house on a frame that stretched the netting in a way that even the smallest holes could be identified. The study did not follow-up to assess whether any of the nets observed with damage were repaired as per study participant claims, and how they were repaired.

Conclusion

There was willingness to both care and repair mosquito nets in Ruangwa district, although net care was more likely to be performed than repair. Promotion of care practices as means to prevent net damage including realistic recommendations for washing frequency need to be included in the BCC messaging to prevent over-washing of nets. Discrepancies were observed between reported intentions to repair mosquito nets and current net condition which further reinforces the findings of previous studies that demonstrated no substantial benefit to promoting net repair. Targeted education through health facilities, particularly workshops for parents and engagement with community change agents were recommended as potential means to overcome barriers to net care by the study community.

Abbreviations

BCC: Behavioural-Change Communication; FGDs: Focus Group Discussions; HBM: Health Belief Model; IDI: In-Depth Interview; IHI: Ifakara Health Institute; LLINs: long-lasting insecticidal net; NMCP: National Malaria Control Programme; PA: participatory activity; PMI: U.S President's Malaria Initiative; SAVVY: Sample Vital registration with Verbal Autopsy; SNP: School Net Programme; SPD: Sentinel Panel of Districts; TNVS: Tanzania National Voucher Scheme; WHO: World Health Organization.

Authors' contributions

ZMM and LML conceived the study. ZMM, GG, KK, AD and LML designed the study. ZMM and AD collected and analyzed the data. ZMM wrote the manuscript. AD, GG, KK, HK and LML critically reviewed the manuscript. All authors read and approved the final manuscript.

Author details

[1] Ifakara Health Institute, Dar-es-Salaam, Tanzania. [2] London School of Hygiene and Tropical Medicine, London, UK. [3] National Malaria Control Programme, Dar-es-Salaam, Tanzania. [4] Swiss Tropical and Public Health Institute, Basel, Switzerland. [5] University of Basel, Petersplatz 1, 4003 Basel, Switzerland. [6] PMI VectorWorks, Johns Hopkins Center for Communication Programs, Baltimore, MD, USA. [7] U.S. President's Malaria Initiative, U.S. Agency for International Development, Dar es Salaam, Tanzania.

Acknowledgements

Ms. Christina Makungu supported the study design. Ms. Herieth Nyange and Mr Christopher Charles supported the data collection and transcription. This manuscript is published with permission of the Director-General of the National Institute of Medical Research (NIMR), Tanzania.

Competing interests

The authors declare that that they have no competing interests.

Funding

The research was made possible by the generous support of the American people through the United States Agency for International Development (USAID) under the terms of USAID/JHU Cooperative Agreement No: AID-OAA-A-14-00057. The contents do not necessarily reflect the views of USAID or the United States Government.

References

1. Bonner K, Mwita A, McElroy PD, Omari S, Mzava A, Lengeler C, et al. Design, implementation and evaluation of a national campaign to distribute nine million free LLINs to children under five years of age in Tanzania. Malar J. 2011;10:73.
2. Hanson K, Marchant T, Nathan R, Mponda H, Jones C, Bruce J, et al. Household ownership and use of insecticide treated nets among target groups after implementation of a national voucher programme in the United Republic of Tanzania: plausibility study using three annual cross sectional household surveys. BMJ. 2009;339:b2434.
3. Renggli S, Mandike R, Kramer K, Patrick F, Brown N, McElroy PD, et al. Design, implementaion and evaluation of a national campaign to deliver 18 million free long-lasting insecticidal nets to uncovered sleeping spaces in Tanzania. Malar J. 2013;12:85.
4. Haji K, Khatib B, Smith S, Ali A, Devine G, Coetzee M, et al. Challenges for malaria elimination in Zanzibar: pyrethroid resistance in malaria vectors and poor performance of long-lasting insecticide nets. Parasit Vectors. 2013;6:82.
5. Scandurra L, Acosta A, Koenker H, Kibuuka D, Harvey S. "It is about how the net looks": a qualitative study of perceptions and practices related to mosquito net care and repair in two districts in eastern Uganda. Malar J. 2014;13:504.

6. Kilian A, Byamukama W, Pigeon O, Gimnig J, Atieli F, Koekemoer L, et al. Evidence for a useful life of more than three years for a polyester-based long-lasting insecticidal mosquito net in Western Uganda. Malar J. 2011;10:299.

7. Kilian A, Byamukama W, Pigeon O, Atieli F, Duchon S, Phan C. Long-term field performance of a polyester-based long-lasting insecticidal mosquito net in rural Uganda. Malar J. 2008;7:49.

8. Mutuku F, Khambira M, Bisanzio D, Mungai P, Mwanzo I, Muchiri E, et al. Physical condition and maintenance of mosquito bed nets in Kwale County, coastal Kenya. Malar J. 2013;12:46.

9. Batisso E, Habte T, Tesfaye G, Getachew D, Tekalegne A, Kilian A, et al. A stitch in time: a cross-sectional survey looking at long lasting insecticide-treated bed net ownership, utilization and attrition in SNNPR, Ethiopia. Malar J. 2012;11:183.

10. WHO. Guidelines for monitoring the durability of long-lasting insecticidal mosquito nets under operational conditions. Geneva: World Health Organization; 2011.

11. Vestergaard. PermaNet 2015. http://www.vestergaard.com/our-products/permanet. Accessed 3 Apr 2015.

12. Leonard L, Diop S, Doumbia S, Sadou A, Mihigo J, Koenker H, et al. Net use, care and repair practices following a universal distribution campaign in Mali. Malar J. 2014;13:435.

13. Loll D, Berthe S, Faye SL, Wone I, Arnold B, Weber R. "You need to take care of it like you take care of your soul": perceptions and behaviours related to mosquito net damage, care and repair in Senegal. Malar J. 2014;13:322.

14. Hunter G, Scandurra L, Acosta A, Koenker H, Obi E, Weber R. "We are supposed to take care of it:" a qualitative observation of care and repair behaviour of long-lasting insecticide-treated nets in Nasarawe State, Nigeria. Malar J. 2014;13:320.

15. Miller J, Jones C, Nduguru S, Curtis V, Lines J. A new strategy for treating nets. Part 2: user's perceptions of efficacy and washing practices and their implications for insecticide dose. Trop Med Int Health. 1999;4:167–74.

16. Chandler C, Beisel U, Hausmann-Muela S, Muela J, Umlauf R. Brief report. Re-imaging malaria: looking into, behind and beyond current priorities, 2–3 September 2014.

17. Ministry of Health Community Development, Gender, Elderly and Children, Ministry of Health Zanzibar, National Bureau of Statistics, Office of the Chief Government Statistician, ICF International. Tanzania Demographic and Health Survey and Malaria Indicator Survey 2015–2016. Dar-es-Salaam, 2016. https://dhsprogram.com/pubs/pdf/fr321/fr321.pdf. Accessed 27 July 2016.

18. National Insecticide-Treated Nets (NATNETS) Tanzania. School Net Programme Dar-es-Salaam: 2015. http://www.natnets.org/index.php/programme-components/school-net-programme.html. Accessed 10 Feb 2015.

19. MoH Tanzania. Tanzanian National Malaria Control Programme Strategy 2014–2020. Dar-es-Salaam, 2014.

20. Lalji S, Ngondi JM, Thawer NG, Tembo A, Mandike R, Mohamed A, et al. School distribution as keep-up strategy to maintain universal coverage of long-lasting insecticidal nets: implementation and results of a program in Southern Tanzania. Glob Health Sci Pract. 2016;4:251–63.

21. Stuck L, Lutambi A, Chacky F, Schaettle P, Kramer K, Mandike R, et al. Can school-based distribution be used to maintain coverage of long-lasting insecticide treated bed nets: evidence from a large scale programme in southern Tanzania? Health Policy Plan. 2017;32:980–9.

22. Kramer K, Mandike R, Nathan R, Mohamed A, Lynch M, Brown N, et al. Effectiveness and equity of the Tanzania National Voucher Scheme for mosquito nets over 10 years of implementation. Malar J. 2017;16:255.

23. Janz NK, Becker MH. The Health Belief Model: a decade later. Health Educ Q. 1984;11:1–47.

24. Koenker HM, Loll D, Rweyemamu D, Ali AS. A good night's sleep and the habit of net use: perceptions of risk and reasons for bed net use in Bukoba and Zanzibar. Malar J. 2013;12:203.

25. Koenker H, Kilian A, Hunter G, Acosta A, Scandurra L, Fagbemi B, et al. Impact of behaviour change intervention on long-lasting insecticidal net care and repair behaviour and net condition in Nasarawe State, Nigeria. Malar J. 2015;14:18.

26. Helinski MH, Namara G, Koenker H, Kilian A, Hunter G, Acosta A, et al. Impact of a behaviour change communication programme on net durability in eastern Uganda. Malar J. 2015;14:366.

27. PMI. U.S. President's Malaria Initiative Technical Guidance. USAID PMI, 2018.

28. Kabadi GS, Geubbels E, Lyatuu I, Smithson P, Amaro R, Meku S, et al. Data Resource Profile: the sentinel panel of districts: Tanzania's national platform for health impact evaluation. Int J Epidemiol. 2014;4:79–86.

29. Huho B, Briët O, Seyoum A, Sikaala C, Bayoh N, Gimnig J, et al. Consistently high estimates for the proportion of human exposure to malaria vector populations occurring indoors in rural Africa. Int J Epidemiol. 2013;42:235.

30. Kaindoa EW, Finda M, Kiplagat J, Mkandawile G, Nyoni A, Coetzee M, et al. Housing gaps, mosquitoes and public viewpoints: a mixed methods assessment of relationships between house characteristics, malaria vector biting risk and community perspectives in rural Tanzania. Malar J. 2018;17:298.

31. Kaindoa EW, Mkandawile G, Ligamba G, Kelly-Hope LA, Okumu FO. Correlations between household occupancy and malaria vector biting risk in rural Tanzanian villages: implications for high-resolution spatial targeting of control interventions. Malar J. 2016;15:199.

32. Russell TL, Lwetoijera DW, Maliti D, Chipwaza B, Kihonda J, Charlwood JD, et al. Impact of promoting longer-lasting insecticide treatment of bed nets upon malaria transmission in a rural Tanzanian setting with pre-existing high coverage of untreated nets. Malar J. 2010;9:187.

33. Tuckett AG. Qualitative research sampling: the very real complexities. Nurse Res. 2004;12:47–61.

34. Lorenz L, Overgaard H, Massue D, Mageni Z, Bradley J, Moore J, et al. Investigating mosquito net durability for malaria control in Tanzania-Attrition, bioefficacy, chemistry, degradation and insecticide resistance (ABCDR): study protocol. BMC Public Health. 2014;14:1266.

35. Massue DJ, Moore SJ, Mageni ZD, Moore JD, Bradley J, Pigeon O, et al. Durability of Olyset campaign nets distributed between 2009 and 2011 in eight districts of Tanzania. Malar J. 2016;15:176.

36. Ritchie J, Spencer L. Qualitative data analysis for applied policy research. In: Analyzing qualitative data. Bryman A, Burges B, eds. Routledge; 2002. p. 246.

37. Braun V, Clarke V. Using thematic analysis in psychology. Qualitative Res Psychol. 2006;3:77–101.

38. Gale NK, Heath G, Cameron E, Rashid S, Redwood S. Using the framework method for the analysis of qualitative data in multi-disciplinary health research. BMC Med Res Methodol. 2013;13:117.

39. Ward DJ, Furber C, Tierney S, Swallow V. Using framework analysis in nursing research: a worked example. J Adv Nurs. 2013;69:2423–31.

40. Srivastava A, Thomson SB. Framework analysis: a qualitative methodology for applied policy research. J Admin Govern. 2009;4:72–9.

41. Harvey SA, Olórtegui MP, Leontsini E, Asayag CR, Scott K, Winch PJ. Trials of improved practices (TIPs): a strategy for making long-lasting nets last longer? Am J Trop Med Hyg. 2013;88:1109–15.

42. Erlanger T, Enayati AA, Hemingway J, Mshinda H, Tami A, Lengeler C. Field issues related to effectiveness of insecticide-treated nets in Tanzania. Med Vet Entomol. 2004;18:153–60.

43. Loll D, Berthe S, Faye SL, Wone I, Koenker H, Arnold B, et al. User-determined end of net life in Senegal: a qualitative assessment of decision-making related to the retirement of expired nets. Malar J. 2013;12:337.

44. Kilian A, Koenker H, Obi E, Selby RA, Fotheringham M, Lynch M. Field durability of the same type of long-lasting insecticidal net varies between regions in Nigeria due to differences in household behaviour and living conditions. Malar J. 2015;14:123.

45. Panter-Brick C, Clarke SE, Lomas H, Pinder M, Lindsay SW. Culturally compelling strategies for behaviour change: a social ecology model and case study in malaria prevention. Soc Sci Med. 2006;62:2810–25.

46. Ernst KC, Erly S, Adusei C, Bell ML, Kessie DK, Biritwum-Nyarko A, et al. Reported bed net ownership and use in social contacts is associated with uptake of bed nets for malaria prevention in pregnant women in Ghana. Malar J. 2017;16:13.

47. Gryseels C, Uk S, Sluydts V, Durnez L, Phoeuk P, Suon S, et al. Factors influencing the use of topical repellents: implications for the effectiveness of malaria elimination strategies. Sci Rep. 2015;5:16847.

48. Management Sciences for Health. Community Health Volunteers Combat Malaria in Madagascar Madagascar: Medium; 2017. https://medium.com/@MSHHealthImpact/community-health-volunteers-combat-malaria-in-madagascar-da598674ad85. Accessed 5 Mar 2018.

4

Prospective comparative multi-centre study on imported *Plasmodium ovale wallikeri* and *Plasmodium ovale curtisi* infections

Gerardo Rojo-Marcos[1]*[iD], José Miguel Rubio-Muñoz[2], Andrea Angheben[3], Stephane Jaureguiberry[4], Silvia García-Bujalance[5], Lina Rachele Tomasoni[6], Natalia Rodríguez-Valero[7], José Manuel Ruiz-Giardín[8], Joaquín Salas-Coronas[9], Juan Cuadros-González[1], Magdalena García-Rodríguez[10], Israel Molina-Romero[11], Rogelio López-Vélez[12], Federico Gobbi[3], María Calderón-Moreno[13], Esteban Martin-Echevarría[14], Matilde Elía-López[15], José Llovo-Taboada[16] and TropNet Plasmodium ovale investigator group

Abstract

Background: Few previous retrospective studies suggest that *Plasmodium ovale wallikeri* seems to have a longer latency period and produces deeper thrombocytopaenia than *Plasmodium ovale curtisi*. Prospective studies were warranted to better assess interspecies differences.

Methods: Patients with imported *P. ovale* spp. infection diagnosed by thick or thin film, rapid diagnostic test (RDT) or polymerase chain reaction (PCR) were recruited between March 2014 and May 2017. All were confirmed by DNA isolation and classified as *P. o. curtisi* or *P. o. wallikeri* using partial sequencing of the ssrRNA gene. Epidemiological, analytical and clinical differences were analysed by statistical methods.

Results: A total of 79 samples (35 *P. o. curtisi* and 44 *P. o. wallikeri*) were correctly genotyped. Males predominate in wallikeri group (72.7%), whereas were 48.6% in curtisi group. Conversely, 74.3% of curtisi group were from patients of African ethnicity, whilst 52.3% of Caucasians were infected by *P. o. wallikeri*. After performing a multivariate analysis, more thrombocytopaenic patients (p = 0.022), a lower number of platelets (p = 0.015), a higher INR value (p = 0.041), and shorter latency in Caucasians (p = 0.034) were significantly seen in *P. o. wallikeri*. RDT sensitivity was 26.1% in *P. o. curtisi* and 42.4% in *P. o. wallikeri*. Nearly 20% of both species were diagnosed only by PCR. Total bilirubin over 3 mg/dL was found in three wallikeri cases. Two patients with curtisi infection had haemoglobin under 7 g/dL, one of them also with icterus. A wallikeri patient suffered from haemophagocytosis. Chemoprophylaxis failed in 14.8% and 35% of curtisi and wallikeri patients, respectively. All treated patients with various anti-malarials which included artesunate recovered. Diabetes mellitus was described in 5 patients (6.32%), 4 patients of wallikeri group and 1 curtisi.

Conclusions: Imported *P. o. wallikeri* infection may be more frequent in males and Caucasians. Malaria caused by *P. o. wallikeri* produces more thrombocytopaenia, a higher INR and shorter latency in Caucasians and suggests a more pathogenic species. Severe cases can be seen in both species. Chemoprophylaxis seems less effective in *P. ovale* spp. infection than in *P. falciparum,* but any anti-malarial drug is effective as initial treatment. Diabetes mellitus could be a risk factor for *P. ovale* spp. infection.

Keywords: *Plasmodium ovale curtisi, Plasmodium ovale wallikeri,* Comparative study, Thrombocytopenia, INR, Antimalarials, Diabetes mellitus

*Correspondence: grojo.hupa@salud.madrid.org
[1] Hospital Universitario Príncipe de Asturias, Ctra de Meco s/n, 28805 Alcalá de Henares, Madrid, Spain
Full list of author information is available at the end of the article

Prospective comparative multi-centre study on imported Plasmodium ovale wallikeri...

37

Background

Malaria remains a global health problem with more than 212 million new cases in 2016 and 429,000 annual deaths worldwide, mostly driven by *Plasmodium falciparum* and *Plasmodium vivax*, to which most of the research resources are devoted [1].

Conversely, *Plasmodium ovale* spp. infection can be considered a neglected disease and little is known on its real incidence, geographic distribution, global disease burden or interactions with other *Plasmodium* species. The main problems for its study have been that it is frequently misdiagnosed because of usual submicroscopic or low parasitaemia levels, low performance of malaria rapid diagnostic tests (RDT) [2] and a majority of mixed infections with other *Plasmodium* spp. [3].

Nowadays, polymerase chain reaction (PCR) techniques have expanded the knowledge on *P. ovale* spp. epidemiology reporting infections in most of sub-Saharan Africa, Southeast Asia, and the Indian subcontinent [4–6], but not in the Americas, with prevalences as high as 15% in zones of Nigeria or Papua New Guinea [3]. In addition, severe complications, such as acute respiratory distress syndrome (ADRS) [7], spleen rupture, severe anaemia, or death may occur in patients with *P. ovale* spp. malaria [8]. Lastly, the incidence of imported *P. ovale* spp. infection seems to be increasing among travellers returning from West Africa [9–11], in whom chemoprophylaxis failed to work more frequently [12] compared to *P. falciparum* or *P. vivax* [13].

Since the study by Sutherland et al. was published in 2010, *P. ovale* is considered to comprise two genetically different subspecies, named *P. ovale curtisi* and *P. ovale wallikeri* that could have diverged 1–2 million years ago in their evolution [4]. They both are morphologically identical and cannot be differentiated by microscopy. Increasing information from different studies in endemic countries support that both subspecies co-circulate in Africa and Asia and are unable to recombine genetically [14–17].

Once established the genetic differences, the next question was to find out if there were any other differences in epidemiology, microbiology or clinical features between both subspecies. *Plasmodium o. curtisi* and *P. o. wallikeri* do not seem to differ in parasitaemia levels [5, 9, 13] and the absence of Schüffner's stippling may be a feature specific to *P. o. wallikeri* but only in 30% of blood samples [9]. Clinical differences between both species have not been clearly established, but *P. o. wallikeri* may have a shorter period of latency [13].

Recently, a multicentre, retrospective study in Spain was reported, comparing 21 imported *P. o. curtisi* and 14 *P. o. wallikeri* infections confirmed by PCR and gene sequencing [5]. The only significant finding was more severe thrombocytopaenia among patients with *P. o. wallikeri* infection than among those with *P. o. curtisi* (p = 0.031). However, non-significant trends showing shorter latency, lower albumin level, higher temperature and markers of more severe haemolysis were found in *P. o. wallikeri* group. Because of the retrospective design and small number of patients, larger, prospective studies were warranted to confirm these findings. Therefore, the results of a multicentre, prospective, comparative study of imported *P. o. wallikeri* and *P. o. curtisi* infections conducted in several European countries during the period 2014–2017 are presented below.

Methods

Study design

A prospective, observational, un-randomized, open-label, multicentre study was performed at European hospitals of TropNet Europe, European Network for Tropical Medicine and Travel Health. Participants were recruited between March 2014 and May 2017. The study was approved by the University Hospital Príncipe de Asturias Ethical Board and at each site as needed. Written informed consent was obtained from the participant or a legal representative before enrolment in the study. The trial was conducted in accord with the Declaration of Helsinki and Good Clinical Practice.

Microbiologic diagnosis

The initial diagnosis of imported *P. ovale* spp. infection was made up by thick and/or thin film and/or second generation RDT and/or PCR available in each hospital. Blood smears were stained by a standard technique with Giemsa solution for 30 min and were reviewed by an expert microbiologist. Parasite count was measured by determining the proportion of parasitized erythrocytes or the number of trophozoites per microlitre. Mixed infections with other *Plasmodium* species were excluded.

Laboratory samples

For cases tested positive, three drops ($\approx$ 50 µL) of full blood left after routine laboratory tests, were dotted on filter paper (Whatman™) and sent by regular mail to the Reference Malaria & Emerging Diseases Laboratory of the National Centre of Microbiology in Madrid. If DNA of *P. ovale* spp. had already been isolated, this was sent into a 1.5 mL screw cap tube with complete closure to the same Reference Laboratory.

Isolation of parasite DNA and molecular diagnosis confirmation

DNA isolation was performed using the QIAamp DNA blood mini kit (QIAGEN®) from whole blood following the manufacturer's protocol. Molecular diagnosis confirmation of *P. ovale* spp. was carried out by semi-nested multiplex malaria PCR [18] which allows to distinguish the four more prevalent human malaria species.

Plasmodium ovale subspecies characterization and confirmation

Characterization of *P. o. curtisi* and *P. o. wallikeri* was performed by partial sequencing of the ssrRNA gene and ssrRNA amplification was performed by a nested PCR assay specific for *Plasmodium* genus. The first reaction included UNR (5′-GACGGTATCTGATCGTCTTC-3′) and PLF (5′-AGTGTGTATCCAATCGAGTTTC-3′) primers [18]. The second PCR reaction incorporates the products of the first reaction along with NewPLFsh (5′-CTATCAGCTTTTGATGTTAG-3′) and NewRevsh (5′-CCTTAACTTTCGTTCTTG-3′) primers. Infection with different malaria species yields products of different sizes between 710 and 740 bp.

The PCR mixture in both reactions consisted of 75 mM TrisHCl (pH 9.0), 2 mM $MgCl_2$, 50 mM KCl, 20 mM $(NH_4)_2SO_4$, 200 µM of dNTP, 0.075 µM of each primers, 1.25 units of *Taq* DNA polymerase (Biotools B&M Labs., S.A., Madrid, Spain), and 5 µL of DNA, extracted by QIAgen kit, was used as template in a reaction volume of 50 µL. For the second reaction mixture, 2 µL of the PCR product of the first reaction was used as template. For both reactions, a GeneAmp® PCR System 2700 thermal cycler (Applied Biosystems Laboratory) was used, beginning with 7 min at 94 °C, followed by (first-round) 40 cycles of 20 s at 94 °C, 20 s at 62 °C, and 30 s at 72 °C, or (second-round) 35 cycles of 20 s at 94 °C, 20 s at 53 °C, and 20 s at 72 °C. The final cycle was followed by an extension time of 10 min at 72 °C.

The amplified products were purified using Illustra DNA and Gel Band Purification Kit (*General Electric Healthcare*) and sequenced with the Big Dye Terminator v3.1 Cycle Sequencing in an ABI PRISM® 3700 DNA Analyzer. All amplified products were sequenced in both directions twice.

In order to confirm *P. ovale* subtyping, a nested PCR amplification plus sequencing targeting cytochrome b was performed in three samples of each group.

Data collection

An anonymized database was designed to input all the medical information and laboratory registries in a prospective way. Data collected included gender, age, ethnicity, underlying diseases, type of patient, dates and purpose of travel, countries visited, malaria chemoprophylaxis, date of admission and diagnosis, presenting clinical signs or symptoms and complications of severe malaria according to criteria of the World Health Organization (WHO) [19] where no threshold of parasitaemia

for *P. ovale* spp. was established. The closest possible date of inoculation was defined as the day of departure from a malaria endemic area. The time between date of arrival and onset of illness or diagnoses was calculated once asymptomatic patients were excluded. Patients were classified as an early immigrant if they had stayed in a country without malaria for less than a year prior to diagnosis. An immigrant was a VFR (visiting friends and relatives) if travelled to a country endemic of malaria after a year of stay in a non-malarial area, and VFR traveller if visited his/her first-degree relative's country of birth having been born in a non-malaria endemic country. Recent *Plasmodium* infection was defined as probable or definite malaria infection in the previous 12 months before *P. ovale* spp. diagnosis.

Laboratory results included microbiological data with parasitaemia count, full blood count with white blood cells, haemoglobin and platelets, values of glucose, creatinine, albumin, transaminases, lactate dehydrogenase (LDH), total bilirubin (tBR) in plasma, the coagulation parameters activated partial thromboplastin time (APTT) and international normalized ratio (INR), glucose-6-phosphate dehydrogenase (G6PDH) activity in red blood cells, as well as serological studies of infection with human immunodeficiency virus (HIV), hepatitis B (HBV) and hepatitis C (HCV). Thrombocytopaenia was defined as a platelet count under 150,000/µL. Treatments, clinical and microbiological evolution and duration of hospital stay of those admitted were recorded. Treatments were performed following the guidelines of each country and health centre without a common recommendation.

Statistical analysis

Differences of proportions were evaluated by the Chi-squared-test if less than 20% of cells had five or less expected values. If more than 20% of cells had five or less expected values we used the Fisher's exact test for categorical variables. Differences of means between groups were calculated by the Student's *t*-test for independent samples if the normal distribution could be assumed. In the Student's t test for independent samples, the Levene's test for homogeneity of variances was used. If normal distribution was not valid, the non-parametric Mann–Whitney *U*-test was performed. To test for normality, either the Shapiro–Wilks for small samples or the Kolmogorov–Smirnov with Lilliefors' correction for large samples were used. Values are reported as number of patients and percentage or, for non-parametric distributions, as median and interquartile range (IQR). A multivariate linear regression analysis was performed for continuous variables and multivariate logistic regression for categorical variables to confirm if real differences were found when non-homogenous population between both groups were identified. A two-sided *p* value of 0.05 or less was considered to indicate statistical significance. Statistical analysis was performed using the SPSS version 21 (SPSS Inc, Chicago, IL, USA).

Results

During the period of the study, a total of 96 blood samples from 29 hospitals were sent to the reference laboratory. Of them, 13 were excluded because of mixed infections (11 with *P. falciparum*, 1 with *P. vivax* and 1 with *Plasmodium malariae*), 2 samples did not get amplified and data from another 2 were not obtained. At the end, 79 correctly genotyped and with complete patient information were included for statistic analysis. Of them, 35 were identified as *P. o. curtisi* and 44 as *P. o. wallikeri.*

Table 1 presents demographic and epidemiological data from both groups. A significant difference in the distribution of gender, ethnicity and type of patients was shown. Males clearly predominate in wallikeri group whereas gender distribution was more evenly matched in the curtisi group. Conversely, on ethnicity, African patients were 74.3% of curtisi group. This ethnic distribution is reflected in the type of patient with a majority of VFR and recent immigrants in the *P. o. curtisi* infection versus a larger number of displaced for working or cooperation in the other species. The remaining epidemiological data did not differ including country of infection, duration of travel, chemoprophylaxis, latency time, time until diagnoses, recent *Plasmodium* infection or underlying diseases. There is a wide range of 21 countries as the place of infection, most of them in West Africa.

Microbiological and laboratory information is reported in Table 2. Several analytical parameters showed statistically significant differences such as total leukocyte and platelet count, number of thrombocytopaenic patients, haemoglobin, creatinine, LDH or INR values. Even after the multivariate study was performed, eliminating the confounding factor of ethnicity, the number of platelets, thrombocytopaenic patients and INR remained significant (Table 3). Latency time was also included in the multivariate analysis because of the significant difference found in a previous report [13]. A statistically shorter latency period also appeared, but only in Caucasians patients with *P. o. wallikeri* compared to those in the curtisi group. On the other hand, no difference in parasitological data including submicroscopic infection, parasitaemia or sensitivity of the common antigen of RDT was seen.

In respect of the clinical manifestations and time of hospitalization no differences were found in (Table 4). Treatments were widely different according to the protocols of each centre. Primaquine was supplied to most

patients in both groups and only three patients showed G6PDH deficiency that contraindicated this treatment. Five patients showed analytical criteria for severe malaria and another one a rare and severe complication (haemophagocytosis). Outcome in nearly all cases was good, although two patients did not receive any anti-malarial treatment due to loss of follow-up.

Discussion

This is the largest prospective study to date on the two species of infection by imported *P. ovale* trying to overcome recruitment difficulties and limitations of previous retrospective studies.

On the results obtained, significant differences were found in the epidemiological characteristics of sex, ethnicity and type of patients between both groups. Ethnic differences may be the main confounding factor since there is a greater probability that African patients retain some semi-immunity against *P. ovale* spp. infection (excluding VFR travellers), which would generally result in less clinical and analytical involvement [20]. On the other hand, the difference in sex distribution and type of patients seems to be clearly related to the ethnic origin since in a subgroup analysis, 16 out of 18 (89%) of the patients with *P. o. wallikeri* who travelled by international cooperation were male and Caucasians, which would bias the characteristics of this group.

This distribution could be a result of chance alone or due to the fact that actually Caucasians patients are more susceptible to infection by wallikeri parasites. However, a previous retrospective study did not show these differences in sex, ethnicity or type of patient [5] and the few studies of imported ovale malaria reporting a significant number of patients showed either equality of sexes (but did not report on ethnicity) [13] or they were nearly all Chinese men who worked in African countries [10].

When performing the multivariate study adjusted by ethnicity to reduce this confounding factor, the number of patients with thrombocytopaenia and two of the analytical alterations remained significant. Thrombocytopaenia was more pronounced in *P. o. wallikeri* and INR values were higher in the wallikeri group. The comparison of the rest of analysis variables were not finally significant, over all those that indicate a greater degree of haemolysis, such as LDH, tBR or haemoglobin level.

In the case of thrombocytopaenia, these results confirm the main finding of a previous retrospective study where the only difference was more severe thrombocytopaenia in *P. o. wallikeri* infection [5]. Thrombocytopaenia is a common finding in patients with malaria of all *Plasmodium* species ranging from 24 to 94% of indicence, although spontaneous haemorrhages are infrequent and limited to very severe cases [21]. Also it is of note that

Table 1 Demographic and epidemiological characteristics

	Plasmodium ovale curtisi (n=35)	*Plasmodium ovale wallikeri* (n=44)	p
Sex			*0.028*
Male	17 (48.6)	32 (72.7)	
Female	18 (51.4)	12 (27.3)	
Age, median years (IQR)	35 (23.0–53.0)	38.5 (22.2–52.7)	0.529
Ethnicity			*0.017*
African	26 (74.3)	21 (47.7)	
Caucasian	9 (25.7)	23 (52.3)	
Type of patient			*0.034*
Early immigrant	11 (31.4)	4 (9.0)	
Visiting friends and relatives	14 (40.0)	17 (38.6)	
VFR traveller	1 (2.9)		
Tourism		3 (6.8)	
Work/cooperation	7 (20.0)	17 (38.6)	
Expatriate, long-term stay	2 (5.7)	3 (6.8)	
Country of infection			0.097
Equatorial Guinea	14 (40.0)	11 (25.0)	
Nigeria	5 (14.3)	6 (13.6)	
Cameroon	1 (2.9)	11 (25.0)	
Togo	1 (2.9)	1 (2.3)	
Liberia	2 (5.7)		
Tanzania		1 (2.3)	
Guinea-Conakry	1 (2.9)	1 (2.3)	
Ivory Coast	3 (8.6)	2 (4.5)	
Mozambique	1 (2.9)	2 (4.5)	
Congo	1 (2.9)	1 (2.3)	
Congo Democratic Republic		1 (2.3)	
Uganda	2 (5.7)		
Chad		2 (4.5)	
Ghana	1 (2.9)	1 (2.3)	
Sierra Leone		1 (2.3)	
Sudan	1 (2.9)		
Burundi	1 (2.9)		
Angola		1 (2.3)	
Mali		1 (2.3)	
Guinea-Bissau		1 (2.3)	
Madagascar	1 (2.9)		
Duration of travel, median days (IQR)	101 (21.0–240.0)	38.5 (26.7–157.5)	0.547
Chemoprophylaxis			0.078
No prophylaxis	14 (60.8)	24 (60.0)	
Incomplete	5 (21.7)	2 (5.0)	
Complete	4 (17.4)	14 (35.0)	
Time from arrival to onset of symptoms, median days (IQR)	34.0 (13.0–181.25)	30.5 (10.0–86.25)	0.171
Time from onset of symptoms to diagnoses, median days (IQR)	3 (0.0–10.0)	3.5 (0.7–8.0)	0.772
Recent *Plasmodium* infection	16 (51.6)	15 (40.5)	0.361
Other underlying conditions			1
G6PDH deficit	1/30 (3.3)	2/37 (5.4)	
Diabetes mellitus	1 (2.9)	4 (9.0)	0.3756
Drepanocytosis	1 (2.9)	1 (2.3)	
Pregnancy	1 (2.9)	0	

Table 1 (continued)

	Plasmodium ovale curtisi (n=35)	Plasmodium ovale wallikeri (n=44)	p
Chronic kidney disease	0	1 (2.3)	
Splenectomy	1 (2.9)	0	
Hepatitis B virus	0	3 (6.8)	
Hepatitis C virus	1 (2.9)	0	
HIV	3 (8.6)	1 (2.3)	

Values are no. (%) or no. positive/total no. (%) and median (interquartile range). Italicface indicates significance

IQR interquartile range, VFR visiting friends and relatives, G6PDH glucose-6-phosphate dehydrogenase, HIV human immunodeficiency virus

Table 2 Microbiological and analytical characteristics

	P ovale curtisi (n = 35)	P ovale wallikeri (n = 44)	p
Positive thick smear	28/34 (82.4)	36/42 (85.7)	0.689
Only PCR positive	5 (18.5)	6 (19.4)	1
Parasitaemia, median × μL (IQR)	2550 (647.5–11,677.5)	946 (600–4450)	0.441
Parasitaemia index			0.275
Very low ≤ 0.01%	3/22 (13.6)	7/28 (25.0)	
Low 0.02–0.1%	8/22 (36.4)	13/28 (46.4)	
Medium > 0.1%	11/22 (50.0)	8/28 (28.6)	
Rapid diagnostic test			
Common antigen positive	6/23 (26.1)	14/33 (42.4)	0.209
P. falciparum antigen positive	0/23 (0.0)	3/33 (9.1)	0.502
Total WBC count, median cells/μL (IQR)	5600 (4600–6270)	4460 (3827–6015)	0.049
Haemoglobin level, median g/dL (IQR)	12.1 (10.1–13.5)	13.2 (11.5–14.1)	0.032
Platelet count, median cells/μL (IQR)	130,000 (81,000–281,000)	105,500 (69,000–141,500)	0.039
Platelet count < 150,000 cells/μL	19 (54.3)	34 (79.1)	0.016
Albumin level, median g/dL (IQR)	3.60 (3.20–4.00)	3.38 (3.02–3.73)	0.139
Creatinine level, median mg/dL (IQR)	0.79 (0.59–1.00)	0.95 (0.75–1.10)	0.030
LDH level, median value × IU/L (IQR)	267.0 (221.2–367.2)	370.0 (256.0–508.7)	0.028
AST level, median IU/L (IQR)	27.00 (20.00–32.50)	25.50 (19.90–43.75)	0.691
ALT level, median IU/L (IQR)	30.00 (18.00–43.20)	24.00 (18.00–48.00)	0.648
Total bilirubin level, median mg/dL (IQR)	0.83 (0.60–1.35)	1.22 (0.70–1.80)	0.086
INR, median (IQR)	1.08 (0.96–1.17)	1.12 (1.10–1.20)	0.019
APTT, median (IQR)	29.50 (25.10–37.07)	30.65 (26.27–32.97)	0.762
Glucose, median mg/dL (IQR)	91.5 (83.0–103.7)	97.0 (82.0–113.0)	0.468

Values are no. (%) or no. positive/total no. (%) and median (interquartile range). Italicface indicates significance

IQR interquartile range, PCR polymerase chain reaction, WBC white blood cells, LDH lactate dehydrogenase, AST aspartate aminotransferase, ALT alanine aminotransferase, INR international normalized ratio, APTT activated partial thromboplastin time

thrombocytopaenia seems to be a very common finding in *P. ovale* spp. infection. Of the 79 patients analysed, 53 (67%) had under 150,000 platelets/μL, which corresponds to our previous series findings of 66.6% in 16 imported ovale infection patients [22] and a retrospective study where 26 out of 35 patients (75.3%) suffered from thrombocytopaenia [5]. Only one patient in each group showed under 50,000 platelets/μL again without any haemorrhagic feature.

The pathogenesis of thrombocytopaenia in malaria is not fully understood but is accepted that encompasses several different mechanisms that lead to increased platelet destruction or consumption, such as increased attachment to endothelium and adherence to Von Willebrand factor, clumping and agglutination of infected and uninfected erythrocytes, consumption into the coagulation process and haemolysis, increased diffuse platelet sequestration, decreased nitric oxide

Table 3 Multivariate linear regression and multivariate logistic regression analysis related to ethnicity of parameters with significant differences in univariate analysis and latency time

	Regression coefficients	95% confidence interval	p
Total WBC count, $\times 10^9$ cells/L	− 850.884	− 1931.456 to 229.689	0.121
Haemoglobin level, g/dL	− 0.903	− 0.085 to 1.891	0.073
Platelet count cells/µL	− 39,707.641	− 71,351.311 to − 8063.972	*0.015*
Creatinine level, mg/dL	0.095	− 0.024 to 0.215	0.117
LDH level, IU/L	12.537	− 160.156 to 185.230	0.885
INR	0.077	0.003–0.151	*0.041*
Time from arrival to onset of symptoms, days			
African patients	− 41.108	− 127.135 to 44.920	0.344
Caucasian patients	− 75.001	− 144.040 to − 5.962	*0.034*
	Odds ratio	95% confidence interval	p
Platelet count < 150,000 cells/µL	0.314	0.117–0.847	*0.022*

Values show the relationship of *P. o. wallikeri* respect to *P. o. curtisi*. Italicface indicates significance

WBC white blood cells, *LDH* lactate dehydrogenase, *INR* international normalized ratio

bioavailability, and immune complexes-mediated destruction [23].

Although thrombocytopaenia is not among the severity criteria of the WHO, evidence is accumulating that it can predict an adverse outcome, which seems to be driven by a greater severity of illness in *P. falciparum* or *P. vivax* [21, 24] and severe thrombocytopaenia can identify an increased risk of death from falciparum or vivax malaria [25]. Therefore, in the case of *P. o. wallikeri* it could indicate a greater intrinsic pathogenicity of this species compared to *P. o. curtisi*, although without evidence of any major significantly worse clinical criteria of severity.

Regarding the other significant finding of this study, the higher INR elevation in *P. o. wallikeri* compared to *P. o. curtisi*, this increase was always mild and in no case exceeded the value of 1.54 nor was related to any bleeding. On the other hand, the APTT values were similar in both groups. No other coagulation factors, fibrinogen levels, fibrin degradation products or D-dimer were measured that could argue in favour of a significant coagulation disorder.

It is well known that *P. falciparum* malaria is associated with significant coagulation activation. The increase in INR or its equivalent, prolongation of prothrombin time, is produced by the activation of the extrinsic pathway of the coagulation cascade and can lead to disseminated intravascular coagulation in the most severe cases of malaria. *Plasmodium falciparum* seems to trigger coagulation activation through multiple different pathways although the mechanisms involved are not well understood [26]. Much less information on coagulation is available in *P. ovale* spp. infection. In the case of INR, the finding of this study might support the hypothesis of

a more pathogenic wallikeri parasite, but does not seem to pose a significant clinical difference or severity.

In the initial analysis, no differences were found in the latency period, but when the multivariate analysis was performed a significant shorter time appeared in *P. o. wallikeri* compared to *P. o. curtisi* infection, but only in Caucasians patients. This difference is more significant since only one of the seven Caucasians patients who suffered infection by *P. o. curtisi* had taken adequate prophylaxis versus 11 out of 22 (50%) of the wallikeri group, which should have lengthened their latency. The retrospective study by Nolder et al. in the UK also found significant shorter latency period in wallikeri cases but did not report the ethnicity or patient characteristics [13]. On the contrary, another study in Chinese people (ethnically homogeneous but with unknown previous exposure to malaria or chemoprophylaxis use) encompassing 109 *P. o. curtisi* and *P. o. wallikeri* [10] imported from Africa, did not find any difference in latency. In a previous retrospective study, only a trend to shorter wallikeri latency was found (p = 0.07) [5].

These results of different latency times in only Caucasians patients suggest a strong influence of the previous partial immunity to malaria in the time of symptoms of *P. ovale* spp. infection. Finally, note that in both species latencies greater than 1 year have been found as described previously [11].

A complete chemoprophylaxis was reported in 22.8% of ovale spp. infections and up to 35% in *P. o. wallikeri*, a high percentage if compared with data from large series of imported malaria as in USA 2014, where only 7.8% of travellers correctly took prophylaxis [11]. If analysed by *Plasmodium* species, these results are similar to the

Table 4 Clinical and therapeutic characteristics

	P ovale curtisi (n=35)	P ovale wallikeri (n=44)	p
Asymptomatic	2 (5.7)	2 (4.5)	1
Fever	32 (91.4)	39 (88.6)	1
Headache	17 (48.6)	29 (65.9)	0.121
Nausea	9 (25.7)	11 (25.0)	0.942
Arthralgia	10 (28.6)	15 (34.1)	0.600
Myalgia	17 (48.6)	18 (40.9)	0.496
Vomitus	4 (11.4)	12 (26.3)	0.082
Abdominal pain	5 (14.3)	3 (6.8)	0.460
Diarrhea	4 (11.4)	5 (11.4)	1
Other (cough, dyspnea, chest pain, dizziness)	9 (25.7)	10 (22.7)	0.758
Duration of hospitalization, median days (IQR)	4 (2.0–6.0)	3 (3.0–6.0)	0.713
Treatment			0.826
Chloroquine	17 (48.6)	18 (40.9)	
Atovaquone/proguanil	12 (34.2)	11 (25.0)	
Quinine + doxycycline		2 (4.5)	
Atovaquone/proguanil + chloroquine	1 (2.9)	1 (2.3)	
Artesunate + artemether–lumefantrine	1 (2.9)		
Dihidroartemisinin–piperaquine	3 (8.6)	7 (15.9)	
Artemether–lumefantrine		1 (2.3)	
Artesunate + chloroquine		1 (2.3)	
Artesunate + atovaquone/proguanil	1 (2.9)		
Artesunate		1 (2.3)	
Lost to follow up, no treatment		2 (4.5)	
Primaquine	25 (71.4)	34 (81.0)	0.325
Severe malaria and complications			1
Total bilirubin > 3 mg/dL and haemoglobin < 7 g/dL	1 (2.9)[a]		
Total bilirubin > 3 mg/dL		3 (6.8)[b]	
Haemoglobin < 7 g/dL	1 (2.9)		
Haemophagocytosis		1 (2.3)	
Exitus	0	0	1

Values are no. (%) or no. positive/total no. (%) and median (interquartile range)

IQR interquartile range

[a] This patient had drepanocytosis

[b] One patient had drepanocytosis and G6PDH deficit and other patient had diabetes

study by Nolder et al. which stated that the proportion of ovale malaria which occurred in patients reporting chemoprophylaxis use (33%) was significantly higher than for *P. falciparum* (6.4%) and *P. vivax* (23.7%) [13]. Also, in a USA and Israel study, up to 73% of imported *P. ovale* spp. used an effective prophylaxis [27]. Moreover, in a recent Spanish study considering only the subgroup of travellers with *P. ovale/P. vivax* malaria, these patients had also taken chemoprophylaxis significantly more frequently than those with non-*P. ovale/P. vivax* malaria (35.5% vs. 2.7%) [28]. These results reinforce the idea that current prophylaxis does not adequately

act on *P. ovale* spp. infection, since it is ineffective against its hypnozoites and, therefore, does not prevent a delayed primary attack or true relapses from occurring when there is no prophylactic medication in blood.

Although the information cannot be completely reliable, over 40% of patients reported an episode of malaria in the previous 12 months. This could have been a primary infection by *P. ovale*, another ovale relapse, a mixed infection with other *Plasmodium* or simply a non-ovale malaria unrelated to the current episode. Since it is not feasible to obtain a previous diagnostic sample, it is impossible to know if the current episode represented a primary infection or a relapse by *P. ovale*. Primary infection could only be diagnosed in the cases of first malarial episode and very short latency period.

Regarding the underlaying conditions, it is worth focusing on diabetes mellitus and drepanocytosis. The prevalence of diabetes mellitus is increasing worldwide, especially in low income countries, as are found in sub-Saharan Africa [29]. The number of diabetics in this study is as high as 6.32% (5/79) in a population with a low average age, especially in wallikeri group. In a retrospective curtisi–wallikeri study up to 8.5% of patients suffered from diabetes [5] and in a previous study of imported *P. ovale* infection 3 out of 16 patients (18.7% with mean age 30.6 years) were also diabetics [22]. A recent Swedish study, reported diabetes in 3.5% of 937 patients with imported *P. falciparum* and 2.5% in 398 imported malaria in a Spanish Tropical Medicine Centre [30]. In a series of 229 *P. falciparum* infections from 2006 to 2015 in Hospital Universitario Príncipe de Asturias (HUPA), 2.6% were diabetics (unpublished data). As diabetes is a known risk factor for malaria due to *P. falciparum* in endemic areas [31], the higher prevalence of this chronic disease in *P. ovale* studies might indicate that would also be a risk factor, and deserves further investigation to confirm this finding.

In endemic areas, carrying the sickle cell trait represents a risk factor for infection by *P. ovale* spp. [20] and a partial protective factor against severe *P. falciparum* infection. In this study, 2 out of 47 African patients (4.2%) had drepanocytosis. Moreover, in the previous comparative retrospective study, 8.3% (2 out of 24) showed drepanocytosis and up to 23% (3/13) in the series of 16 imported *P. ovale* spp. [22]. Gathering African patients from the three studies (7/84) and comparing to 1.35% of patients in 221 African people with imported *P. falciparum* in HUPA during the period 2006–2015 (unpublished data) significant difference can be found (p < 0.005) that would support the results of the study conducted in endemic area.

As in previous studies, no differences were detected in parasitaemias between both groups [6, 9, 32]. Most of them had low parasite counts clearly below 1%, making it even more difficult to find statistically real differences. Surprisingly, two patients reached 2% parasitaemia, a Caucasian traveller without any immunity to malaria and a child with drepanocytosis and intense anaemia that enhanced the proportion of infected red blood cells. Such high parasitaemia has been rarely described, sometimes linked to serious complications such as spleen rupture [33]. Finally, the absence of Schüffner's stippling in blood smear, which has been described as a possible feature specific to *P. o. wallikeri*, was not studied.

There was also no difference in the sensitivity of RDTs, which was low as described in the literature [2] without exceeding 45% in either group. Almost 20% of the cases in both groups were diagnosed only by PCR, as RDT and/ or thick blood smears were negative. In endemic areas this percentage is much higher, especially in asymptomatic patients [3]. Therefore, if the clinical and epidemiological suspicion is high, it would be convenient to repeat the diagnostic tests and request molecular PCR techniques not to miss *P. ovale* spp. diagnosis.

This study confirms that this infection can cause malaria with severity criteria or complications, in this case 7.6% of all patients with no differences between both species. In series of imported malaria by *P. falciparum* the rate of severe cases was around 2–17% [11, 34], but with a much higher incidence of life-threatening complications, such as ADRS, severe anaemia or cerebral malaria than described in *P. ovale* spp. infection [8]. A rare case of haemophagocytosis was included that had been described only in *P. falciparum* and *P. vivax* infection [35], but not in *P. ovale* spp. Analysing the six patients with severe malaria or complications, two had drepanocytosis (which also produces anaemia) and one was diabetic, which might indicate the possible importance of these risk factors in the severity of *P. ovale* spp. infection.

In cases of malaria with tBR > 3 mg/dL, the WHO severity criteria add parasitaemia levels above 100,000/μL in *P. falciparum* and > 20,000/μL in *P. vivax* and *Plasmodium knowlesi*, but is not known in the case of *P. ovale* spp. In this study, all four cases with tBR > 3 mg/dL had parasitaemias over 4000/μL. In addition, four patients received parenteral artesunate, two of them with tBR > 3 mg/dL and one with unusually high parasitaemias of 2%. It is described that host response may reach full strength at lower parasitaemia in *P. vivax* and *P. ovale* spp. infection than in *P. falciparum* [36] so, perhaps it would be also convenient to establish a threshold of parasitaemia with jaundice and hyperparasitaemia in *P. ovale* spp. in the face of treatment decisions and outcome.

The treatments were very varied, including artemisinins alone or in combination, atovaquone/proguanil, chloroquine or quinine-doxycycline, all with good initial clinical evolution, which is compatible with the sensitivity of *P. ovale* spp. described for multiple antimalarials [8]. Over 70% of them received primaquine with good tolerance, although there was no long-term follow-up recorded to assess episodes of relapse or late recrudescence.

The prospective study design has minimized some of the limitations of the previous retrospective study but some of them still remain. First, although it is one of the largest studies carried out worldwide, the number of patients may still lack sufficient statistical power to show other differences between infections with both *P. ovale* species. Second, only strains of *P. ovale* from Africa, and patients from Africa and Europe were analysed; a study of infections and patients from Asia, Oceania or other places might show different results. Third, the behaviour of these species in endemic countries may be different but it would be difficult to gather a significant number of patients with *P. ovale* spp. monoinfection due to the high prevalence of mixed *Plasmodium* infections and malaria reinfections. Fourth, the date of infection is a minimal approximate and it is virtually impossible to distinguish a primary infection from a relapse. Last, a mix of ethnicities, non-immune and semi-immune patients led to heterogeneous study groups, although the multivariate statistical study has reduced this bias.

Conclusions

In this study, imported *P. o. wallikeri* infection was more frequent in males and Caucasian patients than in *P. o. curtisi* group. Malaria caused by *P. o. wallikeri* produced more thrombocytopenic patients, more marked thrombocytopaenia and a higher INR than *P. ovale curtisi*, although without other clinical or severity differences. *Plasmodium o. wallikeri* malaria had shorter latency, but only in Caucasian patients. These findings suggest that wallikeri species might be somewhat more pathogenic than *P. ovale curtisi*. Some cases with severity criteria were seen in both species and required treatment with intravenous artesunate. The clinical evolution with any anti-malarial drug was usually good, however, chemoprophylaxis seemed less effective in *P. ovale* spp. infection than in the case of *P. falciparum*. Diabetes mellitus might also be a risk factor for *P. ovale* spp. infection such as drepanocytosis. Current RDT was shown to have low diagnostic sensitivity in both species and PCR was essential for diagnosis in a significant percentage of cases.

Abbreviations
ADRS: acute respiratory distress syndrome; APTT: activated partial thromboplastin time; DNA: deoxyribonucleic acid; G6PDH: glucose-6-phosphate dehydrogenase; HBV: hepatitis B virus; HCV: hepatitis C virus; HIV: with human immunodeficiency virus; INR: international normalized ratio; IQR: interquartile range; LDH: lactate dehydrogenase; PCR: polymerase chain reaction; RDT: rapid diagnostic test; ssrRNA: small-subunit ribosomal ribonucleic acid; tBR: total bilirubin; VFR: visiting friends and relatives; WHO: World Health Organization.

Authors' contributions
GRM, JMR, JCG and JMRG made substantial contributions to conception and design of this study. GMR, JMR, AA, FG and JCG made substantial contributions to analysis and interpretation of data. SJ, SGB, LRT, NRV, MGR, IMR, MCM, EME, MEG and JLT made substantial contributions to acquisition of data. GRM, JMR, JCG, JSC and RLV were involved in drafting the manuscript. All authors revised the manuscript critically for important intellectual content. All authors read and approved the final manuscript.

Author details
[1] Hospital Universitario Príncipe de Asturias, Ctra de Meco s/n, 28805 Alcalá de Henares, Madrid, Spain. [2] Instituto de Salud Carlos III, Majadahonda, Madrid, Spain. [3] Ospedale Sacro Cuore - Don Calabria, Negrar, Verona, Italy. [4] Hôpital Pitié-Salpêtrière, Assistance Publique des Hôpitaux de Paris (APHP), Paris, France. [5] Hospital Universitario La Paz-Carlos III, Madrid, Spain. [6] Spedali Civili Hospital, University of Brescia, Brescia, Italy. [7] Hospital Clinic, Barcelona, Spain. [8] Hospital Universitario de Fuenlabrada, Madrid, Spain. [9] Hospital del Poniente-El Ejido, Almería, Spain. [10] Hospital General Universitario de Valencia, Valencia, Spain. [11] Hospital Vall D'Hebron-Drassanes, Barcelona, Spain. [12] Hospital Universitario Ramón y Cajal, Madrid, Spain. [13] Hospital Universitario Gregorio Marañón, Madrid, Spain. [14] Hospital Universitario de Guadalajara, Guadalajara, Spain. [15] Complejo Hospitalario de Navarra, Pamplona, Navarra, Spain. [16] Complejo Hospitalario Universitario de Santiago de Compostela, A Coruña, Spain.

Acknowledgements
We thank all patients who kindly participated in this study. We also thank every doctor from 29 hospitals who contributed with their time to enroll patients and collect information: Mar Lago-Nuñez. Hospital Universitario La Paz-Carlos III, Madrid, Spain. Francesco Castelli. Spedali Civili di Brescia, Italy. Jerónimo Jaquetti. Hospital Universitario de Fuenlabrada, Madrid, Spain. Carles Alonso. Hospital General l'Hospitalet - Consorci Sanitari Integral, Barcelona, Spain. Daniel Camprubí. Hospital Clinic, Barcelona, Spain. Miguel Górgolas-Hernández-Mora. Fundación Jiménez Díaz, Madrid, Spain. Guillermo Cuevas-Tascón. Hospital Infanta Leonor, Vallecas, Madrid, Spain. Ana Pérez-Ayala. Hospital Universitario 12 de Octubre, Madrid, Spain. María Teresa Guzmán-GarcíaMonge. Hospital Infanta Cristina, Parla, Spain. Mónica Ribell-Bachs. Hospital General de Granollers, Barcelona, Spain. Nuria Serre-Delcor, Hospital Vall D'Hebron-Drassanes, Barcelona, Spain. Yasmina Martín-Martín. Hospital General de Lanzarote, Las Palmas, Spain. Germán Ramírez-Olivencia. Hospital Gómez Ulla, Madrid, Spain. Rosario Cogollos-Agruña. Hospital Universitario de Móstoles, Madrid, Spain. Francisco Jesús Merino-Fernández. Hospital Universitario Severo Ochoa, Leganés, Madrid, Spain. Antonia García-Castro. Hospital Río Carrión, Palencia, Spain. Purificación Cantudo-Muñoz. Hospital Universitario San Agustín. Linares, Jaén, Spain. Moncef Belhassen-García. Hospital Universitario de Salamanca, Spain. Pablo Martín-Rabadán. Hospital Universitario Gregorio Marañón, Madrid, Spain. Purificación Rubio-Cuevas. Hospital General Universitario de Valencia, Spain. Elena Trigo-Esteban. Hospital Universitario La Paz-Carlos III, Madrid, Spain. Juan Arévalo-Serrano. Hospital Universitario Príncipe de Asturias, Alcalá de Henares, Madrid, Spain.

The authors thank Dr. Francisco Javier Vilar (Consultant in Infectious Diseases, Pennine Acute Hospital NHS Trusts, Manchester, UK) for reviewing the manuscript.

Competing interests
The authors declare that they have no competing interests.

Funding
This study has been funded with a grant FIB-PI14-04 from the Foundation for Biomedical Research of the Hospital Universitario Príncipe de Asturias, Alcalá de Henares, Madrid, Spain.

References

1. WHO. World malaria report 2016. Geneva: World Health Organization; 2015. http://apps.who.int/iris/bitstream/10665/252038/1/9789241511 711-eng.pdf?ua=1. Accessed 26 Nov 2017.
2. Maltha J, Gillet P, Jacobs J. Malaria rapid diagnostic tests in travel medicine. Clin Microbiol Infect. 2013;19:408–15.
3. Mueller I, Zimmerman PA, Reeder JC. *Plasmodium malariae* and *Plasmodium ovale*—the "bashful" malaria parasites. Trends Parasitol. 2007;23:278–83.
4. Sutherland CJ, Tanomsing N, Nolder D, Oguike M, Jennison C, Pukrittayakamee S, et al. Two nonrecombining sympatric forms of the human malaria parasite *Plasmodium ovale* occur globally. J Infect Dis. 2010;201:1544–50.
5. Rojo-Marcos G, Rubio-Muñoz JM, Ramírez-Olivencia G, García-Bujalance S, Elcuaz-Romano R, Díaz-Menéndez M, et al. Comparison of imported *Plasmodium ovale curtisi* and *P. ovale wallikeri* infections among patients in Spain, 2005–2011. Emerg Infect Dis. 2014;20:409–16.
6. Bauffe F, Desplans J, Fraisier C, Parzy D. Real-time PCR assay for discrimination of *Plasmodium ovale curtisi* and *Plasmodium ovale wallikeri* in the Ivory Coast and in the Comoros Islands. Malar J. 2012;11:307.
7. Rojo-Marcos G, Cuadros-González J, Mesa-Latorre JM, Culebras-López AM, de Pablo-Sánchez R. Acute respiratory distress syndrome in a case of *Plasmodium ovale* malaria. Am J Trop Med Hyg. 2008;79:391–3.
8. Groger M, Fischer HS, Veletzky L, Lalremruata A, Ramharter M. A systematic review of the clinical presentation, treatment and relapse characteristics of human *Plasmodium ovale* malaria. Malar J. 2017;16:112.
9. Phuong MS, Lau R, Ralevski F, Boggild AK. Parasitological correlates of *Plasmodium ovale curtisi* and *Plasmodium ovale wallikeri* infection. Malar J. 2016;15:550.
10. Cao Y, Wang W, Liu Y, Cotter C, Zhou H, Zhu G, et al. The increasing importance of *Plasmodium ovale* and *Plasmodium malariae* in a malaria elimination setting: an observational study of imported cases in Jiangsu Province, China, 2011–2014. Malar J. 2016;15:459.
11. Mace KE, Arguin PM. Malaria surveillance—United States, 2014. MMWR Surveill Summ. 2017;66:1–24.
12. Gallien S, Taieb F, Schlemmer F, Lagrange-Xelot M, Atlan A, Sarfati C, et al. Failure of atovaquone/proguanil to prevent *Plasmodium ovale* malaria in traveler returning from Cameroon. Travel Med Infect Dis. 2008;6:128–9.
13. Nolder D, Oguike MC, Maxwell-Scott H, Niyazi HA, Smith V, Chiodini PL, et al. An observational study of malaria in British travellers: *Plasmodium ovale wallikeri* and *Plasmodium ovale curtisi* differ significantly in the duration of latency. BMJ Open. 2013;3(5):e002711.
14. Miller RH, Obuya CO, Wanja EW, Ogutu B, Waitumbi J, Luckhart S, et al. Characterization of *Plasmodium ovale curtisi* and *P. ovale wallikeri* in Western Kenya utilizing a novel species-specific real-time PCR assay. PLoS Negl Trop Dis. 2015;9:e0003469.
15. Fuehrer HP, Habler VE, Fally MA, Harl J, Starzengruber P, Swoboda P, et al. *Plasmodium ovale* in Bangladesh: genetic diversity and the first known evidence of the sympatric distribution of *Plasmodium ovale curtisi* and *Plasmodium ovale wallikeri* in southern Asia. Int J Parasitol. 2012;42:693–9.
16. Lalremruata A, Jeyaraj S, Engleitner T, Joanny F, Lang A, Bélard S, et al. Species and genotype diversity of Plasmodium in malaria patients from Gabon analysed by next generation sequencing. Malar J. 2017;16:398.
17. Oguike MC, Betson M, Burke M, Nolder D, Stothard JR, Kleinschmidt I, et al. *Plasmodium ovale curtisi* and *Plasmodium ovale wallikeri* circulate simultaneously in African communities. Int J Parasitol. 2011;41:677–83.
18. Rubio JM, Post RJ, van Leeuwen WM, Henry MC, Lindergard G, Hommel M. Alternative polymerase chain reaction method to identify Plasmodium species in human blood samples: the semi-nested multiplex malaria PCR (SnM-PCR). Trans R Soc Trop Med Hyg. 2002;96(Suppl 1):S199–204.
19. WHO. Guidelines for the treatment of malaria. 3rd ed. Geneva: World Health Organization; 2015. http://www.who.int/malaria/publications/atoz/9789241549127/en/. Accessed 20 Apr 2018.
20. Faye FB, Spiegel A, Tall A, Sokhna C, Fontenille D, Rogier C, et al. Diagnostic criteria and risk factors for *Plasmodium ovale* malaria. J Infect Dis. 2002;186:690–5.
21. Lacerda MV, Mourão MP, Coelho HC, Santos JB. Thrombocytopenia in malaria: who cares? Mem Inst Oswaldo Cruz. 2011;106(Suppl 1):52–63.
22. Rojo-Marcos G, Cuadros-González J, Gete-García L, Gómez-Herruz P, López-Rubio M, Esteban-Gutierrez G. *Plasmodium ovale* infection: description of 16 cases and a review. Enferm Infecc Microbiol Clin. 2011;29:204–8 **(in Spanish)**.
23. Thachil J. Platelets and infections in the resource-limited countries with a focus on malaria and viral haemorrhagic fevers. Br J Haematol. 2017;177:960–70.
24. Willmann M, Ahmed A, Siner A, Wong IT, Woon LC, Singh B, et al. Laboratory markers of disease severity in *Plasmodium knowlesi* infection: a case control study. Malar J. 2012;11:363.
25. Lampah DA, Yeo TW, Malloy M, Kenangalem E, Douglas NM, Ronaldo D, et al. Severe malarial thrombocytopenia: a risk factor for mortality in Papua, Indonesia. J Infect Dis. 2015;211:623–34.
26. O'Sullivan JM, Preston RJ, O'Regan N, O'Donnell JS. Emerging roles for hemostatic dysfunction in malaria pathogenesis. Blood. 2016;127:2281–8.
27. Schwartz E, Parise M, Kozarsky P, Cetron M. Delayed onset of malaria—implications for chemoprophylaxis in travelers. N Engl J Med. 2003;349:1510–6.
28. Norman FF, López-Polín A, Salvador F, Treviño B, Calabuig E, Torrús D, et al. Imported malaria in Spain (2009–2016): results from the +REDIVI Collaborative Network. Malar J. 2017;16:407.
29. Guariguata L, Whiting DR, Hambleton I, Beagley J, Linnenkamp U, Shaw JE. Global estimates of diabetes prevalence for 2013 and projections for 2035. Diabetes Res Clin Pract. 2014;103:137–49.
30. Ramírez-Olivencia G, Herrero MD, Subirats M, de Juanes JR, Peña JM, Puente S. Imported malaria in adults. Clinical, epidemiological and analytical features. Rev Clin Esp. 2012;212:1–9 **(in Spanish)**.
31. Danquah I, Bedu-Addo G, Mockenhaupt FP. Type 2 diabetes mellitus and increased risk for malaria infection. Emerg Infect Dis. 2010;16:1601–4.
32. Starzengruber P, Fuehrer HP, Ley B, Thriemer K, Swoboda P, Habler VE, et al. High prevalence of asymptomatic malaria in south-eastern Bangladesh. Malar J. 2014;13:16.
33. Facer CA, Rouse D. Spontaneous splenic rupture due to *Plasmodium ovale* malaria. Lancet. 1991;338:896.
34. Seringe E, Thellier M, Fontanet A, Legros F, Bouchaud O, Ancelle T, et al. Severe imported *Plasmodium falciparum* malaria, France, 1996–2003. Emerg Infect Dis. 2011;17:807–13.
35. Ohnishi K, Mitsui K, Komiya N, Iwasaki N, Akashi A, Hamabe Y. Clinical case report: falciparum malaria with hemophagocytic syndrome. Am J Trop Med Hyg. 2007;76:1016–8.
36. Hemmer CJ, Holst FG, Kern P, Chiwakata CB, Dietrich M, Reisinger EC. Stronger host response per parasitized erythrocyte in *Plasmodium vivax* or ovale than in *Plasmodium falciparum* malaria. Trop Med Int Health. 2006;11:817–23.

5

Injectable anti-malarials revisited: discovery and development of new agents to protect against malaria

Fiona Macintyre[1], Hanu Ramachandruni[1], Jeremy N. Burrows[1], René Holm[2,3], Anna Thomas[1], Jörg J. Möhrle[1], Stephan Duparc[1], Rob Hooft van Huijsduijnen[1] [iD], Brian Greenwood[4], Winston E. Gutteridge[1], Timothy N. C. Wells[1*] and Wiweka Kaszubska[1]

Abstract

Over the last 15 years, the majority of malaria drug discovery and development efforts have focused on new molecules and regimens to treat patients with uncomplicated or severe disease. In addition, a number of new molecular scaffolds have been discovered which block the replication of the parasite in the liver, offering the possibility of new tools for oral prophylaxis or chemoprotection, potentially with once-weekly dosing. However, an intervention which requires less frequent administration than this would be a key tool for the control and elimination of malaria. Recent progress in HIV drug discovery has shown that small molecules can be formulated for injections as native molecules or pro-drugs which provide protection for at least 2 months. Advances in antibody engineering offer an alternative approach whereby a single injection could potentially provide protection for several months. Building on earlier profiles for uncomplicated and severe malaria, a target product profile is proposed here for an injectable medicine providing long-term protection from this disease. As with all of such profiles, factors such as efficacy, cost, safety and tolerability are key, but with the changing disease landscape in Africa, new clinical and regulatory approaches are required to develop prophylactic/chemoprotective medicines. An overall framework for these approaches is suggested here.

Keywords: Malaria, *Plasmodium*, Chemoprotection, Prophylaxis, Liver schizont, Intra-muscular, Target candidate profile, Target product profile

Introduction

One of the challenges of malaria control is to be able to provide protection for vulnerable populations. In recent years, there has been great progress in the use of drug regimens to prevent infections in children. However, these require frequent drug administration. One alternative that has been tested is the use of long-acting injectable formulations. Although there are currently no long-acting injectable medicines in development for malaria, new formulation technologies, similar to those developed for prophylaxis against HIV, might point the way to new approaches against this disease. In addition, recent developments in monoclonal antibody technology may be applicable to protect against malaria, especially in vulnerable populations. This paper discusses how such treatments would fit the target product profiles for malaria, and a regulatory pathway for their development. Since they pose similar challenges and possibilities from this perspective, the discussion of small molecules and antibodies was combined.

Background

Over the last decade, there has been a considerable increase in the portfolio of new molecules which are being developed for the treatment of malaria [1, 2]. New paradigms of screening [3–8] have led to another generation of molecules progressing to clinical

*Correspondence: wellst@mmv.org
[1] Medicines for Malaria Venture, Route de Pré Bois 20, 1215 Geneva, Switzerland
Full list of author information is available at the end of the article

development, aimed at producing new medicines which overcome the current problems of multi-drug resistant malaria [9–11] and which also simplify therapy from the current 3-day therapy, to single exposure cures. Protecting vulnerable populations from clinically significant infections is also a key aspect of malaria control and elimination [12]. Although a highly effective vaccine is the ultimate goal of much basic malaria research, the absence of a sterilizing immune response to naturally acquired disease shows how difficult such a target is likely to be [13]; current candidate vaccines provide a protective efficacy in the range of 30–50% [14].

Malaria chemoprophylaxis can be achieved by a variety of different mechanisms. Causal prophylactics target the asexual hepatic stages of malaria. Atovaquone (a *Plasmodium* mitochondrial bc_1 inhibitor binding to the Q_0 site of the complex), pyrimethamine and cycloguanil and its prodrug proguanil (selective inhibitors of dihydrofolate reductase, DHFR), sulfadoxine (an inhibitor of *Plasmodium* dihydropteroate synthase, DHPS) and the 8-aminoquinolines primaquine and tafenoquine are the only causal prophylactics with proven clinical efficacy. In suppressive chemoprophylaxis, the parasite is killed once it enters the erythrocytic stages of the lifecycle, stopping the infection at a low level of parasitaemia before it becomes clinically significant. Inhibitors of beta-haematin formation, such as chloroquine and mefloquine, and (plastid) ribosomal inhibitors, such as doxycycline, are suppressive chemoprophylactics, and must be given for at least 2 weeks after leaving a malaria-endemic area to clear any parasites that emerge from the liver after a person has left the endemic area. Currently, the predominant oral prophylactics used by travelers are (rarely) mefloquine, doxycycline and atovaquone–proguanil. These were initially developed as treatments for uncomplicated malaria [15, 16]. They were subsequently shown to have good protective efficacy when delivered at lower doses on a weekly basis, in the case of mefloquine, and a daily basis in the case of atovaquone–proguanil, respectively [17, 18].

Protective vaccine strategies have focused on developing an immune response which blocks the initial infection, using the parasite antigen CSP-1 (circumsporozoite protein; [19]). Although a high level of protection has not currently been achieved with such vaccine candidate approaches, they have provided a proof of concept that antibodies can be generated that prevent the initial infection of the hepatocyte by sporozoites [20–23]. Efficacious vaccines would hold tremendous promise for prophylaxis, but unlike many viral infections, malaria is not a disease where natural infection results in sterilizing immunity, indicating that the bar to the identification of a highly effective vaccination regimen for malaria remains very high.

Identifying new classes of anti-malarial chemoprotective molecules targeting either blood- or liver-stage has historically been limited by the lack of known molecular targets and of high-throughput screening methods. However, in the last 10 years there has been a dramatic increase in the deployment of high density, phenotypic, cell-based high-throughput screens of *Plasmodium* blood stages [24] and new chemotypes, which are active against the blood stages of *Plasmodium* infection, have been identified [25]. These families of molecules can then be tested for activity against other stages of the parasite life cycle including hepatic schizonts. Examples in the Medicines for Malaria Venture (MMV) pipeline of compounds having both blood and liver stage activity [1] include: the DHODH (dihydroorotate dehydrogenase) inhibitor DSM265 [26, 27], the PI-4 kinase inhibitor MMV048 (MMV390048; [28]) and the EF2 (Elongation Factor 2) inhibitor DDD498 (DDD107498; [29]), now also known as M5717. These molecules have helped identify new molecular targets in liver schizonts. Other scaffolds such as KAF156 [30] have good activity against hepatic schizonts. However, although the main mechanism of resistance generation involves PfCARL, KAF156's molecular site of action is still to be elucidated [31]. More recently, high-throughput screens of the hepatic schizont stages have been carried out for murine parasites [32], increasing the possibility of the identification of compounds which are selectively active against hepatic schizonts. The immediate challenge is to develop high-throughput hepatic schizont stage assays using sporozoites from *Plasmodium falciparum*, and progress in this direction is being made. This is particularly important in order to confirm activity of compounds without asexual blood stage activity, and to avoid a focus on murine-malaria specific prophylaxis.

Work on injectable depot anti-malarials was a key part of the previous malaria eradication campaign with the development of 4-4′-diacetylaminosulphone (DADDS), a long-acting prodrug of the DHPS inhibitor dapsone, and cycloguanil pamoate (CI-501; [33, 34]). Clinical protection over 3–5 months was achieved in the published clinical trial, but the dose had to be delivered deep into the gluteal muscle tissues (350 mg in adults) and caused local discomfort and abscesses [35]. Failure to protect was assumed to be due to cross resistance with pyrimethamine, which was emerging at the time. Interest in long-lasting anti-malarials was renewed in 1976, supported by the UNDP/World Bank/WHO special program for Research and Training in Tropical Disease [WHO CHEMAL/SC(33)77.3 item 1.2] and the US Army Medical Research and Development Command. These groups continued to focus on blood schizonticides for injection, but no molecules were brought forward for testing in field studies. Tafenoquine/WR 238605, an 8-aminoquinoline originally discovered by The Walter Reed Army Institute for Medical Research has recently been approved by the US FDA (Food and Drug Administration) as a weekly oral prophylactic against *Plasmodium vivax* and *P. falciparum* (Arakoda®, 60 Degrees Pharmaceuticals) and for a single-dose radical cure indication (i.e. the treatment of the liver stage, preventing *P. vivax* relapse), as Krintafel®, by GSK. Both uses require a test for a patient's G6PD (glucose-6-phosphate dehydrogenase) deficiency status as a safety measure. No further clinical work on injectables has been reported. In the 1980s, Chinese scientists investigated the use of pyronaridine given by injection, with a total intramuscular dose of 300–400 mg being given in two or three injections. The drug was rapidly absorbed and provided an efficacious concentration that remained for an extended period given the elimination half-life of 60 h [36].

More recently, there has been a significant effort to develop anti-virals that provide protection against HIV infection in high risk individuals using daily oral dosing, termed pre-exposure prophylaxis, PrEP [37]. However, clinical trials have shown variable rates of efficacy with low rates of protection, correlated with non-adherence to the daily oral drug regimen [38]. Long-acting injectables have been developed based on the reverse transcriptase inhibitor cabotegravir (GSK1265744) and the integrase inhibitor rilpivirine. These provide an opportunity for better adherence through protection when administered on a monthly or even less frequent basis [39]. Similar issues have been addressed in the realm of anti-psychotic medicines, where non-adherence to daily oral regimens is also a challenge [39].

When considering new molecules that could be used in chemoprotection, it is important to consider their ultimate use, since this drives the regulatory strategy. As mentioned earlier, previous generations of medicines, such as mefloquine and atovaquone–proguanil, were first approved for case management, and were only subsequently approved for use at lower doses for prophylaxis. However, if the priority is to deliver new medicines for prophylaxis rapidly, one alternative approach would be to pursue a path towards initial registration directly for prophylaxis; this would require a new clinical and regulatory approach. The key question is to define how large and diverse a population will need to be exposed to a new medicine before the risk–benefit balance is established and considered adequate, and this ratio is clearly different between a medicine used for treatment and one for prophylaxis. Another question relevant to development is how to protect the

new drug; any deployment strategy must also take into consideration the need to protect the drug against the emergence of resistance [40]. The assumption made here is that a combination of two molecules with different mode of action would be ideal to protect against the selection of resistance. It is conceivable to use a single molecule, if the case could be made that the potential development and transmission of resistance in human subjects would be minimal [41]. Such a case would be strengthened by targeting non-replicating or low-copy number stages, such as the sporozoite. The key factor in reducing the risk of resistance generation is avoiding exposure of the drug in subjects with existing parasitaemia. At first glance the ideal medicine would prevent development of the blood-stage of the infection, by killing all parasites before they escaped from the liver. However, a subclinical blood-stage infection may also drive some protective immunity, and so could even be advantageous, as long as the prophylactic drug achieved clearance of the blood stage infection.

Previously, targets have been proposed for the characteristics of molecules which could be used as oral medicines in prophylaxis, and a target candidate profile for molecules with hepatic stage activity (TCP-4); [42]). It seemed timely, therefore, to revisit the characteristics of an injectable therapy for prophylaxis for a number of reasons. First, over the last 2 years there has been an increasing interest in the potential for long-acting injectables, perhaps driven by the success in the antiretroviral arena, and also the re-assessment of the difficulty of obtaining a vaccine with high efficacy and a long duration of protection. Second, there has been a renewed interest in the use of monoclonal antibodies to protect against the establishment of a liver stage infection. This is largely driven by the availability of monoclonal antibodies against the Circumsporozoite Antigen-1 (CSP-1), coming from the recent RTS,S clinical trials. Third, there has been dramatic progress in protecting children from infection in the Sahel by Seasonal Malaria Chemoprevention (SMC) since the new strategy was recommended by the WHO in 2012 [43]. Here, administration of full treatment courses of 3 days of amodiaquine and one dose of sulfadoxine–pyrimethamine were delivered to 15 million children in 12 countries in 2016 [44]. This raises the question as to whether such chemo*prevention* could be replaced by a more easily delivered chemo*protection* regimen (chemoprevention is use of a full treatment course for prophylaxis, chemoprotection is using a specifically-designed and tested prophylaxis regimen). A once-per-season injectable regimen would certainly be worth considering. Moving to chemoprotection (prophylaxis), rather than simply using a full treatment course monthly, requires a new regulatory and clinical approach, and early discussions on this strategy have taken place with regulators during the past 2 years.

In a discussion of potential new medicines there are always many moving parts. A common framework for discussion and agreement on the ideal and minimally acceptable protective efficacy and other qualities of new medicines is important, given the lengthy development required from discovery to launch. In the world of injectable chemoprophylaxis, such a discussion is especially important, given the overlap between the potential uses for injectable small molecules, therapeutic antibodies, and vaccines. Based on these insights, the Target Candidate and Product Profiles (TPPs) presented here will need to be refined and updated in discussions within the malaria community, as and when new data become available.

The different modalities for deploying malaria prophylaxis

There are multiple uses for an injectable anti-malarial prophylaxis (Table 1). The first is to protect populations such as migrant workers, soldiers, tourists and university or boarding school students originating from a malaria-free area from becoming infected when they travel to areas with endemic malaria. Historically prophylaxis has been considered as a premium priced market, largely targeting western tourists and the military, who can afford to pay $5/day for protection. However, as the impact of malaria elimination has progressed, there are now many areas, especially in Africa, where it is relatively easy to travel from a low endemic to a high endemic region, such as from Southern to Northern Zambia. This latter group is an important and expanding group in the malaria agenda. With the progress of the elimination agenda there will be a need for affordably-priced protection for Africans who move from low to high transmission areas. Another important group is residents of non-endemic areas, such as Europe or the USA, whose families come from an endemic area and who return to visit their families in a malaria endemic area. This group is responsible for the highest proportion of cases of imported malaria in Europe.

The second use is to protect a non-immune population within their area of residence, who are suddenly exposed to a malaria outbreak or epidemic. This is one of the major concerns late in any eradication effort, in places where 'maintaining zero' is the priority [45]. In a situation where areas are malaria-free, but the mosquito population is still abundant, there may be a need to rapidly protect populations. In such situations both adults and children will need to be protected. It may not be possible to test the population for pregnancy status, so the ultimate challenge here is to have a medicine which has

a high probability of being safe in the first trimester of pregnancy. A variant on this is the protection of populations from malaria during a pandemic outbreak of febrile disease, such as Ebola. During the 2013–2016 outbreak of Ebola in West Africa, many patients who presented with malarial fevers were triaged into the Ebola facilities, where they became infected with Ebola [46–48], resulting in patients not seeking malaria treatment and an increase in deaths due to malaria [49]. Monthly presumptive treatment with artemisinin-based combination therapy (ACT) was used in at-risk populations in Liberia and Sierra Leone. An injectable prophylaxis could be useful in this kind of situation, if it gave a longer period of protection than oral medication.

The third potential use for an anti-malarial chemoprotective agent is to protect vulnerable populations in areas of high malaria incidence, and this is somewhat distinct from the other uses. Over recent years, there has been a massive deployment of sulfadoxine–pyrimethamine plus amodiaquine (SP–AQ) for SMC. Chemoprevention is defined as giving a full curative course of treatment. This is given over 3 days, to each child under 5 years old, monthly throughout the rainy season in the Sahel (to 13 million children in 2016), to reduce the incidence of symptomatic malaria in this vulnerable population. Since a large part of the cost of deployment of SMC is the delivery, a better treatment would be a once-monthly, single oral medication. A longer-acting injectable would have to offer significant advantage, which is why the ideal threshold for this use has been set at 3 months in the target product profile shown in Table 2. The nuance here is that the clinical development strategy of the injectable would be for protection, as discussed below, rather than using a standard treatment dose and, therefore, in theory the dose would be better titrated to the needs of protection.

The regulatory strategy in each case would be to file for an indication of 'Prophylaxis against *Plasmodium falciparum* malaria'. This would be defined as prevention of malaria infection in subjects travelling from geographical areas with no, or very low risk of malaria infection, to geographical areas with significant risk of malaria infection. The clinical development strategy supports the filing by collecting data to demonstrating acceptable efficacy, safety and tolerability in the target populations.

Defining a product profile for injectable prophylaxis

The discussion of a TPP for an injectable prophylactic medicine is informed by the uses described above. The final acceptance of an injectable product is guided by experience with two other therapeutic or preventative approaches. First, site injection tolerability, in terms of

Table 1 Summary of potential uses for injectable prophylactic medicines

Use case	Description	Target population	Comments
(1) Travellers	Residents of regions of very low or no malaria incidence travelling to malaria endemic areas	Initially, all adults and children > 5 years	Increasing numbers of travellers within Africa, given increased GDP; increasing numbers of Africans in areas of low transmission
(2a) Malaria epidemic	Re-emergence of malaria in zones which had been previously declared malaria free	Entire population	Need demonstration of safety in first trimester of pregnancy; deployment during 'maintaining zero'
(2b) Febrile epidemic	Protection of a population from malaria during epidemics such as Ebola	Entire population	Need demonstration of safety in first trimester of pregnancy. Currently maintained as monthly ACT. Value only if injections offer longer protection
(3) Protection from infection of subjects in high transmission zones	Replacing the SMC regimens of monthly protection by SP-AQ given currently to children under 5 in the Sahel with true chemoprotection	Children < 10 years	No requirement for safety demonstration in first trimester of pregnancy; combination would ideally have causal prophylaxis (preventing blood-stage and liver stage activity)

Table 2 TPP for an injectable prophylactic medicine for malaria

Parameter to be clinically evaluated for the combination	Minimum essential	Ideal
Antimalarial effects	Blood schizonticides with at least one molecule also having causal prophylactic activity (killing hepatic schizonts)	Both molecules should have causal prophylactic, blood schizonticidal and transmission-blocking activities
Mechanism of action	Two partner drugs without cross resistance	Two partner drugs have different modes of action, so no cross resistance
Dosing regimen	Once per month, intramuscular, with an acceptable injection volume	Once per 3 months, intramuscular or sub-cutaneous with an acceptable injection volume
Rate of onset of action	Protection, within 72 h of initial injection	Immediate protection (no lag prior to onset of action)
Clinical efficacy	$\geq$ 80% protective efficacy	$\geq$ 95% protective efficacy: reduction in incidence of symptomatic malaria. No drug-resistant parasites identified in volunteer infection studies still capable of transmission
Drug–drug interactions	No unmanageable risk in terms of solid state or PK interactions	No risks in terms of solid state or PK interactions with other co-administered PrEP or therapeutics
Safety and tolerability	No drug-related SAEs; minimal drug-related AEs—i.e., not resulting in clinical study exclusion. No unacceptable pain, irritability of inflammation at injection site, especially injection abscesses	Idem
Use in patients with reduced G6PD activity	Testing not required as no enhanced risk in mild-moderate G6PD deficiency	Testing not required as drugs not linked to haemolytic risk
Use in infants/children	Use in children > 6 months old	Use in infants, children and adults
Formulations	Suitable for intramuscular injection with minimal preparation; maximum volume of 2 mL for adults and 0.5 mL for infants, administered with 27 gauge needle; partner drugs can be injected separately	Liquid pre-filled injection device for intramuscular; maximum volume of 1 mL for adults and < 0.5 mL infants administered with 27–30 gauge needle; fixed dose combination of the drugs; or subcutaneous injection if volumes smaller than above for intramuscular injection
Cost of treatment	< 5 USD per injection	$\leq$ USD 1 for infants, USD 2 for children, USD 4 for adults
Shelf life of formulated product (ICH guidelines for zones/IVb)	$\geq$ 2 years	$\geq$ 3 years

PK pharmacokinetic, *(S)AE* (severe) adverse event, *ICH* International Conference on Harmonization

needle size, and injection volume should be driven by a favourable comparison to vaccines. The most advanced malaria vaccine, Mosquirix® (RTS,S–AS202) has been approved by the European Commission after having been given a positive scientific opinion by the CHMP (Committee for Medicinal Products for Human Use at the EMA (European Medicines Agency), and is about to undergo Phase IV in-country studies. The current course of vaccination involves four 0.5 mL intramuscular injections with a 25-gauge needle, at a cost of around $5 per injection in infants. Second, in HIV infections, where an effective vaccine has also been a major challenge, pre-exposure prophylaxis, or PrEP, using an injectable is being studied [37, 50]. Although large injection volumes and needle have been found acceptable, for example, in the injection of penicillin-G benzoate crystals for bacterial infections, such as mass treatment against yaws [51], a new medicine for children protecting against malaria would need to be more child-friendly to be acceptable

for repeat use. Intravenous injection of the PfSPZ vaccine [52] with a very fine needle has been very well tolerated even in very small children, but i.v. injection would probably not be the ideal route to achieve a prolonged duration of protection. From a formulation and pharmaceutical perspective, intramuscular or subcutaneous depot approaches are preferred to achieve the desired long duration with new chemical entities.

The level of efficacy required for a new product can be gauged by the efficacy of current prophylaxis. In comparative, randomized clinical trials, nonimmune adults, adolescents and children ($\geq$ 11 kg) visiting malaria-endemic regions and receiving once-daily atovaquone/proguanil (250/100 mg in adults and dosage based on body weight in children < 40 kg), had no cases of falciparum malaria for 28 days [53], comparable efficacy was also seen in other studies [54, 55]. Doxycycline provides 84–99% protection (studies cited in [41]). Lessons from the vaccine community also suggest that a protective efficacy of $\geq 80\%$ for a once per 3-month injection might be acceptable. The current working hypothesis is that a molecule either preventing or treating hepatocyte stage infection would be useful when looking at new chemical entities. However, molecules with pure blood stage activity (chloroquine and mefloquine) have been the mainstay of oral prophylaxis and so whether this would be acceptable for an injectable remains a question for further discussion.

The clinical safety requirements of a long-acting injectable for prophylaxis are much more difficult to define precisely in advance of data. The two overriding principles are that first, the drug will be given to subjects with no overt disease, and so the safety thresholds should in general be similar to those required for vaccines. This will inevitably lead to the need for considerable phase IV activities. The second aspect relates to the long plasma residence time of pharmacologically active material. Appropriate safeguards have to be in place for the care of subjects, should a severe adverse event occur, and clearly such an event would preclude further development of the medicine for populations in low-resource settings. However, it is important to underline the fact that the safety considerations related to an injectable drug driving exposure over several months are very similar to the safety considerations related to an oral drug driving exposure over several months. The ideal medicine is one that can be used to protect all ages; however the development of the medicine for children will require particular care, and the availability of substantial safety data in adults before proceeding to the more vulnerable younger populations.

A target product profile (TPP) including other parameters for an injectable prophylactic medicine for malaria is proposed in Table 2.

Approaches to finding and developing new small molecule TCP-4 candidates

Compounds with a TCP-4 profile would normally be shown to be highly potent against the hepatic schizonts of *P. falciparum* parasites. The definition of a hit and a lead still follow the criteria discussed previously [56], with compounds showing an IC_{50} of less than 1 µM being considered as potential starting points for medicinal chemistry, aiming for a final potency of less than 10 nM. The key data however are those that increase our understanding of how well this translates into in vivo efficacy, and allowing an early prediction of the human effective dose.

In vivo measurements of efficacy have been performed traditionally using infection with GFP- (green fluorescent protein) or luciferase-expressing *Plasmodium berghei* sporozoites in mice. This assumes equipotent activity between *P. berghei* and *P. falciparum*. A

newer model is the FRG huHep chimeric mouse model with engrafted human hepatocytes and erythrocytes. FRG stands for the lack of functional Fah, Rag-2 and Interleukin 2 receptor common gamma chain genes in these animals. This model allows an endpoint based on asexual blood stage infection from the liver [57]. Here, the benchmarking with atovaquone shows that a highly efficacious compound should be able to lower the parasite 18S RNA signal in the liver by 10^7-fold, or a 200-fold reduction in the bioluminescence signal [58]. DSM265, a novel PfDHODH inhibitor, with demonstrated activity in humans, shows a 10^4-fold reduction in this model, arguably defining the lower threshold of efficacy. During lead optimization, it is important to be able to assess the human effective dose, i.e. the dose required to produce a similarly effective exposure in humans. In the absence of imaging technologies to determine the time-dependent concentration of a drug within the liver, the definition of the prophylactic concentration has to be based on the plasma concentration, assuming that the plasma to hepatocyte concentration ratio is invariant with plasma exposure. The minimum protective plasma concentration in the mouse model can then be used as the basis for pharmacokinetic modelling of the human exposures. For a pre-clinical orally active compound the ideal threshold is an adult dose of < 100 mg, or < 2 mg/kg. Similar constraints apply to injectables, but driven by a need to be able to deliver the drugs in an acceptable injection volume of < 0.5 mg per drug, as discussed below. Two other biological factors are important. First, the demonstration that clinical selection of mutations is a rare event, or that these mutations are not transmitted. It has been shown that is relatively easy to select for mutations against atovaquone both in vitro and in patients, but that these mutations are difficult to transmit [59]. Second, species selectivity: although 99% of the global burden of disease is currently carried by *P. falciparum*, activity against other species would be an advantage, since many patients have mixed infections that include *P. vivax*, *Plasmodium malariae* and *Plasmodium ovale*.

Selection of a formulation, which may also involve the use of pro-drugs, is critical to enable the maintenance of long-lasting protection. The ideal use case would be a 3-month coverage from a single injection, allowing potential protection for a season in some countries. Thus, compounds having high potency and very low clearance, and with formulations delivering long-term drug release into the systemic circulation are favoured. When considering the product presentation, a number of factors need to be taken into account, including but not limited to: cost of goods, a therapeutic product that can be stored at room temperature in climate zones III and IV, a formulation with a potential for local production, and a formulation that is easy to administer. As such there is no published decision tree that maps the technology path for selecting long-acting injectable formulations. A range of different formulation technologies have been applied in commercial products, such as oil solutions, aqueous micro- and nanosuspensions, in situ forming gels, and micro-particular systems. There is, hence, a good industrial basis to define the most likely options that would fulfil both the technological elements as well as the cost of the product. In resource-limited settings, the first line of formulation will most likely be an oil solution or suspension of the micro- or nano-particulate drug, due to the simplicity of development and production of the formulation, low cost of excipients and potential for thermal sterilization, which would allow local production. The use of an oil-based solution or suspension requires clinically acceptable oils, such as fractionated coconut, castor, corn, cottonseed or olive oils. A key consideration here will be local tolerability [60].

The second option for a long-acting injectable for prophylactic treatment of malaria would probably be an aqueous suspension of either micro- or nanoparticles. The advantage of an aqueous suspension is that there is a well-established relationship between particle size and rate of dissolution. This allows much better control of the rate of release of the drug and, therefore, better matching of the final pharmacokinetics, once the human clearance is known. In the case of oil solutions of the drug, the oil is metabolized by macrophages in the muscle over a period of days to weeks, resulting in an amorphous depot of drug in the tissue. Data from preclinical animal models and in humans have demonstrated that appropriate slow release of a drug can be obtained, although the choice of oil is largely empirical at this stage. The technology associated with aqueous suspensions is well established, i.e. production facilities and capacity are available, however, cost of goods is a bit higher than the oil solutions, and the development complexity the same.

Selection of compounds for long-acting injectable formulations have historically been an afterthought, so the physico-chemical properties needed for success have not been well mapped. The selection criteria depend on the final technology; for an oil based solution, a crystalline material with high solubility (> 75 mg/mL in triglycerides, low aqueous solubility at pH $7.4 < 10$ μM, high lipophilicity (ideally logD > 4) and high melting point of the free form (> 150 °C) are favoured. Ironically, these are properties usually avoided by medicinal chemists when developing an oral product. The definition of the range for logD is under discussion as recent investigations have shown that there is limited correlation between this parameter and the ability to formulate in a lipid based vehicle [61]. The choice of final presentation will be governed by solubility

in oil, aqueous solubility at pH 7.4 and the stability of the formulation under forced-degradation conditions. The molecules for injection can be the parent molecules, or pro-drugs synthesized with increased lipophilicity and oil solubility to fit the parameters described above. However, pro-drugs bring the complexity of requiring the preclinical safety and exposure to both the active molecule and the pro-drug to be determined. The stability of the drug product, especially as a pre-filled sterile solution is particularly critical to ensure adequate shelf-life in tropical conditions, as a cold chain requirement for an injectable TCP-4 prophylactic would not be ideal.

Ideally, the drug should be administered either subcutaneously or intramuscularly. The former has the advantage that it is easier to administer, and requires less training, but there is a greater constraint on the volume that can be delivered. Given that the ultimate product will target the protection of children, infants and adults, the proposed final volume is 0.5 mL for infants and children, and 2.0 mL for adults.

The needle size is provisionally suggested at 27-gauge, to minimize discomfort during the injection. Significantly larger volumes of administration are routinely given, such as the 4 mL of microcrystalline penicillin-G benzoate through a 21-gauge needle [62], which is nevertheless very painful. However, the success of this product will ultimately depend on its acceptability by communities, and so conservative values have been taken. The needle size determines the maximum viscosity of the injected material, which may restrict the uses of certain oil-based vehicles for small molecules, or the maximum protein concentration in the case of an antibody.

Alternatives to injections are implant systems, as used in long-term contraception. These have the potential advantage of controllability, with the possibility of removal should an adverse event occur. But this approach requires potent molecules that allow limited dosage: contraceptive etonogestrel implants only contain 68 mg of drug [63]. Implants have not been developed for paediatric use.

The safety of the molecules is of paramount importance, whether considering long-acting injectables or long-acting oral molecules. In the case of any safety concern, removal of an active drug from plasma would require extensive dialysis, if feasible for the molecule, and lack of access to such a procedure could be life-threatening in resource-poor settings. It is, therefore, important to consider potential long-acting injectables within three tiers of risk:

- The first tier would consist of molecules for which extensive human systemic safety data already exist. This would apply to new formulation or a prodrug of a molecule already used for prophylaxis, such as atovaquone–proguanil. Here the safety and tolerability of the combination is well understood for oral administrations of up to 60 days, enabling an adequate assessment of the risk–benefit balance, and giving a relatively straightforward, albeit cautious path to human studies. In the initial single ascending dose studies in humans, the increase in dose should produce an increase in C_{max} and an increase in the duration of significant plasma concentration. As such, the initial first-in-human study can be de-risked by the selection of an appropriately low starting dose (this group of candidate molecules could also include new monoclonal antibodies, provided that they could be shown to be free of cross-reaction with any host targets and lack target-based enhancement of infectivity or inappropriate immune activation).

- The second tier would be prodrugs of new chemical entities with oral formulation for which initial human safety data can be collected using the oral route, allowing dosing to be halted in case of adverse events of concern. Testing of parenteral formulations could follow, but there would be no understanding of rare serious adverse events until after Phase III trials.

- The third and most difficult tier would be molecules for which no oral formulation of the active parent is possible due the physico-chemical properties of the agent. Given the required long plasma residence time, the starting dose in initial clinical trials would have to be extremely low, and the dose escalation between cohorts extremely conservative.

In some of the uses described above, the population at risk from malaria will include a considerable number of women of childbearing potential, whose pregnancy status may not be determined. For new molecules coming forward for prophylaxis, early analysis of the developmental and reproductive toxicology (DART) would be an essential part of the development strategy. Absence of any signals in such preclinical studies would facilitate the inclusion of women of childbearing age in clinical studies. This could facilitate early use of such an agent in the larger population. As discussed below, monoclonal antibodies offer a considerable advantage, since the materno–fetal transfer of IgG during the first trimester is minimal [64, 65].

The preclinical candidate will be a single molecule. There is still debate within the community as to whether the final product should be a single molecule or a combination. The potential for the selection of resistance is much lower than when a molecule is used for the treatment of uncomplicated malaria, since the molecule encounters far fewer parasites [66]. However, asymptomatic infections with quite high parasitaemias of > 5000/µL are frequently observed, and it is possible that there are pre-existing mutations within the sporozoite population, emphasizing the need for caution [67]. Resistance generation against antibodies is not expected to be a significant problem, provided that the antibodies are generated against conserved non-variant antigens from non-dividing forms, such as sporozoites, unless of course, pre-existing mutations are prevalent.

In this review a conservative approach of taking two active molecules has been adopted. This is important in early development discussions, as early human volunteer studies require the availability of formulations for both molecules that are compatible. The additional twist in this compatibility discussion is that the drug exposure profile of each molecule in the blood needs to be compatible and since this is modulated by the kinetics of release from the initial depot it may be difficult to do this for two individual molecules with different physicochemical properties. Matching pharmacokinetics is important both for duration of efficacy and for mitigating the risk of emergence of resistance during the extended tail of exposure. In theory, separate injections of the two drugs is possible, although this would be a large disadvantage. Seriously mismatched pharmacokinetics would limit the use to applications where subjects are outside of high transmission zones during the tail exposure period; again, this is possible, but not ideal. As such, any preclinical safety and toxicology studies may have to be repeated with the final formulation.

Initial proof of concept in man can be performed in volunteer infection studies with sporozoites. Recent studies with oral small molecule inhibitors of parasite liver stages have demonstrated clinically useful activity with relatively small cohorts, either using direct injections of sporozoites or insect-delivered sporozoites [26, 27]. For small molecules targeting hepatic schizonts, both approaches give similar results, with the direct injection of sporozoites being operationally easier. For antibody therapeutics targeting sporozoite antigens prior to infection of the liver, there is still a need to confirm the best approach.

The TCP-4, for a single molecule suitable for development as part of a new injectable, combination regimen for prophylaxis against malaria is detailed in Table 3.

Monoclonal antibodies for long-acting malaria prophylaxis

An alternative approach to protecting vulnerable populations with an injectable small molecule would be the use of a monoclonal antibody [68]. Even though malaria infection in humans does not lead to a sterilizing immune response, it is still possible that monoclonal antibodies

Table 3 TCP-4 as part of a prophylactic combination

General considerations	Minimum essential	Ideal
Dosing regimen; adult/paediatric dose	Injectable: subcutaneous or intra-muscular, once per month, with injection volumes < 0.25 mL per molecule for infants and < 1 mL for adults via a 27 gauge or smaller needle	Injectable: subcutaneous or intramuscular once per 3 months
Pre-clinical activity	Proven liver schizont stage activity and 100% protective efficacy achieved in vivo, defined as no asexual parasitaemia after 30 days	Proven liver schizont stage activity and 100% protective efficacy achieved in vivo defined as no asexual parasitaemia after 30 days
Susceptibility to loss of efficacy due to acquired resistance	Resistance frequency in culture with erythrocytes < 10^{-5}. Marker identified and no pre-existing resistance determined in the global parasite population	Resistance frequency in culture with erythrocytes < 10^{-9}
Clinical protection from infection	> 80% protective efficacy (positive parasitaemia) predicted from volunteer infection studies	> 95% protective efficacy (positive parasitaemia) predicted from volunteer infection studies
Drug–drug interactions	No unmanageable risks	No interactions with other antimalarial, anti-retroviral or tuberculosis medicines or oral contraception
Safety and tolerability	Therapeutic ratio > tenfold between therapeutic exposure and NOAEL in preclinical studies and easily monitorable adverse event or biomarker for human studies. No unacceptable adverse events associated with pain, irritation or inflammation at injection site	Therapeutic ratio > 50-fold between therapeutic exposure and NOAEL in preclinical studies if not monitorable adverse event or biomarker for human studies. No adverse events associated with pain, irritation or inflammation at injection site
Preclinical DART profile	No signals in EFD and juvenile toxicology studies precluding use in children 6 months old and during 2nd and 3rd trimester pregnancies	No signals in EFD and juvenile toxicology studies precluding use in infants and women with unknown pregnancy status
G6PD deficiency status	Therapeutic dose shows minimal change in haemoglobin concentration in subjects with reduced G6PD activity. New candidate drugs show no enhanced haemolytic risk in preclinical model	Measured—no enhanced risk in subjects with reduced G6PD activity
Injectable formulation	Solutions: soluble in targeted volume based on total dose in clinically acceptable oils Suspensions: particle size controlled to give required compound release profile supporting monthly injection	Idem. Ideal formulation should be delivered in a prefilled injection device for once-in-3-months injection
Cost of single administration	Molecules consistent with a final product cost of < 5 USD per injection	Molecules consistent with a final product cost of ≤ USD 1 for infants, USD 2 for children, USD 4 for adults
Projected stability of final product under zone IVb conditions (30 °C, 75% relative humidity)	≥ 2 years	≥ 3 years

EFD embryo fetal development, NOAEL no-observed-adverse-effect-level with sufficient affinity and prolonged plasma residence times could provide protection from infection [68]. The exquisite selectivity of monoclonal antibodies means there should be no interaction with host targets, and the off-target safety issues can be avoided. Most published work is on antibodies that prevent sporozoite invasion of hepatocytes or merozoites infection of erythrocytes. These antibodies could be compared with small molecules for TCP-4 (hepatic schizonts) or TCP-1 (erythrocytic schizonts) with the subtlety that the antibodies prevent the initial infection of the respective cell types, whereas small molecules prevent the replication of the parasite within the host cells. In both cases the time window for action of an antibody is a critical element which distinguishes the antibody profile from the drug profile. An antibody against sporozoites must be able to act in the short time that it takes for sporozoites to move from the skin to the liver, typically within 30 min. Antibodies against merozoites must exert their effect in the short window when the merozoites are present in free circulation, typically 30 s.

Given the high commercial price of many existing antibody therapies, it is often assumed that the cost of antibody therapy would be prohibitive in most malaria-endemic countries. Provided antibodies are expressed at high levels (4 g/L), and are stable, hence the production costs can drop from around $100–300/g [69] to estimates of around $35–85/g [70], with room for a further decrease in costs, projected to be $20/g at the multi-tonne scale.

As with small molecules, an intramuscular or sub-cutaneous presentation is probably preferable to intravenous injection, and so a limiting factor is the volume of administration. The amount of antibody is, therefore, limited by the achievable concentration. Although concentrations as high as 200 mg/mL have been reported for subcutaneous injection, a more conservative target is 100 mg/mL [71]. Based on a 0.5 mL injection volume for children and 2 mL for adults, this sets a dose ceiling of 50 mg and 200 mg, respectively (Table 2). This in turn sets an optimized cost maximum for the antibody at $1.75 for children and $7 for adults, excluding the costs of vials and distribution. These price estimations are on the borderline of what might be acceptable, in comparison with the pricing for a malaria vaccine. Any decrease in dose, frequency of administration or cost of manufacturing would further bring down these costs.

To achieve long-term prophylaxis, mutations in the Fc region are needed. Monoclonal antibodies tend to be IgGs, with plasma half-lives of 20–25 days [72, 73]. This half-life is partly controlled by FcRn receptor-mediated elimination, and also depends on the antigen abundance. Mutating the IgG Fc region to increase the interaction

with its receptor FcRn, at the acidic pH encountered in the lysosome, prevents elimination of the antibody in the lysosome, favouring its recycling. This can extend the circulation duration of an antibody threefold, as has been achieved for bevacizumab and cetuximab [74], through simple Met428Leu and Asn434Ser mutations. Other approaches to half-life extension make the antibody bulkier by fusion, mulitmerization or pegylation, but these approaches would dramatically increase the cost of goods [75].

An antibody could be compared directly with a small molecule in the animal model. The goal would be an 80% protection from infection, minimally for 1 month and ideally for 3 months. Given the restrictions on injection volume, this would require administration of 2 mg/kg of each active molecule in adults and 2–5 mg/kg in children. As for small molecules, the simplest preclinical model for therapeutic antibodies would be the FRG chimeric mouse model with engrafted human hepatocytes, discussed earlier. Allometric scaling for a series of antibodies [76] suggests that systemic clearance is proportional to the body weight raised to a power of 0.91 ($Cl = a \cdot BW^b$), a much higher number than seen with small molecules. Therefore, allowing for the difference in body weights for humans and mice, this translates approximately into a twofold difference in the mg/kg dose between humans and mice, setting an efficacy threshold in mice of an 80–200 mg total dose. This could be related back to a cellular potency target $EC_{50} < 100$ pM (< 15 ng/mL), based on modelling of various affinity and dissociation rates [77, 78]. It is important to demonstrate in such studies, that there is no risk of stimulating antibody-dependent enhancement [79].

As mentioned above, the exquisite selectivity of antibodies means that off-target effects are minimized. Anti-sporozoite or anti-merozoite antibodies do not target host antigens. Therefore, toxicology studies should be less complicated compared to other indications. Fetal transfer in the first trimester is reported to be minimal; the required Fc receptor for the transfer of IgGs is hardly detectable in the placental syncytiotrophoblast during the first trimester [80]. Specific studies on monoclonal antibodies in pregnancy are rare, given that most antibodies are given for treatment of cancer or autoimmune diseases. Several studies have reported that multiple sclerosis patients in early stages of pregnancy exposed to natalizumab or alemtuzumab did not have an increase in the frequency of abortions [81]. In Inflammatory Bowel Disease, the European evidence-based consensus is to continue treatment with anti-TNF throughout pregnancy, and the practice appears safe [82]. This means that antibody prophylaxis could potentially be given to young women whose pregnancy status is unknown, which is a tremendous advantage over new chemical entities [64].

Antibody discovery tends to be much faster than for small molecules, with a much higher probability that an individual project will deliver a development candidate [83]. However, once a development candidate is defined, the production of high-grade material for the initial clinical trials is much more expensive. Typical costs are in the region of $5 million, which contrasts starkly with around $100 k for a small molecule. This combination of an easier pathway to candidate identification, but a more expensive decision stage gate, means that it is very important to have clear parameters for the TCP.

Clinical and regulatory strategy of long-acting malaria prophylaxis

For new chemical entities and antibodies the Phase I single ascending dose study in healthy volunteers would aim to achieve the plasma concentration predicted from studies using the FRG-mice [84]. At this concentration, prophylactic activity could be assessed in human volunteer malaria infection studies [26, 27]. For new chemical entities, the safety and efficacy in human volunteers should ideally be established initially using an oral formulation, which will help guide the safety recommendations for dose escalation of the injectable in Phase I.

In parallel, it is important to investigate the potential combinations of two molecules that can be brought forward. Simulations using data from preclinical cytochrome P450 and transporter assays can help eliminate combinations with likely problematic drug–drug interactions. Additivity and possible synergy between two molecules can be studied in the FRG SCID mouse. Exposure–response analyses of these studies also allow modelling of the doses proposed for Phase II trials. In addition, the modelling has the potential to demonstrate the contribution of the individual compounds to overall efficacy, addressing the 'combination rule' required by the US FDA. The safety of combinations needs to be investigated in healthy adult volunteers combination studies before moving to Phase II trials in infected but asymptomatic subjects. A flow chart for the selection and optimization of new molecules with potential chemoprotective activity is shown in Fig. 1.

The Phase II and Phase III clinical strategy is based on the lessons learned from the development of atovaquone–proguanil [55, 85, 86] for malaria prophylaxis. Atovaquone–proguanil was first developed as a malaria treatment, and was subsequently shown to be efficacious in prophylaxis, using a daily dosing regimen. However, in the case of a new injectable protective regimen, the goal is to try to achieve registration for a prophylaxis indication *directly*. Such a development plan for

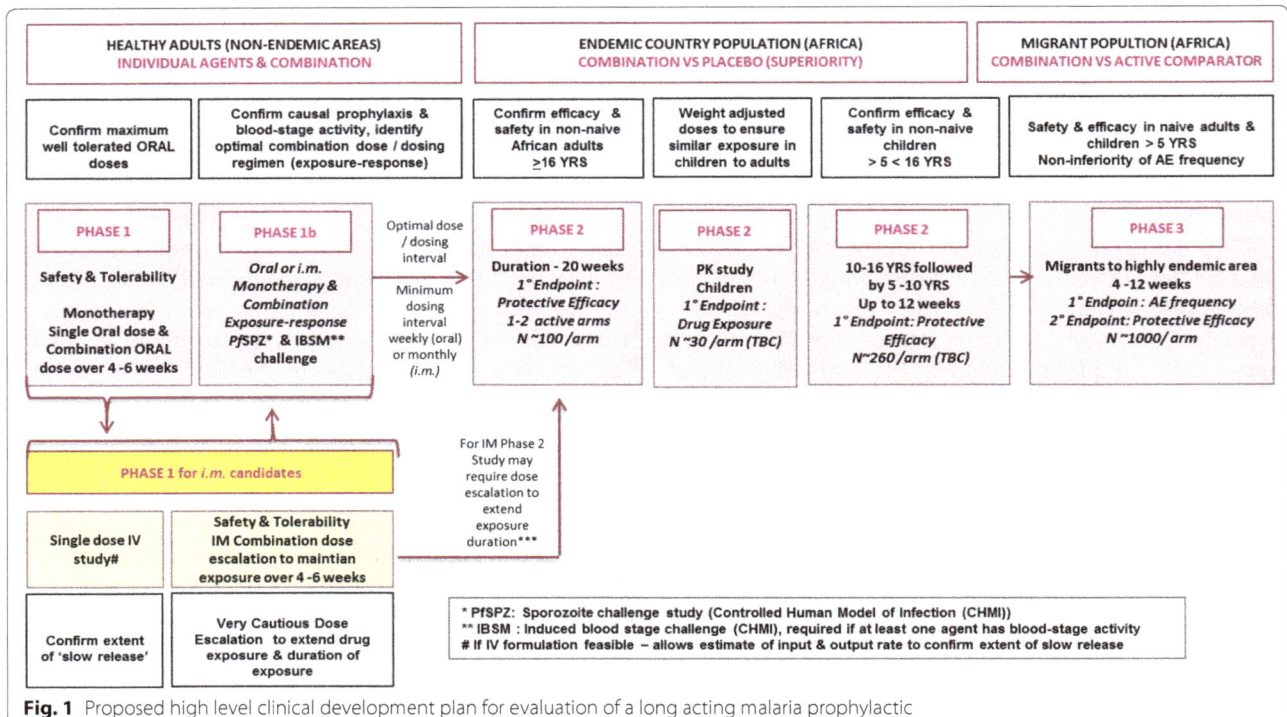

Fig. 1 Proposed high level clinical development plan for evaluation of a long acting malaria prophylactic

prophylaxis was presented for initial discussion with regulators (the UK Medicines and Healthcare products Regulatory Agency, MHRA) in the context of an oral drug combination therapy. Similar considerations would apply for antibodies. Two main clinical trial designs are proposed to support registration for a prophylaxis indication (Fig. 1). Phase II studies would be carried out in subjects resident within an endemic area, and Phase III studies would be undertaken in a genuine migrant population, such as seasonal workers, or boarding school children. Studies would be conducted in highly endemic areas, to obtain sufficient discriminatory power versus comparator to demonstrate efficacy. Since it is thought that relatively few children less than 5 years of age are likely to be travelling from malaria-free to malaria endemic areas, recruitment into clinical trials of this younger population may be problematic. For this reason, the plan would be to seek approval for subjects over 5 years in the first instance. Recruitment of younger children is likely to be easier following approval of the medicine for prophylaxis in the older population, when sufficient evidence of safety and efficacy is available.

To support a stringent regulatory authority registration for prophylaxis, two Phase II studies are proposed in a non-naïve population (Fig. 1), the first carried out over 20 weeks in adults, and the second carried out over 12 weeks in children of 5 years and above. Both studies would be randomized, double-blind placebo-controlled studies to evaluate the prophylactic efficacy, safety and tolerability in non-naïve subjects in regions of Africa with a high incidence of malaria. The primary endpoint would be protective efficacy (PE). A key aspect of this design is that a sterilizing cure is administered to study subjects to clear both blood-stage parasites and gametocytes prior to assessing the prophylactic efficacy of the drugs under investigation. This design is, therefore, a useful model of uninfected populations travelling to endemic areas, although the subjects will have the benefit of partial-immunity from previous infections. From a study design perspective, this approach has the significant advantage of allowing the use of a placebo comparator, thus providing a direct measure of PE (defined as: 1-failure rate active treatment/failure rate of placebo).

In the first of these two studies, two to three combination dose levels or regimens could be evaluated, using an exposure–response approach in a relatively small number of subjects, to identify the optimal dose and frequency of dosing. Following the identification of the dosing regimen that provides the target protective efficacy with a practical dosing frequency, and with acceptable safety and tolerability, a small pharmacokinetic study or Phase II run-in could confirm that the dose adjustments in children achieve the target drug exposures.

This would then be followed by a Phase II study in children which would test the selected regimen in non-naïve school children resident in an endemic area. The design would involve a step-wise, age de-escalation approach. A full safety review would be carried out before enrolling each new cohort, descending via cohorts of approximately 30 10–16 year olds, to 5–10 year olds. The decision to move to Phase III would be based on the likelihood of achieving protection over 3 months. Such protection would ideally be in a population which had no protection supplied by immune memory. The demonstration of activity only in a population with some background immunity could still be useful—for example providing protection in pregnancy, or as a potential replacement for SMC. Since the effect of partial immunity on the efficacy in the Phase II population cannot be estimated directly, a somewhat higher efficacy than required for Phase III could be set as the threshold to move from Phase II to Phase III. The acceptable efficacy for the prophylaxis indication will ultimately depend on the likely use cases and validation in further discussion with the wider community, balancing efficacy and aspects such as deployment practicality, efficacy and cost per Disability Adjusted Life Year (DALY).

The use of a placebo in adults and children in the Phase II studies in areas of high malaria incidence was strongly recommended in initial discussions with regulatory authorities because this is the only circumstance in which the true attack rate is known, and hence the true protective efficacy can be measured. The population enrolled in this study would ordinarily be exposed to sub-clinical malaria infection which would otherwise remain untreated. All subjects would receive an initial sterilizing cure for this sub-clinical malaria, and benefit from close clinical safety monitoring during the study, as well as standard-of-care treatment upon detection of positive parasitaemia during study conduct. The acceptability of placebo controlled trials in adults and in children will need additional discussion with the Ethics Committees at individual sites, to take account of local concerns on this topic. There are sometimes ethical objections to placebo injections, especially if repeated blood sampling was undertaken. An alternative would be to combine the placebo or experimental drug with a proven vaccine against a different disease.

The protective efficacy, safety and tolerability would then be confirmed in a Phase III study in the target population. These are adults and children older than 5 years travelling from geographical areas with no, or a very low risk of malaria infection, to geographical areas of significant risk of malaria infection. Ethically, these studies need to be active controlled studies; oral atovaquone–proguanil being the most likely comparator. The protective efficacy of both atovaquone–proguanil and the NCE (new chemical entity) is expected to be high, therefore a very low rate of malaria infection ('attack rate') would be expected in this population, meaning that very large numbers of subjects would be required to demonstrate non-inferiority of the new medicine. For this reason, in the development of atovaquone–proguanil, the primary endpoint in Phase III studies was the overall frequency of any adverse events assessed at 7 days after leaving the endemic country, with protective efficacy as a secondary endpoint. In these comparator studies, confirmed *P. falciparum* malaria occurred in 0/486 and 0/477 subjects receiving atovaquone–proguanil and mefloquine, respectively [55], and in 0/501 and 3/507 subjects receiving atovaquone–proguanil and chloroquine–proguanil, respectively [87], illustrating the difficulty of this approach. Although atovaquone–proguanil is the best comparator, such studies have the additional complication of a lack of marketing authorization in many of the areas ultimately targeted.

Demonstrating non-inferiority of protective efficacy would as mentioned above require very large trials. Making a number of assumptions about the risk of developing malaria for travellers from Europe, Canada and South Africa to East Africa who do not take prophylaxis, the average duration of travel and the efficacy of a prophylactic treatment, Høgh et al. [87] estimated that assuming a protective efficacy of chloroquine–proguanil of 72%, a study in travellers designed to show that a new anti-malarial drug with 95% efficacy is better than chloroquine–proguanil, assuming a 80% power and a 5% significance level, would require more than 16,000 participants While a number of the assumptions made would not necessarily apply to African migrants traveling for work and for schooling, perhaps for longer periods, and exposed to higher bite rates (due to greater endemicity, and a less protective living environment), nevertheless unrealistically large numbers may be required to test for non-inferiority of efficacy. Indeed, given the reported 98.5–100% efficacy for atovaquone–proguanil, demonstration of non-inferiority would not be expected, but demonstration of high efficacy of the NCE would be required. Therefore, similarly to the development of atovaquone–proguanil, for a long-acting injectable prophylactic trial in adults proposed here (Fig. 1), the primary endpoint would be non-inferior safety and tolerability compared to atovaquone–proguanil, with prophylactic efficacy as a secondary endpoint. Hence the required sample size of any future Phase III studies will be based on the most frequent and clinically relevant adverse event(s) of both test medicine and comparator, and the non-inferiority margin will be set based on a proposed clinically relevant difference in adverse event rate.

In migrant populations a number of potential approaches have been published, including enrolment of subjects in Travel Clinics [55, 87], protection of soldiers on active duty, boarding school children or groups of workers deployed for short periods in hyper endemic regions [88].

In initial discussion with MHRA, a total safety population of approximately 3000 subjects exposed to the clinical dose was deemed a sufficient safety data package for registration of an oral prophylaxis, provided no significant safety signals are detected. The breakdown numbers of adults *versus* children was not considered critical as long as there is a good spread of age across the study.

Conclusions

Several factors have driven a renewed evaluation of the role of prophylaxis in the malaria elimination agenda over the last few years:

- First, the general acceptance that countries that are undergoing elimination will have internal populations migrating from low transmission zones to those of high transmission, for example going from the south to the north of Zambia. In the past, the prophylaxis of migrant populations was considered only to be commercially relevant for protecting western tourists and soldiers. However, it is now clear that cost-effective solutions must be found to protect migratory populations in low- and middle-income countries.

- Second, in countries that have eliminated malaria and are 'maintaining zero' [12], there is the risk of re-introduction and epidemics, and in the absence of a fully effective vaccine, an alternative approach to protection is needed for populations at risk of an epidemic. A special subcategory is the need for malarial prophylaxis during fever outbreaks such as the Ebola crisis in West Africa, to reduce the risk of malaria at the height of the epidemic and to protect health care workers.

- Third, there have been tremendous successes in the last 5 years using SMC, which involves giving a full treatment course of anti-malarials every month. A regimen which was truly optimized for prophylaxis, and available as an injection would have potentially major benefit. This latter point has come into focus recently because of the stagnation in the reduction of malaria incidence globally [44]. One of the strategic responses here is to ask what else can now be done in high-burden countries to achieve significant reductions in morbidity, and new prophylaxis regimens that were simpler to administer than current SMC could have an even bigger impact and which could potentially be given in areas with perennial high transmission.

Several factors lead to some optimism for the future:

- First is the availability of new chemotypes with activity against the malaria parasite, which opens up the possibility of focusing on new medicines specifically designed for prophylaxis. This is an appealing situation since, ideally, the same medicine should not be used for both the protection and the treatment of malaria within the same geographic locale. To date, none of the new molecules has a half-life equivalent to that seen from oral doses of 4-aminoquinolines or the 8-aminoquinoline tafenoquine, hence the need for slow-release injectable formulations, to provide the appropriate duration of cover.
- Second, the availability of better in vitro *P. falciparum* liver stage assays and animal models, including a murine model of the hepatic infection of *P. falciparum* allows the comparison of different molecular classes in vivo. Standardization of protocols for such assays will be an important driving factor over the coming years, allowing head-to-head comparisons of small molecules and monoclonal antibodies.
- Third, in experimental medicine, the arrival of robust supplies of GMP-standardized sporozoites has enabled testing of new chemical series in human volunteer infection studies. These data, or alternatively those obtained in insect-driven infection studies, allow early identification of compounds with activity in humans, and estimation of human effective doses for full-scale clinical studies.
- Finally, new developments in formulation technologies allow the development of some of the molecules with prophylactic activity as long-acting injectables. This can be achieved by formulation of the parent compound or development and formulation of prodrugs. Developments in HIV, oral contraception and antipsychotic medicines have shown that slow release allowing protection for one or even several months is possible, with acceptable dosing volumes and needle sizes. These studies also underline the need for highly potent molecules, to minimize cost, and to maximize acceptability.

Taken together, there are many reasons to be optimistic about the probability of identifying and developing long-acting injectable formulations. What is important is that a common language and common standards are applied to assess the different candidates, and on this basis Target Candidate Profiles are proposed. In addition, the route to registration will be a new one, not necessarily proceeding via the approval of medicines for a treatment indication. As such, new target product profiles and the use cases supporting their delivery in the field are important. This document contains proposals for such profiles, in the full knowledge that over the next few years clinical data will become available providing many lessons that aid in further refinement of the next generation of profiles. More discussion is needed with experts in the field and the bigger malaria community e.g. on the clinically relevant level of efficacy to be targeted. Furthermore, MMV is preparing clinical development strategies for new prophylactic medicines and engaging stringent regulatory authorities in early discussions.

Abbreviations

ACT: artemisinin combination therapy; CHMP: Committee for Medicinal Products for Human Use; CSP-1: Circumsporozoite Antigen-1; DADDS: 4-4'-diacetylaminosulphone; DALY: Disability Adjusted Life Year; DART: developmental and reproductive toxicology; DHFR: dihydrofolate reductase; DHODH: dihydroorotate dehydrogenase; DHPS: dihydropteroate synthase; EF2: Elongation Factor 2; EFD: embryo and fetal development; EMA: European Medicines Agency; FDA: Food and Drug Administration; FRG mice: mice that lack functional Fah, Rag-2 and Interleukin 2 receptor common gamma chain genes; G6PD: glucose-6-phosphate dehydrogenase; GDP: Gross Domestic Product; GSK: GlaxoSmithKline; HIV: human immunodeficiency virus; MHRA: Medicines and Healthcare products Regulatory Agency; MMV: Medicines for Malaria Venture; NCE: new chemical entity; NOAEL: no-observed-adverse-effect-level; *P.: Plasmodium*; PE: protective efficacy; PI-4 kinase: phosphoinositol-4 kinase; PrEP: pre-exposure prophylaxis; (S)AE: (severe) adverse event; SCID: severe combined immunodeficiency; SMC: seasonal malaria chemoprevention; SP–AQ: sulfadoxine–pyrimethamine plus amodiaquine; TCP: target candidate profile; TPP: target product profile; WHO: World Health Organization.

Authors' contributions

JB and TW wrote the initial manuscript draft; JNB, WK, JJM SD and TNCW composed the TCP Tables, HR and RH edited the formulation section, AT, WK SD and FM edited the clinical development and regulatory section. All authors contributed with further edits, comments and discussion. All authors read and approved the final manuscript.

Author details

[1] Medicines for Malaria Venture, Route de Pré Bois 20, 1215 Geneva, Switzerland. [2] Drug Product Development, Janssen R&D, Johnson & Johnson, Turnhoutseweg 30, 2340 Beerse, Belgium. [3] Department of Science and Environment, Roskilde University, 4000 Roskilde, Denmark. [4] Faculty of Infectious and Tropical Diseases, London School of Hygiene and Tropical Medicine, London, UK.

Acknowledgements

We would like to thank all our advisors, past and present, and members of our External Scientific Advisory Committee in particular: John Pottage, Elizabeth Vadas, Dennis Kyle and Dennis Shanks. Thanks to Alain Bernard (AB Consulting), Paul Kellam and Richard Williams (Kymab) for their feedback on the antibody production issues, and to Fred Tonelli and Wim Parys and the team at Janssen; Niya Bowers, Drazen Ostovic at the Bill & Melinda Gates Foundation for constructive discussions. Last, but not least, we wish to acknowledge the insights and input from the MMV R&D team, and the constant support of David Reddy.

Competing interests

The authors declare that they have no competing interests, beyond the fact that MMV is involved in supporting the development of some of these medicines. BG reports a grant to his host institution from Johnson & Johnson to support discussions on the feasibility of the development of long-acting anti-malarial compounds.

Funding

This Report was funded by the Medicines for Malaria Venture. MMV donors are listed on the MMV website (http://www.mmv.org/about-us/our-donors).

References

1. Hooft van Huijsduijnen R, Wells TNC. The antimalarial pipeline. Curr Opin Pharmacol. 2018;42:1471–4892.
2. Phillips MA, Burrows JN, Manyando C, Hooft van Huijsduijnen R, Van Voorhis WC, Wells TNC. Malaria. Nat Rev Dis Primers. 2017;3:17050.
3. Plouffe D, Brinker A, McNamara C, Henson K, Kato N, Kuhen K, et al. In silico activity profiling reveals the mechanism of action of antimalarials discovered in a high-throughput screen. Proc Natl Acad Sci USA. 2008;105:9059–64.
4. Guiguemde WA, Shelat AA, Bouck D, Duffy S, Crowther GJ, Davis PH, et al. Chemical genetics of Plasmodium falciparum. Nature. 2010;465:311–5.
5. Gamo FJ, Sanz LM, Vidal J, de Cozar C, Alvarez E, Lavandera JL, et al. Thousands of chemical starting points for antimalarial lead identification. Nature. 2010;465:305–10.
6. Meister S, Plouffe DM, Kuhen KL, Bonamy GM, Wu T, Barnes SW, et al. Imaging of Plasmodium liver stages to drive next-generation antimalarial drug discovery. Science. 2011;334:1372–7.
7. Spangenberg T, Burrows JN, Kowalczyk P, McDonald S, Wells TN, Willis P. The open access malaria box: a drug discovery catalyst for neglected diseases. PLoS ONE. 2013;8:e62906.
8. Avery VM, Bashyam S, Burrows JN, Duffy S, Papadatos G, Puthukkuti S, et al. Screening and hit evaluation of a chemical library against blood-stage Plasmodium falciparum. Malar J. 2014;13:190.
9. Yeung S. Malaria—update on antimalarial resistance and treatment approaches. Pediatr Infect Dis J. 2018;37:367–9.
10. Haldar K, Bhattacharjee S, Safeukui I. Drug resistance in Plasmodium. Nat Rev Microbiol. 2018;16:156–70.
11. Martin RE, Shafik SH, Richards SN. Mechanisms of resistance to the partner drugs of artemisinin in the malaria parasite. Curr Opin Pharmacol. 2018;42:71–80.
12. The malERA Refresh Consultative Panel on Basic Science and Enabling Technologies. malERA: An updated research agenda for diagnostics, drugs, vaccines, and vector control in malaria elimination and eradication. PLoS Med. 2017;14:e1002455.
13. Doolan DL, Dobano C, Baird JK. Acquired immunity to malaria. Clin Microbiol Rev. 2009;22:13–36.
14. RTS'S Clinical Trials Partnership. Efficacy and safety of the RTS, S/AS01 malaria vaccine during 18 months after vaccination: a phase 3 randomized, controlled trial in children and young infants at 11 African sites. PLoS Med. 2014;11:e1001685.
15. Jiang JB, Li GQ, Guo XB, Kong YC, Arnold K. Antimalarial activity of mefloquine and qinghaosu. Lancet. 1982;2:285–8.
16. Thybo S, Gjorup I, Ronn AM, Meyrowitsch D, Bygberg IC. Atovaquone-proguanil (malarone): an effective treatment for uncomplicated Plasmodium falciparum malaria in travelers from Denmark. J Travel Med. 2004;11:220–3.

17. Tickell-Painter M, Maayan N, Saunders R, Pace C, Sinclair D. Mefloquine for preventing malaria during travel to endemic areas. Cochrane Database Syst Rev. 2017;10:CD006491.
18. Nakato H, Vivancos R, Hunter PR. A systematic review and meta-analysis of the effectiveness and safety of atovaquone proguanil (Malarone) for chemoprophylaxis against malaria. J Antimicrob Chemother. 2007;60:929–36.
19. Dups JN, Pepper M, Cockburn IA. Antibody and B cell responses to Plasmodium sporozoites. Front Microbiol. 2014;5:625.
20. Triller G, Scally SW, Costa G, Pissarev M, Kreschel C, Bosch A, et al. Natural parasite exposure induces protective human anti-malarial antibodies. Immunity. 2017;47:1197–209:e10.
21. Sina BJ, Wright C, Ballou R, Hollingdale M. A protective monoclonal antibody with dual specificity for Plasmodium falciparum and Plasmodium berghei circumsporozoite proteins. Exp Parasitol. 1992;74:431–40.
22. Espinosa DA, Gutierrez GM, Rojas-Lopez M, Noe AR, Shi L, Tse SW, et al. Proteolytic cleavage of the Plasmodium falciparum circumsporozoite protein is a target of protective antibodies. J Infect Dis. 2015;212:1111–9.
23. Foquet L, Hermsen CC, van Gemert GJ, Van Braeckel E, Weening KE, Sauerwein R, et al. Vaccine-induced monoclonal antibodies targeting circumsporozoite protein prevent Plasmodium falciparum infection. J Clin Invest. 2014;124:140–4.
24. Duffy S, Avery VM. Plasmodium falciparum in vitro culture—the highs and lows. Trends Parasitol. 2018;34:812–3.
25. Wells TNC, van Huijsduijnen RH, Van Voorhis WC. Malaria medicines: a glass half full? Nat Rev Drug Discov. 2015;14:424–42.
26. Sulyok M, Ruckle T, Roth A, Murbeth RE, Chalon S, Kerr N, et al. DSM265 for Plasmodium falciparum chemoprophylaxis: a randomised, double blinded, phase 1 trial with controlled human malaria infection. Lancet Infect Dis. 2017;17:636–44.
27. Murphy SC, Duke ER, Shipman KJ, Jensen RL, Fong Y, Ferguson S, et al. A randomized trial of the prophylactic activity of DSM265 against pre-erythrocytic Plasmodium falciparum infection during controlled human malaria infection by mosquito bites and direct venous inoculation. J Infect Dis. 2017;217:693–702.
28. Paquet T, Le Manach C, Cabrera DG, Younis Y, Henrich PP, Abraham TS, et al. Antimalarial efficacy of MMV390048, an inhibitor of Plasmodium phosphatidylinositol 4-kinase. Sci Transl Med. 2017;9:eaad9735.
29. Baragaña B, Hallyburton I, Lee MC, Norcross NR, Grimaldi R, Otto TD, et al. A novel multiple-stage antimalarial agent that inhibits protein synthesis. Nature. 2015;522:315–20.
30. White NJ, Duong TT, Uthaisin C, Nosten F, Phyo AP, Hanboonkunupakarn B, et al. Antimalarial activity of KAF156 in falciparum and vivax malaria. N Engl J Med. 2016;375:1152–60.
31. Kuhen KL, Chatterjee AK, Rottmann M, Gagaring K, Borboa R, Buenviaje J, et al. KAF156 is an antimalarial clinical candidate with potential for use in prophylaxis, treatment and prevention of disease transmission. Antimicrob Agents Chemother. 2014;58:5060–7.
32. da Cruz FP, Martin C, Buchholz K, Lafuente-Monasterio MJ, Rodrigues T, Sonnichsen B, et al. Drug screen targeted at Plasmodium liver stages identifies a potent multistage antimalarial drug. J Infect Dis. 2012;205:1278–86.
33. Thompson PE, Olszewski B, Waitz JA. Laboratory studies on the repository antimalarial activity of 4,4'-diacetylaminodiphenylsulfone, alone and mixed with cycloguanil pamoate (Ci-501). Am J Trop Med Hyg. 1965;14:343–53.
34. Schmidt LH, Rossan RN. Activities of respository preparations of cycloguanil pamoate and 4,4'-diacetyldiaminodiphenylsulfone, alone and in combination, against infections with Plasmodium cynomolgi in rhesus monkeys. Antimicrob Agents Chemother. 1984;26:611–42.
35. Clyde DF. Field trials of repository antimalarial compounds. J Trop Med Hyg. 1969;72:81–5.
36. Chang C, Lin-Hua T, Jantanavivat C. Studies on a new antimalarial compound: pyronaridine. Trans R Soc Trop Med Hyg. 1992;86:7–10.
37. Spinner CD, Boesecke C, Zink A, Jessen H, Stellbrink HJ, Rockstroh JK, et al. HIV pre-exposure prophylaxis (PrEP): a review of current knowledge of oral systemic HIV PrEP in humans. Infection. 2016;44:151–8.
38. Spreen WR, Margolis DA, Pottage JC Jr. Long-acting injectable antiretrovirals for HIV treatment and prevention. Curr Opin HIV AIDS. 2013;8:565–71.

39. Jann MW, Penzak SR. Long-acting injectable second-generation antipsychotics: an update and comparison between agents. CNS Drugs. 2018;32:241–57.

40. Mathews ES, Odom John AR. Tackling resistance: emerging antimalarials and new parasite targets in the era of elimination. F1000Research. 2018;7:1170.

41. Tan KR, Magill AJ, Parise ME, Arguin PM, Centers for Disease Control and Prevention. Doxycycline for malaria chemoprophylaxis and treatment: report from the CDC expert meeting on malaria chemoprophylaxis. Am J Trop Med Hyg. 2011;84:517–31.

42. Burrows JN, Duparc S, Gutteridge WE, van Huijsduijnen RH, Kaszubska W, Macintyre F, et al. New developments in anti-malarial target candidate and product profiles. Malar J. 2017;16:26.

43. Diawara F, Steinhardt LC, Mahamar A, Traore T, Kone DT, Diawara H, et al. Measuring the impact of seasonal malaria chemoprevention as part of routine malaria control in Kita, Mali. Malar J. 2017;16:325.

44. WHO. World malaria report 2017. Geneva: World Health Organization; 2017. http://apps.who.int/iris/bitstream/10665/259492/1/9789241565 523-eng.pdf?ua=1. Accessed 26 Oct 2018

45. Rabinovich RN, Drakeley C, Djimde AA, Hall BF, Hay SI, Hemingway J, et al. malERA: an updated research agenda for malaria elimination and eradication. PLoS Med. 2017;14:e1002456.

46. Parpia AS, Ndeffo-Mbah ML, Wenzel NS, Galvani AP. Effects of response to 2014–2015 Ebola outbreak on deaths from malaria, HIV/AIDS, and tuberculosis, West Africa. Emerg Infect Dis. 2016;22:433–41.

47. Plucinski MM, Guilavogui T, Sidikiba S, Diakite N, Diakite S, Dioubate M, et al. Effect of the Ebola-virus-disease epidemic on malaria case management in Guinea, 2014: a cross-sectional survey of health facilities. Lancet Infect Dis. 2015;15:1017–23.

48. Walker PG, White MT, Griffin JT, Reynolds A, Ferguson NM, Ghani AC. Malaria morbidity and mortality in Ebola-affected countries caused by decreased health-care capacity, and the potential effect of mitigation strategies: a modelling analysis. Lancet Infect Dis. 2015;15:825–32.

49. Pagnoni F, Bosman A. Malaria kills more than Ebola virus disease. Lancet Infect Dis. 2015;15:988–9.

50. Margolis DA, Boffito M. Long-acting antiviral agents for HIV treatment. Curr Opin HIV AIDS. 2015;10:246–52.

51. Rinaldi A. Yaws eradication: facing old problems, raising new hopes. PLoS Negl Trop Dis. 2012;6:e1837.

52. Greenwood B. Progress with the PfSPZ vaccine for malaria. Lancet Infect Dis. 2017;17:463–4.

53. McKeage K, Scott L. Atovaquone/proguanil: a review of its use for the prophylaxis of Plasmodium falciparum malaria. Drugs. 2003;63:597–623.

54. Camus D, Djossou F, Schilthuis HJ, Hogh B, Dutoit E, Malvy D, et al. Atovaquone–proguanil versus chloroquine–proguanil for malaria prophylaxis in nonimmune pediatric travelers: results of an international, randomized, open-label study. Clin Infect Dis. 2004;38:1716–23.

55. Overbosch D, Schilthuis H, Bienzle U, Behrens RH, Kain KC, Clarke PD, et al. Atovaquone–proguanil versus mefloquine for malaria prophylaxis in nonimmune travelers: results from a randomized, double-blind study. Clin Infect Dis. 2001;33:1015–21.

56. Katsuno K, Burrows JN, Duncan K, van Huijsduijnen RH, Kaneko T, Kita K, et al. Hit and lead criteria in drug discovery for infectious diseases of the developing world. Nat Rev Drug Discov. 2015;14:751–8.

57. Ng S, March S, Galstian A, Gural N, Stevens KR, Mota MM, et al. Towards a humanized mouse model of liver stage malaria using ectopic artificial livers. Sci Rep. 2017;7:45424.

58. Flannery EL, Foquet L, Chuenchob V, Fishbaugher M, Billman Z, Navarro MJ, et al. Assessing drug efficacy against Plasmodium falciparum liver stages in vivo. JCI Insight. 2018;3:e92587.

59. Goodman CD, Siregar JE, Mollard V, Vega-Rodriguez J, Syafruddin D, Matsuoka H, et al. Parasites resistant to the antimalarial atovaquone fail to transmit by mosquitoes. Science. 2016;352:349–53.

60. Strickley RG. Solubilizing excipients in oral and injectable formulations. Pharm Res. 2004;21:201–30.

61. Ditzinger F, Price DJ, Ilie AR, Kohl NJ, Jankovic S, Tsakiridou G, et al. Lipophilicity and hydrophobicity considerations in bio-enabling oral formulations approaches—a PEARRL review. J Pharm Pharmacol. 2018;. https://doi.org/10.1111/jphp.12984.

62. Pfizer. Product monograph penicillin G benzathine. 2017. https://www. pfizer.ca/sites/g/files/g10037206/f/201710/Bicillin_PM.pdf. Accessed 26 Oct 2018

63. Winner B, Peipert JF, Zhao Q, Buckel C, Madden T, Allsworth JE, et al. Effectiveness of long-acting reversible contraception. N Engl J Med. 2012;366:1998–2007.

64. Sarno MA, Mancari R, Azim HA Jr, Colombo N, Peccatori FA. Are monoclonal antibodies a safe treatment for cancer during pregnancy? Immunotherapy. 2013;5:733–41.

65. Pentsuk N, van der Laan JW. An interspecies comparison of placental antibody transfer: new insights into developmental toxicity testing of monoclonal antibodies. Birth Defects Res B Dev Reprod Toxicol. 2009;86:328–44.

66. White NJ. Does antimalarial mass drug administration increase or decrease the risk of resistance? Lancet Infect Dis. 2016;17:e15–20.

67. Bousema T, Okell L, Felger I, Drakeley C. Asymptomatic malaria infections: detectability, transmissibility and public health relevance. Nat Rev Microbiol. 2014;12:833–40.

68. Cohen S, Mc GI, Carrington S. Gamma-globulin and acquired immunity to human malaria. Nature. 1961;192:733–7.

69. Kelley B. Industrialization of mAb production technology: the bioprocessing industry at a crossroads. mAbs. 2009;1:443–52.

70. Klutz S, Holtmann L, Lobedann M, Schembecker G. Cost evaluation of antibody production processes in different operation modes. Chem Eng Sci. 2016;141:63–74.

71. Garidel P, Kuhn AB, Schafer LV, Karow-Zwick AR, Blech M. High-concentration protein formulations: how high is high? Eur J Pharm Biopharm. 2017;119:353–60.

72. Glassman PM, Balthasar JP. Mechanistic considerations for the use of monoclonal antibodies for cancer therapy. Cancer Biol Med. 2014;11:20–33.

73. Kontermann RE. Strategies to extend plasma half-lives of recombinant antibodies. BioDrugs. 2009;23:93–109.

74. Kontermann RE. Strategies for extended serum half-life of protein therapeutics. Curr Opin Biotechnol. 2011;22:868–76.

75. Liu JK. The history of monoclonal antibody development—progress, remaining challenges and future innovations. Ann Med Surg (Lond). 2014;3:113–6.

76. Zhao J, Cao Y, Jusko WJ. Across-species scaling of monoclonal antibody pharmacokinetics using a minimal PBPK model. Pharm Res. 2015;32:3269–81.

77. Chimalakonda AP, Yadav R, Marathe P. Factors influencing magnitude and duration of target inhibition following antibody therapy: implications in drug discovery and development. AAPS J. 2013;15:717–27.

78. Davda JP, Hansen RJ. Properties of a general PK/PD model of antibody-ligand interactions for therapeutic antibodies that bind to soluble endogenous targets. mAbs. 2010;2:576–88.

79. Franzén L, Wahlin B, Wahlgren M, Aslund L, Perlmann P, Wigzell H, et al. Enhancement or inhibition of Plasmodium falciparum erythrocyte reinvasion in vitro by antibodies to an asparagine rich protein. Mol Biochem Parasitol. 1989;32:201–11.

80. Azim HA Jr, Azim H, Peccatori FA. Treatment of cancer during pregnancy with monoclonal antibodies: a real challenge. Expert Rev Clin Immunol. 2010;6:821–6.

81. Lycke J. Monoclonal antibody therapies for the treatment of relapsing-remitting multiple sclerosis: differentiating mechanisms and clinical outcomes. Ther Adv Neurol Disord. 2015;8:274–93.

82. Stone RH, Hong J, Jeong H. Pharmacokinetics of monoclonal antibodies used for inflammatory bowel diseases in pregnant women. J Clin Toxicol. 2014;4:e209.

83. Hay M, Thomas DW, Craighead JL, Economides C, Rosenthal J. Clinical development success rates for investigational drugs. Nat Biotechnol. 2014;32:40–51.

84. Kaushansky A, Mikolajczak SA, Vignali M, Kappe SH. Of men in mice: the success and promise of humanized mouse models for human malaria parasite infections. Cell Microbiol. 2014;16:602–11.

85. Lachish T, Bar-Meir M, Eisenberg N, Schwartz E. Effectiveness of twice a week prophylaxis with atovaquone–proguanil (Malarone(R)) in long-term travellers to West Africa. J Travel Med. 2016;23:taw064.

6

Anaemia and malaria

Nicholas J. White[1,2]* (ID)

Abstract

Malaria is a major cause of anaemia in tropical areas. Malaria infection causes haemolysis of infected and uninfected erythrocytes and bone marrow dyserythropoiesis which compromises rapid recovery from anaemia. In areas of high malaria transmission malaria nearly all infants and young children, and many older children and adults have a reduced haemoglobin concentration as a result. In these areas severe life-threatening malarial anaemia requiring blood transfusion in young children is a major cause of hospital admission, particularly during the rainy season months when malaria transmission is highest. In severe malaria, the mortality rises steeply below an admission haemoglobin of 3 g/dL, but it also increases with higher haemoglobin concentrations approaching the normal range. In the management of severe malaria transfusion thresholds remain uncertain. Prevention of malaria by vector control, deployment of insecticide-treated bed nets, prompt and accurate diagnosis of illness and appropriate use of effective anti-malarial drugs substantially reduces the burden of anaemia in tropical countries.

Background

Malaria is the most important parasitic disease of man [1]. It is a major cause of anaemia in endemic areas, and in areas of higher transmission malaria is one of the most common reasons for blood transfusion. Six species of the genus *Plasmodium* infect humans commonly, and all cause anaemia. Most malaria attributable deaths and severe disease are caused by *Plasmodium falciparum*. The majority of fatalities occur in the community. The World Health Organization (WHO) has estimated that there were some 216 million cases and 445,000 deaths from malaria in 2016 [2]. A significant proportion of these deaths resulted directly or indirectly from anaemia.

Epidemiology of malaria and anaemia

The clinical consequences of malaria, and in particular the prevalence of anaemia, depend on the intensity of malaria transmission (Fig. 1). The main determinants of malaria transmission intensity are the density, longevity, biting habits, and efficiency of the local mosquito vectors [1]. In high transmission settings people may receive as much as one infectious bite each day, so the entire population is infected repeatedly, but it is young

children who bear the brunt of the disease, and most are anaemic [3–12]. As the child grows a disease controlling immunity develops such that by adolescence and adulthood nearly all malaria infections are asymptomatic. The prevalence of anaemia declines (Fig. 2). Thus, apparently healthy individuals carry malaria parasites in their blood. These infections can persist for many months. This persistent asymptomatic parasite carriage reduces the operational diagnostic specificity of a positive microscopy or rapid test result as febrile illness in a parasitaemic individual may be caused by other infections. Meta-analyses of the relationship between malaria and anaemia are confounded by the non-specificity of parasitological diagnosis in high transmission settings, widespread self-treatment of febrile illness, inability to characterize preceding infections and thus recurrences in point prevalence surveys, and frequent concomitant haemoglobinopathies, nutritional deficiencies (particularly iron deficiency), and intestinal helminth infections—all of which contribute variably to anaemia [10, 11]. Thus, in higher transmission settings malaria increases the risk of anaemia in the entire population with the greatest impact in young children, and in particular infants [3]. In lower transmission settings symptomatic malaria and resulting anaemia may occur at all ages, although it is children and pregnant women who are more likely to be anaemic. At all levels of transmission malaria (all

*Correspondence: nickw@tropmedres.ac
[1] Faculty of Tropical Medicine, Mahidol University, Bangkok, Thailand
Full list of author information is available at the end of the article

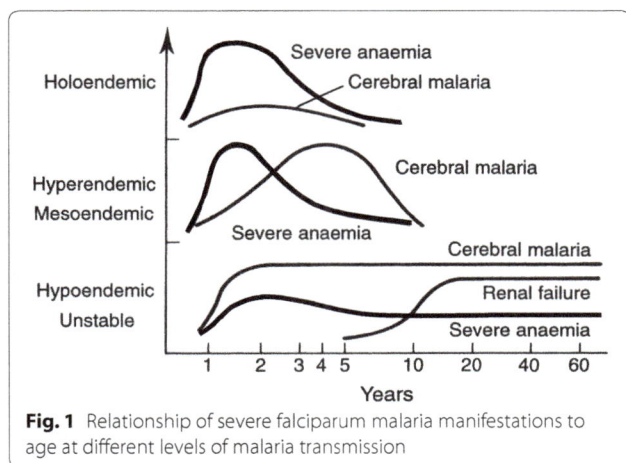

Fig. 1 Relationship of severe falciparum malaria manifestations to age at different levels of malaria transmission

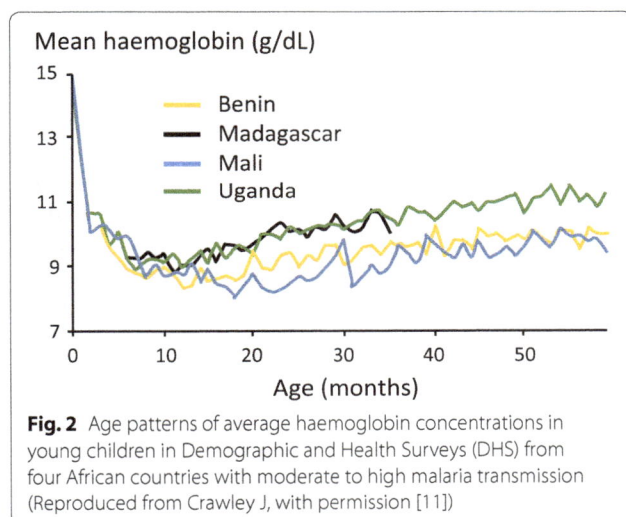

Fig. 2 Age patterns of average haemoglobin concentrations in young children in Demographic and Health Surveys (DHS) from four African countries with moderate to high malaria transmission (Reproduced from Crawley J, with permission [11])

malaria transmission is low, erratic, or focal (often termed *unstable transmission*), protective immunity from malaria is not acquired, and symptomatic malaria may occur at all ages. In such areas changes in environmental, economic, or social conditions, such as heavy rains following drought or large population movements together with a breakdown in malaria control and prevention services (often resulting from conflict) can result in epidemics of malaria with considerable mortality among all age groups [1]. Recent improvements in malaria control have reduced malaria transmission in many areas and increased heterogeneity in malaria epidemiology. Unfortunately, there is evidence that this recent progress has stalled, and malaria incidence in some parts of the tropics has started to rise again.

In areas of moderate or high transmission malaria infections (both *P. falciparum* and *Plasmodium vivax*) in pregnancy cause maternal anaemia, intrauterine growth retardation and prematurity [1]. The newborn starts at a developmental disadvantage with a lowered haemoglobin [15]. The physiological decline in haemoglobin in early infancy is exaggerated and plateaus around 9 g/dL on average around 9 months. Thereafter, there is a slow but steady rise in haemoglobin concentrations punctuated by acute reductions associated with symptomatic malaria infections [11] (Figs. 2 and 3).

Concomitant contributors to anaemia

Poor malaria control is often associated with weak health structures, and high prevalences of other infectious diseases and nutritional deficiencies, all of which contribute to anaemia. In Malawi, where transmission of malaria is moderate to high and childhood malaria is very common, bacterial infections, HIV infection, hookworm and deficiencies in vitamins A and B12 were all independently associated with severe anaemia [10]. Malaria has also selected for haemoglobinopathies and other inherited red cell abnormalities [notably glucose 6 phosphate dehydrogenase (G6PD) deficiency] which provide some protection against the pathological consequences of malaria but themselves contribute to anaemia [12, 16]. Sickle cell anaemia is common in most of sub-Saharan Africa (birth prevalence 1–2%) and is a major cause of severe anaemia, commonly provoked by malaria illness [17]. Patients with G6PD deficiency are also at increased risk of severe malarial anaemia [18]. Dissecting and quantitating the individual contributions of these various genetic factors to malaria anaemia overall is difficult.

Relationship of anaemia to transmission intensity

In most of Asia and the Americas malaria transmission is low and seasonal. In Asia, the prevalences of *P. falciparum* and *P. vivax* malaria overall are approximately equal

species) is an important contributor to maternal anaemia during pregnancy, and poor birth outcomes [13]. Falciparum malaria is a direct cause of maternal mortality in lower transmission settings and an indirect cause by contributing to anemia in higher transmissions settings [14]. Anti-malarial drug resistance causing recrudescent infections increases the prevalence and the severity of malaria anaemia.

Clinical patterns

Constant, frequent, year-round malaria reflects *stable transmission*. In the sub-Sahel region across Africa from Senegal to Sudan there is intense malaria transmission, but this is largely confined to the 3–4 month rainy season. During this period young children are commonly anaemic and frequently present to hospitals and health centres with severe anaemia. In contrast in areas where

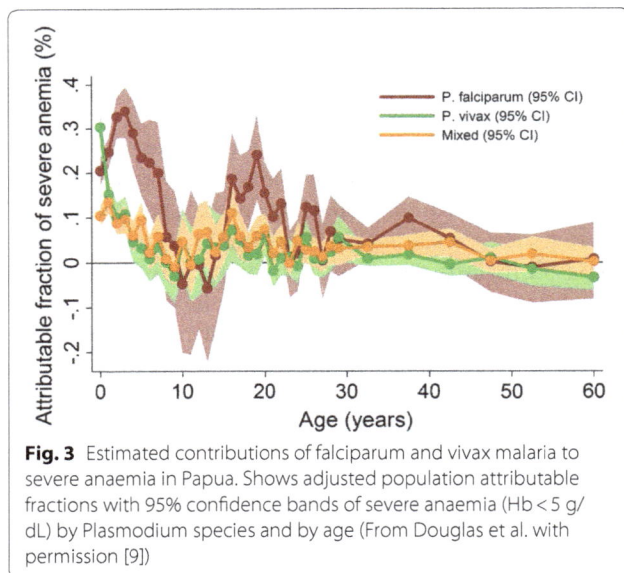

Fig. 3 Estimated contributions of falciparum and vivax malaria to severe anaemia in Papua. Shows adjusted population attributable fractions with 95% confidence bands of severe anaemia (Hb < 5 g/dL) by Plasmodium species and by age (From Douglas et al. with permission [9])

[2]. In the Americas *P. vivax* predominates. In these areas people commonly receive ≤ 1 infectious bite per year (the entomological inoculation rate; EIR). Malaria is usually associated with mild anaemia, although where resources are limited, then even at these low transmission intensities *P. vivax* may still cause severe anaemia in children because each sporozoite inoculation can result in multiple relapses. Transmission intensities are much higher in many parts of sub-Saharan Africa, where *P. falciparum* predominates, and in lowland New Guinea where both *P. falciparum* and *P. vivax* are prevalent (Fig. 3); EIRs may reach as high as 1000/year in some areas of Africa. In such high transmission settings where everyone is infected, morbidity and mortality from malaria are considerable. Newborns have low birthweight and infant mortality is high [1–6]. Babies and young children suffer repeated symptomatic infections with high rates of asymptomatic parasitaemia between these episodes. They are often chronically anaemic with palpably enlarged spleens. There is an increased mortality both from malaria itself, and also indirectly from other infections which repeated malaria predisposes to. If the child survives then by adulthood most malaria infections are asymptomatic.

Contribution of malaria to anaemia

The best estimates of the causal contribution of malaria to anaemia in a particular setting come from randomized trials of malaria control interventions [19, 20]. A review of 29 community-based studies of insecticide-treated nets (ITNs), anti-malarial chemoprophylaxis, and insecticide residual spraying found that among children

< 5 years exposed to between 1 and 2 years of malaria control, mean relative risk for a haemoglobin concentration < 11 g/dL was 0.73 (95% CI 0.64–0.81), and for a haemoglobin < 8 g/dL was 0.40 (95% CI 0.25–0.55) compared with the control groups not exposed to these malaria interventions [20, 21]. The WHO and the Roll Back Malaria (RBM) Partnership have recommended that anaemia be used as an additional indicator to monitor malaria burden at the community level as malaria control interventions are scaled up nationally. This recommendation is based on results of an extensive review conducted by Korenromp et al. [20] showing that, in areas of stable malaria transmission, the prevalence of moderate-to-severe anaemia (haemoglobin < 8 g/dL) is a more sensitive measure of a reduction in malaria exposure than parasite prevalence, and that it may respond more quickly than mortality as coverage of malaria interventions, such as insecticide-treated bed nets (ITNs), malaria chemoprevention and indoor residual spraying are scaled up [20–22]. In randomized controlled trials, the impact of ITNs on anaemia was more pronounced than on the prevalence of malaria parasitaemia or on the incidence of clinical malaria.

Improved control between 2000 and 2015 has resulted in a reduction in malaria in high transmission areas, a substantial reduction in global malaria attributable mortality, and elimination of malaria from several countries [2, 23, 24].

Pathogenesis

The pathogenesis of malarial anaemia is multifactorial [1, 25–34]. Malaria is an intraerythrocytic parasite so there is obligatory destruction of red cells containing parasites at schizont rupture. However, a more important contributor is the accelerated destruction of non-parasitized red cells that parallels disease severity [30]. It has been estimated that loss of unparasitized erythrocytes accounts for approximately 90% of the acute anaemia resulting from a single infection. Parasitaemias in falciparum malaria commonly exceed 1% (of red cells parasitized), and in severe disease may exceed 10%. *Plasmodium knowlesi* may also cause hyperparasitaemia, but parasite densities in the other human malarias very rarely exceed 2% [1]. In severe falciparum malaria there is a heavy parasite burden and anaemia develops rapidly. The main contributor to this usually rapid decline in haematocrit is the haemolysis of unparasitized red cells [30, 35–37]. The ratio of unparasitized red cells to parasitized red cells lost in acute malaria is even higher in *P. vivax* than in *P. falciparum* infections [36].

The haemolytic anaemia of malaria is compounded by bone marrow dyserythropoiesis during and immediately after the acute illness [28, 29, 38, 39]. Bone marrow dyserythropoiesis persists for days or weeks following the start of malaria treatment in acute malaria. As a consequence reticulocyte counts are usually low in the acute symptomatic phase of the disease (Fig. 4). This accounts for the delayed erythropoietic response in acute malaria in low transmission settings. In such settings, the nadir of haemoglobin concentration in acute falciparum malaria is usually around 1 week after presentation with fever [33]. In acute vivax malaria the nadir in haemoglobin is earlier (usually after a few days) [34]. In contrast in higher transmission settings, in the context of some premunition from repeated previous infections, haemoglobin concentrations usually begin to rise immediately following the start of effective anti-malarial treatment. In acute uncomplicated malaria, the resultant anaemia is worse in younger children, and those with protracted infections.

Bone marrow dysfunction in malaria

Dyserythropoiesis in malaria is thought to be related to intramedullary production of mediators which suppress erythropoiesis (proinflammatory cytokines, nitric oxide, lipoperoxides, bioactive aldehydes) and, in some studies, these have been incriminated in causing red cell precursor apoptosis [38–44]. It has long been observed that dyserythropoiesis and anaemia are associated with

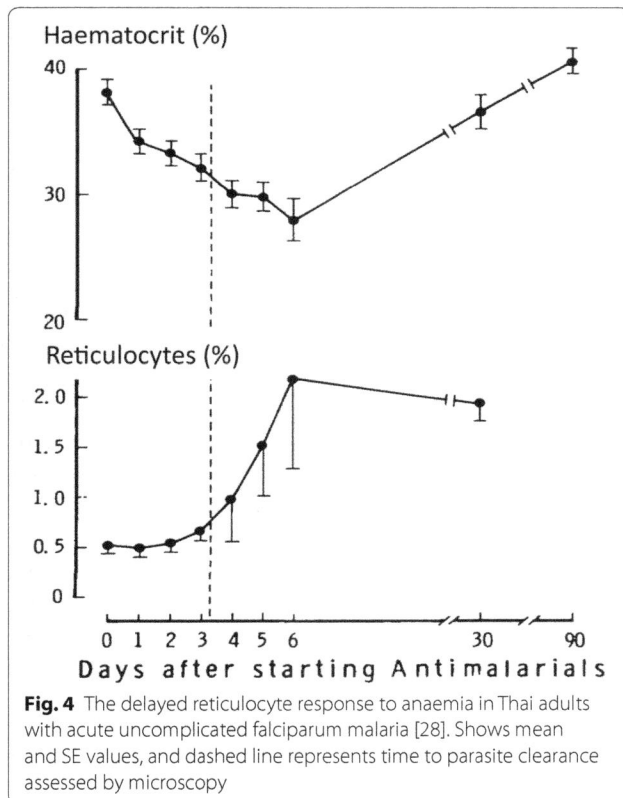

Fig. 4 The delayed reticulocyte response to anaemia in Thai adults with acute uncomplicated falciparum malaria [28]. Shows mean and SE values, and dashed line represents time to parasite clearance assessed by microscopy

intramedullary deposition of malaria pigment (haemozoin). This is the obligatory by-product of intraerythrocytic malaria parasite haemoglobin digestion (and thus haem detoxification). The haemozoin is expelled in the residual body at schizont rupture, and is commonly seen in peripheral blood or bone marrow smears having been phagocytosed by neutrophils and monocytes/macrophages. Indeed high proportions of peripheral blood monocytes containing malaria pigment reflect higher parasite burdens and are associated with anaemia in African children [38, 39]. Native haemozoin comprises a scaffold of crystalline cyclic haem dimers (α-hematin), but it also contains large amounts of associated polyunsaturated fatty acids (PUFA). These PUFA are non-enzymatically peroxidized and broken down by the haemozoin associated iron to bioactive terminal hydroxyaldehydes such as 4-hydroxy 2-nonenal (HNE) [42, 43]. Haemozoin has been shown both to induce and to suppress pro-inflammatory cytokine production in different experimental circumstances. The role of the macrophage in the pathological process has been controversial—while several studies have suggested that macrophages contribute to the inhibition of erythropoiesis either indirectly or directly by generating oxidative stress—others have suggested they exert an overall protective effect against a direct toxic effect of native haemozoin in inducing premature apoptosis of red cell progenitor cells [38, 40, 44]. In a different experimental system inhibition of erythropoiesis rather than apoptosis has been observed. The bioactive aldehyde HNE, generated by the haem iron mediated peroxidation of PUFA, was shown to be an important mediator of this effect [42, 43].

Severe malarial anaemia in African children has been associated with the 238A TNF promoter genetic polymorphism and low levels of the anti-inflammatory cytokine IL-10 [45, 46]. Malaria anaemia in African children is also associated with the haptoglobin 2-2 genotype, an association postulated to reflect the reduced ability of the Hp2-2 polymer to scavenge free haemoglobin-iron following malaria-induced haemolysis [47]. Serum erythropoetin levels are usually elevated in malarial anaemia, although in some series it has been suggested that the degree of elevation was insufficient for the reduction in haemoglobin [31, 32, 48].

Reduced red cell deformability

In severe malaria caused by *P. falciparum* or by *P. knowlesi* the entire red cell population becomes less deformable [49–52]. When red cell deformability was assessed at the shear stresses encountered in the splenic sinusoids (30 Pa) reduced deformability was correlated significantly with the reduction in haemoglobin [49] (Fig. 5). The mechanisms responsible for reduced

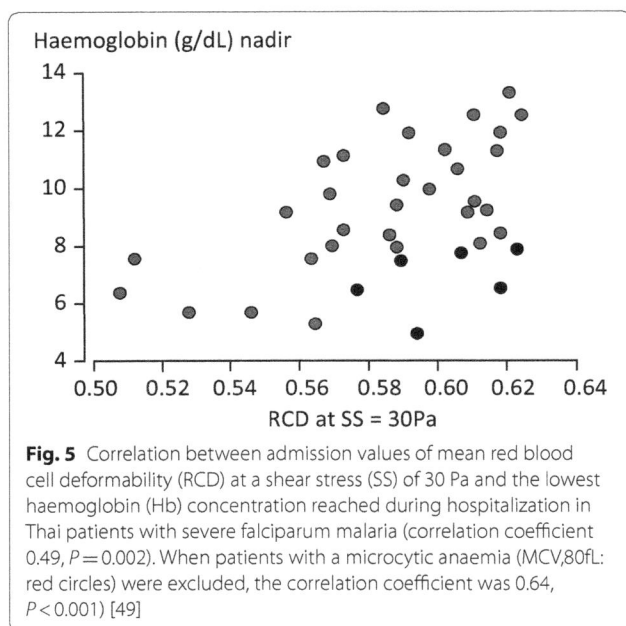

Fig. 5 Correlation between admission values of mean red blood cell deformability (RCD) at a shear stress (SS) of 30 Pa and the lowest haemoglobin (Hb) concentration reached during hospitalization in Thai patients with severe falciparum malaria (correlation coefficient 0.49, $P = 0.002$). When patients with a microcytic anaemia (MCV,80fL: red circles) were excluded, the correlation coefficient was 0.64, $P < 0.001$) [49]

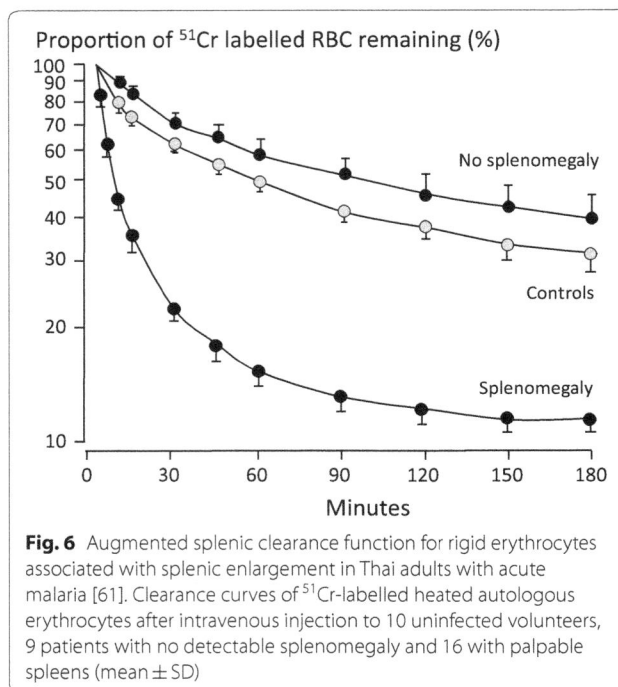

Fig. 6 Augmented splenic clearance function for rigid erythrocytes associated with splenic enlargement in Thai adults with acute malaria [61]. Clearance curves of ^{51}Cr-labelled heated autologous erythrocytes after intravenous injection to 10 uninfected volunteers, 9 patients with no detectable splenomegaly and 16 with palpable spleens (mean ± SD)

uninfected erythrocyte deformability have not been identified with certainty, although there is evidence in acute malaria for increased oxidative damage which might compromise red cell membrane function and reduce deformability [50, 53, 54]. In simian malarias, inversion of the erythrocyte membrane lipid bilayer in uninfected erythrocytes has been reported, but this has not been studied in man [55].

Antibody and complement binding

The role of red cell membrane bound antibody (i.e. Coombs'-positive haemolysis) in malarial anaemia is unresolved. Some studies have shown increased red cell immunoglobulin binding in malaria, whereas others have not [56–58]. In the presence of the malaria associated lowered clearance threshold for splenic red cell removal (Fig. 6), increased antibody or complement binding might be difficult to detect. Nevertheless, studies in Kenyan children with severe anaemia have shown increased surface IgG and immune complexes and also deficiencies in the complement regulatory proteins CR1 and CD55 [59, 60]. The circulating erythrocytes from these children were more susceptible to phagocytosis than were those of controls [59].

The role of the spleen

In acute malaria the spleen reorganizes and enlarges rapidly. This results in increased clearance capacity and a lowered splenic threshold for the clearance of abnormal erythrocytes, whether because of antibody coating or reduced deformability [52, 61–63]. Thus, the spleen

removes large numbers of relatively rigid red cells, which in a healthy uninfected subject would be allowed to remain in the circulation. This results in shortened erythrocyte survival. The reduction in red cell survival is proportional to the severity of the infection. Red cell clearance is unaffected by corticosteroids [64]. The spleen also fulfils its normative function of removing intraerythrocytic particles. In this case, the spleen removes damaged intraerythrocytic parasites (particularly following treatment with an artemisinin derivative) by a process called "pitting" [65]. It then returns the "once parasitized" red cells back to the circulation—but these pitted erythrocytes then have reduced survival [66, 67] (Fig. 7). In non-immune hyperparasitaemic patients the markedly shortened survival of these damaged, once parasitized, erythrocytes may cause a delayed sudden haemolysis, typically 1 to 2 weeks after starting treatment with an artemisinin derivative [67–69]. As it is the killing of these younger circulating parasites which explains much of therapeutic superiority of artesunate over quinine in severe malaria, this deferred haemolysis of once infected erythrocytes may be regarded as the "price" of the life-saving benefit. In higher transmission malaria endemic areas, where most malaria anaemia occurs, clinically significant post-artesunate delayed haemolysis is rare [70] (Fig. 7).

Repeated malaria infections result in splenomegaly and, in some cases, hypersplenism. At its most extreme is a condition called "hyperreactive malarial splenomegaly",

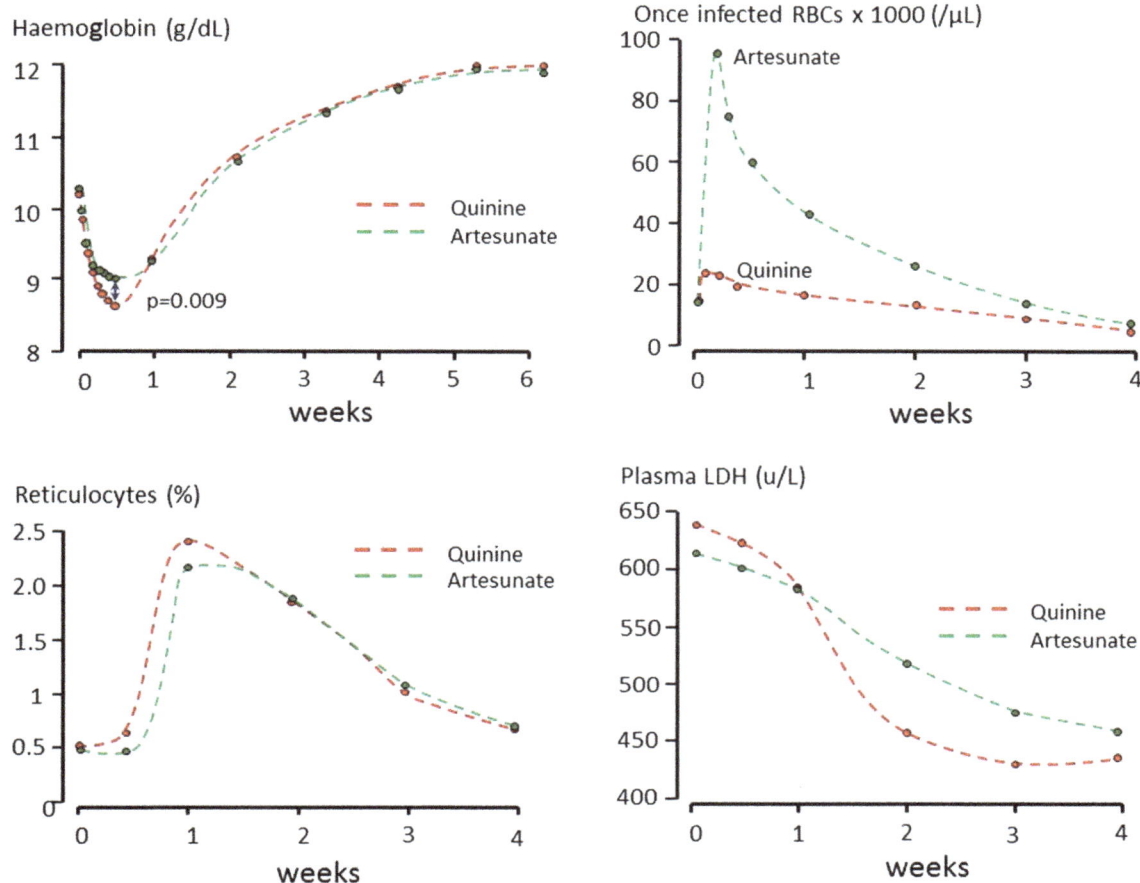

Fig. 7 Reduction in haemoglobin concentrations, corresponding increases in pitted erythrocytes, reticulocyte responses and plasma LDH in relation to anti-malarial drug treatment (artesunate or quinine) in African children in Kinshasa, DRC, admitted to hospital with hyperparasitaemic falciparum malaria [70]

known in the past as "tropical splenomegaly", in which there is massive splenomegaly, hypersplenism and dilutional anaemia. Some cases progress to B cell malignancy. Untreated the mortality is high, but when caused by malaria, the splenomegaly resolves over weeks or months with effective malaria chemoprophylaxis [71–73].

Iron deficiency

The interaction between iron and malaria is complex and controversial. Iron deficiency is very common in malaria endemic areas. It causes anaemia and in young children iron deficiency is associated with neurodevelopmental delay. Malaria does not cause iron deficiency, but iron deficiency does reduce the incidence of severe malaria [74]. Nevertheless, iron deficiency and malaria still often coincide in the same patient. Assessment of iron deficiency in acute malaria is confounded by the associated inflammatory response. In some areas, but not others, routine elemental iron supplementation following

malaria has been shown to promote recovery from anaemia [75, 76]. Secondary folate deficiency is less common. Neither iron nor folate supplementation reduce childhood mortality in areas of high malaria transmission. Much of the controversy has centred on whether iron (and folate) supplementation actually worsen malaria and increase malaria associated mortality. Some large prospective studies, notably a study conducted on Pemba island which was stopped prematurely [77], have shown increased falciparum malaria morbidity and mortality in elemental iron supplemented children [77–80]. So is it good or bad to provide elemental iron supplementation to children in malaria endemic areas? The risk–benefit assessment, and thus the answer to this question, varies and so is likely to be context specific [81]. Currently, the WHO recommends that daily iron supplementation should be given to infants and young children aged 6–23 months, living in settings where the prevalence of anaemia is 40% or higher in that age group [82], a recommendation that may still leave the younger infants vulnerable [83]. This is not widely implemented. Provision of lower quantities of iron within a food matrix, i.e., fortified food, has been proposed as a safer strategy than non-physiological elemental iron supplementation [84]. In acute malaria hepatocyte production of the key iron regulator hepcidin is increased. This reduces iron uptake, and lowers serum iron [85]. Concentrations of serum ferritin, an acute phase reactant, are also raised. The redistribution of iron in malaria is considered a risk factor for supervening bacterial infections which are associated with malaria in endemic areas [86], and particularly with severe malarial anaemia.

Diagnosis of malaria

In the clinical assessment of anaemia a diagnosis of acute malaria requires either demonstration of malaria parasites in a thick or thin blood film, or a positive rapid test (RDT). Microscopy or RDTs have a detection threshold of approximately 50 parasites/µL, which also corresponds approximately with the pyrogenic density in non-immune subjects [1]. The RDTs for falciparum malaria usually identify histidine-rich protein 2 (PfHRP2) as the target antigen. PfHRP2 persists in pitted erythrocytes [87] and so these RDTs commonly remain positive for days or weeks after parasite clearance, whereas the pLDH-based tests become negative as parasitaemia clears. The RDTs for P. falciparum are slightly more sensitive than those for P. vivax malaria. Using sufficient volume blood samples PCR methods can now detect parasite densities 1000 times lower than microscopy or RDTs, but because of the high background rates of asymptomatic parasitaemia, even in low transmission settings [88], they are too sensitive for the diagnosis of acute illness (i.e. their predictive value for identifying malaria as the cause of illness is poor). Serology maybe useful in assessing previous malaria exposure, but not in identifying the cause of an individual's illness [1, 89]. However, in many cases in which malaria causes anaemia the acute infection has resolved or been treated. The epidemiological context is critical to the assessment. In some cases, finding residual malaria pigment in peripheral blood monocytes provides a useful clue to recent infection.

Definitions of anaemia

As the epidemiology of malaria coincides with the epidemiology of inherited red cell abnormalities, nutritional deficiencies and helminth infections, anaemia is often multifactorial, and the distribution of haemoglobin concentrations in healthy people is lower and broader than in temperate countries. Although a wide, and frankly confusing, variety of definitions of anaemia in general have been proposed, the most commonly used definitions in malaria studies, based on haemoglobin concentrations, are as follows.

Mild anaemia ≤ 11 g/dL
Moderate anaemia ≤ 8 g/dL
Severe anaemia ≤ 5 g/dL

Measurement

Pallor is readily recognizable clinically, and village health workers can be trained to recognize it, but anaemia is best quantitated by measurement in a capillary or venous blood sample of either the haemoglobin concentration (most widely assessed using the HemoCue® system-a portable spectrophotometric analyser) or the haematocrit using a microcentrifuge. Well-functioning Coulter counters and other types of cell sorters are rarely found in rural areas of the tropics. The relationship between red cell count and haemoglobin or haematocrit is determined by red cell volume. In many areas microcytosis (either from iron deficiency or thalassaemia) is common. Malaria itself does not affect the relationship. The usual conversion factor of 3 for haemoglobin to haematocrit slightly overestimates the haematocrit [90, 91].

In 1810 patients with acute malaria who provided 3254 simultaneous measurements from various time points (ranging from day 0 to day 63), a good fit was obtained using Haematocrit $= 5.62 + 2.60$ * Haemoglobin [90].

In areas of high malaria transmission where malaria is a major contributor to anaemia in the first years of life the ratio of haemoglobin to haematocrit changes with age [91]. Clinical trials of therapeutic interventions in malaria usually report changes in haemoglobin or haematocrit, whereas large assessments of preventive interventions more commonly report the prevalence of anaemia from cross sectional surveys, or sometimes the incidence of anaemia in cohort studies.

The term moderate anaemia has been used variably in epidemiological studies. For example, in a recent assessment of seasonal chemoprevention in malaria prevention moderate anaemia was defined as < 11 g/dL (and in this study severe anaemia was defined as < 6 g/dL) [92]. In most studies the term anaemia (without specifying severity) refers to < 11 g/dL (although some have also used the < 8 g/dL threshold). The majority of studies have used 5 g/dL to define severe malarial anaemia.

Clinical features
Uncomplicated malaria
Malaria is an acute febrile illness. There are no specific clinical features in uncomplicated infections. Although, in general, higher parasitaemias are associated with more severe clinical disease, the relationship is very variable

[1]. In falciparum malaria there is sequestration of erythrocytes containing mature parasites in the microcirculation. This causes microvascular obstruction and accounts for much of the pathology of severe disease [93, 94]. Thus, the parasites causing pathology in severe infections are not represented directly by those counted in the peripheral blood smear. Patients can have the majority of their parasites circulating, or sequestered. In the latter case, the peripheral parasitaemia can be low (depending on stage of development and synchronicity). However, the peripheral blood film does provide an indication. In patients with a predominance of circulating parasites, most of the parasites seen in the blood smear are young ring stages, whereas those with a predominantly sequestered biomass usually have more mature trophozoites, many of which contain visible malaria pigment [95]. Significant sequestration does not occur in the other human malarias.

Anaemia develops rapidly in acute malaria so the majority of symptomatic patients have already lost at least 1 g of haemoglobin per decilitre (100 mL) of blood before presenting to medical attention. The liver and spleen enlarge rapidly. The anaemia is haemolytic so red cell indices are usually normal, haptoglobin and haemopexin concentrations are reduced, and unconjugated bilirubin may be raised. The leukocyte count is usually in the low-normal range and the platelet count is nearly always reduced. Slight elevations in transaminases may occur—rises in aspartate aminotransferase (AST, SGOT) result both from haemolysis and liver injury whereas alanine aminotransferase (ALT, SGPT) rises reflect liver injury only. With modern treatments (artemisinin-based combination treatments) defervescence occurs rapidly—and most patients have cleared fever and parasitaemia (assessed by microscopy) within 2 days [89]. In higher transmission settings, except in hyperparasitaemic children, the haemoglobin often starts to rise immediately, whereas in lower transmission settings, where patients have little or no immunity, the dyserythropoietic bone marrow is slow to recover, and in most patients the haemoglobin continues to fall reaching a nadir around 7 days after presentation [33] (Fig. 8). Thereafter anaemia gradually resolves and the haemoglobin concentration has returned to steady state values 4–6 weeks after the illness. The reduction in haemoglobin is approximately proportional to disease severity and duration of illness before treatment. Treatment with artemisinin derivatives attenuates the reduction in haemoglobin by providing rapid resolution of the disease and also by returning pitted red cells to the circulation. In a randomised comparison conducted in hyperparasitaemic children in Kinshasa, DRC, the initial fall in haemoglobin concentration following artesunate was less (a difference of 0.4 g/dL) than that following quinine [70] (Fig. 7). In contrast drug resistance is associated with increased anaemia both because of slow initial therapeutic responses and an increased risk of subsequent recrudescence. Both drug resistance

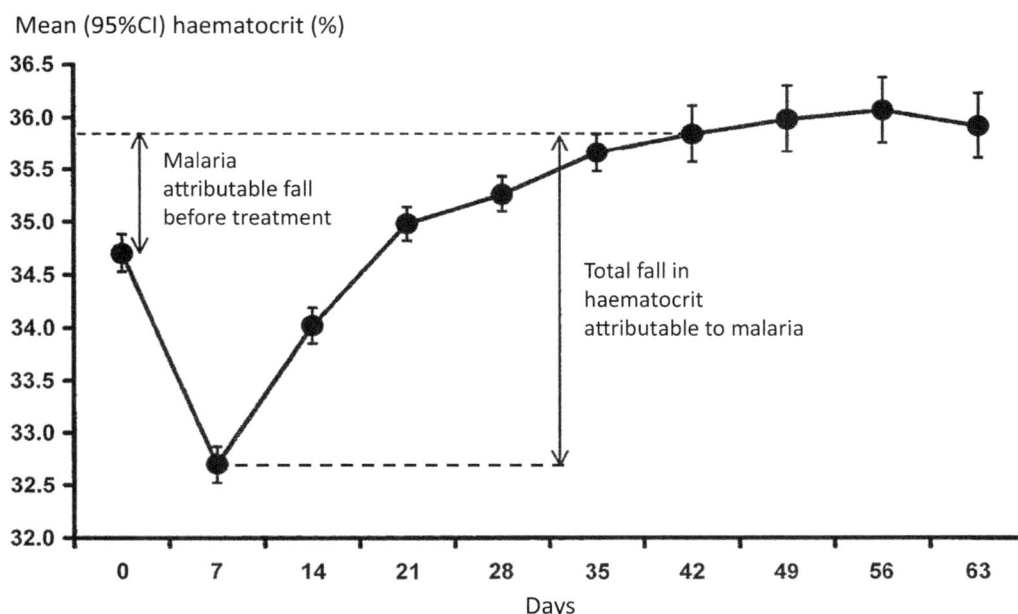

Fig. 8 Development of anaemia and subsequent recovery in Karen patients with acute falciparum malaria treated on the Thailand-Myanmar border [33]

and anaemia are independent risk factors for gameto-cytaemia in *P. falciparum* infections [96, 97], so in a context of worsening anti-malarial drug resistance it is common to see patients (often children) who present with anaemia and patent gametocytaemia.

Anaemia may be regarded a clock of the infection, in that a patient presenting with acute malaria and a normal haematocrit (provided they are not dehydrated) cannot have been ill for many days. The cumulative impact of repeated malaria episodes was documented in detail during the malaria therapy era, which began nearly a century ago, when malaria was used to treat neurosyphilis and also in detailed volunteer studies conducted by the military [98–102]. In volunteers given malaria whose infections were untreated, haemoglobin concentrations declined rapidly initially over 1 to 2 weeks, and then declined more slowly with symptom resolution. Then after 4 to 5 weeks the haemoglobin concentration rose slowly despite persistent parasitaemia [102] (Fig. 9). These extensive and detailed observations demonstrated the important role of illness (manifest by fever) in causing anaemia. They showed how, with continued infection, tolerance to the infecting malaria parasites was induced, so that the inflammatory response subsided, and eventually effective erythropoiesis outstripped haemolysis.

Severe malaria

Severe malaria is usually caused by *P. falciparum*, although *P. knowlesi* and occasionally *P. vivax* may also cause severe disease [93]. Severe malaria is a multi-system disease. Cerebral malaria (a diffuse symmetrical encephalopathy causing coma) is specific for *P. falciparum* infection, but kidney injury, metabolic acidosis, and severe anaemia may occur in all the malarias [93]. The pattern of vital organ dysfunction depends on age, pregnancy status, and, to a lesser extent, the level of transmission intensity [93]. Anaemia develops very rapidly in severe malaria. The initial most rapid decline in haematocrit observed in hospitalized patients reflects rehydration in those who are dehydrated and haemoconcentrated [103]. This has a time course of hours. It is followed by progressive haemolysis over the next few days without a significant erythropoietic response. The haemoglobin concentration commonly reaches a nadir around 1 week after admission [93]. In young children living in higher transmission settings the recovery is more rapid. In severe multisystem disease, the patient may lose 2 or more grams of haemoglobin per decilitre in the first 24 h of treatment. The dyserythropoietic bone marrow does not mount an effective reticulocyte response for several days.

The consequences of severe anaemia are an appropriate increase in cardiac index to maintain oxygen delivery.

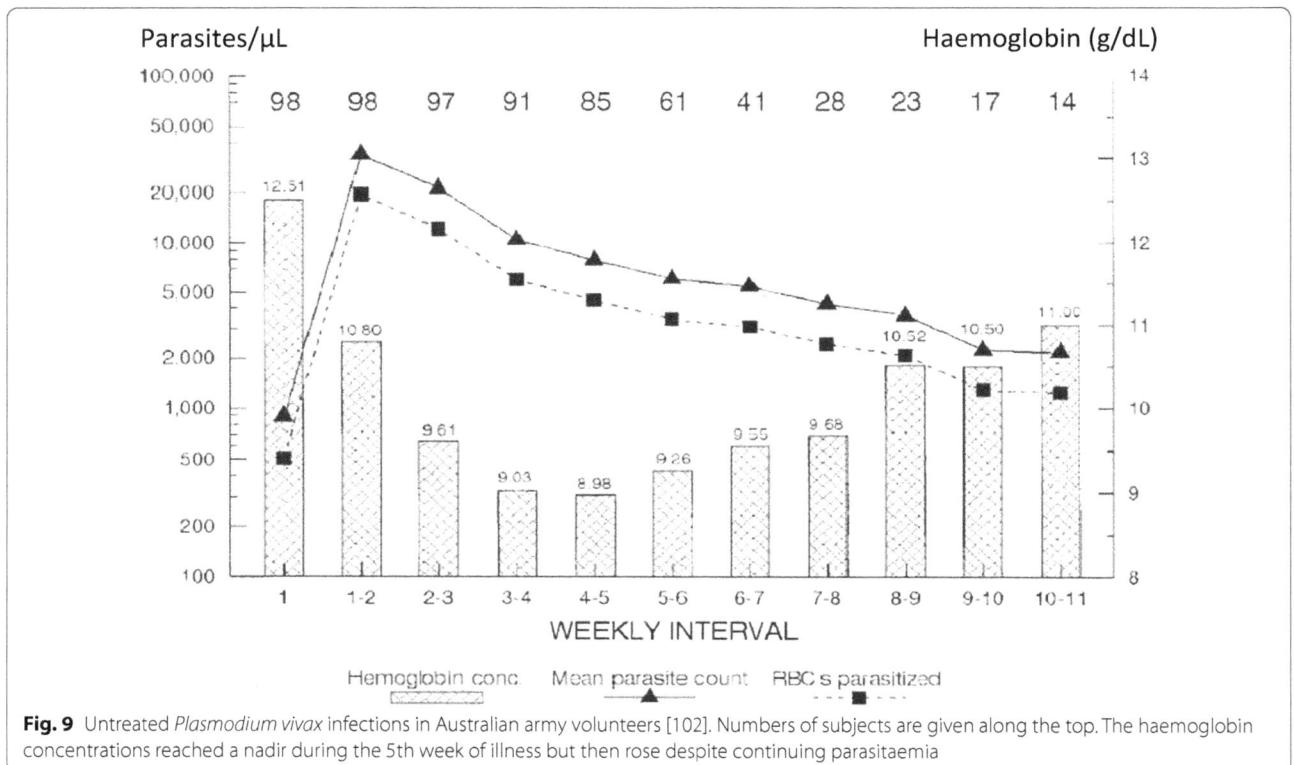

Fig. 9 Untreated *Plasmodium vivax* infections in Australian army volunteers [102]. Numbers of subjects are given along the top. The haemoglobin concentrations reached a nadir during the 5th week of illness but then rose despite continuing parasitaemia

Very severe anaemia ultimately leads to tissue ischaemia and hypoxia, with a rise in lactate production and an increase in the lactate-pyruvate ratio [104–106]. Tissue ischaemia is also caused directly by severe falciparum malaria; the lactate-pyruvate ratio is also increased, and hyperlactataemia correlates strongly with outcome (vide infra), but the pathogenesis is different [93]. In patients with severe falciparum malaria and a high parasite burden the reduction in tissue oxygen delivery results from microvascular obstruction caused by sequestration, compounded by reduced red cell deformability and inter-erythrocytic adhesive forces [107, 108]. Thus, there are two overlapping causes of tissue hypoxia and hyperlactataemia which both occur in malaria:

a. Severe anaemia which may result either from repeated uncomplicated infections with any of the malaria parasites, or a more fulminant haemolytic anaemia which is usually associated with severe falciparum malaria or sometimes blackwater fever.
b. Reduced microvascular perfusion resulting from cytoadherence and inter-erythrocytic adhesion.

The first of these responds rapidly to blood transfusion.

Anaemia and outcome in severe malaria

The relationship between haemoglobin concentration at presentation to hospital and outcome in falciparum malaria suggests that mortality rises sharply at levels below 3 g/dL (independent of other severe manifestations) [109, 110] (Figs. 10, 11). Severe anaemia is a prominent feature of all severe malaria but in areas of high transmission, where severe disease is confined to the first few years of life, it is the predominant manifestation [3, 11]. Consensus definitions of severe malaria have been agreed upon-which for the anaemia criterion is a haemoglobin below 5 g/dL in a patient with at least 10,000 parasites/μL [93]. Patients who fulfil the anaemia criterion for severe falciparum malaria, but have no other manifestations of severe malaria (i.e. cerebral, renal, metabolic or pulmonary dysfunction) have a much better prognosis than patients with one or more of these other manifestations [93]). Although most patients presenting with a parasite density of > 10,000 parasites/μL have malaria as the cause of their illness, this parasitaemia threshold for the "severe malaria" definition still means that some anaemic children with incidental parasitaemia and another infectious disease (usually sepsis) may be diagnosed as having severe malaria. Thus the severe anaemia criterion encompasses a broad range of presentations ranging from a fulminant disease with severe haemolytic anaemia to a sub-acute illness, often from recurrent or inadequately treated malaria, in which there

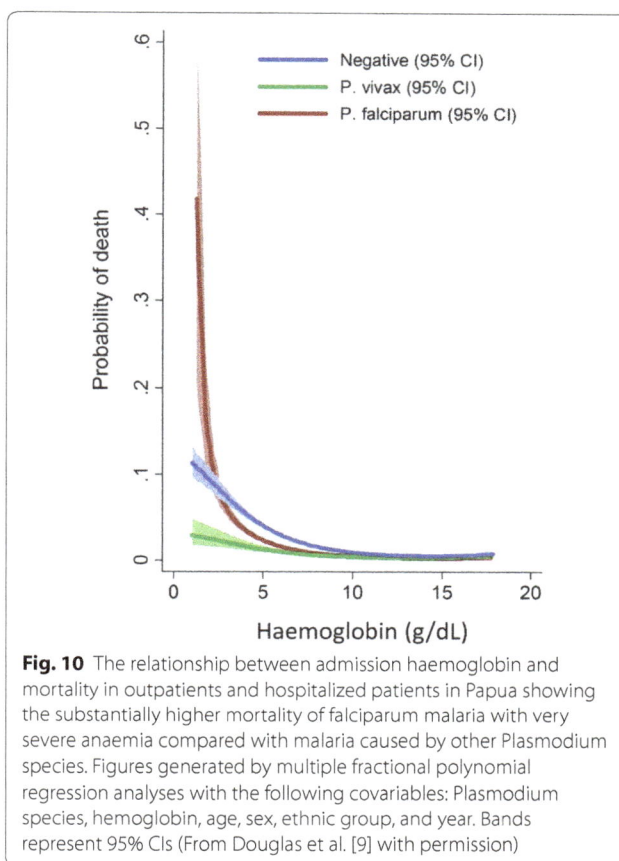

Fig. 10 The relationship between admission haemoglobin and mortality in outpatients and hospitalized patients in Papua showing the substantially higher mortality of falciparum malaria with very severe anaemia compared with malaria caused by other Plasmodium species. Figures generated by multiple fractional polynomial regression analyses with the following covariables: Plasmodium species, hemoglobin, age, sex, ethnic group, and year. Bands represent 95% CIs (From Douglas et al. [9] with permission)

has been progressive anaemia. The prognosis of the sub-acute presentation is much better as there has been time for physiological adaptation to anaemia (right shift of the oxygen dissociation curve) and there is a low risk of other vital organ dysfunction [93, 109]. In addition, the sequestered parasite biomass in these sub-acute presentations is much lower than in patients presenting with acute multi-organ dysfunction [110, 111]. Thus the mortality associated with severe malarial anaemia depends on many factors which include the degree of anaemia, age, transmission intensity, referral practices, access to and quality of health services, availability of safe cross-matched blood and delays in transfusion.

In published series of children admitted to hospital with severe malaria anaemia (including those with other severity manifestations) mortalities range from 2.6 to 10.3%—while mortalities as low as 0.5% have been reported in children with severe anaemia but without any other severity manifestation [106]. Those patients who are admitted with severe anaemia and do not survive succumb quickly, nearly half the deaths are within 12 h of admission (Fig. 12).

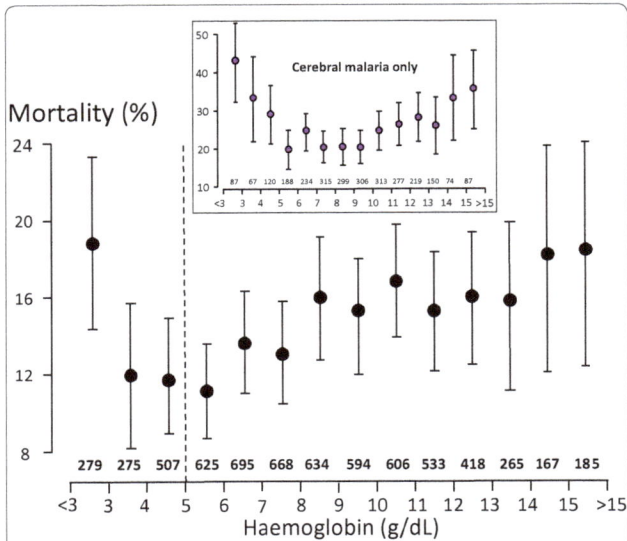

Fig. 11 Overall relationship between haemoglobin concentrations on admission and outcomes in 6451 adults and children with severe falciparum malaria studied in Africa and Asia between 1980 and 2015 who were admitted with a parasite density of > 10,000/μL. Below 5 g/dL (vertical blue dashed line) anaemia itself was a criterion for severe malaria. Inset is shown this same relationship in the subgroup of 2729 patients with cerebral malaria and the same parasitaemia range

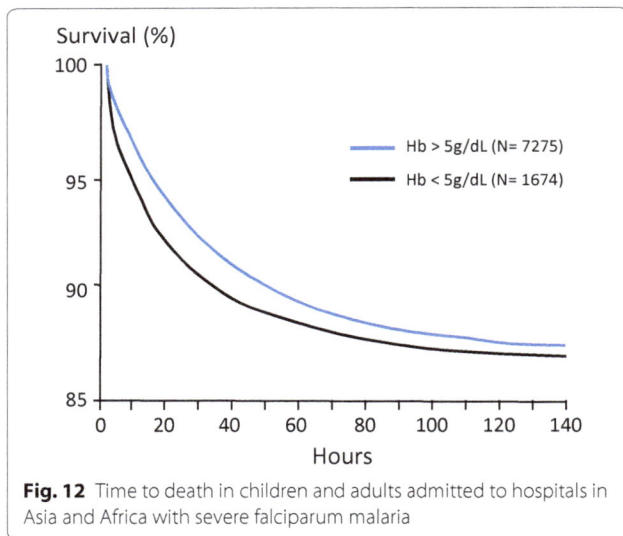

Fig. 12 Time to death in children and adults admitted to hospitals in Asia and Africa with severe falciparum malaria

Above a haemoglobin concentration of 5 g/dL other manifestations are required for a diagnosis of "severe falciparum malaria". In a very large series of over 8000 adults and children with strictly defined severe falciparum malaria studied in Asia and Africa over the past 37 years mortalities rose with increasing admission haemoglobin concentrations above 5 g/dL [112–117] (Fig. 11). A similar pattern was observed in the

subgroup of patients admitted with cerebral malaria (Fig. 11). There are many potential confounders which may explain this finding, but a causal association cannot be excluded. Interestingly in the large FEAST fluid bolus trial [118], which enrolled children with both severe malaria and sepsis, the 8-h mortality of patients with mild anaemia (defined in the trial as haemoglobin 7–9.9 g/dL) was higher among patients who still received a blood transfusion (8/35, 23%) than it was in the patients in the same category who were not transfused (29/808, 4%); a risk ratio of 6.4 (95% CI 3.1–12.9), P < 0.0001 [118]. This large difference was ascribed, very reasonably, to likely severity indicators which prompted a transfusion in mildly anaemic children, in whom it is generally not warranted. But it does raise the possibility of a causal association in patients with severe malaria. If this were confirmed it would mean that mild anaemia reduces the probability of a fatal outcome in patients with severe falciparum malaria (and vital organ dysfunction). It does not mean that anaemia could be beneficial overall—indeed anaemia is clearly harmful—but that within the subgroup of patients with falciparum malaria who have developed vital organ dysfunction it is possible that anaemia protects against death. If a causal association were confirmed then how could it be explained?

The ability of the circulatory system to transport oxygen to tissues and organs is determined by the cardiac index, the rheological properties of blood and the architecture of the microvasculature. Cardiac index is increased in anaemia. Blood, a suspension of cells in proteinaceous fluid, has complex rheological properties with a non-linear relationship between pressure and flow (shear stress and shear rate respectively i.e. non-Newtonian fluid mechanics) which could be altered in severe malaria. Increasing haematocrit is associated with a linear increase in oxygen carriage but a non-linear increase in apparent viscosity. As a consequence there is an optimum haematocrit for oxygen delivery [119]. The dependence of blood viscosity on haematocrit is greatest at the low shear rates encountered in the venous circulation, where sequestration of *P. falciparum* infected erythrocytes begins [120, 121]. Finally, the architecture of the microcirculation is markedly disrupted by sequestration. Cytoadherence, the fundamental pathological process in severe malaria which causes sequestration has been shown to be reduced by haemodilution. In an ex vivo system there was a 5- and 12-fold increase in *P. falciparum* infected erythrocyte rolling and adhesion, respectively, when haematocrit increased from 10 to 30%, as a result of changes in shear rate [122]. The optimum haematocrit is not known in severe malaria, but red cell adherence to vascular endothelium, and to other erythrocytes is likely to lower it, and reduced erythrocyte deformability may reduce it further [121, 123]. Thus reducing the density of erythrocytes (i.e. anaemia) might improve microvascular perfusion in patients with severe malaria. If so that would increase oxygen delivery, until it was outweighed by the reduction in oxygen carriage.

Alternatively there is no causal relationship. Severe anaemia may simply reflect duration of illness, and thus control of a severe infection or series of infections without intervening lethal vital organ dysfunction. The observed relationship between admission haematocrit and outcome of severe malaria might be explained entirely by other covariate relationships. Clearly this is an important question requiring further study to inform treatment guidelines and patient management.

Blackwater fever

This condition is well described but still poorly understood [93]. Blackwater fever means sudden massive haemolysis with fever and haemoglobinuria. The urine is black and, if the haemolysis is extensive, the patient has a pale, slate-grey appearance. Blackwater fever may be part of severe malaria [124–126]. Death may occur from severe anaemia or from acute renal failure. Haemoglobinuria may also occur in otherwise uncomplicated infections. Blackwater fever has historically been linked to quinine use, and it may occur in glucose-6-phosphate dehydrogenase deficiency with febrile illnesses such as malaria or following ingestion of oxidants (notably radical cure primaquine regimens) [127].

Post-artesunate haemolytic anaemia

There are several reports, mainly from temperate countries describing returned travellers, of late haemolytic anaemia occurring 1–3 weeks after parenteral artesunate treatment of hyperparasitaemic falciparum malaria. Most cases followed intravenous artesunate, although some were reported after intramuscular artemether, intrarectal artesunate and oral artemisinin derivatives. No deaths have been reported, but blood transfusion was often required. A recent review of published data, from non-immune and semi-immune patients, estimated the incidence of late haemolysis after intravenous artesunate to be 13% (95% CI 9–18%) and the requirement for a blood transfusion at 9% (95% CI 6–14%). Most of the data are from case reports and case definitions have varied substantially [67–69, 128]. However, in African children post-artesunate haemolytic anaemia occurs in less than 1% of cases [70] (Fig. 7). Post-artesunate haemolytic anaemia has been attributed to the pitting of drug-damaged malaria parasites from infected erythrocytes [67]. These once-infected red blood cells (oi-RBC) have a much shorter survival time (7–14 days) compared with normal erythrocytes in healthy subjects

(120 days) or in patients following severe malaria (44 days) [66, 128]. In the French series, a threshold of 180 once-infected erythrocytes/µL discriminated patients with delayed haemolysis with 89% sensitivity and 83% specificity [67]. The shorter survival of oi-RBC following artesunate probably reflects drug killing and then pitting of developed ring form parasites whereas background (and quinine associated) pitting may only occur for very young ring stages shortly after merozoite invasion with correspondingly less damage to the erythrocytes. The rapid and synchronous elimination of these oi-RBC from the circulation 1 to 2 weeks after the start of anti-malarial treatment results in haemolytic anaemia, which in some cases can be marked [67].

Management
Severe malaria

Severe anaemia (haemoglobin < 5 g/dL) requires blood transfusion which can be life-saving [129, 130]. The lower the haemoglobin the greater the need for transfusion. If there are other features of severe malaria such as acidotic breathing (respiratory distress) or coma, together with severe anemia then transfusion is more urgent. Respiratory distress with severe anaemia is often a sign of impending death [93, 131]. The rate of transfusion is titrated according to vital signs. In children, the WHO recommends 20 mls/kg of whole blood to be given over 4 h, or 10mls/kg of packed cells (although this is often unavailable). In low transmission settings malaria treatment guidelines recommend transfusion in severe malaria if the haemoglobin is < 7 g/dL (haematocrit 20%), whereas in higher transmission settings the recommended threshold is 5 g/dL (haematocrit 15%) [93]. The haemoglobin transfusion thresholds for acute malaria differ slightly from other WHO guidelines for the clinical use of blood. These recommend transfusion if the haemoglobin concentration is 4 g/dL or less (or haematocrit 12%), whatever the clinical condition of the patient, but they also recommend transfusion for haemoglobin concentrations of 4–6 g/dL (or haematocrits of 13–18%) if clinical features of any the following are present: hypoxia, acidosis, impaired consciousness or hyperparasitaemia (> 20%) [132, 133]. None of these transfusion recommendations are based on solid evidence [134]. Transfusion thresholds in malaria were set intentionally slightly higher than for some other conditions [135] because haemoglobin concentrations usually fall rapidly in severe malaria. Thus, to avoid falling into the danger zone it has been thought better to order blood for transfusion sooner rather than later. But what is the danger zone? And are these pragmatic thresholds correct? Retrospective observations have the disadvantage that many factors determine whether or not a patient with severe malaria receives a timely blood transfusion, and several of these factors could affect outcomes independently, so prospective randomized trials are under way to try and answer these questions [134].

The anti-malarial treatment of choice for severe malaria is parenteral artesunate [89, 93, 114, 116]. When the patient can swallow reliably this should be followed by a full course of an oral artemisinin-based combination therapy. Anti-malarial treatment should not be delayed by transfusion.

In areas where the HIV prevalence is high severe anaemia with malaria is more likely in HIV positive patients [136], and in high malaria transmission settings concomitant HIV exacerbates the anaemia that occurs in infancy after 3 months of age [137]. In these high transmission settings children admitted to hospital with severe anaemia have an increased risk of readmission with severe anaemia, and they also have an increased risk of dying in the following months [10]. Prevention of malaria reinfection with slowly eliminated anti-malarial drugs reduces these risks [138].

Blackwater fever

Blackwater fever results from massive haemolysis sufficient to cause haemoglobinuria. The management of blackwater fever anaemia is with blood transfusion [93]. Anti-malarial treatment should not be withheld. Steroids are ineffective. Some cases result from oxidant haemolysis in G6PD deficiency. In these cases the precipitant should be withdrawn and adequate hydration ensured. Blackwater fever patients, who are not G6PD deficient, are notoriously difficult to cross match. Acute kidney injury is an important complication.

Anaemia in uncomplicated malaria

A promptly treated discrete episode of malaria in a patient with a pre-morbid normal haemoglobin is unlikely to result in clinically significant anaemia. It is the cumulative impact of repeated illness from recurrent malaria that is the main cause. In areas where *P. vivax* is endemic frequently recurring illness caused by repeated relapse is the main contributor to malarial anaemia in childhood [8, 9]. In areas where *P. falciparum* is endemic frequent infections or repeated treatment failure cause anaemia. The prevalence of anaemia therefore increases with transmission intensity, and where anti-malarial drug resistance compromises drug efficacy [139]. In areas of high transmission the greatest burden is in infants [3]. Prompt effective artemisinin combination treatment is currently the cornerstone of management of the individual acute illness [89], but prevention of repeated or recurrent infection is the key to reducing malarial anaemia at the community level.

Malaria in pregnancy

Anaemia is common in pregnancy in tropical regions. Malaria is a major contributor to anaemia in pregnancy [13, 14, 139]. The risks of anaemia increase as the pregnancy progresses although severe haemolytic anaemia may occur during the middle trimester in high transmission settings. Concomitant HIV infection exacerbates malarial anaemia in pregnancy. High maternal parasitaemias are associated with fetal and newborn anaemia [6]. Even asymptomatic infection in the mother is harmful for the fetus and reduces birthweight. Symptomatic infections need prompt treatment, but prevention is better for both mother and baby. This can be achieved by chemoprophylaxis, although there is currently no satisfactory safe drug for falciparum malaria prevention. Chloroquine is regarded as safe in pregnancy and is still effective in preventing the non-falciparum malarias in most areas. The more widely used approach in higher transmission settings is intermittent preventive treatment which involves giving treatment doses at approximately 1 month intervals starting from 13 weeks gestation, or initial presentation at the antenatal clinic—whichever is later [89]. Sulfadoxine–pyrimethamine is the most widely used drug although this is increasingly challenged by resistance. The WHO recommends that in malaria-endemic areas of Africa, intermittent preventive treatment with SP should be provided to all pregnant women (SP-IPTp) as part of antenatal care, unless they are HIV coinfected and already receiving co-trimoxazole prophylaxis. Dosing should start in the second trimester and doses should be given at least 1 month apart, with the objective of ensuring that at least three doses are received [89]. Pregnant women in malaria endemic areas should also receive iron and folate supplementation according to standard guidelines.

Authors' contributions
The author read and approved the final manuscript.

Author details
[1] Faculty of Tropical Medicine, Mahidol University, Bangkok, Thailand. [2] Centre for Tropical Medicine and Global Health, Nuffield Department of Medicine, University of Oxford, Oxford, UK.

Acknowledgements

I am a Wellcome Trust Principal Fellow. I am very grateful to my colleagues in the Mahidol Oxford Research Unit for all their advice and help.

Competing interests

The author declare no competing interests.

Funding

Wellcome Trust (Grant Number 089179/Z/09/Z) Principal Fellowship.

References

1. White NJ, Pukrittayakamee S, Hien TT, Faiz MA, Mokuolu OA, Dondorp AM. Malaria. Lancet. 2014;383:723–35.
2. WHO. Word malaria report 2017. Geneva: World Health Organization; 2017.
3. Schellenberg D, Menendez C, Kahigwa E, Font F, Galindo C, Acosta C, et al. African children with malaria in an area of intense *Plasmodium falciparum* transmission: features on admission to the hospital and risk factors for death. Am J Trop Med Hyg. 1999;61:431–8.
4. Kahigwa E, Schellenberg D, Sanz S, Aponte JJ, Wigayi J, Mshinda H, et al. Risk factors for presentation to hospital with severe anaemia in Tanzanian children: a case-control study. Trop Med Int Health. 2002;7:823–30.
5. Mulenga M, Malunga P, Bennett S, Thuma PE, Shulman C, Fielding K, et al. Factors associated with severe anaemia in Zambian children admitted with *Plasmodium falciparum* malarial anaemia. Ann Trop Paediatr. 2005;25:87–90.
6. Accrombessi M, Ouédraogo S, Agbota GC, Gonzalez R, Massougbodji A, Menéndez C, et al. Malaria in pregnancy is a predictor of infant haemoglobin concentrations during the first year of life in Benin, West Africa. PLoS ONE. 2015;10:e0129510.
7. Moraleda C, Aguilar R, Quintó L, Nhampossa T, Renom M, Nhabomba A, et al. Anaemia in hospitalised preschool children from a rural area in Mozambique: a case control study in search for aetiological agents. BMC Pediatr. 2017;17:63.
8. Kenangalem E, Karyana M, Burdarm L, Yeung S, Simpson JA, Tjitra E, et al. *Plasmodium vivax* infection: a major determinant of severe anaemia in infancy. Malar J. 2016;15:321.
9. Douglas NM, Lampah DA, Kenangalem E, Simpson JA, Poespoprodjo JR, Sugiarto P, et al. Major burden of severe anemia from non-falciparum malaria species in Southern Papua: a hospital-based surveillance study. PLoS Med. 2013;10:e1001575.
10. Calis JC, Phiri KS, Faragher EB, Brabin BJ, Bates I, Cuevas LE, et al. Severe anemia in Malawian children. N Engl J Med. 2008;358:888–99.
11. Crawley J. Reducing the burden of anemia in infants and young children in malaria-endemic countries in Africa: from evidence to action. Am J Trop Med Hyg. 2004;71(Suppl 2):25–34.
12. Weatherall DJ. Genetic variation and susceptibility to infection: the red cell and malaria. Br J Haematol. 2008;141:276–86.
13. Desai M, ter Kuile FO, Nosten F, McGready R, Asamoa K, Brabin B, et al. Epidemiology and burden of malaria in pregnancy. Lancet Infect Dis. 2007;7:93–104.
14. Brabin BJ, Hakimi M, Pelletier D. An analysis of anemia and pregnancy-related maternal mortality. J Nutr. 2001;131:604S–14S.
15. Brabin B. Fetal anaemia in malarious areas: its causes and significance. Ann Trop Paediatr. 1992;12:303–10.
16. Casanova JL. Human genetic basis of interindividual variability in the course of infection. Proc Natl Acad Sci USA. 2015;112:e7118–27.
17. Williams TN. Sickle cell disease in sub-Saharan Africa. Hematol Oncol Clin North Am. 2016;30:343–58.
18. Uyoga S, Ndila CM, Macharia AW, Nyutu G, Shah S, Peshu N, et al. Glucose-6-phosphate dehydrogenase deficiency and the risk of malaria and other diseases in children in Kenya: a case-control and a cohort study. Lancet Haematol. 2015;2:e437–44.
19. Shanks GD, Hay SI, Bradley DJ. Malaria's indirect contribution to all-cause mortality in the Andaman Islands during the colonial era. Lancet Infect Dis. 2008;8:564–70.
20. Korenromp EL, Armstrong-Schellenberg JR, Williams BG, Nahlen BL, Snow RW. Impact of malaria control on childhood anaemia in Africa—a quantitative review. Trop Med Int Health. 2004;9:1050–65.
21. Mathanga DP, Campbell CH Jr, Vanden Eng J, Wolkon A, Bronzan RN, Malenga GJ, et al. Comparison of anaemia and parasitaemia as indicators of malaria control in household and EPI-health facility surveys in Malawi. Malar J. 2010;9:107.
22. Aregawi MW, Ali AS, Al-mafazy AW, Molteni F, Katikiti S, Warsame M, et al. Reductions in malaria and anaemia case and death burden at hospitals following scale-up of malaria control in Zanzibar, 1999–2008. Malar J. 2011;10:46.
23. Gitonga CW, Edwards T, Karanja PN, Noor AM, Snow RW, Brooker SJ. Plasmodium infection, anaemia and mosquito net use among school children across different settings in Kenya. Trop Med Int Health. 2012;17:858–70.
24. Gething PW, Casey DC, Weiss DJ, Bisanzio D, Bhatt S, Cameron E, et al. Mapping *Plasmodium falciparum* mortality in Africa between 1990 and 2015. N Engl J Med. 2016;375:2435–45.
25. Zuckerman A. Recent studies on factors involved in malarial anaemia. Milit Med. 1966;131(supplement):1201–16.
26. Abdallah S, Weatherall DJ, Wickramasinghe SN, Hughes M. The anaemia of *P. falciparum* malaria. Br J Haematol. 1980;46:171–83.
27. Perrin LH, Mackey LJ, Miecher PA. The hematology of malaria in man. Semin Hematol. 1982;19:70–82.
28. Phillips RE, Looareesuwan S, Warrell DA, Lee SH, Karbwang J, Warrell MJ, et al. The importance of anaemia in cerebral and uncomplicated falciparum malaria: role of complications, dyserythropoiesis and iron sequestration. Quart J Med. 1986;58:305–23.
29. Knuttgen HJ. The bone marrow of non-immune Europeans in acute malaria infection: a topical review. Ann Trop Med Parasitol. 1987;81:567–76.
30. Looareesuwan S, Davis TME, Pukrittayakamee S, Supanaranond W, Desakorn V, Silamut K, et al. Erythrocyte survival in severe falciparum malaria. Acta Trop. 1991;48:263–70.
31. Burgmann H, Looareesuwan S, Kapiotis S, Viravan C, Vanijanonta S, Hollenstein U, et al. Serum levels of erythropoietin in acute *Plasmodium falciparum* malaria. Am J Trop Med Hyg. 1996;54:280–3.
32. Vedovato M, De Paoli Vitali E, Dapporto M, Salvatorelli G. Defective erythropoietin production in the anaemia of malaria. Nephrol Dial Transplant. 1999;14:1043–4.
33. Price RN, Simpson J, Nosten F, Luxemburger C, Hkirjaroen L, ter Kuile F, et al. Factors contributing to anemia in uncomplicated falciparum malaria. Am J Trop Med Hyg. 2001;65:614–22.
34. Douglas NM, Anstey NM, Buffet PA, Poespoprodjo JR, Yeo TW, White NJ, et al. The anaemia of *Plasmodium vivax* malaria. Malar J. 2012;11:135.
35. Looareesuwan S, Merry AH, Phillips RE, Pleehachinda R, Wattanagoon Y, Ho M, et al. Reduced erythrocyte survival following clearance of malarial parasitaemia in Thai patients. Br J Haematol. 1987;67:473–8.
36. Collins WE, Jeffery GM, Roberts JM. A retrospective examination of anemia during infection of humans with *Plasmodium vivax*. Am J Trop Med Hyg. 2003;68:410–2.
37. Jakeman GN, Saul A, Hogarth WL, Collins WE. Anaemia of acute malaria infections in non-immune patients primarily results from destruction of uninfected erythrocytes. Parasitology. 1999;119:127–33.
38. Casals-Pascual C, Kai O, Cheung JO, Williams S, Lowe B, Nyanoti M, et al. Suppression of erythropoiesis in malarial anemia is associated with hemozoin in vitro and in vivo. Blood. 2006;108:2569–77.
39. Aguilar R, Moraleda C, Achtman AH, Mayor A, Quintó L, Cisteró P, et al. Severity of anaemia is associated with bone marrow haemozoin in children exposed to *Plasmodium falciparum*. Br J Haematol. 2014;164:877–87.
40. Lamikanra AA, Theron M, Kooij TW, Roberts DJ. Hemozoin (malarial pigment) directly promotes apoptosis of erythroid precursors. PLoS ONE. 2009;4:e8446.

41. Perkins DJ, Were T, Davenport GC, Kempaiah P, Hittner JB, Ong'echa JM. Severe malarial anemia: innate immunity and pathogenesis. Int J Biol Sci. 2011;7:1427–42.

42. Skorokhod OA, Caione L, Marrocco T, Migliardi G, Barrera V, Arese P, et al. Inhibition of erythropoiesis in malaria anemia: role of hemozin and hemozoin-generated 4-hydroxynonenal. Blood. 2010;116:4328–37.

43. Schwarzer E, Arese P, Skorokhod OA. Role of the lipoperoxidation product 4-hydroxynonenal in the pathogenesis of severe malaria anemia and malaria immunodepression. Oxid Med Cell Longev. 2015;2015:638416.

44. Lamikanra AA, Merryweather-Clarke AT, Tipping AJ, Roberts DJ. Distinct mechanisms of inadequate erythropoiesis induced by tumor necrosis factor alpha or malarial pigment. PLoS ONE. 2015;10:e0119836.

45. McGuire W, Knight JC, Hill AV, Allsopp CE, Greenwood BM, Kwiatkowski D. Severe malarial anemia and cerebral malaria are associated with different tumor necrosis factor promoter alleles. J Infect Dis. 1999;179:287–90.

46. Kurtzhals JA, Adabayeri V, Goka BQ, Akanmori BD, Oliver-Commey JO, Nkrumah FK, et al. Low plasma concentrations of interleukin 10 in severe malarial anaemia compared with cerebral and uncomplicated malaria. Lancet. 1998;351:1768–72.

47. Atkinson SH, Rockett K, Sirugo G, Bejon PA, Fulford A, O'Connell MA, et al. Seasonal childhood anaemia in West Africa is associated with the haptoglobin 2-2 genotype. PLoS Med. 2006;3:e172.

48. Burchard GD, Radloff P, Philipps J, Nkeyi M, Knobloch J, Kremsner PG. Increased erythropoietin production in children with severe malarial anemia. Am J Trop Med Hyg. 1995;53:547–51.

49. Dondorp AM, Angus BJ, Chotivanich K, Silamut K, Ruangveerayuth R, Hardeman MR, et al. Red blood cell deformability as a predictor of anemia in severe falciparum malaria. Am J Trop Med Hyg. 1999;60:733–7.

50. Griffiths MJ, Ndungu F, Baird KL, Muller DP, Marsh K, Newton CR. Oxidative stress and erythrocyte damage in Kenyan children with severe *Plasmodium falciparum* malaria. Br J Haematol. 2001;113:486–91.

51. Barber BE, Russell B, Grigg MJ, Zhang R, William T, Amir A, et al. Reduced red blood cell deformability in *Plasmodium knowlesi* malaria. Blood Adv. 2018;2:433–43.

52. Duez J, Holleran JP, Ndour PA, Pionneau C, Diakité S, Roussel C, Dussiot M, Amireault P, Avery VM, Buffet PA. Mechanical clearance of red blood cells by the human spleen: potential therapeutic applications of a biomimetic RBC filtration method. Transfus Clin Biol. 2015;22:151–7.

53. Nuchsongsin F, Chotivanich K, Charunwatthana P, Omodeo-Salè F, Taramelli D, Day NP, et al. Effects of malaria heme products on red blood cell deformability. Am J Trop Med Hyg. 2007;77:617–22.

54. Matthews K, Duffy SP, Myrand-Lapierre ME, Ang RR, Li L, Scott MD, et al. Microfluidic analysis of red blood cell deformability as a means to assess hemin-induced oxidative stress resulting from *Plasmodium falciparum* intraerythrocytic parasitism. Integr Biol (Camb). 2017;9:519–28.

55. Joshi P, Alam A, Chandra R, Puri SK, Gupta CM. Possible basis for membrane changes in non parasitised erythrocytes of malaria infected animals. Biochim Biophys Acta. 1986;862:220–2.

56. Facer CA, Bray RS, Brown J. Direct Coombs' antiglobulin reactions in Gambian children with *Plasmodium falciparum* malaria. I. Incidence and class specificity. Clin Exp Immunol. 1979;35:119–27.

57. Facer CA. Direct Coombs' antiglobulin reactions in Gambian children with *Plasmodium falciparum* malaria. II. Specificity of erythrocyte bound IgG. Clin Exp Immunol. 1980;39:279–88.

58. Merry AH, Looareesuwan S, Phillips RE, Chanthavanich P, Supanaranond W, Warrell DA, et al. Evidence against immune haemolysis in falciparum malaria in Thailand. Br J Haematol. 1986;64:187–94.

59. Waitumbi JN, Opollo MO, Muga RO, Misore AO, Stoute JA. Red cell surface changes and erythrophagocytosis in children with severe *Plasmodium falciparum* anemia. Blood. 2000;95:1481–6.

60. Stoute JA, Odindo AO, Owuor BO, Mibei EK, Opollo MO, Waitumbi JN. Loss of red blood cell-complement regulatory proteins and increased levels of circulating immune complexes are associated with severe malarial anemia. J Infect Dis. 2003;187:522–5.

61. Looareesuwan S, Ho M, Wattanagoon Y, White NJ, Warrell DA, Bunnag D, et al. Dynamic alteration in splenic function during acute falciparum malaria. N Engl J Med. 1987;317:675–9.

62. Lee SH, Looareesuwan S, Wattanagoon Y, Ho M, Wuthiekanun V, Vilaiwanna N, et al. Antibody-dependent red cell removal during P.

63. falciparum malaria: the clearance of red cells sensitized with an IgG anti-D. Br J Haematol. 1989;73:396–402.

63. Ho M, White NJ, Looareesuwan S, Wattanagoon Y, Lee SH, Walport MJ, et al. Splenic Fc receptor function in host defense and anemia in acute *Plasmodium falciparum* malaria. J Infect Dis. 1990;161:555–61.

64. Charoenlarp P, Vanijanonta S, Chat-Panyaporn P. The effect of prednisolone on red cell survival in patients with falciparum malaria. Southeast Asian J Trop Med Public Health. 1979;10:127–31.

65. Angus B, Chotivanich K, Udomsangpetch R, White NJ. In-vivo removal of malaria parasites from red cells without their destruction in acute falciparum malaria. Blood. 1997;90:2037–40.

66. Newton PN, Chotivanich K, Chierakul W, Ruangveerayuth R, Teerapong P, Silamut K, et al. A comparison of the in vivo kinetics of *Plasmodium falciparum* ring-infected erythrocyte surface antigen-positive and -negative erythrocytes. Blood. 2001;98:450–7.

67. Jaureguiberry S, Ndour PA, Roussel C, Ader F, Safeukui I, Nguyen M, et al. Post artesunate delayed haemolysis is a predictable event related to the lifesaving effect of artemisinins. Blood. 2014;124:167–75.

68. Rehman K, Lotsch F, Kremsner PG, Ramharter M. Haemolysis associated with the treatment of malaria with artemisinin derivatives: a systematic review of current evidence. Int J Infect Dis. 2014;29:268–73.

69. Rolling T, Agbenyega T, Krishna S, Kremsner PG, Cramer JP. Delayed haemolysis after artesunate treatment of severe malaria—review of the literature and perspective. Travel Med Infect Dis. 2015;13:143–9.

70. Fanello C, Onyamboko M, Lee SJ, Woodrow C, Setaphan S, Chotivanich K, et al. Post-treatment haemolysis in African children with hyperparasitaemic falciparum malaria; a randomized comparison of artesunate and quinine. BMC Infect Dis. 2017;17:e575.

71. Crane GG. Hyperreactive malarious splenomegaly (tropical splenomegaly syndrome). Parasitol Today. 1986;2:4–9.

72. Bedu-Addo G, Bates I. Causes of massive tropical splenomegaly in Ghana. Lancet. 2002;360:449–54.

73. Leoni S, Buonfrate D, Angheben A, Gobbi F, Bisoffi Z. The hyper-reactive malarial splenomegaly: a systematic review of the literature. Malar J. 2015;14:e185.

74. Gwamaka M, Kurtis JD, Sorensen BE, Holte S, Morrison R, Mutabingwa TK, Fried M, et al. Iron deficiency protects against severe *Plasmodium falciparum* malaria and death in young children. Clin Infect Dis. 2012;54:1137–44.

75. van Hensbroek MB, Morris-Jones S, Meisner S, Jaffar S, Bayo L, Dackour R, et al. Iron, but not folic acid, combined with effective antimalarial therapy promotes haematological recovery in African children after acute falciparum malaria. Trans R Soc Trop Med Hyg. 1995;89:672–6.

76. Schellenberg D, Kahigwa E, Sanz S, Aponte JJ, Mshinda H, Alonso P, et al. A randomized comparison of two anemia treatment regimens in Tanzanian children. Am J Trop Med Hyg. 2004;71:428–33.

77. Sazawal S, Black RE, Ramsan M, Chwaya HM, Stoltzfus RJ, Dutta A, et al. Effects of routine prophylactic supplementation with iron and folic acid on admission to hospital and mortality in preschool children in a high malaria transmission setting: community-based, randomised, placebo-controlled trial. Lancet. 2006;367:133–43.

78. Soofi S, Cousens S, Iqbal SP, Akhund T, Khan J, Ahmed I, et al. Effect of provision of daily zinc and iron with several micronutrients on growth and morbidity among young children in Pakistan: a cluster-randomised trial. Lancet. 2013;382:29–40.

79. Zlotkin S, Newton S, Aimone AM, Azindow I, Ammenga-Etego S, Tchum K, et al. Effect of iron fortification on malaria incidence in infants and young children in Ghana: a randomized trial. JAMA. 2013;310:938–47.

80. Veenemans J, Milligan P, Prentice AM, Schouten LR, Inja N, van der Heijden AC, et al. Effect of supplementation with zinc and other micronutrients on malaria in Tanzanian children: a randomised trial. PLoS Med. 2011;8:e1001125.

81. English M, Snow RW. Iron and folic acid supplementation and malaria risk. Lancet. 2006;367:90–1.

82. WHO. Guideline: daily iron supplementation in infants and children. Geneva: World Health Organization; 2016.

83. Moraleda C, Rabinovich R, Menendez C. Are infants less than 6 months of age a neglected group for anemia prevention in low-income countries? Am J Trop Med Hyg. 2018;98:647–9.

84. Prentice AM, Mendoza YA, Pereira D, Cerami C, Wegmuller R, Constable A, et al. Dietary strategies for improving iron status: balancing safety and efficacy. Nutr Rev. 2017;75:49–60.

85. Drakesmith H, Prentice AM. Hepcidin and the iron-infection axis. Science. 2012;338:768–72.

86. Church J, Maitland K. Invasive bacterial co-infection in African children with Plasmodium falciparum malaria: a systematic review. BMC Med. 2014;12:e31.

87. Ndour PA, Larréché S, Mouri O, Argy N, Gay F, Roussel C, et al. Measuring the Plasmodium falciparum HRP2 protein in blood from artesunate-treated malaria patients predicts post-artesunate delayed hemolysis. Sci Transl Med. 2017;9:397.

88. Imwong M, Nguyen TN, Tripura R, Peto TJ, Lee SJ, Lwin KM, et al. The epidemiology of subclinical malaria infections in South-East Asia: findings from cross-sectional surveys in Thailand-Myanmar border areas, Cambodia, and Vietnam. Malar J. 2015;14:e381.

89. WHO. Guidelines for the treatment of malaria. 3rd ed. Geneva: World Health Organization; 2015.

90. Lee SJ, Stepniewska K, Anstey N, Ashley E, Barnes K, Binh TQ, et al. The relationship between the haemoglobin concentration and the haematocrit in Plasmodium falciparum malaria. Malar J. 2008;7:149.

91. Quintó L, Aponte JJ, Menéndez C, Sacarlal J, Aide P, Espasa M, et al. Relationship between haemoglobin and haematocrit in the definition of anaemia. Trop Med Int Health. 2006;11:1295–302.

92. Cissé B, Ba EH, Sokhna C, NDiaye JL, Gomis JF, Dial Y, et al. Effectiveness of seasonal malaria chemoprevention in children under ten years of age in Senegal: a stepped-wedge cluster-randomised trial. PLoS Med. 2016;13:1002175.

93. WHO. Severe malaria. Trop Med Int Health. 2014;19(Supplement 1):1–131.

94. Davis TME, Krishna S, Looareesuwan S, Supanaranond W, Pukrittayakamee S, Attatamsoothorn K, et al. Erythrocyte sequestration and anaemia in severe falciparum malaria. Analysis of acute changes in venous haematocrit using a simple mathematical model. J Clin Invest. 1990;865:793–800.

95. Silamut K, White NJ. Relation of the stage of parasite development in the peripheral blood to prognosis in severe falciparum malaria. Trans R Soc Trop Med Hyg. 1993;87:436–43.

96. Price RN, Nosten F, Luxemburger C, Phaipun L, ter Kuile F, van Vugt M, et al. Risk factors for gametocyte carriage in uncomplicated falciparum malaria. Am J Trop Med Hyg. 1999;60:1019–23.

97. Stepniewska K, Price RN, Sutherland CJ, Drakeley CJ, von Seidlein L, Nosten F, et al. Plasmodium falciparum gametocyte dynamics in areas of different malaria endemicity. Malar J. 2008;7:e249.

98. James SP, Nichol WD, Shute PG. A study of induced malignant tertian malaria. Proc R Soc Med. 1932;25:1153–86.

99. Kitchen SF. Symptomatology: general considerations and falciparum malaria. In: Boyd MF, editor. Malariology, vol. 2. Philadelphia: WB Saunders; 1949. p. 996–1017.

100. Kitchen SF. Vivax malaria. In: Boyd MF, editor. Malariology, vol. 2. Philadelphia: WB Saunders; 1949. p. 1027–45.

101. Fairley NH. Sidelights on malaria in man obtained by subinoculation experiments. Trans R Soc Trop Med Hyg. 1947;40:521–676.

102. Bickerton-Blackburn CR. Observations on the development of resistance to Plasmodium vivax. Trans R Soc Trop Med Hyg. 1948;42:117–62.

103. Hanson JP, Lam SW, Mohanty S, Alam S, Pattnaik R, Mahanta KC, et al. Fluid resuscitation of adults with severe falciparum malaria: effects on acid-base status, renal function, and extravascular lung water. Crit Care Med. 2013;41:972–81.

104. Cain SM. Appearance of excess lactate in anesthetized dogs during anemic and hypoxic hypoxia. Am J Physiol. 1965;209:604–10.

105. Neill WA, Jensen PE, Rich GB, Werschkul JD. Effect of decreased O_2 supply to tissue on the lactate:pyruvate ratio in blood. J Clin Invest. 1969;48:1862–9.

106. Brand NR, Opoka RO, Hamre KE, John CC. Differing causes of lactic acidosis and deep breathing in cerebral malaria and severe malarial anemia may explain differences in acidosis-related mortality. PLoS ONE. 2016;11:e0163728.

107. Hanson J, Lam SW, Mahanta KC, Pattnaik R, Alam S, Mohanty S, et al. Relative contributions of macrovascular and microvascular dysfunction to disease severity in falciparum malaria. J Infect Dis. 2012;206:571–9.

108. Ishioka H, Ghose A, Charunwatthana P, Maude R, Plewes K, Kingston H, et al. Sequestration and red cell deformability as determinants of hyperlactatemia in falciparum malaria. J Infect Dis. 2015;213:788–93.

109. von Seidlein L, Olaosebikan R, Hendriksen IC, Lee SJ, Adedoyin OT, Agbenyega T, et al. Predicting the clinical outcome of severe falciparum malaria in African children: findings from a large randomized trial. Clin Infect Dis. 2012;54:1080–90.

110. Kiguli S, Maitland K, George EC, Olupot-Olupot P, Opoka RO, Engoru C, et al. Anaemia and blood transfusion in African children presenting to hospital with severe febrile illness. BMC Med. 2015;13:e21.

111. Hendriksen IC, Mwanga-Amumpaire J, von Seidlein L, Mtove G, White LJ, Olaosebikan R, et al. Diagnosing severe falciparum malaria in parasitaemic African children: a prospective evaluation of plasma PfHRP2 measurement. PLoS Med. 2012;9:e1001297.

112. Waller D, Krishna S, Crawley J, Miller K, Nosten F, Chapman D, et al. The clinical features and outcome of severe malaria in Gambian children. Clin Infect Dis. 1995;21:577–87.

113. Hien TT, Day NPJ, Phu NH, Mai NTH, Chau TTH, Loc PP, et al. A controlled trial of artemether or quinine in Vietnamese adults with severe falciparum malaria. N Engl J Med. 1996;335:76–83.

114. Dondorp A, Nosten F, Stepniewska K, Day N, White N, South East Asian Quinine Artesunate Malaria Trial Group. Artesunate versus quinine for treatment of severe falciparum malaria: a randomised trial. Lancet. 2005;366:717–25.

115. Phu NH, Tuan PQ, Day N, Mai NT, Chau TT, Chuong LV, et al. Randomized controlled trial of artesunate or artemether in Vietnamese adults with severe falciparum malaria. Malar J. 2010;9:e97.

116. Dondorp AM, Fanello CI, Hendriksen IC, Gomes E, Seni A, Chhaganlal KD, et al. Artesunate versus quinine in the treatment of severe falciparum malaria in African children (AQUAMAT): an open-label, randomised trial. Lancet. 2010;376:1647–57.

117. Newton PN, Stepniewska K, Dondorp A, Silamut K, Chierakul W, Krishna S, et al. Prognostic indicators in adults hospitalized with falciparum malaria in Western Thailand. Malar J. 2013;12:229.

118. Maitland K, Kiguli S, Opoka RO, Engoru C, Olupot-Olupot P, Akech SO, et al. Mortality after fluid bolus in African children with severe infection. N Engl J Med. 2011;364:2483–95.

119. Crowell JW, Smith EE. Determinant of the optimal hematocrit. J Appl Physiol. 1967;22:501–4.

120. Reinhart WH. The optimum hematocrit. Clin Hemorheol Microcirc. 2016;64:575–85.

121. Piety NZ, Reinhart WH, Stutz J, Shevkoplyas SS. Optimal hematocrit in an artificial microvascular network. Transfusion. 2017;57:2257–66.

122. Flatt C, Mitchell S, Yipp B, Looareesuwan S, Ho M. Attenuation of cytoadherence of Plasmodium falciparum to microvascular endothelium under flow by hemodilution. Am J Trop Med Hyg. 2005;72:660–5.

123. Schmalzer EA, Lee JO, Brown AK, Usami S, Chien S. Viscosity of mixtures of sickle and normal red cells at varying haematocrit levels. Implications for transfusion. Transfusion 1987;27:228–33.

124. Tran TH, Day NP, Ly VC, Nguyen TH, Pham PL, Nguyen HP, et al. Blackwater fever in southern Vietnam: a prospective descriptive study of 50 cases. Clin Infect Dis. 1996;23:1274–81.

125. Bodi JM, Nsibu CN, Longenge RL, Aloni MN, Akilimali PZ, Tshibassu PM, et al. Blackwater fever in Congolese children: a report of clinical, laboratory features and risk factors. Malar J. 2013;12:e205.

126. Olupot-Olupot P, Engoru C, Uyoga S, Muhindo R, Macharia A, Kiguli S, et al. High frequency of blackwater fever among children presenting to hospital with severe febrile illnesses in Eastern Uganda. Clin Infect Dis. 2017;64:939–46.

127. Recht J, Ashley EA, White NJ. Safety of 8-aminoquinoline antimalarial medicines. Geneva: World Health Organization; 2014.

128. Jauréguiberry S, Thellier M, Ndour PA, Ader F, Roussel C, Sonneville R, et al. Delayed-onset hemolytic anemia in patients with travel-associated severe malaria treated with artesunate, France, 2011–2013. Emerg Infect Dis. 2015;21:804–12.

129. Lackritz EM, Campbell CC, Ruebush TK II, Hightower AW, Wakube W, Steketee RW, et al. Effect of blood transfusion on survival among children in a Kenyan hospital. Lancet. 1992;340:524–8.

130. Lackritz EM, Hightower AW, Zucker JR, Ruebush TK 2nd, Onudi CO, Steketee RW, et al. Longitudinal evaluation of severely anemic children in Kenya: the effect of transfusion on mortality and hematologic recovery. AIDS. 1997;11:1487–94.

131. Bojang KA, van Hensbroek MB, Palmer A, Banya WA, Jaffar S, Greenwood BM. Predictors of mortality in Gambian children with severe malaria anaemia. Ann Trop Paediatr. 1997;17:355–9.

132. WHO; Blood Transfusion Safety Team. The clinical use of blood: handbook. Geneva: World Health Organization; 2001. http://www.who.int/iris/handle/10665/42396. Accessed 15 Aug 2018.

133. WHO. Management of the child with a serious infection or severe malnutrition: guidelines for care at the first-referral level in developing countries. Geneva: World Health Organization; 2000.

134. Mpoya A, Kiguli S, Olupot-Olupot P, Opoka RO, Engoru C, Mallewa M, et al. Transfusion and treatment of severe anaemia in African children (TRACT): a study protocol for a randomised controlled trial. Trials. 2015;16:e593.

135. Kyeyune FX, Calis JC, Phiri KS, Faragher B, Kachala D, Brabin BJ, et al. The interaction between malaria and human immunodeficiency virus infection in severely anaemic Malawian children: a prospective longitudinal study. Trop Med Int Health. 2014;19:698–705.

136. van Eijk AM, Ayisi JG, ter Kuile FO, Misore AO, Otieno JA, Kolczak MS, et al. Malaria and human immunodeficiency virus infection as risk factors for anemia in infants in Kisumu, western Kenya. Am J Trop Med Hyg. 2002;67:44–53.

137. Phiri K, Esan M, van Hensbroek MB, Khairallah C, Faragher B, ter Kuile FO. Intermittent preventive therapy for malaria with monthly artemether-lumefantrine for the post-discharge management of severe anaemia in children aged 4–59 months in southern Malawi: a multicentre, randomised, placebo-controlled trial. Lancet Infect Dis. 2012;12:191–200.

138. Zucker JR, Ruebush TK 2nd, Obonyo C, Otieno J, Campbell CC. The mortality consequences of the continued use of chloroquine in Africa: experience in Siaya, western Kenya. Am J Trop Med Hyg. 2003;68:386–90.

139. Fleming AF. Tropical obstetrics and gynaecology. 1. Anaemia in pregnancy in tropical Africa. Trans R Soc Trop Med Hyg. 1989;83:441–8.

7

Characterization and monitoring of deltamethrin-resistance in *Anopheles culicifacies* in the presence of a long-lasting insecticide-treated net intervention

Madhavinadha Prasad Kona[1], Raghavendra Kamaraju[1]*[iD], Martin James Donnelly[2], Rajendra Mohan Bhatt[1], Nutan Nanda[1], Mehul Kumar Chourasia[1], Dipak Kumar Swain[1], Shrity Suman[1], Sreehari Uragayala[1], Immo Kleinschmidt[3] and Veena Pandey[4]

Abstract

Background: Deltamethrin-impregnated, long-lasting insecticidal nets (LLINs) were distributed in the study area from November 2014 to January 2015 to evaluate their impact on malaria transmission in the presence of insecticide-resistant vectors. Studies were carried out in 16 selected clusters in Keshkal sub-district, Chhattisgarh State, India to monitor and characterize deltamethrin resistance in *Anopheles culicifacies* sensu lato.

Results: Deltamethrin susceptibility of *An. culicifacies* decreased in a post-LLIN survey compared to a pre-LLIN survey and was not significant ($p > 0.05$) while, the knockdown values showed significant increase ($p < 0.05$). Pre-exposure to piperonyl butoxide, triphenyl phosphate showed synergism against deltamethrin ($p < 0.001$). Biochemical assays showed significantly ($p < 0.05$) elevated monooxygenases in 3 of 5 clusters in post-LLIN survey-I that increased to 10 of 11 clusters in post-LLIN survey-II, while esterases were found significantly elevated in all clusters and both enzymes were involved in conferring pyrethroid resistance, not discounting the involvement of *kdr* (L1014L/S) gene that was heterozygous and at low frequency (4–5%).

Conclusion: This field study, in a tribal district of India, after distribution of deltamethrin-impregnated LLINs showed decrease in deltamethrin susceptibility in *An. culicifacies*, a major vector of malaria in this study area and in India. Results indicated development of resistance as imminent with the increase in insecticide selection pressure. There is an urgent need to develop new vector control tools, with insecticide classes having novel mechanisms of resistance, to avoid or delay the onset of resistance. Regular insecticide resistance monitoring and mechanistic studies should be the priority for the malaria control programmes to suggest strategies for insecticide resistance management. The global commitment to eliminate malaria by 2030 needs various efforts that include development of combination vector control products and interventions and few are becoming available.

Keywords: *Anopheles culicifacies*, Deltamethrin, Long-lasting insecticidal nets (LLINs), Piperonyl butoxide (PBO), Triphenyl phosphate (TPP), Monooxygenase, Esterase, Knockdown resistance (*kdr*)

*Correspondence: kamarajur2000@yahoo.com
[1] ICMR-National Institute of Malaria Research, Sector-8, Dwarka, New Delhi 110077, India
Full list of author information is available at the end of the article

Background

In 2016, an estimated 216 million malaria cases were reported worldwide [1] with India contributing ≈ 1.1 million cases and 384 deaths [2]. The absence of an effective anti-malarial vaccine, spread of anti-malarial drug resistance in parasites and development of multi-insecticide resistance in mosquito vectors are key reasons for inadequate control of malaria [3].

During the years 2012–2017, a World Health Organization (WHO)-coordinated, Bill and Melinda Gates Foundation-sponsored project was conducted in 80 village clusters of community health centre (CHC) Keshkal, a tribal sub-district of district Kondagaon, Chhattisgarh State. The primary aim of the study was to find out the impact of insecticide resistance in malaria vectors on malaria burden, with a secondary aim to quantify how insecticide resistance patterns change in response to insecticide-based interventions. Chhattisgarh is a malaria-endemic state with just 2% of India's population, but which contributed 14% of annual malaria cases in 2016 and 17% in 2017 [2]. In CHC Keshkal, deltamethrin-impregnated, long-lasting insecticide-treated nets [(LLINs) Vestergaard PermaNet 2.0] were distributed from November 2014 to January 2015. Following the distribution, 98.4% of households had at least one LLIN; 80% of households were in possession of two or more LLINs, but only 38.7% of the households met the WHO universal coverage criterion of one LLIN per two persons. LLIN usage in children under 5 years old was 81.2% and in 5–14 years age range, it was 69.8%. LLIN use by adults was lower than that of children, probably due to an inadequate number of LLINs per household [4].

Anopheles culicifacies (Diptera: Culicidae) is reportedly the major malaria vector in Chhattisgarh State with *Anopheles fluviatilis* of more localized importance in hilly, forested regions [5]. In Chhattisgarh State, the National Malaria Control Programme has implemented DDT and pyrethroid-based indoor residual spraying (IRS) as the primary anti-malaria vector intervention [3]. Across India continuous use of DDT in IRS for the last 5 decades led to widespread resistance in *An. culicifacies*. Malathion (organophosphate) and pyrethroids were introduced into the IRS programme in 1970s and 1990s, respectively, in this State [5] and LLINs in 2009/10. Using the recent standard WHO-criteria [6], *An. culicifacies* in most districts of Chhattisgarh State were triple resistant to DDT, malathion and deltamethrin [3]. In the study area, the deltamethrin mortality in *An. culicifacies* across the 80 clusters was 97.01% in 2014–2015, and following the LLIN distribution the mortality decreased to 83.83% in 2015–2016 (KR, pers. comm.).

For proper management of insecticide resistance and better control of malaria through vector control interventions, early detection and accurate information on status of insecticide resistance and underlying resistance mechanisms in vectors are important. The present study was conducted in 16 clusters among the abovementioned 80 study clusters. The study coincided with LLIN distribution from November 2014 to January 2015. Deltamethrin susceptibility data were generated in 16 clusters by WHO tube test during the pre-LLIN distribution period in 2014 (pre-LLIN survey) and two surveys were conducted: post-LLIN survey-I in March/April 2015 and post-LLIN survey-II in October/November 2015. Synergistic bioassays were conducted with monooxygenases, carboxylesterases and esterases specific inhibitors piperonyl butoxide (PBO), triphenyl phosphate (TPP) and S,S,S-tributylphosphorotritioate (DEF), respectively, to explore the involvement of these detoxification enzyme families in phenotype resistance to insecticide deltamethrin (0.05%), alpha-cypermethrin (0.01%) and malathion (5%). Molecular studies were performed to evaluate the association between mutations in the voltage-gated sodium channel (*kdr*, L1014F/S) and deltamethrin resistance phenotype. Previous molecular studies on *An. culicifacies* showed very low frequencies of *kdr* mutations [7, 8]. Biochemical-based enzyme assays were performed to detect the target insensitive acetylcholinesterase (*i*AChE) and detoxification enzymes esterases, and monooxygenases activities in individual mosquitoes. Combined cytological and insecticide susceptibility studies were conducted in two seasons for detecting the prevalence of sibling species composition in *An. culicifacies,* a complex of 5 species which differ in seasonal prevalence, distribution patterns, host feeding preference, and vectorial potential [9].

The overall aim of the study was to assess the impact of LLINs on deltamethrin susceptibility and to inform insecticide resistance management planning.

Methods

Study area and survey periods

The study was conducted in 16 clusters of CHC Keshkal (20°5′1N and 81°35′12E) sub-district of Kondagaon district, Chhattisgarh State, India. The 16 clusters were selected among the 80 clusters included in the project, 4 from each primary health centre based on the mosquito productivity. Malaria transmission occurs primarily during the rainy season (June to October). Vector control for the past 20 years has been a twice yearly IRS application of alphacypermethrin @ 25 mg/m^2. The major agricultural crop in the study area is rice and pesticides used in this area include organophosphates (OP), pyrethroids and carbamates. The population in the selected 16 clusters ranged from 150 to 1100 and their geographical locations are shown in Fig. 1. Polyester LLINs (PermaNet 2.0)

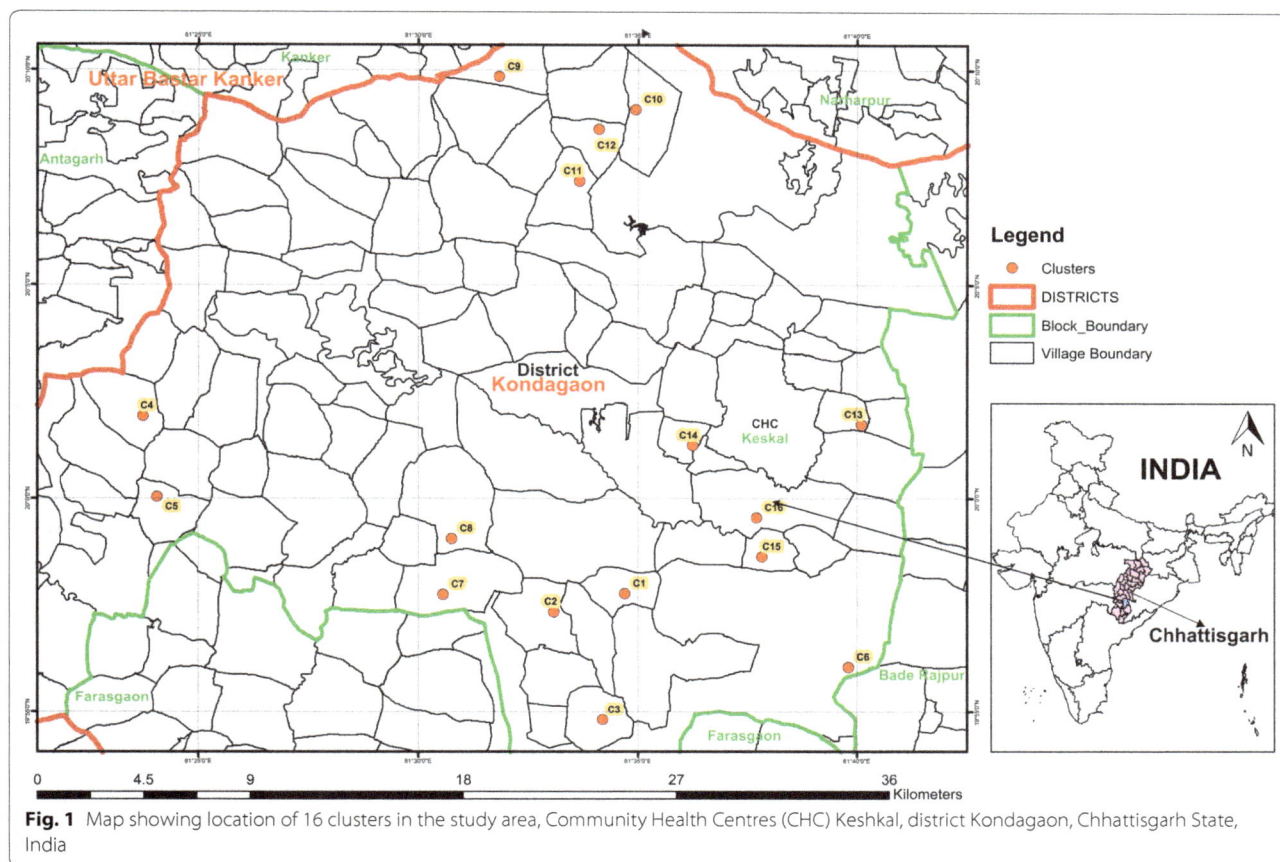

Fig. 1 Map showing location of 16 clusters in the study area, Community Health Centres (CHC) Keshkal, district Kondagaon, Chhattisgarh State, India

impregnated with deltamethrin (55 mg/m²) manufactured by M/s. Vestergaard Frandsen (Switzerland) were distributed in the study area from November 2014 to January 2015 in collaboration with the State health department [4]. In the present study 3 surveys were conducted in selected 16 clusters. One survey before LLIN distribution (pre-LLIN survey) in March, 2014 and two surveys after LLIN distribution in March/April, 2015 (post-LLIN survey-I) and October/November, 2015 (post-LLIN survey-II).

Adult susceptibility tests

Adult susceptibility tests were performed following WHO protocols [6]. The blood-fed female *An. culicifacies* mosquitoes were collected by aspirator during the early hours of the day and brought to the field laboratory in cloth cages (≈30 cu cm) covered with wet towels. Mosquitoes were identified based on morphological characters using a standard key [10]. The WHO diagnostic dose insecticide deltamethrin 0.05%-impregnated papers were obtained from the Vector Control Research Unit (VCRU), Universiti Sains Malaysia, Malaysia (http://www.usm.my). The fully fed mosquitoes were exposed to insecticide-impregnated papers for 1 h in 3–5 replicates (15–25 mosquitoes/replicate) along with appropriate controls. Number knocked down was noted at 3- or 5-min time intervals up to 1 h exposure. After exposure mosquitoes were transferred to holding tubes with glucose-soaked cotton pad for a 24-h holding period. The holding tubes were kept in a thermocol box with wet filter paper at the bottom to maintain relative humidity (70–80%) and temperature (27 ± 2 °C). After 24 h of holding, per cent mortality was scored. The corrected per cent mortality was calculated by applying Abbott's formula [11], if the mortality in control replicates was between 5 and 20% and if the control mortality is more than 20% the test was discarded. The susceptibility or resistance in mosquito populations was defined based on WHO criteria: 98–100% mortality indicates susceptibility, 90–97% mortality requires further confirmation of possible resistance, and below 90% mortality indicates resistance [6]. Statistical analysis was performed to determine knock-down time for 50 (KdT_{50}) using log-time probit regression analysis (PASW 16.0 version) and R statistical software version 3.4.1 for further analysis of adult susceptibility data and knockdown times. Data were fitted using generalized linear mixed effects statistical models (GLMMs) to describe the effects of collection round on deltamethrin mortality and median knockdown time. For mortality data, a binomial distribution model was used. The outcomes were assessed as a function of round as a fixed effect, and collection village as a random factor. Models were chosen based upon Akaike Information Criterion.

Synergist bioassay

Synergist bioassays were performed to assess possible involvement of insecticide resistance mechanisms in field-collected, blood-fed, female *An. culicifacies* from study clusters. Three synergists were used in this study, namely PBO (Sigma, USA) an inhibitor of monooxygenases [12], TPP (Sigma, USA) an inhibitor of carboxylesterases [13, 14] and DEF (Sigma, USA) an inhibitor of esterases [12]. Three insecticides were used deltamethrin (0.05%), alpha-cypermethrin (0.01%) and malathion (5%). The synergist (10%)-impregnated papers (12 cm × 15 cm Whatman No. 1 filter papers) were prepared in laboratory and insecticide-impregnated papers were procured from VCRU. Two treatments were compared for each test: insecticide alone and synergist + insecticide combination. In the insecticide alone, test mosquitoes were exposed to insecticide-impregnated papers for 1 h and during the synergist + insecticide combination assay mosquitoes were exposed for first 1 h to synergist-impregnated papers followed by 1 h to the insecticide-impregnated papers. After exposures mosquitoes were transferred to holding tubes for 24-h holding period and analysed as above to determine per cent mortality.

Isolation of mosquito DNA

After the adult deltamethrin susceptibility test, live and dead mosquitoes were separated and were preserved in isopropanol for DNA extraction. Mosquito DNA was isolated by DNAzol method (Invitrogen) essentially following manufacturer's instructions.

L1014F/S kdr genotyping

The point mutation [Leucine (L) to Phenylalanine (F)] in codon 1014 of the voltage-gated sodium channel (VGSC) was identified by Amplification Refractory Mutation System (ARMS) following the method described by Singh et al. [15] with minor modifications. Another point mutation Leucine (L) to Serine (S) in the same codon was identified by Primer Induced Restriction Analysis PCR (PIRA-PCR) following method developed by Singh et al. [7] with minor modifications. Products were visualized on 2% agarose gel and stained with ethidium bromide (0.5 µg/ml).

DNA sequencing

In order to validate PCR-based *kdr* genotyping, DNA sequence was performed. A part of IIS4-IIS5 linked to IIS-6 segment of VGSC was amplified by two separate PCRs following published protocol by Singh et al. [15]. Purified amplicons were sequenced by Central Instrumentation Facility (CIF), South Campus, University of Delhi, New Delhi.

Biochemical assays

Blood-fed female *An. culicifacies* mosquitoes were collected from the study area in post-LLIN surveys-I and -II and transported to National Institute of Malaria Research (NIMR) field unit to obtain F_1 progeny. Two- to 3-day old, sugar-fed, female mosquitoes were transported in liquid nitrogen to NIMR, New Delhi. Acetylcholinesterase, esterase and monooxygenase enzyme assays were performed following WHO guidelines [16]. Assay reaction absorbance was measured by NanoQuant Infinite® M200 PRO ELISA reader (Tecan Group Ltd, Switzerland) with inbuilt Magellan 7.2 software. The results were analysed by Mann–Whitney U test.

Native-PAGE

Native-PAGE was performed for determining α- and β-esterase profile of the susceptible laboratory and field strains of *An. culicifacies* following the procedure described by Prasad et al. [14]. The imageJ (Wayne Rasband, ImageJ 1.50i, National Institutes of Health, USA, http://imagej.nih.gov/ij/) software was used to carry out densitometry analysis of the stained native gels for estimating esterase activity.

Sibling species identification

Field collected *An. culicifacies* sibling species were identified based on cytological method. The ovaries were removed from individual semi-gravid female mosquitoes and were stored in Carnoy's fixative (1:3 acetic acid: methanol). Then overies were processed for preparing polytene chromosomes described by Green and Hunt [17]. The complex of *An. culicifacies* sibling species A, B, C, and D was identified based on paracentric inversions on the X-chromosome and chromosome arm 2 [9].

To study the susceptibility of sibling species to insecticides deltamethrin (0.05%) and malathion (5%), semi-gravid females were exposed to insecticide-impregnated papers for 1 h [18]. After 1-h exposure, ovaries were extracted from dead (malathion)/knockdown (deltamethrin) and live mosquitoes separately and processed as above. The per cent mortality of given sibling species was calculated based on formula given below. Susceptibility or resistance in sibling species were determined based on WHO criteria [6].

$$\% \text{ mortality in given sibling species}$$
$$= \frac{\text{No dead of given species}}{\text{Total alive + dead of given species}} \times 100$$

Results

Adult susceptibility test

The cluster-wise data of per cent mortality and knock-down (KdT_{50}) values are given in Table 1. The cluster-specific mortalities for *An. culicifacies* to deltamethrin ranged from 62 to 100%. There was a small but non-significant ($p > 0.05$) decrease in mortality over the 3 surveys, pre- and post-LLIN surveys-I and -II (Fig. 2a). The knockdown indices (KdT_{50}) calculated from the data in

Table 1 Susceptibility status of *Anopheles culicifacies* to deltamethrin (0.05%) collected from 16 clusters of three surveys, once in before LLIN distribution (Pre LLIN survey) and twice after LLIN distribution (Post LLIN-survey I and II)

Clusters	Pre LLIN survey (March, 2014)		Post LLIN survey-I (March/April, 2015)		Post LLIN survey-II (October/November, 2015)	
	% Mortality (n)	KdT$_{50}$ (min)	% Mortality (n)	KdT$_{50}$ (min)	% Mortality (n)	KdT$_{50}$ (min)
C1	100 (91)	30	96 (113)	57	97 (103)	50
C2	95 (103)	40	97 (112)	54	98 (102)	56
C3	100 (33)	36	96 (77)	43	92 (84)	45
C4	98 (100)	33	97 (79)	27	87 (95)	59
C5	99 (105)	31	99 (115)	41	92 (81)	41
C6	99 (98)	43	97 (63)	39	91 (81)	50
C7	98 (83)	38	84 (100)	67	97 (78)	42
C8	84 (100)	62	89 (104)	57	93 (82)	48
C9	97 (67)	43	90 (70)	37	77 (91)	53
C10	99 (103)	33	97 (71)	35	82 (60)	55
C11	93 (29)	53	92 (53)	46	83 (104)	60
C12	100 (94)	31	93 (44)	37	99 (78)	39
C13	96 (98)	44	100 (49)	31	92 (94)	54
C14	99 (120)	36	89 (56)	38	62 (101)	77
C15	98 (101)	43	86 (48)	38	96 (82)	44
C16	90 (100)	36	100 (59)	42	96 (72)	40

C cluster, *n* number of samples, *min* minutes, *KdT$_{50}$* 50% knockdown in mosquitoes population

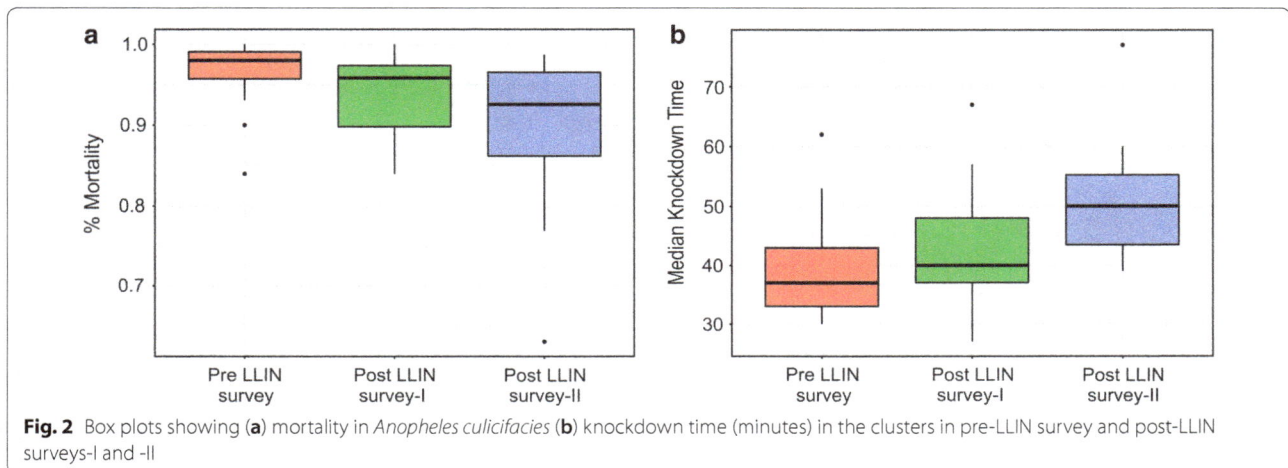

Fig. 2 Box plots showing (**a**) mortality in *Anopheles culicifacies* (**b**) knockdown time (minutes) in the clusters in pre-LLIN survey and post-LLIN surveys-I and -II

1-h exposure showed a trend in increase in KdT_{50} values. The median knockdown time increased significantly ($p < 0.05$) over the 3 surveys (Fig. 2b).

Synergistic assay

Synergistic data of exposure to synergist PBO, TPP and DEF are depicted in Fig. 3. Field-collected *An. culicifacies* mosquitoes were pre-exposed to the monooxygenases-specific synergist, PBO showed synergism to insecticides deltamethrin and alpha-cypermethrin. The average deltamethrin per cent mortalities significantly increased from 90 ± 7 to 99 ± 1 in PBO + deltamethrin exposed population compared to deltamethrin alone ($p < 0.001$, χ^2 test). The knockdown times (KdT_{50}) in these assays decreased from 53 ± 2 min (mean $\pm$ SD) to 24 ± 4 min at 95% CI. Against alpha-cypermethrin, the per cent mortalities significantly increased from 63 ± 14 to 95 ± 4 ($p < 0.001$, χ^2 test) and was higher than those recorded for deltamethrin exposure, and KdT_{50} values decreased from 159 ± 95 to 39 ± 4 min. The PBO showed antagonism to malathion and the mean per cent mortalities slightly decreased from 73 ± 9 to 63 ± 14 ($p > 0.05$, χ^2 test), and KdT_{50} values increased from 50 ± 6 to 59 ± 12 min.

Carboxylesterase-specific inhibitor TPP showed synergism to insecticides deltamethrin, alpha-cypermethrin and malathion. TPP showed similar kind of synergistic effect as PBO on deltamethrin and the average per cent

mortalities increased significantly from 90 ± 7 to 99 ± 1 ($p < 0.001$, χ^2 test) and KdT_{50} values decreased from 53 ± 2 min to 34 ± 7 min. For alpha-cypermethrin the per cent mortalities slightly increased from 63 ± 14 to 70 ± 0 ($p > 0.05$, χ^2 test) and KdT_{50} values decreased from 159 ± 95 to 68 ± 0 min. The TPP synergism in pyrethroids may be due to esterase bonds in the structure. The average malathion per cent mortalities increased significantly from 73 ± 9 to 85 ± 11 in TPP + malathion exposed population compared to malathion alone exposed population ($p < 0.001$, χ^2 test) and KdT_{50} values decreased from 50 ± 6 to 35 ± 8 min.

The non-specific esterases inhibitor DEF showed strong synergism against alpha-cypermethrin and malathion in *An. culicifacies* compared to synergist TPP. The per cent mortalities increased significantly from 63 ± 4 to 83 ± 0 for alpha-cypermethrin and 73 ± 9 to 95 ± 0 for malathion ($p < 0.05$, χ^2 test) and KdT_{50} values decreased from 159 ± 95 to 76 ± 0 and 50 ± 6 to 30 ± 0, respectively.

Knockdown resistance gene (*kdr*) frequency

The live and dead *An. culicifacies* mosquitoes from deltamethrin susceptibility tests were genotyped for two *kdr* mutations Leu-Phe (L1014F) and Leu-Ser (L1014S). Genotype association studies showed L1014F and L1014S *kdr* mutations conferred significant protection against deltamethrin in both the surveys. In post-LLIN survey-I, 408 mosquitoes (25 alive and 383 dead) were examined and there was a significant difference in codon 1014 genotypes between categories (Fisher's exact test $p < 0.0002$). The 1014F and 1014S allele frequencies were, respectively, 0.12 and 0.10 in alive mosquitoes and 0.03 for both the alleles in dead mosquitoes. In post-LLIN survey-II, 490 mosquitoes (72 alive and 418 dead) were examined and again there was a significant difference in codon 1014 genotypes between categories (Fisher's exact test $p < 1.15 \times 10^{-6}$) of the 1014F and 1014S alleles were 0.12 and 0.10 in live mosquitoes and 0.05 and 0.02 in dead mosquitoes, respectively (Table 2). The *kdr* mutations in the genome were also confirmed by DNA sequencing in 9 sequences of DNA from individual field-collected mosquitoes.

Acetylcholinesterase assay

The mean % inhibition of AChE was 98 ± 1.1 (% inhibition $\pm$ Standard Deviation) in susceptible *An. culicifacies* laboratory population. The AChE inhibition studies were conducted in field-collected *An. culicifacies* from 5 clusters in post-LLIN survey-I and 11 clusters in post-LLIN survey-II. The mean % AChE inhibition values during the post-LLIN survey-I were between 82 ± 7.1 and 99 ± 1 and during the post-LLIN survey-II values were between 96 ± 4.2 and 98 ± 1.2, indicating decrease in % AChE

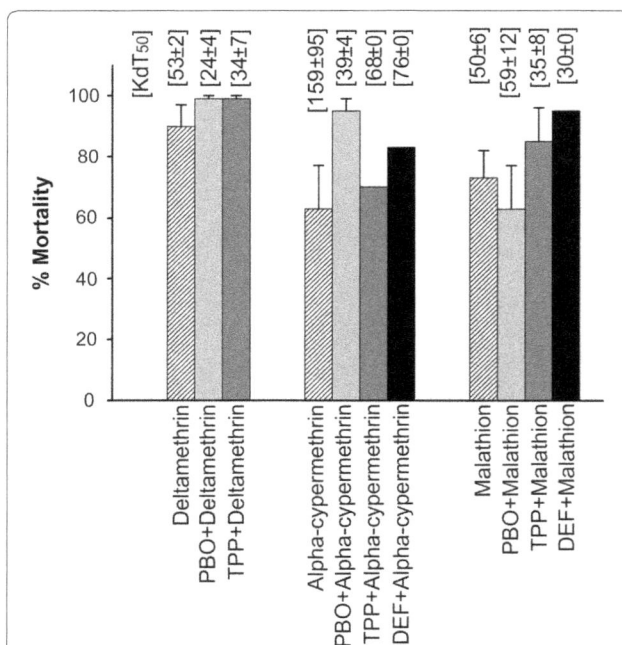

Fig. 3 Synergistic bioassay data of pre-exposure to PBO, TPP followed by deltamethrin exposure, and pre-exposure to PBO, TPP, DEF followed by alpha-cypermethrin, and malathion exposure. Calculated KdT_{50} values in minutes

Table 2 Distribution of L1014, 1014F and 1014S knockdown resistance (*kdr*) alleles frequency in *An. culicifacies* collected from 16 clusters

Survey	n	Phenotype	Genotypes						Allele frequency			p value (Fisher exact test)		
			L/L	L/F	F/F	L/S	S/S	F/S	L	F	S	L vs F	L vs S	Post LLIN survey-I vs Post LLIN survey-II
Post LLIN survey-I	408	Alive	15	6	0	3	1	0	0.78	0.12	0.10	0.002	0.053	0.015
		Dead	336	21	0	26	0	0	0.94	0.03	0.03			
Post LLIN survey-II	490	Alive	48	10	3	7	3	1	0.78	0.12	0.10	0.008	0.001	
		Dead	362	38	0	17	0	1	0.93	0.05	0.02			

n number of samples, *p* probability value

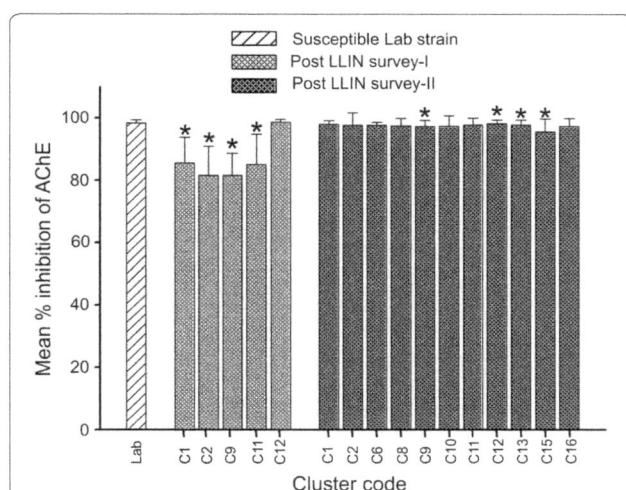

Fig. 4 Inhibition of AChE activity by propoxur in *Anopheles culicifacies* collected from study area and susceptible laboratory strain. Asterisk % inhibition is significantly low compared to susceptible strain

inhibition in field *An. culicifacies* population at very low frequency (Fig. 4).

Detoxification enzymes esterases and monooxygenases

The detoxification enzymes esterases and monooxygenases, activities were determined on *An. culicifacies* samples from 5 to 11 clusters in post-LLIN surveys-I and −II, respectively. The mean α- and β-esterases and monooxygenases enzyme activities in susceptible laboratory and field populations are shown in Table 3. The results of α- and β-esterases showed significantly (p < 0.05, Mann–Whitney U test,) higher activity in *An. culicifacies* field populations in both the surveys except in one cluster (C11) for β-esterase in post-LLIN survey-II. The maxim α- and β-esterase activity in susceptible lab strain was considered as the threshold activity and was 0.92 and 0.74 mmol/min/mg. The population beyond threshold α- and β-esterase activity value were 67 and 71% in post-LLIN survey-I and 61 and 58% in post-LLIN survey-II (Fig. 5). For monooxygenases,

significantly increased activity (p < 0.05, Mann–Whitney U test) levels were found in mosquito population in 3 and 9 clusters in post-LLIN surveys -I and −II, respectively. The maximum monooxygenase activity in susceptible lab strain was considered as the threshold activity and was 0.0039 mmol/mg. In post-LLIN survey-I, 33% of the population showed monooxygenase activities beyond threshold, while it was 60% in post-LLIN survey-II (Fig. 5). The results indicated elevated levels of α- and β-esterases and monooxygenases in the field population compared to susceptible counterpart.

Native-PAGE

The electrophoretic migration pattern of esterase activity in female *An. culicifacies* of susceptible laboratory strain and field population from selected clusters aged between 1 and 4-day post-eclosion are shown in Fig. 6. In susceptible laboratory strain, 3 bands (designated as Band-1, Band-2, Band-3), while in field populations, 2 bands (designated as Band-A and Band-B) were localized on PAGE by staining with α- and β-naphthol acetate. The calculated R_f (retention factor) values for Band-1, -2 and -3 were 0.63, 0.54 and 0.30, respectively, while Band-A and -B were 0.56 and 0.17. The esterase bands were characterized as alpha/or beta esterases by the appearance of brown or purple bands on the native-PAGE. Band-1, -2 and -3 and Band-A and -B, all hydrolyze generally both alpha- and beta- naphthyl acetates though Band-2 and Band-A seems more specific to beta-naphthyl acetate hydrolysis as seen in purple colour on native-PAGE. On analysis with Image J software, the Band-A intensity of field-collected *An. culicifacies* was 2.5–10 times more than that of Band-2 intensity of susceptible laboratory *An. culicifacies*, as shown in Fig. 6, indicating possible overexpression of Band-A in field population.

Sibling species prevalence

Distribution of *An. culicifacies* sibling species was examined among the 16 clusters, during post-LLIN surveys-I

Table 3 Mean α- and β-esterase and monooxygenases activities in field collected _An. culicifacies_

Survey	Site	n	α-Esterases, mmol/min/mg ± SD	β-Esterases, mmol/min/mg ± SD	Monooxygenases, mmol/mg ± SD
	Susceptible lab strain	47	0.62 ± 0.08	0.50 ± 0.09	0.0026 ± 0.0005
Post LLIN survey-I	C1	60	1.14 ± 0.56*	1.04 ± 0.53*	0.0030 ± 0.0011
	C2	60	1.27 ± 0.55*	1.27 ± 0.61*	0.0034 ± 0.0014*
	C9	53	1.50 ± 0.72*	1.38 ± 0.70*	0.0027 ± 0.0011
	C11	123	1.37 ± 0.65*	1.38 ± 0.70*	0.0031 ± 0.0013*
	C12	30	1.39 ± 0.64*	1.14 ± 0.67*	0.0064 ± 0.0024*
Post LLIN survey-II	C1	47	1.78 ± 0.79*	1.39 ± 0.68*	0.0047 ± 0.0017*
	C2	47	0.91 ± 0.47*	0.74 ± 0.43*	0.0042 ± 0.0020*
	C6	47	1.05 ± 0.57*	0.86 ± 0.52*	0.0075 ± 0.0045*
	C8	34	1.57 ± 0.77*	1.12 ± 0.70*	0.0052 ± 0.0015*
	C9	47	0.91 ± 0.54*	0.81 ± 0.52*	0.0040 ± 0.0020*
	C10	47	1.35 ± 0.72*	0.98 ± 0.62*	0.0058 ± 0.0024
	C11	47	0.90 ± 0.60*	0.72 ± 0.57	0.0051 ± 0.0016*
	C12	47	1.20 ± 0.58*	0.87 ± 0.54*	0.0040 ± 0.0022*
	C13	47	0.96 ± 0.55*	0.82 ± 0.56*	0.0045 ± 0.0016*
	C15	47	1.05 ± 0.60*	0.91 ± 0.52*	0.0034 ± 0.0013*
	C16	47	2.25 ± 1.00*	2.21 ± 1.08*	0.0065 ± 0.0018*

_n_ number of samples, _SD_ standard deviation

* Levels of enzyme activity significantly increased compared with susceptible lab strain

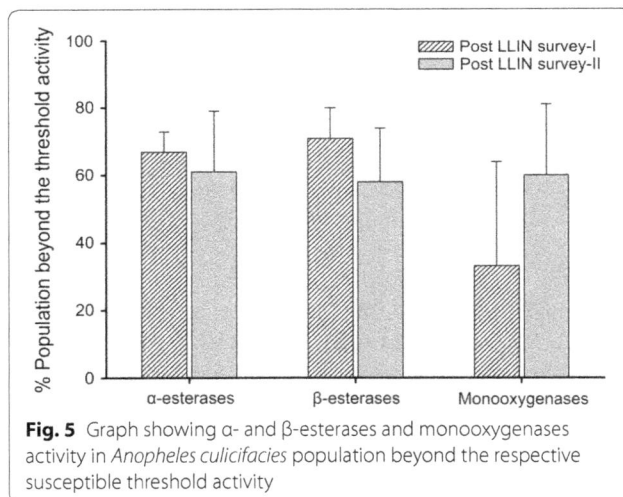

Fig. 5 Graph showing α- and β-esterases and monooxygenases activity in _Anopheles culicifacies_ population beyond the respective susceptible threshold activity

and -II. Species B and C were present in this area and % distribution of the sibling species is given in Additional file 1: Table S1. The overall sibling species B was dominant over species C (90.2 vs 9.8% in post-LLIN survey-I; 89.6 vs 10.4% in post-LLIN survey-II).

In post-LLIN survey-I the 1-h percent mortality to malathion in species B was 77% and in post-LLIN survey-II it was 66%, while in species C 1-h percent mortality was 25 and 71%, respectively (Additional file 1: Table S2). The response to malathion between two sibling species

was significant during the post-LLIN survey-I ($p < 0.05$, χ^2 test) while in post-LLIN survey-II, it was insignificant. Overall, it can be stated that both species B and C developed resistance to malathion.

The deltamethrin 24-h percent mortalities ranged from 62 to 100% in 16 clusters in both the surveys (Table 1). In post-LLIN survey-I the 1-h % knockdown of species B was 71 and in post-LLIN survey-II it was 100, while species C registered 67 and 100% knockdown, respectively (Additional file 1: Table S2). Thus, both species showed similar susceptibility status.

Discussion

Development of deltamethrin resistance and resistance mechanisms were studied in the major malaria vector _An. culicifacies_ from 16 clusters in tribal sub-district Keshkal of Kondagaon district in Chhattisgarh State, central India. Cohort-based active case surveillance (ACS) studies conducted in these LLIN-distributed 80 clusters by Chourasia et al. [19] reported 84% reduction in malaria incidence and sub-clinical malaria significantly in children under 14 years old. Continued use of LLINs was ensured through regular monitoring by village level, women, health volunteers and the usage of LLINs in children under 5 years old was 81.2% and children between 5 and 14 years old was 69.8% [4].

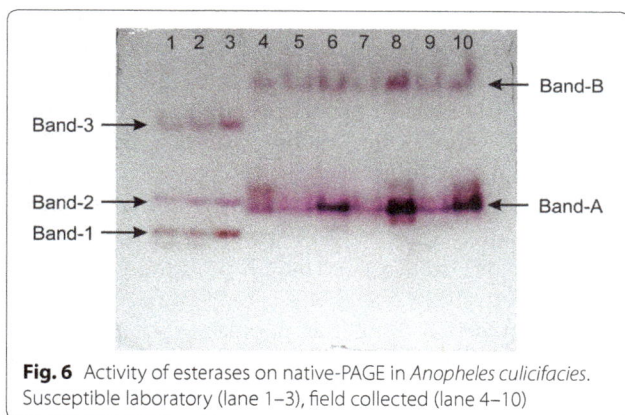

Fig. 6 Activity of esterases on native-PAGE in *Anopheles culicifacies*. Susceptible laboratory (lane 1–3), field collected (lane 4–10)

In the 16 study clusters selected for the study, adult susceptibility tests against WHO diagnostic dosage of deltamethrin (0.05%) showed decrease in susceptibility in both the surveys after LLIN distribution compared to before LLIN distribution, and was not significant ($p > 0.05$), while, the knockdown time values (KdT_{50}) showed significant increase ($p < 0.05$). A 10-year study (1998–2007) in Western Uganda to assess the impact of conventionally treated insecticide-treated nets (ITNs), deltamethrin (25 mg/sq m), cyfluthrin (50 mg/sq m), and alpha-cypermethrin (50 mg/sq m) on development of resistance in *Anopheles gambiae* showed 4-fold increase in KdT_{50} values with about 1.5-fold decrease in susceptibility [20]. However, a 3-year study by Vulule et al. [21] in Western Kenya on the impact of permethrin-treated nets and curtains stated 2.4-fold increase in tolerance in the first year that did not sustain in subsequent years although reduction in parous rate and malaria transmission was observed. Such observations on variations in deltamethrin phenotypic resistance among study villages was observed owing to selection from IRS and ITNs [22]. There are conflicting observations on sustainability of pyrethroid resistance in time and space owing to selection by vector control interventions.

In this study, *An. culicifacies* showed 20–76% mortality to another pyrethroid insecticide, 0.01% alpha-cypermethrin, during post-LLIN survey-I which could be due to alpha-cypermethrin IRS in these areas in past 20 years. *An. culicifacies* registered 63–84% mortality to malathion (5%). The species has shown resistance to malathion and variable susceptibility to alpha-cypermethrin and deltamethrin. The development of deltamethrin resistance in *An. culicifacies* was earlier reported from different tribal districts of Chhattisgarh State, during studies in 2009 and 2010 by Bhatt et al. [5] with mortality in the range of 42–99% while to malathion it was 10–73%. In studies conducted during the same period (2009–2010) in 32 tribal districts of other four states: Andhra Pradesh,

Jharkhand, Odisha, and West Bengal, *An. culicifacies* registered deltamethrin resistance in 4 districts, to malathion in 14 districts, while in some districts this species reported susceptibility to both the insecticides [23]; 9 tribal districts of Madhya Pradesh showed resistance to deltamethrin in 2 districts and to malathion in 7 districts [24]. In another study in 2014 in 5 tribal districts of southern Odisha, this species showed resistance to both insecticides [25]. *An. culicifacies* in the study area in district Kondagaon and other districts of Chhattisgarh State and congruent states, Odisha and Madhya Pradesh showed variable susceptibility status to deltamethrin and malathion. The pyrethroid resistance in these areas was likely due to selection by pyrethroid IRS and LLINs and possibly agriculture.

Cytogenetic studies in the study area in 2 surveys (post-LLIN surveys-I and -II) indicated prevalence of species B (90%) and C (10%). Sibling species B and C were characterized as resistant to deltamethrin in post-LLIN survey-I but susceptible in post-LLIN survey-II. In the present study the % knockdown in *An. culicifacies* increased by 12% in post-LLIN survey-II (from 71% in post-LLIN survey-I to 83% in post-LLIN survey-II) (Additional file 1: Table S2) at the end of 1 h exposure, stating an increase in susceptibility which is also reflected in sibling species. However, the proportionate increase in the sibling species could not be seen as the sample size was low for cytotaxonomical studies as only readable polytene chromosome plates could be examined that resulted in loss of samples. The sample size for species C was very low. Species B showed trend for susceptibility. Both the species were resistant to malathion in the surveys and without differences between the species. In a study conducted in Andhra Pradesh in 1980s in cash crop cultivated areas, *An. culicifacies* developed malathion resistance in the absence of malathion IRS. Species C reportedly developed resistance (4–6% mortality) to malathion faster than species B (48–76% mortality) [18]. Agricultural use of insecticides has been suggested as one of the major drivers of insecticide resistance in malaria vectors *An. gambiae* [26, 27] and *An. culicifacies* [28].

In the present study, preliminary information on metabolic resistance mechanisms was obtained using synergist bioassays; PBO showed synergism against pyrethroid insecticides, deltamethrin and alpha-cypermethrin with mortalities increased by 9% against deltamethrin and 32% against alpha-cypermethrin, and KdT_{50} values decreased 2 times and 4 times, respectively. Previous studies showed PBO synergistic effect against deltamethrin resistance in *Anopheles stephensi* from India [29], *An. gambiae* from Cameroon, Central Africa [12], *Anopheles arabiensis* from rural southeastern Tanzania [30], and *Anopheles hyrcanus* from Thailand [31].

In the present study, PBO showed antagonistic effect against organophosphate insecticide malathion and mortalities decreased by 10% and increased KdT_{50} values by 9 min in mosquitoes exposed to PBO+ malathion compared to malathion alone, exposures indicating non-involvement of monooxygenase in conferring malathion resistance in *An. culicifacies* in the study area. The current observation is consistent with previous PBO synergist studies conducted with malathion-resistant *An. culicifacies* population from Surat [13] and in *An. stephensi* from Pakistan [32].

Synergistic bioassays with TPP showed synergism against pyrethroids and organophosphate insecticides. The mortalities increased by 9% for deltamethrin, 7% for alpha-cypermethrin and by 12% for malathion, and KdT_{50} values decreased by 1.5, 2.3 and 1.5 times, respectively, in *An. culicifacies* pre-exposed to TPP. Synergist DEF for non-specific esterases showed synergism against alpha-cypermethrin and malathion insecticides and the mortalities increased by 20% against alpha-cypermethrin and by 22% against malathion, and the KdT_{50} values decreased by 2.1 and 1.6 times, respectively. DEF showed stronger synergistic effect than TPP for malathion. A study by Raghavendra et al. [13] showed carboxylesterase-mediated malathion resistance mechanism in *An. culicifacies* from Surat by TPP. In another study, Matowo et al. [30] showed moderate synergism of TPP against pyrethroid in *An. arabiensis* from rural southeastern Tanzania. In another study, significant increase in deltamethrin activity was reported in *An. hyrcanus*-resistant population from Thailand by pre-exposure to 4% PBO and 0.25% DEF [32]. In a study by Akiner and Eksi [33], PBO and DEF synergistic studies with *Culex pipiens L* showed decrease in toxicity of malathion and pyrethroids, permethrin and deltamethrin from 4 different locations in Turkey. Esterases can mediate resistance to organophosphates, carbamates and pyrethroids which are rich with ester-bonds [34]. Similarly, in the present study, pyrethroid and organophosphate resistant-*An. culicifacies* showed involvement of carboxylesterase and other non-specific esterases in conferring resistance as probable minor mechanisms.

Identification of biochemical-based resistance mechanisms using microplate enzyme assays in a single mosquito is more informative and could be of value in early detection of insecticide resistance in field population [13, 35–37]. Target site insensitive AChE assay and detoxification enzymes, α- and β-esterases and monooxygenases assays were conducted in F1-female *An. culicifacies* in a few selected clusters in post-LLIN surveys-I and -II. The biochemical enzyme assay results of field samples were compared with susceptible laboratory strain of *An. culicifacies*. The AChE assay results indicated low level of AChE activity in the population. AChE is a target of 2 major classes of insecticides: OP and carbamates. In the study area, *An. culicifacies* is susceptible to carbamate insecticide bendiocarb (93 to 100%). The activities of α- and β-esterases and monooxygenases significantly increased in post-LLIN surveys compared to susceptible mosquitoes. In post-LLIN survey-I, 67 and 71% of population showed α- and β-esterases activity beyond the susceptible threshold value while it decreased to 61 and 58%, respectively, in post-LLIN survey-II. For monooxygenases activity, 33% of the population in post-LLIN survey-I showed activity beyond susceptible threshold value while it increased to 60% in post-LLIN survey-II. The role of esterases and cytochrome P450s in pyrethroid resistance was reported in *An. stephensi* from Dubai and India [38, 39]. Hemingway [32] reported quantitative increase of esterases in malathion-resistant *An. stephensi* from Pakistan. Safi et al. [40] reported metabolic-based mechanisms, including esterases, P450s and glutathione S-transferase (GSTs) combined with insensitive AChE in *An. stephensi* from Kunar and Nangarhar provinces of Afghanistan, and further stated that the high level of resistance was found in the Nangarhar population compared to the Kunar population due to selection of different pesticides in agriculture, and, more importantly, higher number of deltamethrin-treated LLINs were distributed in the Nangarhar population. Esterases can provide resistance to organophosphates, carbamates and pyrethroids which are rich with ester-bonds [34]. Thus, it can be stated that cytochrome P450s can mediate resistance to all classes of insecticides, increased enzyme activity can be brought about by gene amplification, upregulation, coding sequence mutations, or by a combination of these mechanisms.

Genotyping results demonstrated a significant association between *kdr* genotype and deltamethrin phenotype. Overall *kdr* frequencies were low (4-5%) but suggest that *kdr* plays a role in evolving deltamethrin resistance in *An. culicifacies* in addition to mixed-function oxidases (MFOs) and esterases. Similarly, studies by Dykes et al. [8] on *An. culicifacies* from different states in India, namely Gujarat, Chhattisgarh, Haryana and Rajasthan, *kdr* mutations were in low frequency (1.2–7.4%) and mostly in heterozygous condition, and exhibited significant protection against deltamethrin.

In the present field studies in a tribal area, the multiple insecticide-resistant *An. culicifacies* has shown a decrease in deltamethrin susceptibility owing to the use of deltamethrin-impregnated LLINs. Involvement of MFOs as major mechanism associated with esterases in conferring deltamethrin resistance in *An. culicifacies* was observed as supported by synergistic bioassays.

Conclusion

This field study in a tribal district of India, after distribution of deltamethrin-impregnated LLINs, showed a decrease in deltamethrin susceptibility in the major vector of malaria *An. culicifacies*. Among 16 study clusters, the observed variations in mortality were not significant although the knockdown times were found to increase significantly. Monooxygenases as a major mechanism associated with esterases were found to confer deltamethrin resistance and synergized by specific synergists. The *kdr* gene frequencies was mostly in heterozygous condition and showed significant protection against deltamethrin. To suggest appropriate insecticide-reliant stratagies for insecticide resistance management in disease vectors, information on insecticide-specific biochemical resistance mechanism/s is important. This is to avoid the introduction of insecticides that have similar insecticide resistance mechanism/s that could confer cross resistance to the replaced insecticide. Results of the main study in 80 clusters suggested the continued use of LLINs in spite of developing resistance, which is imminent with the increase in insecticide selection pressure, with a caution for pro-active efforts to develop new vector control tools especially with insecticide classes with novel mechanisms of resistance [41]. To avoid or delay the onset of resistance, various strategies are propounded by Global Plan for Insecticide Resistance Management (GPIRM) [42]. The global commitment to eliminate malaria by 2030 needs immediate efforts that include establishment of infrastructure for regular insecticide resistance monitoring, development of combination vector control products and interventions for effective vector control.

Abbreviations

LLINs: long-lasting insecticidal nets; IRS: indoor residual spraying; ITN: insecticide-treated net; IIR: implications of insecticide resistance; PHC: Primary Health Centres; CHC: Community Health Centres; WHO: World Health Organization; SD: standard deviation; DDT: dichlorodiphenyltrichloroethane; kdr: knock down resistance; iAChE: insensitive acetylcholinesterase; AChE: acetylcholinesterase; PBO: piperonyl butoxide; TPP: triphenyl phosphate; DEF: S,S,S-tributylphosphorotritioate; OP: organophosphate; KdT: knock-down time; GLMMs: generalized linear mixed effects statistical models; GPIRM: global plan for insecticide resistance management; VCRU: Vector Control Research Unit; PCR: polymerase chain reaction; ARMS: amplification-refractory mutation system; PIRA: primer-introduced restriction analysis; VGSC: voltage-gated sodium channels; DNA: deoxyribonucleic acid; NIMR: National Institute of Malaria Research; ELISA: enzyme-linked immunosorbent assay; PAGE: polyacrylamide gel electrophoresis; MFOs: mixed-function oxidases; CIF: Central Instrumentation Facility.

Authors' contributions

KR, KMP, RMB, MJD, IK and VP designed the study. KMP and DKS field work and bioassays, KMP and SS conducted biochemical and molecular experiments. MKC and MJD performed statistical tests. NN and KMP performed cytotaxonomical work. KR, KMP, and MJD analysed the data. KMP and KR drafted the manuscript. KR, RMB, MKC, MJD, SU, IK and VP reviewed the manuscript. All authors made intellectual input to the study. All authors read and approved the final manuscript.

Author details

[1] ICMR-National Institute of Malaria Research, Sector-8, Dwarka, New Delhi 110077, India. [2] Liverpool School of Tropical Medicine, Liverpool, UK. [3] Department of Infectious Disease Epidemiology, London School of Hygiene and Tropical Medicine, London, UK. [4] Department of Biotechnology, Kumaun University, Nainital, India.

Acknowledgements

The authors express sincere thanks to the Director, ICMR-National Institute of Malaria Research for the continuous encouragement for this study and support for providing laboratory facilities. The authors sincerely thank technical assistance rendered by Mr. Krishna Gopal, Mr. Udayveer Singh, Mr. Rajan K. Reddiar and insect collectors. We would also like to thank technical and laboratory staff of IIR Project Field Site at Kondagaon, NIMR Field Unit, Raipur and NIMR HQ, New Delhi for their support in undertaking field and laboratory activities. We would also like to thank CEO, Chhattisgarh Infotech Promotion Society (CHiPS) and Mr. Abhishek Dewangan (CHiPS) for their support in map preparation.

Competing interests

The authors declare that they have no competing interests.

Funding

Funding was provided by the Bill and Melinda Gates Foundation (Grant Number OPP 1062754), which has no role in the planning, study design, data collection or writes up. This research forms part of a multi-country study coordinated by the Global Malaria Programme of the World Health Organization, Geneva.

References

1. World Health Organization. World malaria report 2017. Geneva: World Health Organization; 2017.
2. National Vector Borne Disease Control Programme. Malaria situation in India. http://www.nvbdcp.gov.in/Doc/malaria-situation.pdf. Accessed 3rd Jun 2018.
3. Raghavendra K, Velamuri PS, Verma V, Elamathi N, Barik TK, Bhatt RM, et al. Temporo-spatial distribution of insecticide-resistance in Indian malaria vectors in the last quarter-century: need for regular resistance monitoring and management. J Vector Borne Dis. 2017;54:111–30.
4. Raghavendra K, Chourasia MK, Swain DK, Bhatt RM, Uragayala S, Dutta GDP, et al. Monitoring of long-lasting insecticidal nets (LLINs) coverage versus utilization: a community-based survey in malaria endemic villages of Central India. Malar J. 2017;16:467.
5. Bhatt RM, Sharma SN, Barik TK, Raghavendra K. Status of insecticide resistance in malaria vector, Anopheles culicifacies in Chhattisgarh state, India. J Vector Borne Dis. 2012;49:36–8.
6. WHO. Test procedures for insecticide resistance monitoring in malaria vector mosquitoes (second edition). Geneva: World Health Organization; 2016. (http://www.who.int/malaria/publications/atoz/9789241511575/en/).
7. Singh OP, Dykes CL, Das MK, Pradhan S, Bhatt RM, Agrawal OP, et al. Presence of two alternative kdr-like mutations, L1014F and L1014S, and a novel mutation, V1010L, in the voltage gated Na+ channel of Anopheles culicifacies from Orissa, India. Malar J. 2010;9:146.
8. Dykes CL, Kushwah RBS, Das MK, Sharma SN, Bhatt RM, Veer V, et al. Knockdown resistance (kdr) mutations in Indian Anopheles culicifacies populations. Parasit Vectors. 2015;8:333.
9. WHO, Regional Office for South-East Asia. 1998. Anopheline species complexes in South-East Asia. WHO Regional Office for South-East Asia. http://www.who.int/iris/handle/10665/204780.
10. Christophers SR. The fauna of British India including Ceylon and Burma. London: Taylor and Francis; 1933.

11. Abbott WS. A method of computing the effectiveness of an insecticide. J Econ Entomol. 1925;18:265–7.

12. Nwane P, Etang J, Chouaïbou M, Toto JC, Koffi A, Mimpfoundi R, et al. Multiple insecticide resistance mechanisms in *Anopheles gambiae* populations from Cameroon, Central Africa. Parasit Vectors. 2013;6:41.

13. Raghavendra K, Subbarao SK, Pillai MKK, Sharma VP. Biochemical mechanisms of malathion resistance in Indian *Anopheles culicifacies* (Diptera: Culicidae) sibling species A, B, and C: microplate assays and synergistic studies. Ann Entomol Soc Am. 1998;91:834–9.

14. Prasad KM, Raghavendra K, Verma V, Velamuri PS, Pande V. Esterases are responsible for malathion resistance in *Anopheles stephensi*: a proof using biochemical and insecticide inhibition studies. J Vector Borne Dis. 2017;54:226–32.

15. Singh OP, Bali P, Hemingway J, Subbarao SK, Dash AP, Adak T. PCR-based methods for the detection of L1014 kdr mutation in *Anopheles culicifacies* sensu *lato*. Malar J. 2009;8:154.

16. WHO. Techniques to detect insecticide resistance mechanisms (field laboratory mannual). Geneva: World Health Organization; 1998. http://www.who.int/malaria/publications/atoz/who_cds_cpc_mal_98_6/en/.

17. Green CA, Hunt RH. Interpretation of variation in ovarian polytene chromosomes of *Anopheles funestus* Giles, *A. parensis* Gillies, and *A. aruni*. Genetica. 1980;51:187–95.

18. Raghavendra K, Vasantha K, Subbarao SK, Pillai MKK, Sharma VP. Resistance in *Anopheles culicifacies* sibling species B and C to malathion in Andhra Pradesh and Gujarat States. India. J Am Mosq Control Assoc. 1991;7:255–9.

19. Chourasia MK, Raghavendra K, Kleinschmidt I, Bhatt RM, Swain DK, Knox TB, et al. Impact of long-lasting insecticidal nets on prevalence of subclinical malaria among children in the presence of pyrethroid resistance in *Anopheles culicifacies* in Central India. Int J Infect Dis. 2017;57:123–9.

20. John R, Ephraim T, Andrew A. Reduced susceptibility to pyrethroid insecticide treated nets by the malaria vector *Anopheles gambiae s.l.* in western Uganda. Malar J. 2008;7:92.

21. Vulule JM, Beach RF, Atieli FK, Mount DL, Roberts JM, Mwangi RW. Longterm use of permethrin-impregnated nets does not increase Anopheles gambiae permethrin tolerance. Med Vet Entomol. 1996;10:71–9.

22. Yahouédo GA, Cornelie S, Djègbè I, Ahlonsou J, Aboubakar S, Soares C, et al. Dynamics of pyrethroid resistance in malaria vectors in southern Benin following a large scale implementation of vector control interventions. Parasit Vectors. 2016;9:385.

23. Raghavendra K, Barik TK, Sharma SK, Das MK, Dua VK, Pandey A, et al. A note on the insecticide susceptibility status of principal malaria vector *Anopheles culicifacies* in four states of India. J Vector Borne Dis. 2014;51:230–4.

24. Mishra AK, Chand SK, Barik TK, Dua VK, Raghavendra K. Insecticide resistance status in *Anopheles culicifacies* in Madhya Pradesh, central India. J Vector Borne Dis. 2012;49:39–41.

25. Sahu SS, Gunasekaran K, Vijayakumar T, Jambulingam P. Triple insecticide resistance in *Anopheles culicifacies*: a practical impediment for malaria control in Odisha State, India. Indian J Med Res. 2015;142:59–63.

26. Chouaibou M, Etang J, Brevault T, Nwane P, Hinzoumbe CK, Mimpfoundi R, et al. Dynamics of insecticide resistance in the malaria vector *Anopheles gambiae s.l.* from an area of extensive cotton cultivation in Northern Cameroon. Trop Med Int Health. 2008;13:476–86.

27. Diabate A, Baldet T, Chandre F, Akoobeto M, Guiguemde TR, Darriet F, et al. The role of agricultural use of insecticides in resistance to pyrethroids in *Anopheles gambiae s.l.* in Burkina Faso. Am J Trop Med Hyg. 2002;67:617–22.

28. Subbarao Y. Susceptibility status of *Anopheles culicifacies* to DDT, dieldrin and malathion in village Mangapeta, District Warangal, Andhra Pradesh. J Commun Dis. 1979;11:41–3.

29. Raghavendra K, Barik TK, Sharma P, Bhatt RM, Srivastava HC, Sreehari U, et al. Chlorfenapyr: a new insecticide with novel mode of action can control pyrethroid resistant malaria vectors. Malar J. 2011;10:16.

30. Matowo NS, Munhenga G, Tanner M, Coetzee M, Feringa WF, Ngowo HS, et al. Fine-scale spatial and temporal heterogeneities in insecticide resistance profiles of the malaria vector, *Anopheles arabiensis* in rural south-eastern Tanzania. Wellcome Open Res. 2017;2:96.

31. Sumarnrote A, Overgaard HJ, Marasri N, Fustec B, Thanispong K, Chareonviriyaphap T, et al. Status of insecticide resistance in *Anopheles* mosquitoes in Ubon Ratchathani province, Northeastern Thailand. Malar J. 2017;16:299.

32. Hemingway J. The biochemical nature of malathion resistance in *Anopheles stephensi* from Pakistan. Pest Biochem Physiol. 1982;17:149–55.

33. Akıner MM, Ekşi E. Evaluation of insecticide resistance and biochemical mechanisms of *Culex pipiens L.* in four localities of east and middle mediterranean basin in Turkey. Int J Mosq Res. 2015;2:39–44.

34. Feyereisen R. Insect cytochrome P450. Compr Mol Insect Sci. 2005;4:1–77.

35. Hemingway J. A note on simple biochemical methods for resistance detection and their field application in Sri Lanka. Pest Manag Sci. 1989;27:281–5.

36. Brogdon WG. Biochemical resistance detection: an alternative to bioassay. Parasitol Today. 1989;5:56–60.

37. Cordón-Rosales C, Beach RF, Brogdon WG. Field evaluation of methods for estimating carbamate resistance in *Anopheles albimanus* mosquitos from a microplate assay for insensitive acetylcholinesterase. Bull World Health Organ. 1990;68:323.

38. Enayati AA, Vatandoost H, Ladonni H, Townson H, Hemingway J. Molecular evidence for a kdr-like pyrethroid resistance mechanism in the malaria vector mosquito *Anopheles stephensi*. Med Vet Entomol. 2003;17:138–44.

39. Ganesh KN, Urmila J, Vijayan VA. Pyrethroid susceptibility and enzyme activity in two malaria vectors, *Anopheles stephensi* (Liston) and *A. culicifacies* (Giles) from Mysore, India. Indian J Med Res. 2003;117:30–8.

40. Safi NHZ, Ahmadi AA, Nahzat S, Ziapour SP, Nikookar SH, Fazeli-Dinan M, et al. Evidence of metabolic mechanisms playing a role in multiple insecticides resistance in *Anopheles stephensi* populations from Afghanistan. Malar J. 2017;16:100.

41. Kleinschmidt I, Knox TB, Mnzava AP, Kafy HT, Mbogo C, Ismail BA, et al. Implications of insecticide resistance for malaria vector control with longlasting insecticidal nets: a WHO-coordinated, prospective, international, observational cohort study. Lancet Infect Dis. 2018;18:640–9.

42. WHO. Global plan for insecticide resistance management in malaria vectors.). Geneva: World Health Organization; 2012. http://www.who.int/malaria/publications/atoz/gpirm/en/.

8

Low uptake of malaria testing within 24 h of fever despite appropriate health-seeking among migrants in Myanmar: a mixed-methods study

Kyaw Thu Hein[1]*[iD], Thae Maung Maung[1], Kyaw Ko Ko Htet[1], Hemant Deepak Shewade[2,3], Jaya Prasad Tripathy[2,3], Swai Mon Oo[4], Zaw Lin[5] and Aung Thi[6]

Abstract

Background: There is limited information on uptake of malaria testing among migrants who are a 'high-risk' population for malaria. This was an explanatory mixed-methods study. The quantitative component (a cross sectional analytical study-nation-wide migrant malaria survey in 2016) assessed the knowledge; health-seeking; and testing within 24 h of fever and its associated factors. The qualitative component (descriptive design) explored the perspectives of migrants and health care providers [including village health volunteers (VHV)] into the barriers and suggested solutions to increase testing within 24 h. Quantitative data analysis was weighted for the three-stage sampling design of the survey. Qualitative data analysis involved manual descriptive thematic analysis.

Results: A total of 3230 households were included in the survey. The mean knowledge score (maximum score 11) for malaria was 5.2 (0.95 CI 5.1, 5.3). The source of information about malaria was 80% from public health facility staff and 21% from VHV. Among 11 193 household members, 964 (8.6%) had fever in last 3 months. Health-seeking was appropriate for fever in 76% (0.95 CI 73, 79); however, only 7% (0.95 CI 5, 9) first visited a VHV while 19% (0.95 CI 16, 22) had self-medication. Of 964, 220 (23%, 0.95 CI 20, 26) underwent malaria blood testing within 24 h. Stable migrants, high knowledge score and appropriate health-seeking were associated with testing within 24 h. Qualitative findings showed that low testing within 24 h despite appropriate health-seeking was due to lack of awareness among migrants regarding diagnosis services offered by VHV, delayed health-seeking at public health facilities and not all cases of fever being tested by VHV and health staff. Providing appropriate behaviour change communication for migrants related to malaria, provider's acceptance for malaria testing for all fever cases and mobile peer volunteer under supervision were suggested to overcome above barriers.

Conclusions: Providers were not testing all migrant patients with fever for malaria. Low uptake within 24 h was also due to poor utilization of services offered by VHV. The programme should seriously consider addressing these barriers and implementing the recommendations if Myanmar is to eliminate malaria by 2030.

Keywords: Malaria diagnosis and treatment, Knowledge, health-seeking, Barriers, Suggestion, Uptake of malaria testing, Myanmar, SORT IT

*Correspondence: hein.z.ze@gmail.com
[1] Department of Medical Research, Ministry of Health and Sports, Yangon, Myanmar
Full list of author information is available at the end of the article

Background

To decrease the risk of severe complications and onward transmission of malaria, World Health Organization has emphasized early diagnosis and prompt treatment within 24–48 h of onset of symptoms [1]. The advent and scale up of rapid diagnostic test kits has made early and accurate diagnosis of malaria possible at primary health care and community settings [1, 2].

Myanmar is one of the five countries in south-east Asia (Cambodia, Laos, Thailand, Vietnam, and Myanmar) with artemisinin resistance [3]. Myanmar reported more than 152 thousand confirmed cases in 2015, accounting over 70% of total cases in the greater Mekong sub-region [3, 4]. It has high malaria morbidity and mortality rates, third highest in the south-east Asia region and highest in the greater Mekong sub-region [5].

With the countrywide scale-up of malaria prevention and control measures under the National malaria control programme (NMCP), the malaria morbidity significantly reduced from 11.2 to 4.1 cases per 1000 population and malaria deaths reduced from 1707 to 92 between 2005 and 2014, respectively [4].

Malaria is now largely concentrated among hard-to-reach and other 'populations at risk', including internal migrants (henceforth called as migrants) who also work as forest goers and outdoor night-time workers [4, 5]. Ensuring universal access to malaria diagnosis and treatment among migrants is central to eliminating malaria by 2030 and Myanmar is no exception [4]. To eliminate malaria from the greater Mekong sub-region and prevent the spread of artemisinin drug resistant malaria, regional artemisinin-resistance initiative (RAI) project was launched in Myanmar with the support of the Global Fund in 2014. One of the objectives was to provide access to prevention, diagnosis and treatment for migrants [6, 7].

Previously, there have been studies on awareness of malaria, health-seeking behaviour and testing within 24 h of fever among general population in the endemic regions of Myanmar and treatment-seeking preferences within the public sector amongst migrant workers. However malaria testing among migrants has not been reported yet [8–10].

A nation-wide migrant malaria survey was conducted jointly by the department of medical research (DMR) and NMCP in 2016 to understand the knowledge, attitude and health-seeking behaviour towards malaria and the ownership and utilization of insecticide-treated bed nets among the migrant population in the selected townships of RAI supported areas. This provides us a unique opportunity to study the uptake of malaria testing (within 24 h) among migrant population and the associated factors. Secondly, a systematic qualitative enquiry into the perspective of migrants and health care providers including village health volunteers (VHV) into barriers to access malaria testing despite availability of rapid diagnostic test kits at village level would aid the programme in designing specific interventions or modify existing intervention to suit the needs of migrants.

Hence, this mixed-methods study was conducted to assess the knowledge; health-seeking; and malaria testing within 24 h of fever and its barriers among migrant population in RAI supported areas in Myanmar.

Methods
Study design

This was an explanatory mixed-methods study involving a quantitative component (a cross sectional analytical study-nation-wide migrant malaria survey 2016) followed by a descriptive qualitative component where the findings from the quantitative component fed into the qualitative component [11].

General study setting

In the south-east Asian region, the Republic of the Union of Myanmar is neighboured by countries like Bangladesh, India, China, Laos and Thailand in the North and East [5]. It is divided into seven states, seven regions and one capital territory (Nay Pyi Taw Council territory). There are 74 districts with 330 townships [12]. In 2014, 9.4 million people were internal migrants, which is approximately 20% of the total population. Myanmar has grown to be the largest migration source country in greater Mekong sub-region [13].

Specific study setting
Health care services in Myanmar

Township hospitals provide health care services including laboratory, dental and also major surgical procedures and act as the first referral health institutions. Station hospitals including sub-township hospitals are basic medical units with essential curative elements, such as general medical, surgical and obstetric facilities. Basic health staff (BHS) are the major community-based health workforce responsible for providing comprehensive health care services and are stationed at rural health centre (RHC) or the sub-centres under RHCs. RHC is staffed by health assistant, one lady health visitor, five midwives and five public health supervisors. Sub-centre is staffed by one midwife and one public health supervisor. VHVs work under the supervision of midwife at sub-centre [12].

National malaria control programme (NMCP)

In Myanmar, 291 out of 330 townships are malaria endemic with about 44 million at risk of the disease. All cases of fever should undergo a rapid diagnostic test

Low uptake of malaria testing within 24 h of fever despite appropriate health-seeking among migrants...

95

(SD-Bioline malaria Ag P.f/P.v combo 25) within 24 h for detection of *Plasmodium falciparum* and/or non-*falciparum* infections. It is available at all public health facilities including township/station hospitals and RHCs. The same has also been decentralized at the level of BHS and VHV. All malaria diagnostic and treatment services are offered free of cost [14].

RAI supported area

Of the 291 endemic townships, 52 were covered under RAI project in 2015 and 76 were covered in 2016. In RAI areas, migrant clusters were divided into three categories: permanent or semi-permanent work settings with high social capital, where substantial results can be achieved for malaria control (category I); semi-permanent settings with moderate social capital, where substantial community-based results can be achieved for malaria control (category II); and small, often temporary work sites, with low social capital and resource availability (category III) [8].

Study population
Quantitative component

The migrant populations covered in the nation-wide migrant malaria survey 2016 (August to December) were included. A migrant was a male or female of any age who temporarily lived in the selected townships for less than 3 years duration of stay and not registered as a native villager in the village census.

The planning for the nation-wide migrant malaria survey 2016 was done based on the 2015 data profile. As 52 townships were part of the RAI areas in 2015, it was decided in 2015 to implement the 2016 survey in these 52 townships.

A multistage sampling procedure was employed. Out of 52 townships in RAI areas, 13 townships were excluded as they were geographically hard-to-reach. Among 39 townships, 27 were selected by probability proportional to size (Fig. 1). In each selected township, migrant clusters were mapped and five migrant clusters were randomly (simple random sampling) selected. A

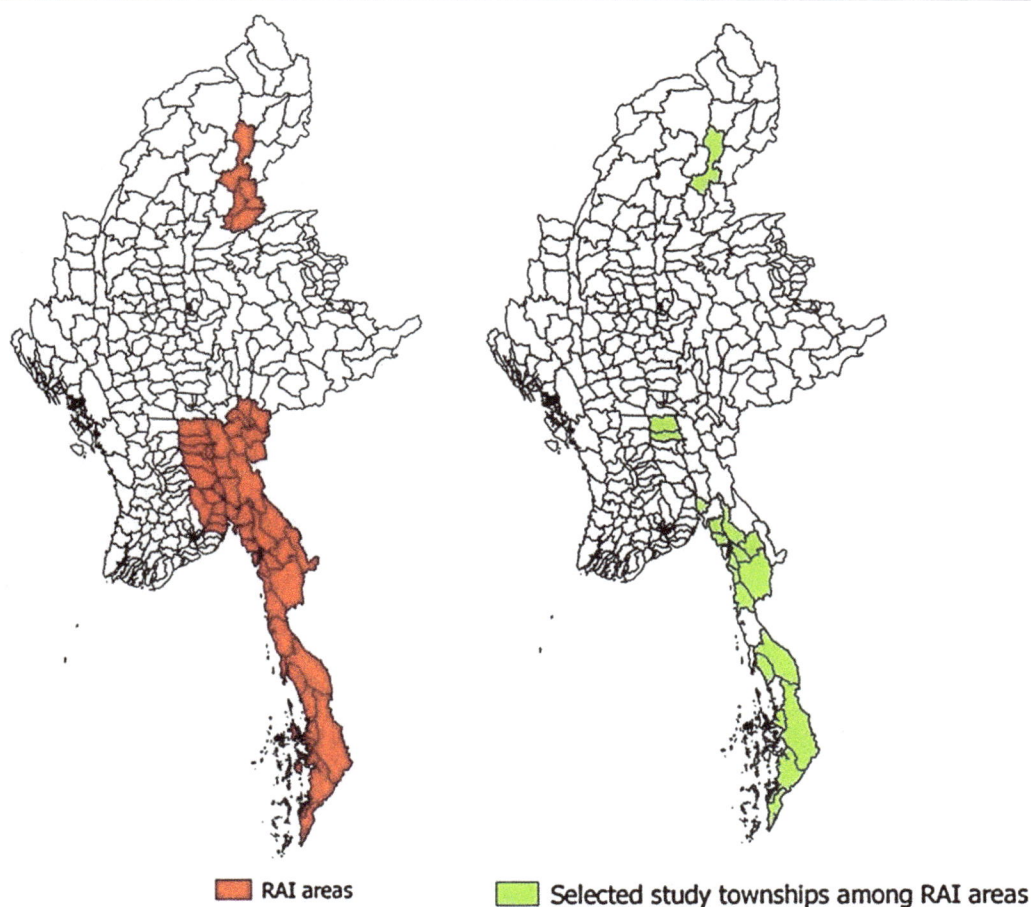

Fig. 1 Map of Myanmar showing regional artemisinin-resistance initiative (RAI) townships and selected RAI townships for nation-wide migrant malaria survey in 2016

list of households in these five clusters was prepared. A total of 125 households were selected from 5 clusters in each township and the number of households sampled from each cluster was proportional to the total number of households in that migrant cluster.

Qualitative component

Two state/regions (Bago and Sagaing) that contained the RAI areas and had large sites of migrant population with wide variations in occupational characteristic were purposively selected. In each state/region, two RAI townships that were part of the nation-wide migrant malaria survey 2016 were selected (Taungoo and Yedashe Townships in Bago, Homalin and Kalay Townships in Sagaing).

Programmatic challenges in early diagnosis and treatment of malaria among migrants and their suggested solutions were explored. Provider side (VHV, BHS, local vector-borne disease control staff, regional medical officer) and client side participants (migrant people of varying occupation with or without history of fever in last 3 months) were selected based on their availability at the time of visits by the research team—December 2017 to January 2018 (convenience sampling).

Data collection

Quantitative component

Under migrant malaria survey 2016, face-to-face interview was conducted with preferably the female adult respondent or any other adult using a semi-structured questionnaire by a trained interviewer (see Additional file 1).

Questionnaires were pre-tested and all interviewers were well trained in each state/region by NMCP and DMR. The questionnaires included household characteristics, household level knowledge regarding malaria (cause, transmission, risk groups, signs/symptoms, prevention and treatment) and household level sources of information. Among individuals in the household who had fever in last 3 months, health-seeking for fever and testing for malaria diagnosis within 24 h was assessed.

Qualitative component

One-to-one interviews among key informants and focus group discussion-FGD among migrant people were conducted. Two researcher officers from DMR who were medical doctors conducted the qualitative enquiry. They were trained in qualitative research. Though they were not part of NMCP, they were knowledgeable and understood the implementation of NMCP and the RAI project.

One-to-one interviews and FGDs were arranged at the place convenient to participants: health facility or residence for key informants, work sites for migrants. Participants were informed the purpose of the study before the

visit. Interview and FGD guides were pilot-tested before implementation in field (see Additional files 2 and 3). Audio recording (after consent) and verbatim notes were taken during the interview. After the interview/FGD was over, the summary was read back to the participants to ensure participant validation. Field notes (if any) from observations during data collection were also made.

Data management and analysis

Quantitative component

Survey data was double-entered and validated using Epi-Data entry software (version 3.1, EpiData Association, Odense, Denmark) and analysed using STATA (version 12.1 STATA Corp., College Station, TX, USA).

The household and individual characteristics were described by using means (95% confidence interval (CI)) for continuous variables and frequencies and proportions (95% CI) for categorical variables. Questions related to knowledge about malaria—its cause, transmission, signs and symptoms, vulnerable groups, severity, prevention were scored as 1 (yes) and 0 (no). Specific scores were summed up to get overall knowledge score for each individual in the survey (see Additional file 4). The maximum and minimum scores were 0 and 11. The score were then categorized into high (>5) and low (≤ 5) based on the mean cut-off value. Health-seeking was considered 'appropriate' if the visit was made to a VHV or any public health facility or private clinics of doctor/health assistant/auxiliary midwife.

The factors associated with malaria testing within 24 h of fever were determined using multivariable log-binomial regression analysis. Variables having a p-value less than 0.2 in unadjusted analysis were included. Prevalence ratio (unadjusted and adjusted) along with 95% CI were calculated.

The quantitative analysis was weighted for the multi-stage sampling design and hence, weighed estimates have been provided [15]. The probability of selection of townships and selection of the migrant cluster were used to derive the weights. Information on probability of selection of households within clusters was not available and not included in the weights.

Qualitative component

The transcripts were made based on the verbatim notes and listening to the audio records. The transcripts obtained were compiled and the principal investigator (KTH) read the transcripts to become familiar with the data. Manual descriptive thematic analysis was used to analyze the transcripts [11, 16]. It was reviewed by a second investigator (KKKH) to reduce bias and interpretive credibility. The decision on coding rules and theme generation was done by using standard procedures and in consensus [17]. Any differences between the two were resolved by discussion. This approach in health-care research is flexible and appropriate for determining solutions to real-world problems. Both inductive and deductive codes were generated. Similar codes were combined into themes [11]. The codes/themes were related back to the original data to ensure that the results are a reflection of the data [18]. The themes were and relevant quotes were summarized in a table. The findings were reported by using 'Consolidated Criteria for Reporting Qualitative Research' [19].

Results

Quantitative findings

Migrant household characteristics

A total of 3230 households were included and their characteristics have been summarized in Table 1. The mean household size was 3.4, 40% (n = 1294) stayed in temporary shelters made by themselves, 39% (n = 1251) belonged to migrant category III.

Knowledge regarding malaria among migrant households

The mean (0.95 CI) knowledge score (maximum score 11) among households was 5.2 (5.1, 5.3) (Table 1). The knowledge on cause, transmission, vulnerable groups, symptoms, prevention and treatment regarding malaria has been summarized in Figs. 2, 3. Though 89% knew that malaria is caused by mosquito bites, 31% did not mention mosquitoes as a source of transmission. Fourteen percent recognized under-five children as a vulnerable group for malaria, while 42% did not know anything about vulnerable groups. Fever and chills/rigors were mentioned as symptoms of malaria by 61% and 67% household, respectively. Malaria was preventable and treatable according to 91% and 96% household, respectively. Western medicine was identified as a treatment option for malaria by 86% of the households.

Sources of information regarding malaria among migrant households

The sources of information regarding malaria are depicted in Fig. 4. Public health facility staff and VHV were the sources for 80% and 21% households, respectively.

Migrants with fever: characteristics and health-seeking

Of 11,193 household members, 964 (8.6%) had fever in last 3 months. The individual, household and health-seeking characteristics of these 964 individuals have been summarized in Table 2. Mean age was 24.6 years and 55% were males. After the onset of fever, health care was first sought from the sub-centre/RHC, township/

Table 1 Background characteristics of the migrant households in regional artemisinin resistance initiative (RAI) areas of Myanmar, 2016 [N = 3230]

Variables	N	Proportion[a]	(95% CI)
Total	3230	100	–
House hold size			
1–2	1153	35.7	(33.8, 37.5)
3–4	1254	38.8	(36.9, 40.7)
5–6	600	18.5	(17.1, 20.1)
>6	223	6.9	(5.9, 7.8)
Mean	3230	3.4	(3.3, 3.5)
Housing status			
Own house	1294	40.1	(38.2, 41.9)
Rental	40	1.2	(0.8, 1.6)
Employer allowed place	1624	50.3	(48.3, 52.2)
Not known	272	8.4	(7.2, 9.7)
Main occupation of family			
Farming/gardening/rubber plantation work	1231	38.1	(36.2, 40.0)
Stone mining work/brick kiln work	817	25.3	(23.5, 27.0)
Merchant	38	1.2	(0.8, 1.5)
Daily wage labourer	572	17.7	(16.3, 19.2)
Not known	572	17.7	(16.2, 19.2)
Migrant category[b]			
Category I	756	23.4	(21.8, 24.9)
Category II	982	30.4	(28.6, 32.2)
Category III	1251	38.7	(36.8, 40.6)
Not known	241	7.5	(6.3, 8.6)
Duration of intention to stay			
Less than 6 months	415	12.8	(11.4, 14.3)
6 months to 1 year	204	6.3	(5.3, 7.3)
More than 1 year	366	11.3	(10.2, 12.5)
Not known	2245	69.5	(67.7, 71.4)
Location of intent to go back			
Native place	1263	39.1	(37.2, 41.0)
Another workplace within township	195	6.1	(5.2, 6.9)
Another workplace another township	72	2.2	(1.7, 2.8)
Not known	1700	52.6	(50.7, 54.6)
Knowledge score			
Mean	3230	5.2	(5.1, 5.3)

Weighted estimates given taking into account the sampling design

CI confidence interval

[a] Column percentages

[b] Permanent or semi-permanent work settings with high social capital, where substantial results can be achieved for malaria control (category I); semi-permanent settings with moderate social capital, where substantial community-based results can be achieved for malaria control (category II); and small, often temporary work sites, with low social capital and resource availability (category III)

station hospital, private clinic of midwife or health assistant and private clinic of doctor by 39%, 10%, 9%, and 7%, respectively. Seven percent first visited a VHV while

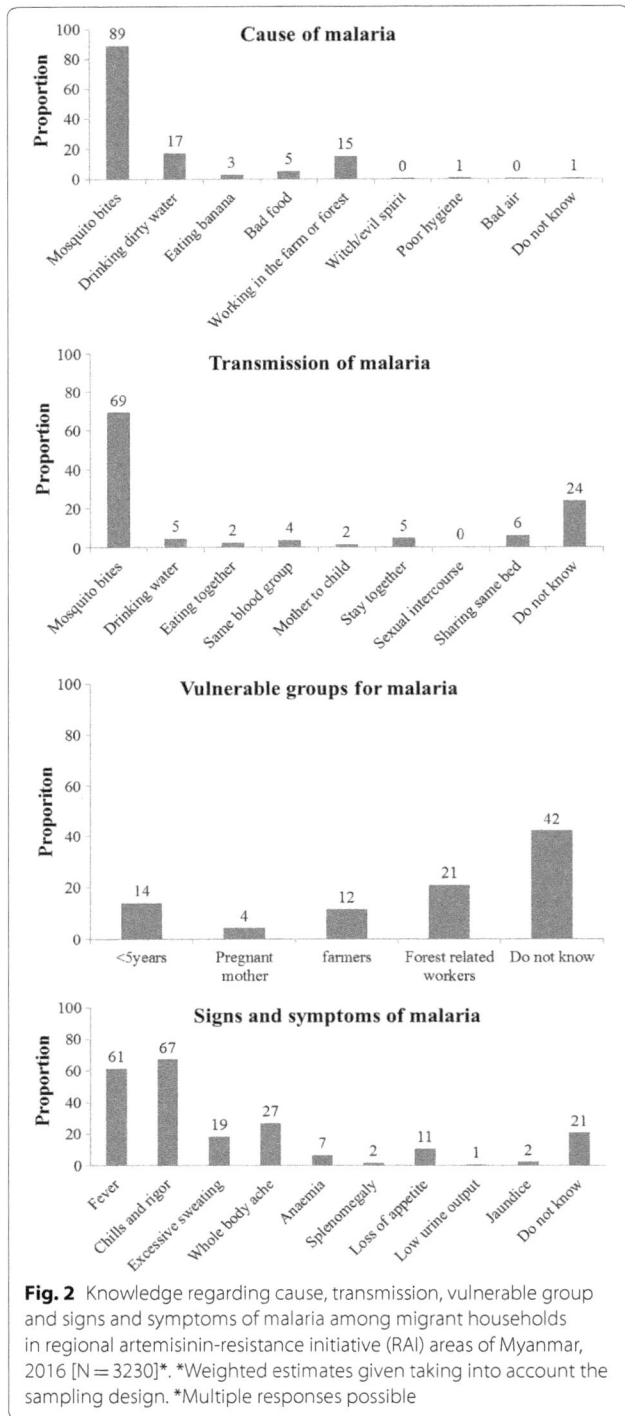

Fig. 2 Knowledge regarding cause, transmission, vulnerable group and signs and symptoms of malaria among migrant households in regional artemisinin-resistance initiative (RAI) areas of Myanmar, 2016 [N = 3230]*. *Weighted estimates given taking into account the sampling design. *Multiple responses possible

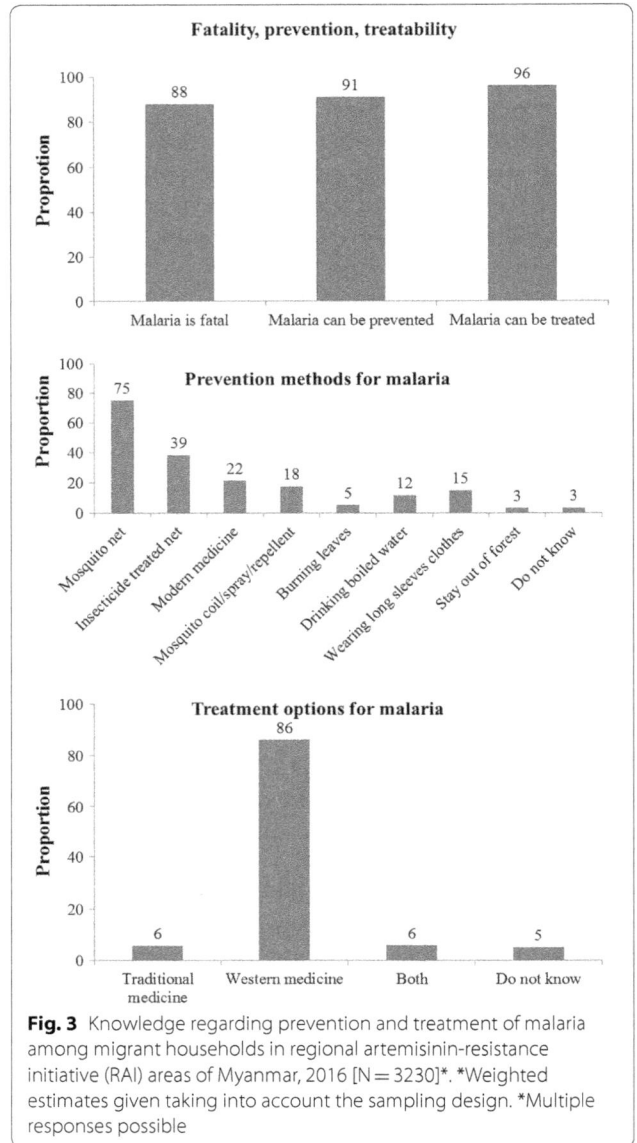

Fig. 3 Knowledge regarding prevention and treatment of malaria among migrant households in regional artemisinin-resistance initiative (RAI) areas of Myanmar, 2016 [N = 3230]*. *Weighted estimates given taking into account the sampling design. *Multiple responses possible

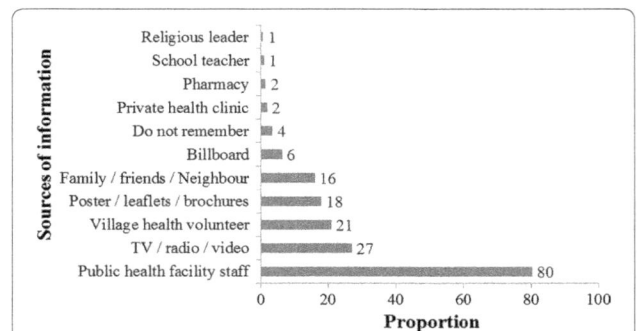

Fig. 4 Sources of information for knowledge regarding malaria among migrant households in regional artemisinin-resistance initiative (RAI) areas of Myanmar, 2016 [N = 3230]*. *Weighted estimates given taking into account the sampling design. *Multiple responses possible

self-medication was done by 19%. There was a question on 'difficulty to visit a VHV' in the migrant malaria survey; however, data was missing for majority.

Table 2 Background characteristics andhealth-seeking for malaria among migrants with fever in last 3 months in regional artemisinin-resistance initiative (RAI) areas of Myanmar, 2016 [N = 964]

Variables	N	Proportion[a]	(95% CI)
Total	964	100	–
Individual level			
Age n years			
<5	175	18.2	(15.5, 20.9)
5–14	196	20.3	(17.4, 23.1)
15–59	538	55.8	(52.2, 59.4)
≥60	22	2.3	(1.2, 3.4)
Not known	33	3.4	(1.9, 4.9)
Mean	964	24.6	(22.9, 26.3)
Sex			
Male	526	54.5	(50.9, 58.2)
Female	438	45.5	(41.8, 49.1)
Household level			
House hold size			
1–2	149	15.5	(12.7, 18.3)
3–4	372	38.6	(35.0, 42.1)
5–6	332	34.5	(31.0, 37.9)
>6	111	11.5	(9.2, 13.8)
Mean	964	4.4	(4.2, 4.5)
Housing status			
Own house	433	44.9	(41.3, 48.5)
Rental	10	1.0	(0.3, 1.7)
Employer allowed place	467	48.5	(44.8, 52.1)
Not known	54	5.6	(3.7, 7.6)
Main occupation of family			
Farming/gardening/rubber plantation work	285	29.6	(26.2, 33.0)
Stone mining work/brick kiln work	236	24.4	(21.3, 27.6)
Merchant	20	2.1	(1.2, 3.0)
Daily wage labourer	212	22.0	(19.0, 25.0)
Not known	212	22.0	(19.0, 25.0)
Migrant category[b]			
Category I	329	34.1	(30.6, 37.6)
Category II	222	23.0	(19.9, 26.0)
Category III	369	38.3	(34.6, 41.8)
Not known	45	4.7	(2.8, 6.5)
Duration of intention to stay			
Less than 6 months	92	9.6	(7.3, 11.9)
6 months to 1 year	81	8.4	(6.2, 10.5)
More than 1 year	167	17.3	14.7, 19.9)
Not known	624	64.8	(61.3, 68.3)
Knowledge score[c]			
Mean	964	5.1	(4.9, 5.3)

Table 2 (continued)

Variables	N	Proportion[a]	(95% CI)
Total	964	100	–
Health-seeking			
Inappropriate	209	21.7	(18.6, 24.7)
No medication	16	1.7	(0.6, 2.7)
Self-medication	186	19.3	(16.4, 22.2)
Quack	7	0.7	(0.1, 1.3)
Appropriate	734	76.1	(73.0, 79.2)
Trained VHV	67	6.9	(5.0, 8.9)
RHC/sub-centre	380	39.4	(35.8, 42.9)
Township/station hospital	95	9.9	(7.7, 12.1)
Private clinic	68	7.0	(5.2, 8.8)
Private clinic of midwife/HA	88	9.1	(6.9, 11.3)
AMW	36	3.8	(2.3, 5.3)
Not known	21	2.2	(1.3, 3.1)

Weighted estimates given taking into account the sampling design

VHV village health volunteer, *RHC* rural health centre, *HA* health assistant, *AMW* auxiliary midwife; *CI* confidence interval

[a] Column percentages

[b] Permanent or semi-permanent work settings with high social capital, where substantial results can be achieved for malaria control (category I); semi-permanent settings with moderate social capital, where substantial community-based results can be achieved for malaria control (category II); and small, often temporary work sites, with low social capital and resource availability (category III)

[c] Maximum knowledge score is 11

Migrants with fever: testing for malaria within 24 h

Of 964, 734 (76.1%) sought appropriate care and 347 (36.0%) underwent malaria blood testing. Among 347, malaria was diagnosed in 47 (13.5%). Testing within 24 h among migrants with fever was seen in 220 [22.8% (0.95 CI: 19.9%, 25.8%)] (Fig. 5). Factors associated with testing within 24 h have been shown in Table 3. The factors were: age 5–59 years, migrant category I, long (> 1 year) intention to stay, high (> 5) knowledge score and appropriate health-seeking.

Qualitative findings

A total of 17 one-to-one interviews and 17 FGDs (involving 121 migrants) were done. The characteristics of key informants and FGD participants have been summarized in Table 4. The perceived barriers and suggested solutions along with the relevant quotes have been summarized in Table 5.

Under perceived barriers, 11 themes were identified and broadly grouped into two categories: migrant level (eight themes) and provider level (three themes). The

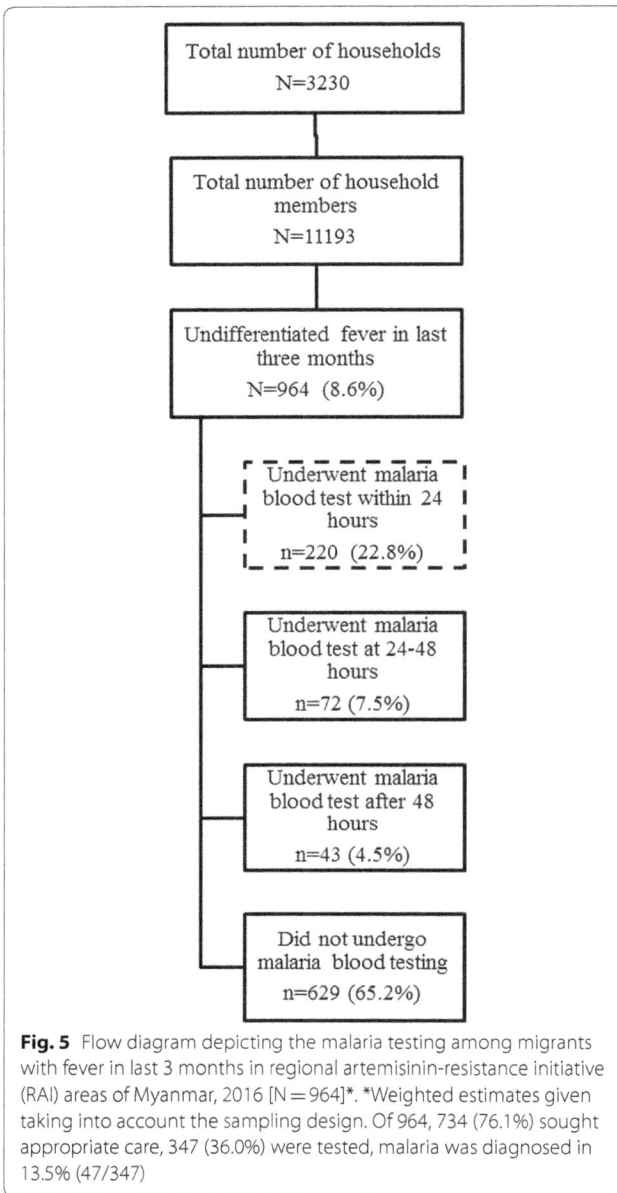

Fig. 5 Flow diagram depicting the malaria testing among migrants with fever in last 3 months in regional artemisinin-resistance initiative (RAI) areas of Myanmar, 2016 [N = 964]*. *Weighted estimates given taking into account the sampling design. Of 964, 734 (76.1%) sought appropriate care, 347 (36.0%) were tested, malaria was diagnosed in 13.5% (47/347)

Discussion

This is the first study reporting the extent of malaria testing within 24 h of fever among migrants in Myanmar. There were some key findings.

First, around one in five migrants with fever received a malaria blood test within 24 h. Around two-thirds did not receive a test at all which is concerning. However, testing within 24 h among migrants was significantly higher than general population in Myanmar (12.3%, year 2015) [10]. This was heartening to know because malaria is concentrated among migrants that are one of the high-risk populations. The Myanmar national guidelines recommend detection/treatment and notification of malaria, whether symptomatic or not, within 24 h [4].

Second, factors associated with testing within 24 h were identified. Stable migrants (those belonging to Category I and long intentions to stay) were more likely to be tested within 24 h. This could be explained by relatively better health-seeking among this group of migrants when compared to unstable migrants (data not known). Association with stable migrants (Category I) and appropriate health-seeking from public sector has also been reported among migrants previously [9]. In this study, satisfactory knowledge and appropriate health-seeking also independently contributed to testing within 24 h.

Children less than 5 years are a vulnerable group in high transmission areas; belonging to migrant households further increases their vulnerability to malaria. This group had lower chances of testing within 24 h when compared to other age groups and is of serious concern. The knowledge regarding vulnerable groups was poor among migrant households especially related to this sub-group. Factors for testing within 24 h have not been studied in previous studies either in migrant or in general population. These studies limited themselves to assessing the reasons for health-seeking in public health sector [9, 10].

Third, health-seeking was appropriate in three-fourths of migrants with fever. Knowledge regarding prevention and treatment for malaria was also satisfactory. Despite this, testing within 24 h was seen in one-fifth. The qualitative findings revealed that it was common among migrants to seek appropriate care after 24 h. Many sought care when the fever did not subside. This has also been reported previously among migrants in Myanmar [20]. Few did not get assessed for malaria despite seeking care within 24 h. There were some provider related factors for non-testing which included providing tests preferentially for those who are more ill, fear of stock out and additional paper work. It is possible that in transmission reduction areas, health staff might not have tested some cases of fever. Some migrants also expected symptomatic

migrant level themes were: inappropriate health care seeking, self-medication, not giving importance to fever, transportation difficulty, not affordable, previous experiences of no timely testing, uninformed about VHV or activities of VHV and lack of symptomatic treatment from a VHV. The provider level themes were: lack of practices for malaria testing, afraid of paper workload and waste of test kits in no burden area.

Under suggested solutions, 'provider acceptance for malaria testing' and 'mobile peer volunteer with supervision' were the key themes.

Table 3 Association of background characteristics and health-seeking with malaria testing within 24 h of fever among migrants in regional artemisinin-resistance initiative (RAI) areas of Myanmar, 2016 [N = 964]

Variables	Total	Test within 24 h N (%)[a]	PR (95% CI)	aPR (95% CI)
Total	**964**	**220 (22.8)**		
Individual level				
Age n years				
< 5	175	31 (17.8)	Ref	Ref
5–14	196	53 (27.1)	1.51 (0.99, 2.31)	1.51 (1.01, 2.25)[b]
15–59	538	127 (23.7)	1.32 (0.90, 1.92)	1.57 (1.09, 2.26)[b]
≥ 60	22	5 (21.2)	1.18 (0.44, 3.21)	1.49 (0.66, 3.36)
Not known	33	3 (10.5)	0.58 (0.17, 1.98)	0.98 (0.34, 2.81)
Sex				
Male	526	113 (21.5)	Ref	Ref
Female	438	107 (24.4)	1.14 (0.88, 1.47)	1.09 (0.86, 1.38)
House hold level				
House hold size				
1–2	149	20 (13.5)	Ref	Ref
3–4	372	81 (21.9)	1.62 (1.01, 2.61)	1.04 (0.65, 1.68)
5–6	332	97 (29.1)	2.16 (1.35, 3.47)	1.56 (0.98, 2.49)
>6	111	22 (19.8)	1.47 (0.80, 2.69)	1.22 (0.67, 2.20)
Housing status				
Own house	433	112 (25.9)	1.15 (0.89, 1.49)	–[c]
Rental	10	3 (29.6)	1.31 (0.47, 3.65)	–[c]
Employer allowed place	467	105 (22.5)	Ref	Ref
Not known	54	0 (0.0)	–	–
Main occupation of family				
Farming/garden/rubber	285	77 (26.9)	1.56 (1.04, 2.34)	1.20 (0.83,1.74)
Stone mining work/brick kiln	236	41 (17.3)	ref	ref
Merchant	20	3 (15.3)	0.88 (0.36, 2.19)	0.94 (0.35, 2.50)
Daily wage labourer	212	51 (24.1)	1.40 (0.91, 2.13)	1.07 (0.72, 1.59)
Not known	212	49 (22.9)	1.33 (0.86, 2.04)	1.28 (0.87, 1.89)
Migrant category[d]				
Category I	329	113 (34.3)	1.86 (1.39, 2.49)	1.83 (1.39, 2.41)[b]
Category II	222	39 (17.6)	0.95 (0.64, 1.42)	0.95 (0.65, 1.41)
Category III	369	68 (18.5)	Ref	Ref
Not known	45	0 (0.0)	–	–
Knowledge score[e]				
≤5	485	83 (17.0)	Ref	Ref
>5	479	138 (28.7)	1.69 (1.28, 2.22)	1.42 (1.09, 1.85)[b]
Duration of intention to stay				
Less than 6 month	92	7 (7.4)	Ref	Ref
6 month to 1 year	81	9 (10.8)	1.46 (0.51, 4.22)	1.37 (0.48, 3.91)
More than 1 year	167	36 (21.5)	2.90 (1.25, 6.74)	2.54 (1.07, 6.01)[b]
Not known	624	169 (27.0)	3.64 (1.63, 8.10)	3.27 (1.41, 7.54)[b]
Health seeking				
Inappropriate	209	13 (6.1)	Ref	Ref
Appropriate	734	204 (27.8)	4.56 (2.60, 8.00)	4.25 (2.41, 7.49)[b]
Not known	21	3 (15.8)	2.60 (0.96, 7.06)	2.54 (1.00, 6.42)[b]

All the estimates are weighted estimates taking into account the sampling design

PR prevalence ratio, *aPR* adjusted prevalence ratio (log binomial regression), *CI* confidence interval

[a] Row percentages

Table 3 (continued)

[b] $p < 0.05$

[c] Not included in the model as unadjusted p value for association with testing within 24 h was > 0.2

[d] Permanent or semi-permanent work settings with high social capital, where substantial results can be achieved for malaria control (category I); semi-permanent settings with moderate social capital, where substantial community-based results can be achieved for malaria control (category II); and small, often temporary work sites, with low social capital and resource availability (category III)

[e] Maximum knowledge score is 11

Table 4 Socio-demographic details of the key informants involved in one-to-one interviews and migrants involved in focus group discussions (FGDs) in four regional artemisinin-resistance initiative (RAI) townships of Myanmar (Dec 2017–Jan 2018)

	FGD participants N (%)	Key informants N (%)
Total	121 (100)	17 (100)
Gender		
Male	77 (64)	14 (82)
Female	44 (36)	3 (18)
Age group (years)		
15–24	26 (21)	1 (6)
25–44	67 (55)	9 (53)
45–64	27 (22)	6 (35)
65 years and above	1 (1)	1 (6)
Years of service (years)		
0–5	–	8 (47)
6–10	–	2 (12)
More than 10 years	–	5 (29)
Missing	–	2 (12)

FGD participants were bamboo cutters (n = 15), bridge construction workers (n = 15), charcoal makers (n = 11), fishermen (n = 13), gold miners (n = 16), oil diggers (n = 19), stone mine workers (n = 12), forest worker (n = 3), teak plantation workers (n = 6), others (n = 11)

Key informants were health assistant (n = 2), malaria assistant (n = 2), malaria supervisor (n = 3), public health supervisor (n = 2), village health volunteers (n = 8); the FGDs (n = 17) and one-to-one interviews (n = 17) were done in four townships namely Homalin, Kalay, Yay Tar Shay, Taungoo in two regions Bago and Sagaing

treatment to be provided by VHV in case malaria was ruled out (this was not done or provided with out of pocket payment).

The presence of VHV is to ensure testing within 24 h. Though there was a question in the migrant malaria survey related to this point (difficulty to visit a VHV), data was missing for majority of migrants with fever. However, there were other findings which pointed towards suboptimal benefit from VHVs. VHVs were the source of information regarding malaria only in one in five households. Health care was first sought from VHV only in 7% cases while in half it was first sought in township hospital or station hospital or RHC which itself could be far away.

The study has some policy and practice implications. There is a need to improve testing within 24 h. First, there

is a need for improving the knowledge related to malaria in general especially the need for testing within 24 h of fever and the option of testing by the nearest available VHV. The existing behaviour change communication strategy for migrants as well as providers should be reviewed for this aspect. Second, the staff at public health facility and VHV should test every case of fever as per guidelines and provide symptomatic treatment as well. The later has been started since 2017 where the VHV has been mandated to provide oral rehydration solution and antipyretics [21]. Finally, the programme may consider peer volunteers trained as VHV among identified mobile population. The same may be linked to the nearest VHV for malaria diagnosis.

Strengths and limitations

The strengths of the study were as follows (i) the policy and practice implications are from the suggested solutions to address the barriers and the mixed methods design helped us in exploring these, (ii) double data entry and validation of quantitative data minimized data entry errors and (iii) quantitative analysis was weighted for sampling designing making the estimates reliable and robust.

There were some limitations. The following variables were not included in the study as they were not part of the migrant malaria survey 2016: rural–urban status, education status of each individual, availability and distance of VHV for the migrant cluster. Thirteen hard-to-reach townships were excluded and their inclusion would have resulted in lower estimates for testing within 24 h than what has been reported. In the qualitative enquiry, in depth exploration was not done into migrants not visiting the VHV despite knowing that the diagnosis services were available with them and into factors related to not testing among the providers.

Conclusion

The mixed-methods study identified that blood testing for malaria within 24 h of fever was low among migrants in RAI supported areas of Myanmar. However, this was better than the general population. Satisfactory knowledge, appropriate health care seeking and stable migrant status were associated with undergoing testing within

Table 5 Provider level and migrant level perceived barriers and suggested solutions to increase timely malaria testing among migrants in regional artemisinin-resistance initiative (RAI) areas of Myanmar (Dec 2017–Jan 2018)

Categories	Theme	Verbatim quotes
Migrant level	Inappropriate health care seeking	"He [Quack] is specialized in malaria. We usually go to him when face with sickness [fever]" (28 year old female stone mine worker)
	Self-medication	"We will go for health care provider if we cannot stand because of fever. [We take] some traditional medicines for mild fever" (49 year male fisherman)
	Not giving importance to fever	"I have no idea to say for timely testing of every fever cases. Actually we sleep when having fever and when feel recovered, go to work." (36 year male construction worker) "We will not go for health care and will go when not recovering from sickness" (24 year male charcoal maker)
	Transportation difficulty	"Going to the bottom of this mountain [to rural health centre or village health volunteer] is mainly difficult, especially in rainy season, the only possible way is walking." (52 year male oil digger)
	Not affordable	"Even the blood testing is free of charges but needed to pay for the treatment for the fever." (30 year female charcoal maker)
	Previous experiences of no timely testing	"The health care providers, here is midwives from public clinics, asking previous history of experiencing malaria and what medication taking when we go with fever. No experiences on malaria blood testing" (45 year male fisherman)
	Uninformed about VHV or activities of VHV	"Firstly, it [malaria blood test] can be done at Pauk Taw [sub centre] then also possible at Inn Din [private clinic] and finally we can go Kalay [hospital or private clinic]." (28 year male oil digger) "We didn't know and not heard about malaria volunteer [VHV]". (39 year female oil digger, 36 year male oil digger and 51 year male oil digger)
	Lack of symptomatic treatment from a VHV	"Only malaria diagnosis is not sufficient. There should be treatment for other symptoms as well" (33 year male fisherman)
Provider level	Lack of practices for malaria testing	"If the symptoms is as malaria, then giving blood test and not undergo blood test for the simple sickness [fever]." (34 year male BHS)
	Afraid of paper workload	"Because VHV afraid to fill in the needed forms, some are not trying to do blood testing" (39 year male vector borne disease control staff)
	Waste of test kits in no burden area	"They [BHS and VHV] not try to do blood testing because of low burden in the area and also worrying about stock out of malaria test kits [rapid diagnostic tests kits]." (39 year male vector borne disease control staff)
Suggestion to improve timely blood testing among migrants		
Providing needed health message Provider acceptance for malaria testing		"Everybody will do blood testing timely when the clinics or services available in easily accessible places for example the Dam Gate and needed such kind of health message for timely malaria testing."(33 year male charcoal maker) "However, I would like to suggest the health care providers or volunteer also need to be patient and accept for coming request to do blood testing in every fever cases." (33 year male charcoal maker)
Providing peer volunteer with supervision		"They have [Migrants] need to have the information about timely testing within 24 h of fever. Also providing volunteer in their working site because they will not coming if available sources are far away even they know the information" (60 year male vector borne disease control staff)
		"After providing the person who knows well and well trained for malaria in our working places, we suggest community to do timely testing even the fever seems to be malaria or not." (51 year male oil digger) "It is the best to provide Working site leader or other one volunteer from village near work site or in our work site for the purpose of training on blood testing" (29 year male bamboo cutter)
		"Peer volunteer is the best and they are always closest one for them. But needs supervision for not becoming quack." (56 year male BHS)

24 h. Though many sought care appropriately for fever, it was mostly after a few days of fever. This was possibly due to poor utilization of diagnosis services offered by VHV. Barriers and suggested solutions were explored both from the provider as well as migrant perspective. The programme should seriously consider addressing these barriers and implementing the recommendations if Myanmar is to eliminate Malaria by 2030 [4].

Additional files

> **Additional file 1.** Questionnaire of nation-wide migrant malaria survey 2016.
>
> **Additional file 2.** One-to-one interview guide used in the nation-wide migrant malaria survey 2016.
>
> **Additional file 3.** Focus group discussion guide used in the study.
>
> **Additional file 4.** Questions from the nation-wide migrant malaria survey 2016 that contributed to the knowledge score.

Abbreviations

NMCP: National malaria control programme; RAI: Regional artemisinin-resistance initiative; DMR: Department of medical research; VHV: village health volunteer; BHS: basic health staff; RHC: rural health centre; FGD: focus group discussion; CI: confidence interval.

Authors' contributions

KTH is the principal investigators; KKKH, HDS, TMM are SORT IT mentors; ZL and AT are the senior authors. All authors were involved in conception and design of the study, inference of results, providing critical review and approval to the manuscript as an output of this protocol. KTH and TMM were involved in data collection; KTH, KKKH, TMM, HDS and JPT were involved in data analysis; KTH, KKKH and HDS prepared first draft of the manuscript. All authors read and approved the final manuscript.

Author details

[1] Department of Medical Research, Ministry of Health and Sports, Yangon, Myanmar. [2] International Union Against Tuberculosis and Lung Disease (The Union), South-East Asia Office, New Delhi, India. [3] International Union Against Tuberculosis and Lung Disease (The Union), Paris, France. [4] Population Services International, Yangon, Myanmar. [5] Vector Borne Disease Control Program, Ministry of Health and Sports, Nay Pyi Taw, Myanmar. [6] National Malaria Control Program, Ministry of Health and Sports, Nay Pyi Taw, Myanmar.

Acknowledgements

We would like to thanks the NMCP for sharing and giving permission to use the dataset used in this study. This research was conducted through the Structured Operational Research and Training Initiative (SORT IT), a global partnership led by the Special Programme for Research and Training in Tropical Diseases at the World Health Organization (WHO/TDR). The model is based on a course developed jointly by the International Union Against Tuberculosis and Lung Disease (The Union) and Médecins sans Frontières (MSF/Doctors Without Borders). The specific SORT IT program which resulted in this publication was jointly organized and implemented by The Centre for Operational Research, The Union, Paris, France; The Department of Medical Research, Ministry of Health and Sports, Myanmar; The Department of Public Health, Ministry of Health and Sports, Myanmar; The Union Country Office, Mandalay, Myanmar; The Union South-East Asia Office, New Delhi, India; and Burnet Institute, Australia. We are also gratefully thankful to Ministry of Health and Sports for supporting Implementation Research Grant to conduct our study.

Competing interests

The authors declare that they have no competing interests.

Funding

For the data collection of this study, the quantitative component was funded by the Global Fund and the qualitative component was funded by Implementation Research Grant, Ministry of Health and Sports. The training program, within which this paper was developed, and the open access publication costs were funded by the Department for International Development (DFID), UK and La Fondation Veuve Emile Metz-Tesch (Luxembourg). The funders had no role in study design, data collection and analysis, decision to publish, or preparation of the manuscript.

References

1. WHO. Guideline for the treatment of malaria. 3rd ed. Geneva: World Health Organization; 2015.
2. WHO. World malaria report 2017. Geneva: World Health Organization; 2017.
3. WHO. World malaria report 2016. Geneva: World Health Organization; 2016.
4. National Malaria Control Programme (NMCP), Department of Public Health. National plan for malaria elimination in Myanmar 2016–2030. Nay Pyi Taw: National Malaria Control Programme (NMCP) and Department of Public Health; 2016.
5. WHO. External Evaluation of the National Malaria Control Programme. New Delhi: World Health Organization, Regional Office for South-East Asia; 2012.
6. Global fund to fight AIDS tuberculosis and malaria (GFATM), United Nation Office for Project Services (UNOPS). Addendum to programme management and procedural manual, regional artemisinin containment initiative grant (RAI), monitoring and evaluation plan (2014–2016). Geneva: Global fund to fight AIDS tuberculosis and malaria (GFATM) and United Nation Office for Project Services (UNOPS); 2016.
7. The Global Fund. New global fund grant aims for malaria elimination in the Mekong. 2017. https://www.theglobalfund.org/en/news/2017-04-25-new-global-fund-grant-aims-for-malaria-elimination-in-the-mekong/. Accessed 11 Aug 2017.
8. Hlaing T, Wai KT, Oo T, Sint N, Min T, Myar S, et al. Mobility dynamics of migrant workers and their socio-behavioral parameters related to malaria in Tier II, Artemisinin Resistance Containment Zone, Myanmar. BMC Public Health. 2015;15:886.
9. Win AYN, Maung TM, Wai KT, Oo T, Thi A, Tipmontree R, et al. Understanding malaria treatment-seeking preferences within the public sector amongst mobile/migrant workers in a malaria elimination scenario: a mixed-methods study. Malar J. 2017;16:462.
10. Naing PA, Maung TM, Tripathy JP, Oo T, Wai KT, Thi A. Awareness of malaria and treatment-seeking behaviour among persons with acute undifferentiated fever in the endemic regions of Myanmar. Trop Med Health. 2017;45:31.
11. Cameron R. Mixed methods research. Deakin University, Melbourne; 2015. p. 53. https://www.deakin.edu.au/__data/assets/pdf_file/0020/681023/Dr-r-cameron_mixed-methodology.pdf. Accessed 21 May 2018.
12. Ministry of Health and Sports. Health in Myanmar, 2014. Myanmar: Nay Pyi Taw; 2014.
13. International Organization for Migration. Movement, emergency and post-crisis migration management, Myanmar. 2017. https://www.iom.int/countries/myanmar. Accessed 11 Aug 2017.
14. National Malaria Control Programme, Department of Public Health. National strategic plan for intensifying malaria control and accelerating progress towards malaria elimination (2016–2020). Nay Pyi Taw: National Malaria Control Programme and Department of Public Health; 2016.
15. Pitblado J. Survey data analysis in Stata. 2009. p. 28. http://www.stata.com/meeting/canada09/ca09_pitblado_handout.pdf. Accessed 10 Mar 2018.
16. Kvale S. Doing interviews London United Kingdom. California: Sage Publications Ltd; 2007.
17. Saldana J. The coding manual for qualitative researchers. California: Sage Publications Ltd; 2010.

18. Robert Wood Johnson Foundation. Qualitative research guidelines project: Lincoln and Guba's evaluative criteria. 1985. http://www.qualres.org/HomeLinc-3684.html. Accessed 21 May 2018.

19. Tong A, Sainsbury P, Craig J. Consolidated criteria for reporting qualitative research (COREQ): a 32-item checklist for interviews and focus groups. Int J Qual Health Care. 2007;19:349–57. https://doi.org/10.1093/intqhc/mzm042

20. Wai KT, Kyaw MP, Oo T, Zaw P, Nyunt MH, Thida M, et al. Spatial distribution, work patterns, and perception towards malaria interventions among temporary mobile/migrant workers in artemisinin resistance containment zone. BMC Public Health. 2014;14:463.

21. National Malaria Control Programme, Department of Public Health, WHO, UNOPS. Manual for integrated community malaria volunteer. Nay Pyi Taw: Ministry of Health And Sports; 2017.

9

First report of natural *Wolbachia* infection in wild *Anopheles funestus* population in Senegal

El Hadji Amadou Niang[1,2,3]* ⓘ, Hubert Bassene[3,4], Patrick Makoundou[5], Florence Fenollar[4], Mylène Weill[5] and Oleg Mediannikov[1]

Abstract

Background: Until very recently, *Anopheles* were considered naturally unable to host *Wolbachia*, an intracellular bacterium regarded as a potential biological control tool. Their detection in field populations of *Anopheles gambiae* sensu lato, suggests that they may also be present in many more anopheline species than previously thought.

Results: Here, is reported the first discovery of natural *Wolbachia* infections in *Anopheles funestus* populations from Senegal, the second main malaria vector in Africa. Molecular phylogeny analysis based on the 16S rRNA gene revealed at least two *Wolbachia* genotypes which were named *wAnfu-A* and *wAnfu-B*, according to their close relatedness to the A and B supergroups. Furthermore, both *wAnfu* genotypes displayed high proximity with *wAnga* sequences previously described from the *An. gambiae* complex, with only few nucleotide differences. However, the low prevalence of infection, together with the difficulties encountered for detection, whatever method used, highlights the need to develop an effective and sensitive *Wolbachia* screening method dedicated to anopheline.

Conclusions: The discovery of natural *Wolbachia* infection in *An. funestus*, another major malaria vector, may overcome the main limitation of using a *Wolbachia*-based approach to control malaria through population suppression and/or replacement.

Keywords: *Wolbachia*, *Plasmodium*, *An. funestus*, *wAnfu*, Malaria, Biological control Senegal

Background

Wolbachia are intracellular bacteria found in the cytoplasmic vacuoles of different cells of a wide range of invertebrates, including multiple insect species [1]. The success of *Wolbachia* spp. becoming the most widespread intracellular bacterium, originates from their ability to manipulate the biology of their host to facilitate their maternal transmission to offspring [2, 3]. The most common of these host reproductive manipulation phenotypes, known as cytoplasmic incompatibility (CI), is considered as a potential biological control alternative or complement to traditional vector control measures [4].

Over the past decade, two research groups have reported that *Wolbachia* infection protects against viral RNA infections in *Drosophila melanogaster* [5, 6]. Subsequently, the successful trans-infection of *Aedes aegypti* with a *Drosophila Wolbachia* strain has opened a new era for environmental-friendly control strategies of main mosquitoes-borne diseases using *Wolbachia*-based strategies [7]. Moreover, successful releases of *Wolbachia*-infected *Aedes aegypti* in Australia has provided experimental validation of previous theoretical models of *Wolbachia* population dynamics and demonstrated the viability of *Wolbachia*-based vector control strategies [8]. For decades, anopheline mosquitoes that transmit human malaria have been considered resistant or less susceptible to *Wolbachia* infections due to the failure to detect native *Wolbachia* infection in 38 species of anopheles [9, 10], and the impossibility to obtain stable *Wolbachia*

*Correspondence: eaniang1@yahoo.fr
[1] Aix Marseille Univ, IRD, AP-HM, MEPHI, IHU-Méditerranée Infection, Marseille, France
Full list of author information is available at the end of the article

trans-infected anopheline lines [11, 12]. Although, *Wolbachia* trans-infections have been attempted with success in both *Anopheles gambiae* [11, 13] and *Anopheles stephensi* [14], respectively major vectors of human malaria in Africa and the Middle East, and South Asia [15, 16], their impact on *Plasmodium* development were not always conclusive. The dogma of the absence of native *Wolbachia* infection in anopheline mosquito has recently changed with the first report of *Wolbachia* in *Anopheles gambiae* sensu lato (s.l.) from Burkina Faso [17, 18]; and more recently from Mali [10].

Recent advances in the molecular biology area, including sequencing of 16S rRNA, have revolutionized the characterization of several fastidious microorganisms. This is particularly true for intracellular bacteria of the members of the *Wolbachia* genus [19]. Indeed, phylogenetic analyses of the 16S rRNA gene have revealed that *Wolbachia pipientis*, the *nomen* species of the genus, forms a monophyletic clade within the *Alphaproteobacteria* class, closely related to the *Anaplasma*, *Ehrlichia* and *Neorickettsia* genera of the *Anaplasmataceae* family [20]. Further phylogenetic analysis based on the 16S rRNA of newly discovered anopheline *Wolbachia* strains revealed that they belong to a new phylogenetic group called *wAnga* related to, but distinct from *Wolbachia* infecting other arthropods [9, 10, 17]. Baldini et al. [17], explain previous failure of detecting *Wolbachia* in anopheline mosquitoes as possibly due to the lack of sufficiently sensitive detection systems and developed a nested amplification method. In addition, the new *wAnga* genotypes display a low degree of sequence conservation compared to previously described genotypes isolated in other insects leading to unsuccessful amplification of several genes commonly used for Multi-Locus Sequence Typing (MLST) *Wolbachia* universal genotyping tool [17]. These discoveries suggest that more anopheline species, including others major malaria vectors, may also be infected by *Wollbachia*.

In this study, is reported the first discovery of natural *Wolbachia* infections in *Anopheles funestus* in Senegal, the second main malaria vector in Africa.

Methods
Study area and mosquito collection
A total of 247 adult females of *An. funestus* collected during the raining season of the year 2014 were screened. Samples were randomly selected from an existing mosquito collection from the longitudinal cohort study conducted since 1990 in the village of Dielmo [Senegal]. Detail of the study village and mosquito collection methods are described elsewhere [21, 22]. All specimens were identified morphologically as *An. funestus* using the taxonomic key of Gillies and Meillon [23] prior to molecular detection and genotyping of *Wolbachia* spp.

Molecular detection and phylogenetic genotyping of *Wolbachia*
Genomic DNA was extracted from the abdomen of individual mosquito using the Biorobot EZ1 System with the EZ1 DNA tissue kit [Qiagen, Court a boeuf, France] following the manufacturer's instructions. Individual mosquitoes were screened as described in Shaw et al. [18] using both the standard [W16S-Spec] [24] and the nested PCR [W16S-Nested] [17] protocols. A third qPCR assay [W16S-qPCR] recently developed [10] was used to confirm *Wolbachia* infection in *An. funestus*.

The nested-16S rDNA *Wolbachia* primers were used to generate a 340–412-bp fragment according to Baldini et al. [17]. The PCR products of all *Wolbachia*-positive samples were purified by filtration using NucleoFast® 96 PCR DNA purification plate then amplified using the BigDye™ Terminator v3.1 Cycle Sequencing Kit [Applied Biosystems, Foster City, CA]. The BigDye PCR products were purified on the Sephadex G-50 Superfine gel filtration resin prior the sequencing on the ABI Prism 3130XL.

Phylogenetic analysis of *Wolbachia*
Nucleotide sequences were edited using ChromasPro 2.0.0, then aligned against close reference sequences of *wMel* [LC108848] and *wAlb*, [AM999887], respective representatives of the A and B supergroups; and three *wAnga* genotypes, previously described in field populations of *An. gambiae* s.l. from Burkina [KJ728749 and KJ728744] and from Mali [MF944114]. All the reference sequences were retrieved from the GenBank database and the alignment was performed using the ClustalW application within Bioedit v.7.2.5. [25]. Nucleotides conservation between the *An. funestus Wolbachia* sequences comparatively to reference sequences was visualized on CLC Sequence Viewer 7 (CLC Bio Qiagen, Aarhus, Denmark).

The maximum likelihood phylogenetic tree was inferred on Topali v2.5 [26], based on the Kimura three-substitution-type substitution model [27].

Results
Wolbachia infection in wild *Anopheles funestus* populations from Senegal
Wolbachia DNA was detected in three specimens out of 247 females of *An. funestus* tested, which corresponds to a frequency of infection of 1.21%. This is the first report of *Wolbachia* infection among natural population of *An. funestus* in Senegal. Despite several attempt, the quantitative PCR developed by Gomez et al. [10] failed to

amplify the three positive samples amplified with the nested PCR.

Phylogenetic analysis of *Wolbachia* infecting *Anopheles funestus*

Phylogenetic analysis of the16S rRNA gene revealed that the *An. funestus* samples from Senegal infected with at least two *Wolbachia* genotypes which cluster with the A or B clades (Figs. 1, 2), and were named *wAnfu*-A and *wAnfu*-B. Further sequences comparisons showed the identity of *wAnfu*-A to *wMel* and *wAnga*-BF VK7; and the close relatedness of *wAnfu*-B sequence to *wAlb* and *wAnga*-BF VK5 (Fig. 2). Noteworthy, despite their proximity, slight levels of divergence were found between the *wAnfu* genotypes of *An. funestus* and *wAnga* strains previously found in the *An. gambiae* complex. Furthermore, mutations differentiating the two *wAnfu* variants suggest further diversification within *Wolbachia* strain infecting *An. funestus*.

Discussion

This is the first report of *Wolbachia* infection among natural population of *An. funestus* in Senegal, the second main malaria vector in the African continent [15]. This extends the presence of *Wolbachia* to another anopheline species since its first discovery in field populations of *An. gambiae*, *Anopheles coluzzii* and *Anopheles arabiensis* from Burkina Faso [17, 18] and in *An. gambiae* and *An. coluzzii* from Mali [10]. However, the prevalence of *Wolbachia* in *An. funestus* is lower compared to the previous reports, with 46% (275/602) in 2014 in Burkina Faso and varying spatially and temporally in Mali with a minimal infection rate of 45% in Dangassa in 2015 reaching 95% (38/40) in Kenieroba in 2016. Such differences in prevalence may be explained by lower infection rates in *An. funestus* compared to *An. gambiae* species [10, 17, 18] due to biological, immunological or any other factors. Another hypothesis could be a weaker infection density in *An. funestus* [quantity of *Wolbachia* per cell] that could prevent its correct detection. The failure of the qPCR assay developed by Gomez et al. [10] to amplify the three positive samples, confirmed independently in two laboratories (in Marseille and Montpellier), suggests such an explanation, since the sequences of the primers designed for this qPCR are conserved in the *Wolbachia* of *An. funestus*. Thus, the *wAnfu* prevalence detected in Senegal is minimal and could be higher with a more efficient detection system. Moreover, a certain level of divergence

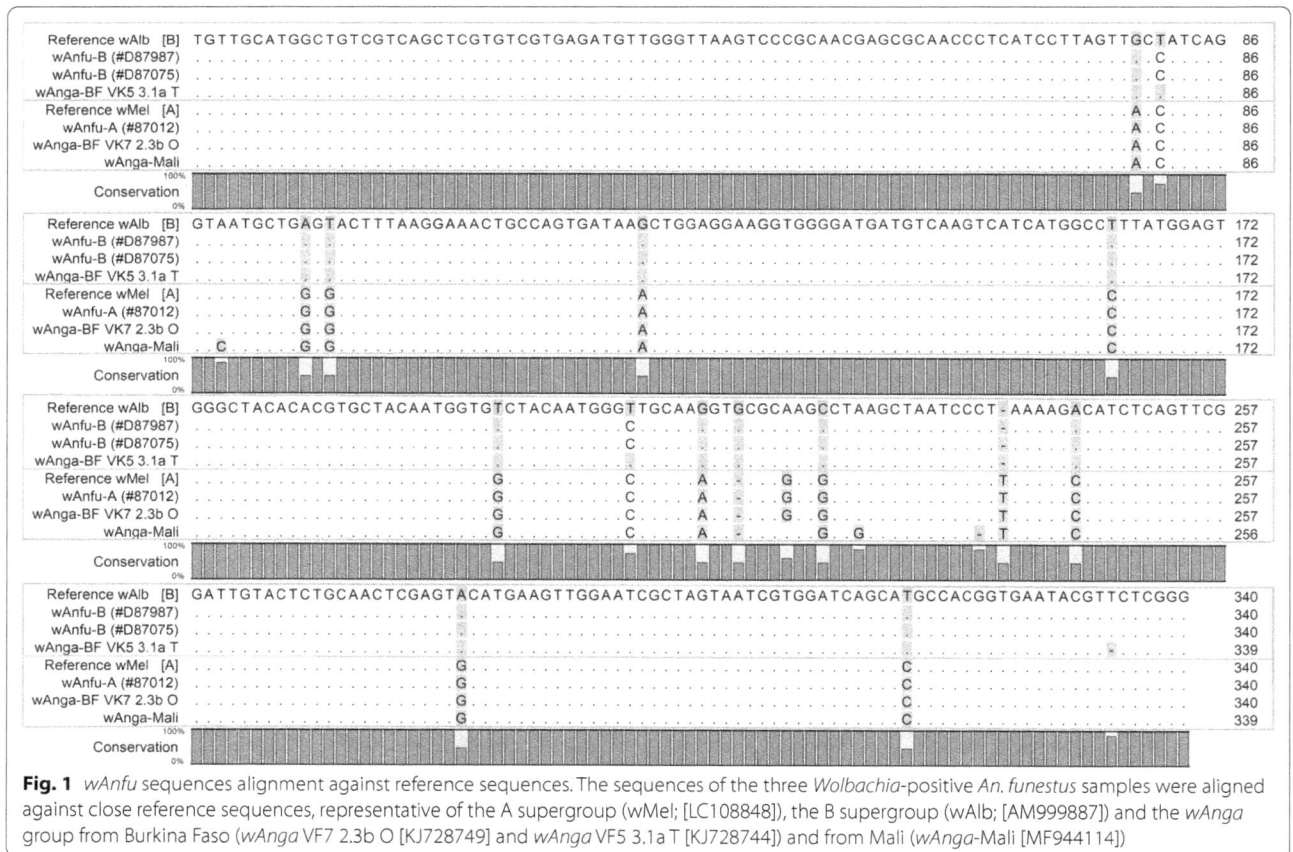

Fig. 1 *wAnfu* sequences alignment against reference sequences. The sequences of the three *Wolbachia*-positive *An. funestus* samples were aligned against close reference sequences, representative of the A supergroup (wMel; [LC108848]), the B supergroup (wAlb; [AM999887]) and the *wAnga* group from Burkina Faso (*wAnga* VF7 2.3b O [KJ728749] and *wAnga* VF5 3.1a T [KJ728744]) and from Mali (*wAnga*-Mali [MF944114])

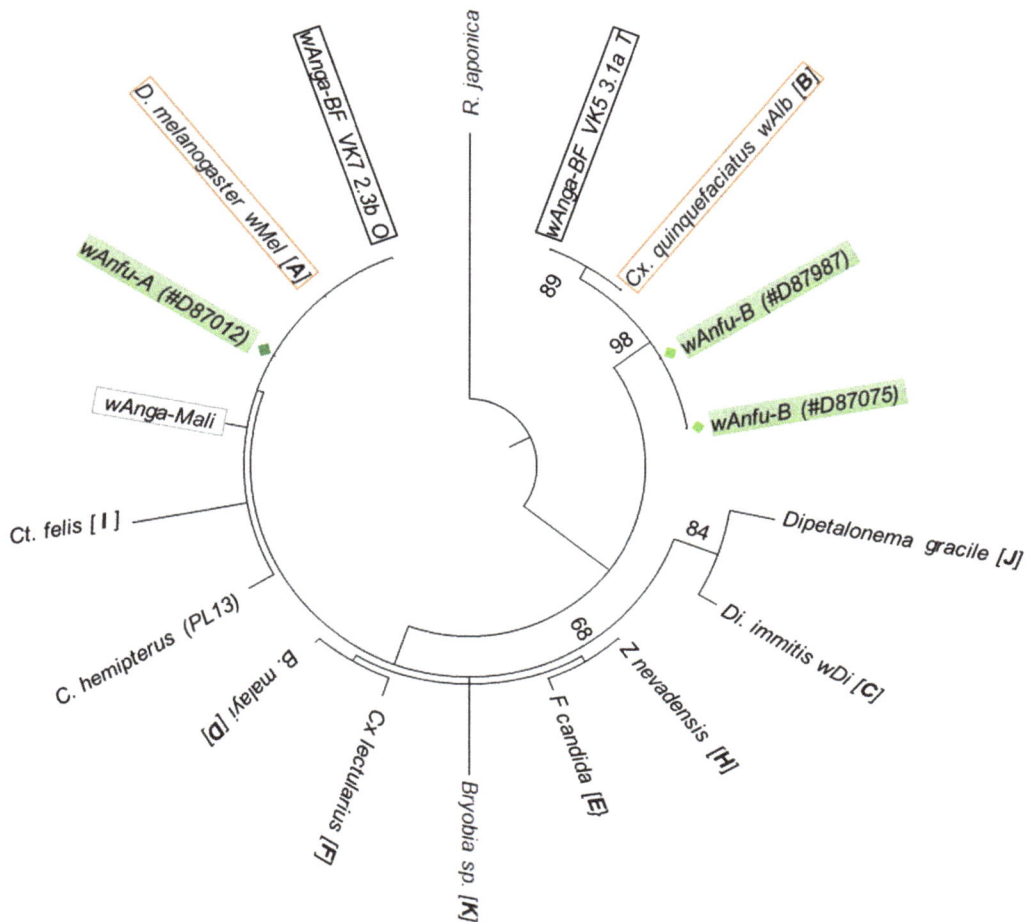

Fig. 2 Molecular Phylogenetic analysis by the Maximum Likelihood method. The evolutionary history based on the 340 bp sequence of the partial *Wolbachia* 16S rRNA gene was inferred using the Maximum Likelihood method based on the Kimura three-substitution-type model [27]. *Wolbachia* genotypes of *An. funestus* are highlighted by green shaded boxes. The two red boxes show the A and B supergroups reference sequences. The *wAnga* genotypes from Burkina Faso are highlighted with black boxes and *wAnga*-Mali is illustrated by a grey box. The different *Wolbachia* supergroups are mentioned in brackets after each reference genotype name

between *wAnfu* and *wAnga* sequences previously found in the *An. gambiae* complex [10, 17, 18] could also prevent efficient amplification and thus detection. Indeed, Baldini et al. [17], also attributed the previous failure to detect *Wolbachia* infection in wild anopheline populations by non-optimal detection tools, due to the genetic divergence of the new *wAnga* strain from *Wolbachia* found in other insects. Finally, because of the low prevalence (1.2%) of *Wolbachia* infection in *An. funestus*, probably due to the low infection level that can lead to qPCR failures, and in the absence of vertical transmission history, we cannot exclude the possibility of an occasional unstable infection.

Phylogenetic analysis showed that natural populations of Senegalese *An. funestus* harbour at least two distinct *Wolbachia* genotypes; clustering respectively with the clade A and B commonly encountered in the *Arthropoda* phylum [3]. The new genotypes were therefore named *wAnfu-A* and *wAnfu-B*, according to their respective relatedness to the A and B supergroups. Indeed, further analyses revealed the similarity of *wAnfu*-A to *wMel* and *wAnga*-BF VK7; while *wAnfu*-B was closer to *wAlb* and *wAnga*-BF VK5. However, multi-sequence alignment revealed that despite their proximity, the *An. funestus Wolbachia* genotypes were slightly different from the previously described *wAnga* infecting several species of the *An. gambiae* complex [17, 18].

Moreover, the appearance of some mutations also favours diversification between *Wolbachia* in *An. funestus*, with at least two variants. Given the suspected further divergence between anopheline *Wolbachia* groups, some genotypes may have been missed. It is, therefore, critical to vary detection methods targeting more genes. A classic approach to characterize *Wolbachia* genotypes and clades is based on the MLST system using internal fragments of five ubiquitous genes (*gatB, coxA, hcpA, fbpA,* and *ftsZ*) [28]. However, as shown by Baldini et al. [17], their newly identified *wAnga* genotype was highly divergent from groups isolated in other insects, leading potentially to the presence of null alleles if mutations have occurred in the region targeted to design the standard primers of the MLST universal genotyping tool. This seems to be corroborated by Gomes et al. [10], who failed to successfully amplify the *gatB* and *ftsZ* genes. There is, therefore, an urgent need to develop an optimal screening method, but also a specific MLST system for anopheline *Wolbachia*. A critical and challenging step for this would be the isolation and whole genome sequencing of, as much as possible, *Wolbachia* genotypes infecting anopheline mosquitoes to come-up with a specific MLST system and potentially a more efficient screening system. Then, more data on *Wolbachia* prevalence will be required to further assess their potential role in impeding the development of *Plasmodium* or any other parasites.

This is the first report of the presence of *Wolbachia* spp. in *An. funestus* from Senegal. Stable natural *Wolbachia* carriage among main malaria vectors may overcome the main limitation of using a *Wolbachia*-based approach to control malaria through population suppression and/or replacement. However, further studies are needed to better characterize the diverse *Wolbachia* groups infecting anopheline mosquitoes prior they could be efficiently used as control tool.

Abbreviations

DNA: deoxyribonucleic acid; MLST: multilocus sequence typing; PCR: polymerase chain reaction; qPCR: quantitative polymerase chain reaction; RNA: ribonucleic acid.

Authors' contributions

EAN, FF, MW and OM designed research; EAN, HB and PM performed the field collection and the lab work. All the authors have drafted and reviewed the manuscript. All authors read and approved the final manuscript.

Author details

[1] Aix Marseille Univ, IRD, AP-HM, MEPHI, IHU-Méditerranée Infection, Marseille, France. [2] Laboratoire d'Ecologie Vectorielle et Parasitaire, Faculté des Sciences et Techniques, Université Cheikh Anta Diop, Dakar, Senegal. [3] VITROME, Campus International, UCAD-IRD, Dakar, Senegal. [4] Aix Marseille Univ, IRD, AP-HM, SSA, VITROME, IHU-Méditerranée Infection, Marseille, France. [5] Institut des Sciences de l'Evolution (ISEM), CNRS-Université de Montpellier-IRD-EPHE, Montpellier, France.

Acknowledgements

The authors gratefully acknowledge the field team and the population of Dielmo.

Competing interests

The authors declare that they have no competing interests.

Funding

This work was supported by IHU Méditerranée Infection, Marseille, France, the French Government under the « Investissements d'avenir » (Investments for the Future) program managed by the Agence Nationale de la Recherche (ANR, fr: National Agency for Research), (reference: Méditerranée Infection 10-IAHU-03), and by the Région Provence Alpes Côte d'Azur and European funding FEDER PRIMI.

References

1. Ilinsky Y, Kosterin OE. Molecular diversity of *Wolbachia* in Lepidoptera: prevalent allelic content and high recombination of MLST genes. Mol Phylogenet Evol. 2017;109:164–79.
2. Werren JH, Baldo L, Clark ME. *Wolbachia*: master manipulators of invertebrate biology. Nat Rev Microbiol. 2008;6:741–51.
3. Glowska E, Dragun-Damian A, Dabert M, Gerth M. New *Wolbachia* supergroups detected in quill mites (Acari: Syringophilidae). Infect Genet Evol. 2015;30:140–6.
4. Brelsfoard CL, Dobson SL. *Wolbachia*-based strategies to control insect pests and disease vectors. As Pac J Mol Biol Biotechnol. 2009;17:55–63.
5. Hedges LM, Brownlie JC, O'Neill SL, Johnson KN. *Wolbachia* and virus protection in insects. Science. 2008;322:702.
6. Teixeira L, Ferreira Á, Ashburner M. The bacterial symbiont *Wolbachia* induces resistance to RNA viral infections in *Drosophila melanogaster*. PLoS Biol. 2008;6:e1000002.
7. Moreira LA, Iturbe-Ormaetxe I, Jeffery JA, Lu G, Pyke AT, Hedges LM, et al. A *Wolbachia* symbiont in *Aedes aegypti* limits infection with Dengue, Chikungunya, and Plasmodium. Cell. 2009;139:1268–78.
8. Jiggins FM, Smidler A, Catteruccia F, Snoeck K, Day J, Jiggins F. The spread of *Wolbachia* through mosquito populations. PLoS Biol. 2017;15:e2002780.
9. Joshi D, Pan X, McFadden MJ, Bevins D, Liang X, Lu P, et al. The maternally inheritable *Wolbachia* wAlbB induces refractoriness to *Plasmodium berghei* in *Anopheles stephensi*. Front Microbiol. 2017;8:1–11.
10. Gomes FM, Hixson BL, Tyner MDW, Ramirez JL, Canepa GE, Alves e Silva TL, et al. Effect of naturally occurring *Wolbachia* in *Anopheles gambiae* s.l. mosquitoes from Mali on *Plasmodium falciparum* malaria transmission. Proc Natl Acad Sci USA. 2017;114:12566–71.
11. Kambris Z, Blagborough AM, Pinto SB, Blagrove MSC, Godfray HCJ, Sinden RE, et al. *Wolbachia* stimulates immune gene expression and inhibits Plasmodium development in *Anopheles gambiae*. PLoS Pathog. 2010;6:e1001143.
12. Murdock CC, Blanford S, Hughes GL, Rasgon JL, Thomas MB. Temperature alters Plasmodium blocking by *Wolbachia*. Sci Rep. 2014;4:3932.
13. Hughes GL, Koga R, Xue P, Fukatsu T, Rasgon JL. *Wolbachia* infections are virulent and inhibit the human malaria parasite *Plasmodium falciparum* in *Anopheles gambiae*. PLoS Pathog. 2011;7:e1002043.

14. Bian G, Joshi D, Dong Y, Lu P, Zhou G, Pan X, et al. *Wolbachia* invades *Anopheles stephensi* populations and induces refractoriness to Plasmodium infection. Science. 2013;340:748–50.
15. Sinka ME, Bangs MJ, Manguin S, Coetzee M, Mbogo CM, Hemingway J, et al. The dominant Anopheles vectors of human malaria in Africa, Europe and the Middle East: occurrence data, distribution maps and bionomic precis. Parasit Vectors. 2010;3:117.
16. Sinka ME, Bangs MJ, Manguin S, Rubio-Palis Y, Chareonviriyaphap T, Coetzee M, et al. A global map of dominant malaria vectors. Parasit Vectors. 2012;5:69.
17. Baldini F, Segata N, Pompon J, Marcenac P, Robert Shaw W, Dabiré RK, et al. Evidence of natural *Wolbachia* infections in field populations of *Anopheles gambiae*. Nat Commun. 2014;5:3985.
18. Shaw WR, Marcenac P, Childs LM, Buckee CO, Baldini F, Sawadogo SP, et al. *Wolbachia* infections in natural Anopheles populations affect egg laying and negatively correlate with Plasmodium development. Nat Commun. 2016;7:11772.
19. Werren JH, O'Neill SL. The evolution of heritable symbionts. In: O'Neill SL, Hoffmann AA, Werren JH, editors. Influential passengers: inherited microorganisms and invertebrate reproduction. Oxford: Oxford University Press; 1997.
20. La Scola B, Bandi C, Raoult D. *Wolbachia*. Bergey's Manual of Systematics of Archaea and Bacteria. Chichester: Wiley; 2015.
21. Trape JF, Tall A, Diagne N, Ndiath O, Ly AB, Faye J, et al. Malaria morbidity and pyrethroid resistance after the introduction of insecticide-treated bednets and artemisinin-based combination therapies: a longitudinal study. Lancet Infect Dis. 2011;11:925–32.
22. Trape JF, Tall A, Sokhna C, Ly AB, Diagne N, Ndiath O, et al. The rise and fall of malaria in a west African rural community, Dielmo, Senegal, from 1990 to 2012: a 22 years longitudinal study. Lancet Infect Dis. 2014;14:476–88.
23. Gillies MT, De Meillon B. The Anophelinae of Africa south of the Sahara (Ethiopian Zoogeographical Region). Johannesburg: South African Institute for Medical Research; 1968.
24. Werren JH, Windsor DM. *Wolbachia* infection frequencies in insects: evidence of a global equilibrium? Proc R Soc Lond B. 2000;267:1277–85.
25. Hall TA. BioEdit: a user-friendly biological sequence alignment editor and analysis program for Windows 95/98/NT. Vol. 41, Nucleic Acids Symposium Series. 1999. p. 95–8.
26. Milne I, Lindner D, Bayer M, Husmeier D, McGuire G, Marshall DF, et al. TOPALi v2: a rich graphical interface for evolutionary analyses of multiple alignments on HPC clusters and multi-core desktops. Bioinformatics. 2009;25:126–7.
27. Kimura M. Estimation of evolutionary distances between homologous nucleotide sequences (molecular evolution/comparison of base sequences/base substitution rate/neutral mutation-random drift hypothesis). Genetics. 1981;78:454–8.
28. Baldo L, Hotopp JCD, Jolley KA, Bordenstein SR, Biber SA, Choudhury RR, et al. Multilocus sequence typing system for the endosymbiont *Wolbachia pipientis*. Appl Environ Microbiol. 2006;72:7098–110.

A single nucleotide polymorphism in the *Plasmodium falciparum atg18* gene associates with artemisinin resistance and confers enhanced parasite survival under nutrient deprivation

Kimberly F. Breglio[1,2*], Roberto Amato[3], Richard Eastman[1], Pharath Lim[4], Juliana M. Sa[4], Rajarshi Guha[1,5], Sundar Ganesan[4], David W. Dorward[6], Carleen Klumpp-Thomas[1], Crystal McKnight[1], Rick M. Fairhurst[4], David Roberts[7†], Craig Thomas[1†] and Anna Katharina Simon[8†]

Abstract

Background: Artemisinin-resistant *Plasmodium falciparum* has been reported throughout the Greater Mekong sub-region and threatens to disrupt current malaria control efforts worldwide. Polymorphisms in *kelch13* have been associated with clinical and in vitro resistance phenotypes; however, several studies suggest that the genetic determinants of resistance may involve multiple genes. Current proposed mechanisms of resistance conferred by polymorphisms in *kelch13* hint at a connection to an autophagy-like pathway in *P. falciparum*.

Results: A SNP in *autophagy-related gene 18 (atg18)* was associated with long parasite clearance half-life in patients following artemisinin-based combination therapy. This gene encodes PfAtg18, which is shown to be similar to the mammalian/yeast homologue WIPI/Atg18 in terms of structure, binding abilities, and ability to form puncta in response to stress. To investigate the contribution of this polymorphism, the *atg18* gene was edited using CRISPR/Cas9 to introduce a T38I mutation into a *k13*-edited Dd2 parasite. The presence of this SNP confers a fitness advantage by enabling parasites to grow faster in nutrient-limited settings. The mutant and parent parasites were screened against drug libraries of 6349 unique compounds. While the SNP did not modulate the parasite's susceptibility to any of the anti-malarial compounds using a 72-h drug pulse, it did alter the parasite's susceptibility to 227 other compounds.

Conclusions: These results suggest that the *atg18* T38I polymorphism may provide additional resistance against artemisinin derivatives, but not partner drugs, even in the absence of *kelch13* mutations, and may also be important in parasite survival during nutrient deprivation.

Keywords: Artemisinin resistance, Autophagy, Fitness, Drug resistance, atg18

*Correspondence: Kimberly.breglio@nih.gov
†David Roberts, Craig Thomas and Anna Katharina Simon contributed equally to this work
[1] National Center for Advancing Translational Sciences, National Institutes of Health, Bethesda, MD, USA
Full list of author information is available at the end of the article

Background

Artemisinin (ART)-resistant *Plasmodium falciparum* has been reported in the Greater Mekong Subregion since 2007. Artemisinin-based combination therapy (ACT), which pairs a short-acting ART derivative with a long-acting partner drug, is the mainstay of anti-malarial treatment and is likely to have been partly responsible for significantly decreasing malaria-related morbidity and mortality over the past 15 years. The slow parasite clearance rates following ACT suggest resistance to ART derivatives. This resistance places increasing selective pressure for variants or traits that confer resistance to ACT partner drugs and has led to the rapid failure of several artemisinin-based combinations, including dihydroartemisinin-piperaquine in Cambodia [1, 2]. Single nucleotide polymorphisms (SNPs) in *kelch13* (*k13*) have been associated with slow parasite clearance rates in response to ACT [3] and increased in vitro parasite survival in response to ART derivatives [4, 5].

In clinical isolates, *k13* polymorphisms appear on a genetic background comprising polymorphisms in *apicoplast ribosomal protein S10* (*arps10*), *chloroquine resistance transporter* (*crt*), *ferrodoxin* (*fd*), and *multidrug-resistance protein 2* (*mdr2*) [6]. Although parasites with *k13* mutations have been found elsewhere in the world, including Africa, they are not always associated with long parasite clearance half-life in response to ACT [7–12]. Therefore, the genetic background specific to some areas in Southeast Asia may be responsible for some of the drug resistance phenotype. Alternatively, these background mutations may be important in transmission or confer a survival advantage over parasites without this array of SNPs. Indeed, overcoming the cellular stress response following ART treatment may underlie the parasite resistance mechanism. Autophagy is one such cellular stress response that may be employed by a parasite and therefore may not only be modified by genetic variants that promote survival but also may represent a potential target pathway for novel anti-malarial compounds.

Autophagy, an intracellular process that degrades and recycles damaged organelles, has been well-characterized in many organisms, but is not well-described in *P. falciparum*. A limited set of putative autophagy-related proteins is encoded by the *P. falciparum* genome, but the functions of most of these proteins have yet to be defined. Two of these autophagy-related proteins, autophagy-related protein 8 (PfAtg8) and autophagy-related protein 18 (PfAtg18), have been shown to co-localize with the apicoplast and to be involved in apicoplast inheritance [13]. Homologous Atg8 and Atg18 proteins in yeast and mammals have been shown to form puncta during the upregulation of autophagy [14]. Autophagy was investigated as a possible mechanism related to ART resistance due to several connections between an autophagy-like pathway in *P. falciparum* and known mechanisms of ART action and resistance [15]. Indeed, ART can damage cells by reactive oxygen species (ROS) [16] and ROS are potent activators of autophagy [17]. This would indicate that ARTs, even in the absence of resistance, could induce an autophagy-like pathway. Several possible resistance mechanisms have been posited wherein the resistant isolate is able to withstand the deleterious effects of ART based on an ability to withstand oxidative stress. Another hint at a connection to autophagy is through increased levels of phosphatidylinositol 3-phosphate (PI3P), a lipid regulating autophagy, that occur in ART-resistant isolates [18]. Lastly, the upregulation of the unfolded protein response (UPR), a process that induces autophagy, is associated with resistance [19]. Therefore, an ostensible connection between an autophagy-like pathway and ART resistance in *P. falciparum* was investigated.

Several polymorphisms were found in autophagy-related genes that associate with drug-resistant phenotypes, most interestingly a T38I SNP in *autophagy-related gene 18* (*atg18*), which associates with long parasite clearance half-life following ACT. The protein encoded by this gene has similar structural domains, binding capabilities, and behaviour as mammalian and yeast homologues. A T38I CRISPR-edited line was created that determined that the SNP confers increased parasite survival in a nutrient-limited setting, as well as differential susceptibility to over 200 compounds in a 72-h assay that measures the half-maximal inhibitory concentration (IC_{50}) values for ART derivatives.

Methods

Bioinformatics of autophagy-related genes

Putative autophagy-related genes in the *P. falciparum* genome were found through the conversion of a previously published list of human autophagy-related genes from Behrends et al. [20] and supplemented with autophagy-related genes appearing on the PlasmoDB and Malaria Parasite Metabolic Pathways (MPMP) websites.

A sub-analysis of a previously performed genome-wide association study (GWAS) on 782 isolates from Southeast Asia was performed to determine if any SNPs in genes involved in autophagy were associated with slow parasite clearance rates following ART treatment or partner drug resistance (IC_{50} values). The resistance phenotype was a quantitative trait in a linear mixed model. A Bonferroni correction was applied, placing statistical significance at p-values less than 5E−6.

IC_{50} experiments for chloroquine, piperaquine, quinine, artesunate, and DHA were performed ex vivo in Cambodia on a subset of isolates from the GWAS, namely those isolates from in the NIH Cambodian research sites, as previously described [21] and used a SYBR green fluorescence readout [22], assessed using a FLUOstar OPTIMA. IC_{50} calculations were performed using the online IVART IC50 analysis, Worldwide Antimalarial Resistance Network (http://www.wwarn.org/tools-resources/toolkit/analyse/ivart).

These data were pooled and matched with sequencing data from whole genome sequencing (WGS). Samples were excluded from the IC_{50} analyses if data were missing for either *atg18* (n = 265) or *k13* (n = 311) or both (n = 196) or if the final sequence was heterogeneous for that locus (*atg18*: n = 22; *k13*: n = 37). In total, 334 isolates were excluded, making the final cohort of 448 samples. Data were analysed using GraphPad Prism 6, unpaired *t* test.

Plasmodium falciparum line production

The homology region sequences were designed to include the *atg18* SNP, changing the 38th amino acid from a threonine to an isoleucine (T38I). The protospacer adjacent motif (PAM) guide sequence was edited to include multiple synonymous SNPs to prevent cutting of the new sequence via the PAM-directed Cas9. PciI sites flank the sequences for later infusion reactions. The pL6 plasmid with human dihydrofolate reductase (*hDHFR*) was modified as described by Ghorbal and colleagues using In-Fusion cloning (Clontech) to include the desired single guide RNA (sgRNA) [4]. A DNA construct for the homology repair region was made by gene synthesis (GENEWIZ) and added to the pL6 plasmid via In-Fusion. sgRNA and homology region sequences were confirmed using DNA sequencing (GENEWIZ). The pUF1-Cas9 plasmid was used for Cas9 expression with yeast dihydroorotate dehydrogenase (*yDHODH*) resistance cassette [4].

The plasmid backbone for pDC2 AttP BSD was obtained from Dr. Richard Eastman at the National Center for Advancing Translational Sciences (NCATS). The sequence for *atg18* with an N-terminal green fluorescent protein (GFP) was made by Integrated DNA Technologies and inserted into pDC2 AttP plasmid with a BSD resistance cassette and ef1α promoter. Plasmid sequences were confirmed by PCR and DNA sequencing (GENEWIZ).

Uninfected erythrocytes were electroporated in the presence of plasmids using a Bio-Rad Gene Pulser Xcell and Percoll-isolated late-stage parasites were allowed to invade as previously described [23–25]. Selection for pUF1-Cas9 plasmids was with 1.5 µM DSM1, selection for pL6 was with 2 nM WR99210, and selection for pDC2 AttP BSD was with 4 µM blasticidin (BSD). Drug selection media was changed every day for 1 week until all parasites appeared dead by microscopy. Media was then changed three times a week and blood was added once weekly. Smears were checked three times a week for parasites until day 60 post-transfection. Parasites were detected by Giemsa-stained smears and were screened for editing by PCR. Cultures with positive PCR products associated with editing were sequenced, then cloned by limiting dilution and sequence verified (GENEWIZ). The *atg18* T38I locus of Dd2^{R539T}, a laboratory line (Dd2) with a R539T Kelch13 mutation [5], was edited to create the mutant Dd2$^{R539T/T38I}$.

Drug screen

Isogenic parasite lines Dd2^{R539T} and Dd2$^{R539T/T38I}$ were screened at NCATS against Mechanism Interrogation Plate (MIPE) 4.1 library [26] and NPACT library (https://ncats.nih.gov/preclinical/core/compound/npact). MIPE 4.1 contained 1978 compounds, which were screened against the lines at 11 concentrations. NPACT contained 5632 compounds, which were screened at seven concentrations. Because NPACT and MIPE contain some of the same compounds, the total screened were 6349 unique compounds. Concentrations screened were three-fold dilutions for MIPE from 29 µM to 0.5 nM, or five-fold dilutions for NPACT from 29 µM to 1.86 nM. Parasite lines were diluted to 0.3% parasitaemia at 4% Hct and dispensed using a Multidrop Combi in 5 µL volume and 3 µL complete media into 1536-well black clear cyclo-olefin polymer plate plates for a final hematocrit of 2.5%. Compounds were plated with 23 nL of each compound using a pin tool [27]. Plates were incubated for 72 h at 37 °C to allow for 1.5 generations of intraerythrocytic parasite growth [28].

Cells were lysed with SYBR Green I in lysis buffer and incubated overnight (approximately 18 h) in the dark [29, 30]. Fluorescence was measured using an EnVision plate reader at 485/14 nm excitation and 535/25 nm emission. The dose response data was fitted to the 4-parameter Hill equation using a grid-based algorithm developed in house [31]. For compounds with valid curve fits, an IC_{50} value was obtained. In addition, fits were classified into curve classes, a heuristic scheme that allows one to easily categorize fits as good quality (i.e., well defined upper and lower asymptotes, greater than 80% efficacy), inconclusive (missing an asymptote or displaying activity at the highest dose) or inactive (no dose response). Statistical analysis to identify statistically significant differences in the responses at the maximum dose (MaxR) was done using ANOVA followed by Tukey post hoc test. Determination of class enrichment was assessed using Fishers test with Benjamini–Hochberg correction for multiple comparisons.

Atg18 alignment with homologues

Genes for proteins in the WIPI family were aligned using MegAlign version 12.2.0 using protein sequences from *Homo sapiens* WIPI1 (AAH39867.1), WIPI2a-d (NP_056425.1, NP_057087.2, NP_001028690.1, NP_00102891.1) and *P. falciparum* Atg18 (XP_001347411.1). Analysis was performed using the Clustal V method, although relevant findings did not differ when Clustal W or Jotun Hein methods were used.

Using the sequence from PlasmoDB to the currently available crystal structure of Hsv2 in *K. lactis*, a model of PfAtg18 was created with UCSF Chimera version 1.10.1. The sequence for PI3P binding, FRRG, was highlighted in addition to the SNP of interest, T38I, and Atg16 binding site. The phosphorylation site score of T38 was determined using NetPhos 3.1 server to predict the likelihood of the threonine being a phosphorylation site for one of 17 kinases [32].

PIP binding assay

The ability of Dd2^{R539T} to bind to various lipids, including PI3P, was assessed using a PIP Strip (Echelon). A GFP-trap_M (Chromotek) was used to isolate GFP-tagged Atg18 from Dd2^{R539T} parasites with Atg18-GFP, according to the manufacturer's instructions. The PIP Strip membrane was then prepared according to the manufacturer's instructions using the isolated Atg18-GFP, then stained with anti-GFP antibody (Abcam, ab290) at 1:2000 for 1 h at room temperature. Anti-rabbit HRP secondary antibody was used at 1:2000 for 1 h at room temperature followed by incubation with K-TMBP (Echelon) for development for 10 min. The membrane was then imaged to detect binding. The resulting image was processed using ImageJ. Briefly, the image was converted to 32-bit grayscale, background was subtracted with a radius set to 25 pixels, and the image was inverted. A circular selection was created and the integrated density of the center of each dot on the membrane was measured. The value of the blank on the membrane was subtracted out and anything below the blank was recorded as zero.

Confocal slide production

Dd2^{R539T} lines with GFP-tagged Atg18 were used for confocal imaging studies. Cultures were washed three times with PBS, then were fixed with 0.0075% glutaraldehyde, 2% paraformaldehyde in PBS at room temperature for 30 min, washed with PBS three times, and permeabilized with 0.1% Triton X-100 (Sigma) in PBS for 10 min at room temperature. Parasites were washed with PBS three times and then stained with anti-GFP rabbit polyclonal (Abcam ab290) primary antibody overnight at 4 °C,

washed with PBS three times, then stained with goat polyclonal to rabbit secondary antibody (Abcam ab150079, AF647) for 2 h at room temperature. Cells were washed three times with PBS and slides were made using Prolong Gold mounting solution with 4′,6-diamidino-2-phenylindole (DAPI) (ThermoFisher). Coverslips were placed on top of each slide, slides were covered with tin foil, and left to dry overnight at room temperature. Slides were stored at 4 °C before imaging. Images were collected on a Leica SP5 inverted confocal microscope with a 63 × oil immersion objective NA 1.4 (Leica Microsystems, Buffalo Grove, IL). Post-processing and image analysis were performed using Huygens (SVI imaging, Nederland) and Imaris software (Bitplane Inc., South Windsor, CT).

Electron microscopy

Parasite culture Dd2^{R539T} with GFP-labelled Atg18 were synchronized to trophozoite and schizont stages using a Percoll gradient separation and then exposed to 700 nM DHA for 10 min, 1 h, or left unexposed. Cultures were pelleted and washed with PBS then pelleted and resuspended in 4% paraformaldehyde and 0.1% glutaraldehyde. Samples were stored at 4 °C before being shipped to Rocky Mountain Laboratories for processing and imaging.

For transmission electron microscopy of immune-labelled sections, samples were prepared essentially as previously described [33] with several adaptations as follows. For embedment, LR White acrylic resin (Electron Microscopy Sciences, Hatfield, PA) was used rather than Araldite epoxy resin. Silver sections were mounted on nickel grids, then dried overnight at 45 °C. The treatments with formic acid and sodium meta-periodate were omitted. Before labeling, grids were immersed in 100% ethanol for 10 s, then quickly rinsed with deionized water, and placed into blocking buffer. Primary and secondary antibodies were used at 1:50 dilution in blocking buffer. A rabbit anti-eGFP polyclonal primary antibody (Thermofisher OSE00003G) was used overnight at 4 °C following microwave irradiation.

Nutrient deprivation assays

The ability of parasite lines Dd2, Dd2^{R539T}, and Dd2$^{R539T/T38I}$ to survive under nutrient deprivation was assessed using growth studies. Parasitaemia of the three lines were assessed by FACS and then diluted down to approximately 0.5% parasitaemia. Lines were then plated in flat-bottomed plates in various nutrient restriction conditions at 5% Hct and incubated in a gassed incubator. Complete media was titrated with a basal salt solution (Additional file 1) to create 100%, 85%, 75%, 65%, 50%, and 20% complete media with and without glucose. Parasitaemia was assessed at 48 h by FACS.

Ring-stage survival assays to dihydroartemisinin or piperaquine pulse

Ring-stage survival assay (RSA) and piperaquine survival assay (PSA) were performed based on the methodologies described by Kite et al. and Duru et al. respectively [2, 34]. Briefly, Dd2, Dd2^{R539T}, and Dd2$^{R539T/T38I}$ parasites were cultivated in 20 mL cultures at 5% hematocrit cultures and synchronized every 46–48 h by a 10 min incubation with 5% sorbitol at 37 °C. After at least two sorbitol synchronizations, 0–3 h ring-stage 1 mL cultures at 2% hematocrit and 1% initial parasitaemia were incubated with either DMSO (Sigma, vehicle), 700 nM DHA (Sigma) in DMSO, 3% methanol (Sigma, vehicle), or 200 nM piperaquine in 3% methanol (kindly provided by Erin Coonahan). DMSO and DHA cultures were washed with 10 mL complete RPMI twice (2500 rpm, 3 min, 9/10 acceleration, 4/10 deacceleration) after 6 h incubation; methanol and piperaquine cultures were washed after 48 h incubation. Thin blood films were prepared from all cultures after a total of 72 h from beginning of each drug or vehicle incubation. Percentage parasite survival was calculated dividing the parasitaemia from a drug-treated culture by the parasitaemia of the culture incubated with the respective drug vehicle, then multiplying the result by 100. To determine parasitaemia, an estimated 10,000 red blood cells from methanol-fixed and 20% Giemsa-stained blood films were counted with oil immersion in a light microscope.

Results

A SNP in *atg18* is associated with ART-resistance phenotypes

A GWAS of 782 isolates from Southeast Asia significantly associated a nonsynonymous SNP in *PF3D7_1012900-* (encoding a T38I substitution) with slow parasite clearance rate in patients treated with an ART derivative (p = 5.89E−7) and non-significantly associated with chloroquine resistance (p = 0.0002) (Table 1). This gene putatively encodes *P. falciparum* autophagy-related protein 18 (PfAtg18). Other polymorphisms in autophagy-related genes, putatively encoding Atg7, Atg11, and Atg14, were non-significantly associated with drug resistance phenotypes, but the presence of multiple polymorphisms in the pathway points to parasite modulation of the autophagy pathway as a possible mechanism of drug resistance.

PfAtg18 is similar in structure and behaviour to yeast and mammalian homologues

To understand the role of the mutation in PfAtg18 in drug resistance, its structure and behaviour in *Plasmodium* were investigated further. An alignment of the protein sequence from *PF3D7_1012900* with the homologous WD-repeat protein Interacting with Phosphoinositides (WIPI) proteins confirmed that sequences important for the function of WIPI proteins are also present in PfAtg18 (Fig. 1a). The binding of WIPI to PI3P is one of its principal functions and is facilitated by the FRRG domain. This sequence (highlighted in Fig. 1a) is also present in PfAtg18. WIPI also interacts with Atg16 via its two arginine domains (also highlighted in Fig. 1a). Although PfAtg18 has only one arginine, the function of the second

Table 1 SNPs in autophagy-related genes from the Tracking Resistance to Artemisinin Collaboration (TRAC) study

Gene	Annotation	Protein	Position	Amino acid change	Mutation type	p value	Phenotype
PF3D7_1343700	Kelch protein K13	Kelch13	1,725,259	X	N	4E−26	Parasite clearance half-life
PF3D7_1012900	Autophagy-related protein 18 (Atg18), putative	Atg18	497,461	T38I	N	5.89E−07	Parasite clearance half-life
PF3D7_1239800	Conserved *Plasmodium* protein, unknown function	Atg11	1,669,294	D2948E	N	3.92E−05	Parasite clearance half-life
PF3D7_1012900	Autophagy-related protein 18 (Atg18), putative	Atg18	497,461	T38I	N	0.0002	Chloroquine IC$_{50}$
PF3D7_1239800	Conserved *Plasmodium* protein, unknown function	Atg11	1,670,910	N3487S	N	0.0002	Parasite clearance half-life
PF3D7_0709400	Cg7 protein	Atg14	426,753	V161E	N	0.0007	Chloroquine IC$_{50}$
PF3D7_1239800	Conserved *Plasmodium* protein, unknown function	Atg11	1,674,565	N4705K	N	0.0007	Piperaquine IC$_{50}$
PF3D7_1126100	ThiF family protein, putative	Atg7	1,018,965	I177C	S	0.0044	Chloroquine IC$_{50}$
PF3D7_1126100	ThiF family protein, putative	Atg7	1,018,965	I177C	S	0.0129	Quinine IC$_{50}$

Proteins listed are putative proteins as annotated by PlasmoDB or through BLAST searches. Kelch13 has been included as a reference, since polymorphisms in this gene have been previously associated with drug resistance phenotypes. The amino acid change for Kelch13 is denoted as "X" to represent several different SNPs that have been found within this gene. Mutation types "N" and "S" indicate non-synonymous and synonymous mutations, respectively. The p values are unadjusted for multiple comparisons. All SNPs that associated with long parasite clearance half-life in the TRAC study were published by Miotto et al. [6]

a

```
Majority         M-NLASQSGEAGAGQLLFA--NFNQDNT------------------SLAVGSKSGYKFFSLSSVDKLEQIYECTDTE---
                          10        20        30        40        50        60        70        80
XP_001347411.1_PfAtg18   MVSLRLDNNR---------YISFNQDYG------------------CLCMANEKGFKIYN---TNPFTQTYSRDLTDRNK 50
NP_056425.1_WIPI2a       M-NLASQSGEAGAGQLLFA--NFNQDNTEVKGASRAAGLGRRAVVWSLAVGSKSGYKFFSLSSVDKLEQIYECTDTE--- 74
NP_057087.2_WIPI2b       M-NLASQSGEAGAGQLLFA--NFNQDNT------------------SLAVGSKSGYKFFSLSSVDKLEQIYECTDTE--- 56
NP_001028690.1_WIPI2c    M-NLASQSGEAGAGQLLFA--NFNQDNTEVKGASRAAGLGRRAVVWSLAVGSKSGYKFFSLSSVDKLEQIYECTDTE--- 74
NP_001028691.1_WIPI2d    M-NLASQSGEAGAGQLLFA--NFNQDNT------------------SLAVGSKSGYKFFSLSSVDKLEQIYECTDTE--- 56
AAH39867.1_WIPI1         M-EAEAADAPPGGVESALSCFSFNQDCT------------------SLAIGTKAGYKLFSLSSVEQLDQVHGSNEIP--- 58

Majority         -DVCIVERLFSSSLVAIVSLKAPRK-------LKVCHFKKGTEICNYSYSNTILAVKLNRQRLIVCLEESLYIHNIRDMK
                          90       100       110       120       130       140       150       160
XP_001347411.1_PfAtg18   NGLYLAEMLYRCNILAITGNKNDKKGKWAKNVLIIWDDRQMREIAKLTFSSNIIGVRLLREIIVVILEYKLCIYRLKDII 130
NP_056425.1_WIPI2a       -DVCIVERLFSSSLVAIVSLKAPRK-------LKVCHFKKGTEICNYSYSNTILAVKLNRQRLIVCLEESLYIHNIRDMK 146
NP_057087.2_WIPI2b       -DVCIVERLFSSSLVAIVSLKAPRK-------LKVCHFKKGTEICNYSYSNTILAVKLNRQRLIVCLEESLYIHNIRDMK 128
NP_001028690.1_WIPI2c    -DVCIVERLFSSSLVAIVSLKAPRK-------LKVCHFKKGTEICNYSYSNTILAVKLNRQRLIVCLEESLYIHNIRDMK 146
NP_001028691.1_WIPI2d    -DVCIVERLFSSSLVAIVSLKAPRK-------LKVCHFKKGTEICNYSYSNTILAVKLNRQRLIVCLEESLYIHNIRDMK 128
AAH39867.1_WIPI1         -DVYIVERLFSSSLVVVVSHTKPRQ-------MNVYHFKKGTEICNYSYSNILSIRLNRRLVLCLEESIYIHNIRKDMK 130

Majority         VLHTIRETPPNPAGLCALSINNDNCYLAYPGSAT-IGEVQVFDT-----------INLRAANMIPAHDSPLAALAFDAS
                         170       180       190       200       210       220       230       240
XP_001347411.1_PfAtg18   LLETL-NTSKNVSGLCCLSNIDKNIIIAYLSPIKGRVNIHIFEINSSENIHEELPYINFKTNLSIYAHDNSIGCINLSND 209
NP_056425.1_WIPI2a       VLHTIRETPPNPAGLCALSINNDNCYLAYPGSAT-IGEVQVFDT-----------INLRAANMIPAHDSPLAALAFDAS 213
NP_057087.2_WIPI2b       VLHTIRETPPNPAGLCALSINNDNCYLAYPGSAT-IGEVQVFDT-----------INLRAANMIPAHDSPLAALAFDAS 195
NP_001028690.1_WIPI2c    VLHTIRETPPNPAGLCALSINNDNCYLAYPGSAT-IGEVQVFDT-----------INLRAANMIPAHDSPLAALAFDAS 213
NP_001028691.1_WIPI2d    VLHTIRETPPNPAGLCALSINNDNCYLAYPGSAT-IGEVQVFDT-----------INLRAANMIPAHDSPLAALAFDAS 195
AAH39867.1_WIPI1         LLKTLLDIPANPTGLCALSINHSNSYLAYPGSLT-SGEIVLYDG-----------NSLKTVCTIAAHEGTLAAITFNAS 197

Majority         GTKLATASEKGTVIRVFSIPEGQKLFEFRRGVKRCVSICSLAFSMDGMFLSASSNTETVHIFKLETVKEKPPEEPTTWTG
                         250       260       270       280       290       300       310       320
XP_001347411.1_PfAtg18   GKLLVTSSTKGTIIRLFNTFDGTLLNEFRRGTKN-AKILSLNISEDNNWLCLTSSRNTVHVFSI--------------- 272
NP_056425.1_WIPI2a       GTKLATASEKGTVIRVFSIPEGQKLFEFRRGVKRCVSICSLAFSMDGMFLSASSNTETVHIFKLETVKEKPPEEPTTWTG 293
NP_057087.2_WIPI2b       GTKLATASEKGTVIRVFSIPEGQKLFEFRRGVKRCVSICSLAFSMDGMFLSASSNTETVHIFKLETVKEKPPEEPTTWTG 275
NP_001028690.1_WIPI2c    GTKLATASEKGTVIRVFSIPEGQKLFEFRRGVKRCVSICSLAFSMDGMFLSASSNTETVHIFKLETVKEKPPEEPTTWTG 293
NP_001028691.1_WIPI2d    GTKLATASEKGTVIRVFSIPEGQKLYEFRRGVKRCVSICSLAFSMDGMFLSASSNTETVHIFKLETVKEKPPEEPTTWTG 275
AAH39867.1_WIPI1         GSKLASASAEKGTVIRVFSVPDGQKLYEFRRGVKRYVTISSLVFSMDSQFLCASSNTETVHIFKLEQVTNSRPEEPSTWSG 277

Majority         YFGKVLMASTSYLPSQVTEMFNQGRAFATVRLPFCGHKNICSLATIQKIPRLLVGAADGYLYMYNLDPQEGGECALMKQH
                         330       340       350       360       370       380       390       400
XP_001347411.1_PfAtg18   --------------------YKKKRPLRKVDI-ICKGKNVSP--------PALLN---------YEKESKN-------KKS 308
NP_056425.1_WIPI2a       YFGKVLMASTSYLPSQVTEMFNQGRAFATVRLPFCGHKNICSLATIQKIPRLLVGAADGYLYMYNLDPQEGGECALMKQH 373
NP_057087.2_WIPI2b       YFGKVLMASTSYLPSQVTEMFNQGRAFATVRLPFCGHKNICSLATIQKIPRLLVGAADGYLYMYNLDPQEGGECALMKQH 355
NP_001028690.1_WIPI2c    YFGKVLMASTSYLPSQVTEMFNQGRAFATVRLPFCGHKNICSLATIQKIPRLLVGAADGYLYMYNLDPQEGGECALMKQH 373
NP_001028691.1_WIPI2d    YFGKVLMASTSYLPSQVTEMFNQGRAFATVRLPFCGHKNICSLATIQKIPRLLVGAADGYLYMYNLDPQEGGECALMKQH 355
AAH39867.1_WIPI1         YMGKMFMAATNYLPTQVSDMMHQDRAFATARLNFSGQRNICTLSTIQKLPRLLVASSSGHLYMYNLDPQDGGECVLIKTH 357

Majority         RLDGSLETTNEILDSASHDCPLVTQTYGAAAGKXX-XXX--X--AYTDDLGAVGGACLEDE---ASALRLDEDSEHPPMI
                         410       420       430       440       450       460       470       480
XP_001347411.1_PfAtg18   SLK-CLLPCHPYLNSEWS-----FASYKLPGKKISSIC------AFVNDQNCIIVICSNGIIYK---LRFNEHIGGDMFK 373
NP_056425.1_WIPI2a       RLDGSLETTNEILDSASHDCPLVTQTYGAAAGKGTYVPSSPTRLAYTDDLGAVGGACLEDE---ASALRLDEDSEHPPMI 450
NP_057087.2_WIPI2b       RLDGSLETTNEILDSASHDCPLVTQTYGAAAGKGTYVPSSPTRLAYTDDLGAVGGACLEDE---ASALRLDEDSEHPPMI 432
NP_001028690.1_WIPI2c    RLDGSLETTNEILDSASHDCPLVTQTYGAAAGK-----------AYTDDLGAVGGACLEDE---ASALRLDEDSEHPPMI 439
NP_001028691.1_WIPI2d    RLDGSLETTNEILDSASHDCPLVTQTYGAAAGK-----------AYTDDLGAVGGACLEDE---ASALRLDEDSEHPPMI 421
AAH39867.1_WIPI1         SLLGS-GTTEENKENDLR--PSLPQSYAATVARPS-ASSASTVPGYSEDGGALRGEVIPEHEFATGPVCLDDENEFPPII 433

Majority         L---------RTD
                         490
XP_001347411.1_PfAtg18   I------SSHSFD         380
NP_056425.1_WIPI2a       L---------RTD         454
NP_057087.2_WIPI2b       L---------RTD         436
NP_001028690.1_WIPI2c    L---------RTD         443
NP_001028691.1_WIPI2d    L---------RTD         425
AAH39867.1_WIPI1         LCRGNQKGKTKQS         446
```

b Atg16 binding · T38I SNP · PI3P binding

c Score (1.0, 0.8, 0.6, 0.4, 0.2, 0.0) vs Threonine Location (0, 100, 200, 300)

d Phosphatidylserine, Lysophosphatidic acid, Lysophosphocholine, PI, PI(4,5)P2, PI(3,4)P2, Phosphatidylethanolamine, PI(3,4,5)P3, PI(3,5)P2, Phosphatidylcholine, PI(4)P, Phosphatidic acid, PI(3)P, PI(4)P, PI(5)P — Integrated Density (0, 1000, 2000, 3000, 4000)

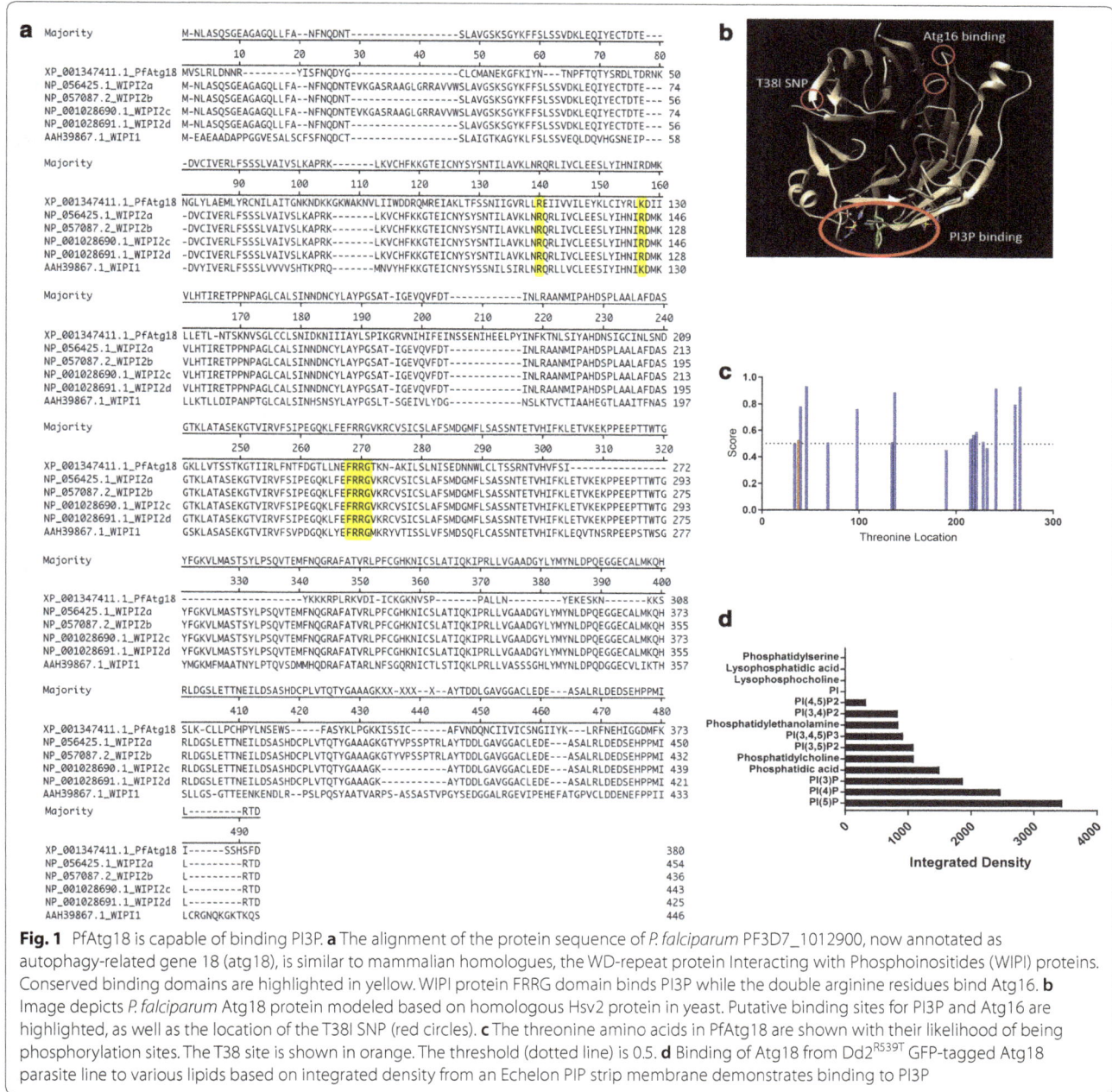

Fig. 1 PfAtg18 is capable of binding PI3P. **a** The alignment of the protein sequence of *P. falciparum* PF3D7_1012900, now annotated as autophagy-related gene 18 (atg18), is similar to mammalian homologues, the WD-repeat protein Interacting with Phosphoinositides (WIPI) proteins. Conserved binding domains are highlighted in yellow. WIPI protein FRRG domain binds PI3P while the double arginine residues bind Atg16. **b** Image depicts *P. falciparum* Atg18 protein modeled based on homologous Hsv2 protein in yeast. Putative binding sites for PI3P and Atg16 are highlighted, as well as the location of the T38I SNP (red circles). **c** The threonine amino acids in PfAtg18 are shown with their likelihood of being phosphorylation sites. The T38 site is shown in orange. The threshold (dotted line) is 0.5. **d** Binding of Atg18 from Dd2^R539T GFP-tagged Atg18 parasite line to various lipids based on integrated density from an Echelon PIP strip membrane demonstrates binding to PI3P

arginine is likely performed by lysine, which is another basic amino acid. A model for PfAtg18 was generated by comparing it structurally to the homologous yeast protein Hsv2, as the human WIPI proteins have not been crystalized. This comparison revealed multiple putative blades on PfAtg18 (Fig. 1b). The PI3P- and Atg16-binding motifs are circled in Fig. 1b, where the FRRG domain is shown to form a pocket, and the arginine/lysine domains are on adjacent blades for protein binding. The SNP of interest was determined to be outside of the binding region for both PI3P and Atg16; however, this does not preclude the possibility that the SNP disrupts binding of PfAtg18 to another protein or lipid. It has been proposed that this area of the homologous human WIPI protein binds to several regulatory proteins [35]. Alternatively, the SNP that mutated threonine to isoleucine (T38I) may impact the function of PfAtg18 through phosphorylation, as a threonine can be phosphorylated and an isoleucine cannot, although protein analysis indicates that the T38 site has a low likelihood of being a phosphorylation site, with a phosphorylation score (0.526) that is just above the threshold (0.500) (Fig. 1c).

Homologous Atg18 proteins bind PI3P as one of the first steps in initiating an autophagy cascade; therefore, in determining possible functions of PfAtg18, it is important to assess if this protein also has these binding capabilities. An Echelon phosphatidylinositol phosphate (PIP) Strip membrane was used to assess binding of PfAtg18 with eight phosphoinositides and seven other lipids. The protein was detected in 10 of the 15 spots, including seven of the eight phosphoinositides (Fig. 1d). Similarly to other Atg18 proteins, PfAtg18 bound PI5P and PI3P at high levels [36].

Homologues of Atg18 are important in the initiation of the autophagy cascade and denote the start of autophagy through the formation of puncta on the nascent autophagosome. (GFP)-Atg18-expressing parasites were generated and transmission electron microscopy (TEM) and confocal microscopy imaging was performed to investigate parasite response to dihydroartemisinin (DHA) as a cellular stressor, known to induce PfAtg8 puncta [37]. Under normal culture conditions, the GFP-Atg18 protein appears diffuse throughout the cytoplasm of late-stage parasites by TEM (Fig. 2A1) and confocal (Fig. 2B1iii) imaging. However, following 700 nM DHA treatment, PfAtg18 proteins start to coalesce within 10 min (Fig. 2A2, B2iii). After 1 h of such treatment, PfAtg18 proteins have formed many puncta, scattered throughout the cytoplasm (Fig. 2A3, B3iii). These results were congruent with previous studies demonstrating rapid puncta formation of WIPI/Atg18 following cellular stressors in mammalian cells [38], thus suggesting that GFP-Atg18 could be used to observe the activation of an autophagy-like pathway in *P. falciparum*. Furthermore, the fact that DHA induces puncta formation of both PfAtg8 and PfAtg18, suggests that DHA may have pro-autophagy effects on parasites.

An *atg18* SNP is associated with faster growth in nutrient-limited conditions

Given that *atg18* in homologous organisms is important in the autophagy pathway, which is used for nutrient acquisition, the role of PfAtg18 under nutrient-limited conditions was investigated. To determine whether *atg18* T38I, without the variable genetic background found in some contemporary clinical isolates, modulates parasite

fitness, the *atg18* T38I locus of Dd2^{R539T} was compared to the *atg18*-edited line, Dd2$^{R539T/T38I}$. The mutation was confirmed by sequencing (Additional file 1). To investigate if the T38I mutation confers a survival advantage to parasites, growth rates of Dd2, Dd2^{R539T}, and Dd2$^{R539T/T38I}$ were assessed in a 48-h growth assay with parasitaemia measured by a two-color flow cytometry-based assay using SYBR Green and MitoTracker Deep Red co-staining, as previously described [39]. SYBR Green stains DNA while MitoTracker Deep Red stains intact mitochondria; therefore, double-positive cells represent live parasites. All parasites grew equally well in complete medium (Fig. 3a). A variety of nutrient-limited media were made by titrating complete media with a basal salt solution lacking amino acids, vitamins, and Albumax. Parasites were grown in these nutrient-restricted media and parasitaemia was assessed at 48 h (Fig. 3). In media with 50% reduced nutrients, Dd2$^{R539T/T38I}$ parasites grew significantly faster than their wild-type counterparts (Fig. 3a; vs. Dd2^{R539T}, p = 0.02; vs. Dd2, p = 0.002). All parasite lines were still able to grow in 25% complete media; however, Dd2$^{R539T/T38I}$ also outgrew the other lines at this very low concentration of nutrients (vs. Dd2^{R539T}, p = 0.0002; vs. Dd2, p < 0.0001) (Fig. 3a). To further understand if the mutation also confers a survival advantage in limiting glucose, the same experiment was performed with and without glucose. When glucose was a limiting nutrient, wild-type parasites struggled to survive in 65% and 50% complete media, and all died in 25% complete media (Fig. 3b). In 50% complete media, Dd2$^{R539T/T38I}$ showed near-normal growth, while Dd2 and Dd2^{R539T} grew significantly slower than Dd2$^{R539T/T38I}$ (both p < 0.0001).

An *atg18* mutation associates with ex vivo resistance even in the absence of k13 mutations

Clinical isolates with any *k13*-propeller mutation and the *atg18* T38I mutation had higher ex vivo IC$_{50}$ values for artesunate (t-test, p < 0.0001) and DHA (p < 0.0001) than parasites with wild-type alleles for both *k13*-propeller and *atg18* (Fig. 4a, b). Interestingly, parasites with wild-type *k13*-propeller sequences and the *atg18* T38I mutation had higher IC$_{50}$ values for artesunate (p < 0.001) and DHA (p < 0.01) than parasites with wild-type alleles for both *k13*-propeller and *atg18* (Fig. 4a, b). While this pattern also holds true for chloroquine (t-test, p < 0.0001)

(See figure on next page.)

Fig. 2 PfAtg18 forms puncta following DHA exposure **a** TEM images of Dd2^{R539T} GFP-Atg18 parasites that were untreated (1) or exposed to 700 nM DHA for 10 min (2) or 1 h (3). Antibodies to GFP were gold-labelled (dots). Labels that congregate to form puncta are highlighted (circles). **b** Late-stage Dd2^{R539T} Atg18-GFP parasites stained with DAPI (blue) and anti-GFP antibody (red). Rows depict images with (i) DAPI only, (ii) DIC only, (iii) anti-GFP only, and (iv) a merged image with all channels. Columns depict parasites that were untreated (1) or exposed to 700 nM DHA for 10 min (2) or 1 h (3)

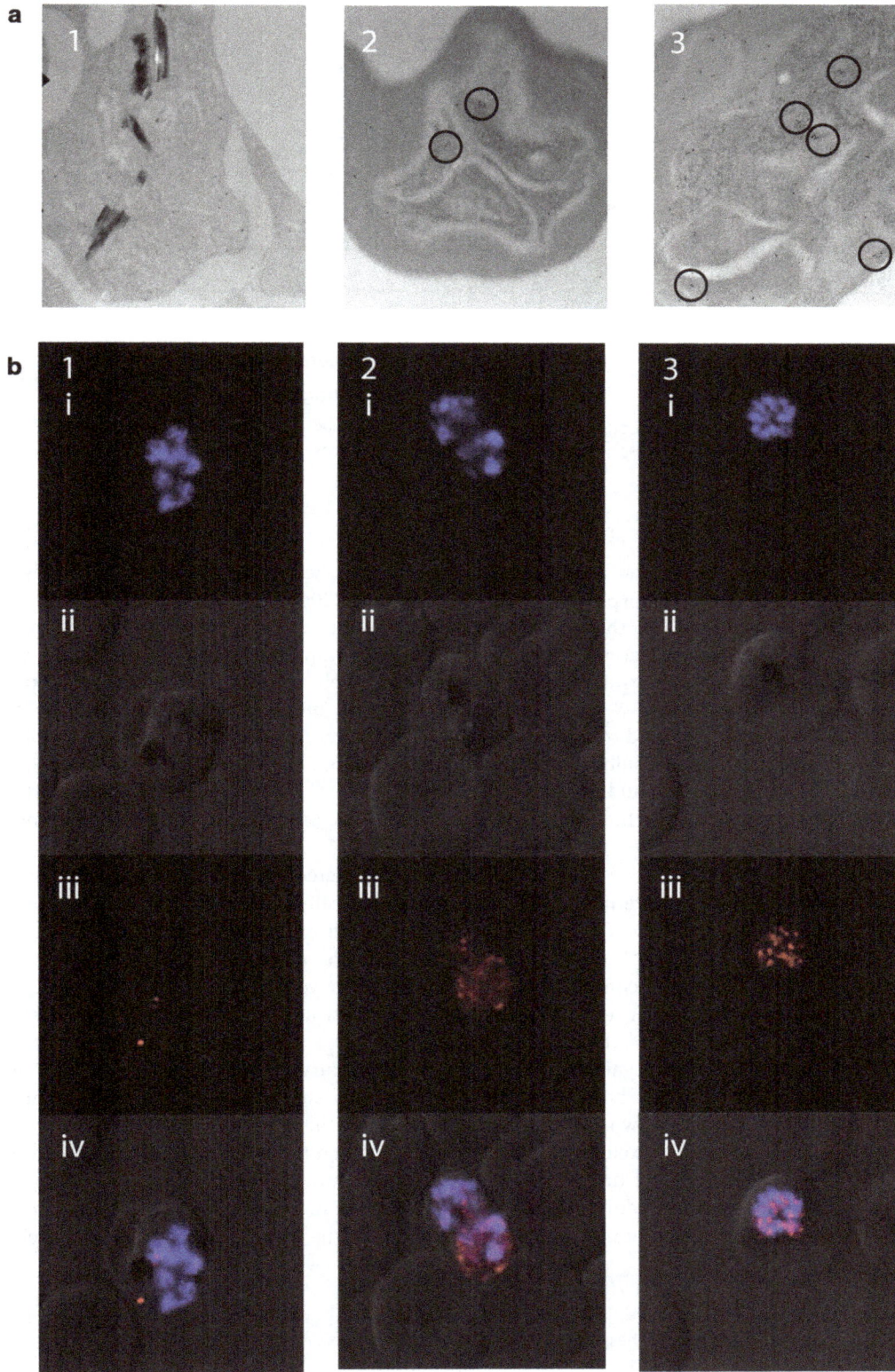

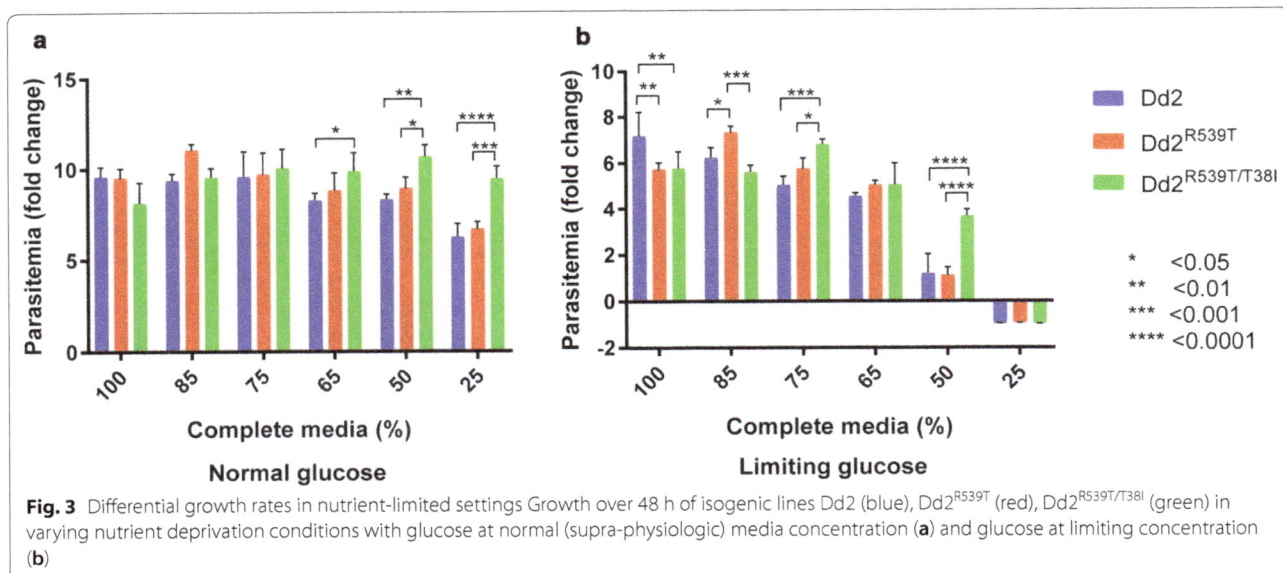

Fig. 3 Differential growth rates in nutrient-limited settings Growth over 48 h of isogenic lines Dd2 (blue), Dd2^{R539T} (red), Dd2$^{R539T/T38I}$ (green) in varying nutrient deprivation conditions with glucose at normal (supra-physiologic) media concentration (**a**) and glucose at limiting concentration (**b**)

and piperaquine (p < 0.0001) when the samples are grouped by *atg18* SNP and *k13* polymorphisms (Additional file 1), the pattern disappears when the samples are grouped by *atg18* SNP and the genetic variant associated with that specific drug's resistance pattern (*crt* polymorphism for chloroquine or *plasmepsins 2–3* copy number for piperaquine). The pattern did not hold true for mefloquine in either case (Fig. 4c–e). These results suggest that the *atg18* T38I mutation may provide additional resistance against ART derivatives, but not partner drugs, even in the absence of *k13* mutations.

An atg18 mutant parasite line shows differential susceptibility to over 200 compounds

The Dd2^{R539T} parent and Dd2$^{R539T/T38I}$ mutant lines were screened against 6349 unique compounds. Of the 6349 unique compounds, 90 were at least 5× more active against Dd2$^{R539T/T38I}$ than Dd2^{R539T} (Fig. 5a). Most of these compounds were not active against Dd2^{R539T} but were active against Dd2$^{R539T/T38I}$; however, eight compounds had a shift in IC$_{50}$ value. Two of these had unconvincing curves and were thus excluded, leaving six compounds that were active against both lines, but more active against the mutant line (Additional file 1). The six compounds to which the mutant was more

susceptible were benzethonium chloride, elesclomol, sapitinib, R306465, YM022, and vincristine. A subset of the compounds was annotated (n = 29). Of the 29 differential compounds that were annotated, 41.4% of them acted on cell signaling, 20.7% on transcriptional regulation, 13.8% on a cell surface protein; three compounds were traditional antimicrobials (Fig. 5b). Conversely, 137 compounds were less active against Dd2$^{R539T/T38I}$ than Dd2^{R539T}. Sixteen of these had a shift in IC$_{50}$ value (Fig. 5a). Again, a subset of the compounds was annotated (n = 62). Of the 62 differential compounds that were annotated, 46.8% acted on cell signaling, representing statistically significant enrichment (p = 0.006), while 16.1% acted on a cell surface protein, 8.1% on metabolism, 8.1% on physiological homeostasis and again, three compounds were traditional antimicrobials (Fig. 5b). The annotated drug library was organized based on mechanism of action and demonstrated no differences in area under the curve (AUC) between Dd2^{R539T} and Dd2$^{R539T/T38I}$ for any superclass or class of mechanism of action (Fig. 5c). These results indicate that the parent and mutant had differential responses to 227 compounds, and that 24 compounds had a shift in IC$_{50}$ value. Several of these drugs induced ROS or were autophagy modulators, including the metal-chelating drug elesclomol, whose

(See figure on next page.)

Fig. 4 An atg18 T38I SNP is associated with higher IC$_{50}$ values to ART derivatives ex vivo IC$_{50}$ values for six anti-malarial drugs according to the presence of the atg18 T38I polymorphism and/or the polymorphism associated with resistance for that particular drug. **a** DHA and **b** artesunate are synthetic ART derivatives. IC$_{50}$ values for ART derivatives are displayed against any K13-propeller mutation. **c** Mefloquine in the presence or absence of mdr copy number variations. **d** Piperaquine in the presence or absence of plasmepsins 2–3 copy number variations. **e** Chloroquine in the presence or absence of crt mutations. Given the single value in crt^{WT}/atg18^{MT}, it was not possible to statistically test for differences between this and the other groups. SCN denotes single copy number; ICN denotes increased copy number

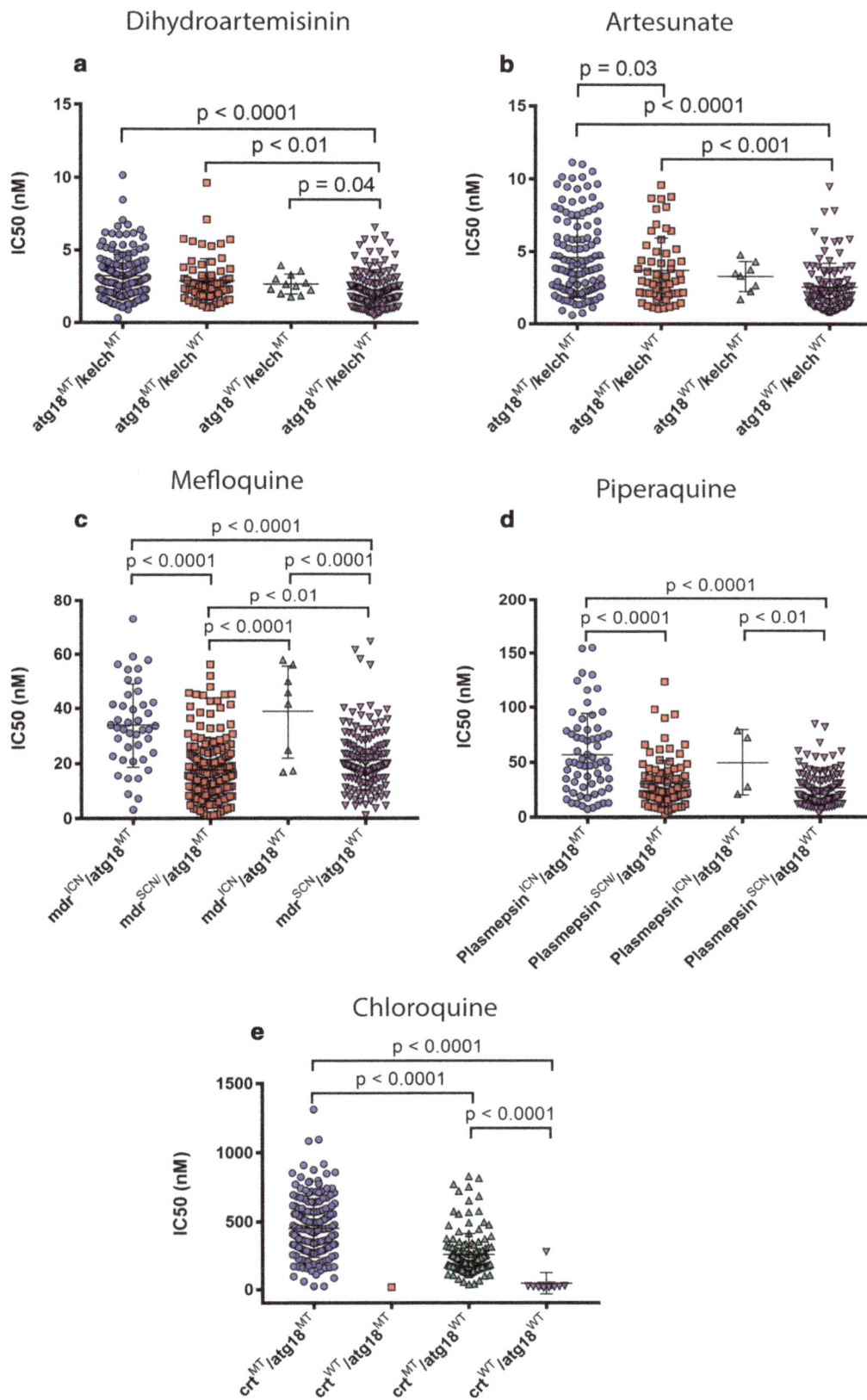

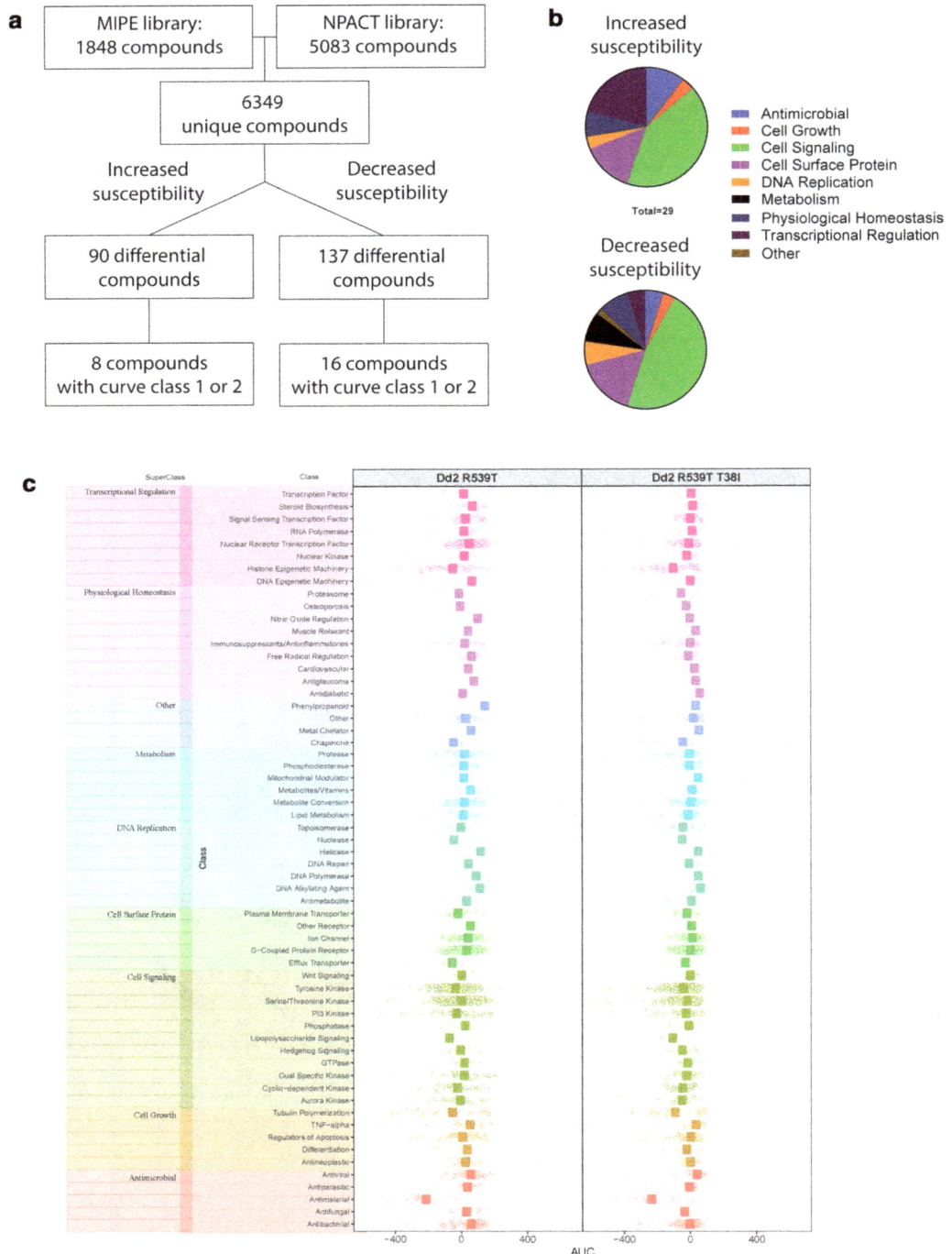

Fig. 5 Overview of drug screen against atg18 isogenic lines. **a** NCATS libraries MIPE and NPACT were used to screen 6349 unique compounds. The atg18 T38I SNP was associated with increased susceptibility to 90 compounds. Of these, 8 compounds demonstrated curves in curve classes 1 or 2, demonstrating a shift in susceptibility. On the other hand, this SNP was associated with decreased susceptibility to 137 compounds, 16 of which showed curve classes 1 or 2. **b** The atg18 T38I SNP was associated with increased susceptibility to 90 compounds, 29 of which have known mechanisms of action. The SNP caused decreased susceptibility to 137 compounds, of which 62 were annotated. Drugs are categorized into antimicrobial (blue), cell growth (red), cell signaling (green), cell surface protein (purple), DNA replication (orange), metabolism (black), physiological homeostasis (navy), transcriptional regulation (crimson), or other (tan). **c** AUC values for parent (Dd2^{R539T}) and mutant (Dd2$^{R539T/T38I}$) lines organized by superclasses: transcriptional regulation (pink), physiological homeostasis (purple), other (periwinkle blue), metabolism (sky blue), DNA replication (aqua), cell surface protein (green), cell signaling (olive), cell growth (orange), and antimicrobial (coral). These are further broken down into classes by line

mechanism of action is linked to disruption of oxidative phosphorylation and ROS generation [40, 41].

The compound library also included 36 anti-malarial compounds; however, none of their IC_{50} values differed between the parent and mutant lines. Drug response curves of the anti-malarial compounds used in the Greater Mekong Subregion, including ART, two ART derivatives, chloroquine, mefloquine, and piperaquine, are displayed in Fig. 6. Ring-stage survival assay (RSA) and piperaquine survival assay (PSA) did not show a difference in survival in parent or mutant lines, though both $Dd2^{R539T}$ and $Dd2^{R539T/T38I}$ showed increased survival above Dd2 in the RSA (p = 0.02 and p = 0.04, respectively) and PSA (p = 0.04 and p = 0.03, respectively) (Additional file 1). These findings suggest that either this SNP does not directly impact parasite response to these anti-malarials or that a change in IC_{50} value is not suitable to detect the impact of the atg18 T38I SNP on resistance.

Discussion

The proposed mechanisms of ART resistance suggest that an autophagy-like mechanism could play a role in modulating resistance in P. falciparum. Several SNPs in autophagy-related proteins were associated with drug resistance phenotypes; however, this study chose to focus on atg18 based on the level of significance of its SNP in the GWAS. A second report associated a similar SNP in atg18 with ART derivative and piperaquine resistance phenotypes in an independent cohort in the border region of China and Myanmar, confirming the potential relevance of this SNP in conferring anti-malarial resistance [42].

PfAtg18 is likely a homologue of WIPI/Atg18 with a similar binding capacity and behaviour pattern following stress. The ability of PfAtg18 to bind to PI3P is significant. Homologous Atg18/WIPI proteins also bind PI3P and, therefore, the conservation of binding suggests potential preservation of part of the autophagy pathway.

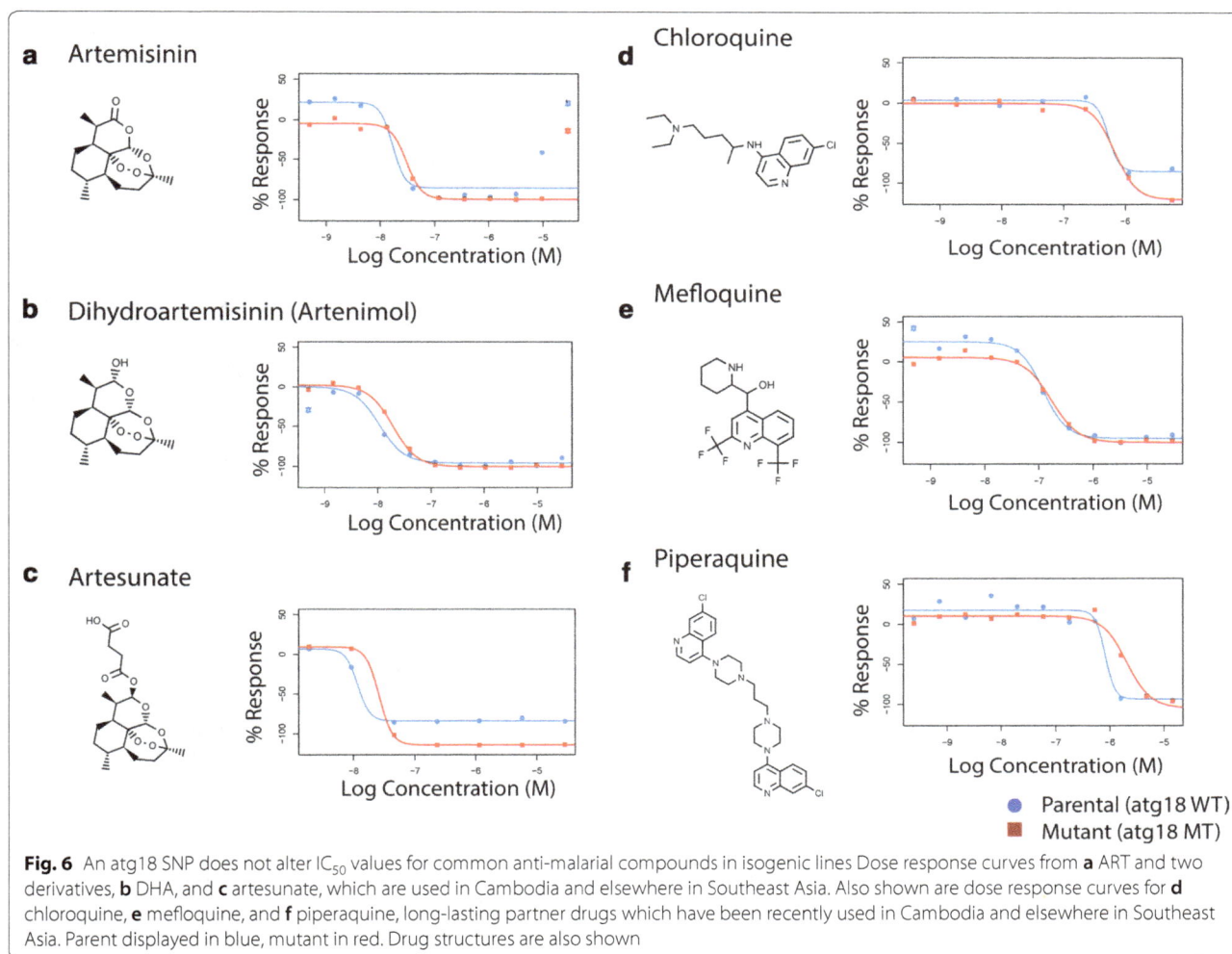

Fig. 6 An atg18 SNP does not alter IC_{50} values for common anti-malarial compounds in isogenic lines Dose response curves from **a** ART and two derivatives, **b** DHA, and **c** artesunate, which are used in Cambodia and elsewhere in Southeast Asia. Also shown are dose response curves for **d** chloroquine, **e** mefloquine, and **f** piperaquine, long-lasting partner drugs which have been recently used in Cambodia and elsewhere in Southeast Asia. Parent displayed in blue, mutant in red. Drug structures are also shown

Further, PI3P been implicated in drug resistance in *P. falciparum* from work by Mbengue and colleagues [18], who suggested there is a relationship between PI3P and artemisinin resistance. While autophagy-related proteins are involved in apicoplast inheritance [13], the results of this study indicate that autophagy-related proteins may have alternative functions outside of the apicoplast, as the only apparently essential function of the apicoplast is to provide isopentyl pyrophosphate (IPP) [43].

If PfAtg18 is involved in an autophagy-like pathway in *Plasmodium*, this SNP may modulate its activity. A number of mutations in homologous WIPI proteins have been described in various cancers [44]. The diversity of mutations found in WIPI proteins in cancer suggests that these mutations provide a survival advantage. For a mutation to be advantageous in cancer, it must facilitate cancer cell growth, for example through nutrient acquisition, dealing with cellular stress or several other pro-survival mechanisms [45, 46]. Thus, the plasmodial *atg18* T38I mutation may similarly offer a survival benefit. Given the ability of the Dd2$^{R539T/T38I}$ mutant to survive better in nutrient-limited settings than either its parent Dd2^{R539T} line or the original Dd2 line, the T38I SNP may therefore represent a fitness advantage by growing more effectively in the nutrient-limited setting of parasite infection and acute malaria. This alone or in addition to a drug-resistance phenotype, could select for the T38I SNP. Despite allowing for increased survival of early ring-stage parasites, *k13* polymorphisms have been shown to cause growth deficits in vitro [47]. The T38I mutation could, therefore, compensate for the loss of fitness caused by *k13* or other unknown polymorphisms in the parasite population. DHA-resistant isolates have been shown to grow more rapidly in stressful conditions, as evidenced by a decreased growth rate for sensitive parasites at high parasitaemia [48]. At higher parasitaemia, growth media, which is normally supra-physiologic, may become rapidly depleted, thus creating a nutrient-limited media. Therefore, these results align with the finding that efficient growth in nutrient deprivation may be driving selection. Further, these stressful, oxidative stress-inducing conditions would typically slow parasite growth [49]. One possible explanation is that if a parasite is better equipped to handle damage by oxidative stress, perhaps by employing autophagy-like mechanisms, that parasite would likely outcompete other parasites in a population.

Growth of *Plasmodium* parasites appears to be susceptible to changes in the immediate host environment. Dietary restrictions in mice have been shown to be protective against cerebral malaria by *Plasmodium berghei* [50, 51]. Refeeding of patients with *P. falciparum* in the hospital setting has been associated with an increase in parasitaemia [52]. In culture supplemented with sera from calorie-restricted mice as compared to fed mice, parasites formed fewer merozoites during schizogony, thus reducing overall parasitaemia [53]. Thus, parasitaemia is intricately tied to host nutrition status. The serine/threonine kinase KIN, which is putatively homologous to AMP-activated kinase (AMPK), has been implicated in nutrient sensing in *Plasmodium* in the absence of TOR proteins [53]. AMPK is another regulator of autophagy along with mTOR [54]. An autophagy-like pathway may therefore play a role in nutrient sensing in *Plasmodium* and may modulate parasite virulence based on the ability of the parasite to obtain limited nutrients.

Many anti-malarial drugs target metabolic pathways [55]. An improvement in a parasite's ability to survive low nutrient conditions not only benefits the parasite in terms of its growth rate, but also enables a parasite to evade drugs that may target various metabolic pathways. While a drug may block one metabolic pathway, another pathway that was previously redundant may become essential. The ability to grow more efficiently in nutrient-limited media suggests changes in the metabolism of parasites carrying this mutation, which could allow the parasite to survive drug treatment. Again, the ability to survive a drug pulse based on the parasite's ability to employ alternate metabolic pathways may appear inconsequential in a drug screen in complete media, where nutrient limitation is not a factor. Experiments examining parasite responses to drugs in a variety of media are ongoing.

The drug screen revealed that the mutant line is differentially susceptible to > 200 compounds, including a number of compounds that would likely modulate autophagy, including vincristine [56], sapitinib [57, 58], and gefitinib [59, 60], whereas others modulate ROS, including elesclomol [41, 61], olmesartan [62], and paeoniflorin [63]. Despite these effects on the parasite's susceptibility to other compounds, the *atg18* T38I SNP did not change IC$_{50}$ values for the tested anti-malarial compounds. This was surprising given the results of the ex vivo IC$_{50}$ experiments and GWAS. It is possible that, like *k13* polymorphisms, the contribution of the *atg18* polymorphism to resistance cannot be detected using a 72-h assay [64, 65]. Thus, studies are underway to determine if this SNP modulates several other phenotypes including those measured by dormancy assays. Additionally, the effects of the SNP may be important only in the context of other background mutations, which are absent in the Dd2^{R539T} line.

It is possible that the T38I SNP changes the function of PfAtg18 to promote more efficient nutrient acquisition through an autophagy-like pathway. This could allow for either increased fitness leading to expansion within

A single nucleotide polymorphism in the Plasmodium falciparum atg18 gene associates with artemisinin...

125

the parasite population or the ability of a parasite to survive drug treatment by utilizing its autophagy-like pathway to survive in the absence of a blocked metabolic pathway. Further studies, including a more detailed characterization of the function of PfAtg18, are necessary to determine if this is indeed the case.

Abbreviations
AMPK: AMP-activated kinase; *arps10: apicoplast ribosomal protein S10*; AUC: area under the curve; ART: artemisinin; ACT: artemisinin-based combination therapy; *atg18: autophagy-related gene 18*; PfAtg8: autophagy-related protein 8; BSD: blasticidin; *crt: chloroquine resistance transporter*; DAPI: 4',6-diamidino-2-phenylindole; *fd: ferrodoxin*; GWAS: genome-wide association study; GFP: green fluorescent protein; IC$_{50}$: half-maximal inhibitory concentration; hDHFR: human dihydrofolate reductase; IPP: isopentyl pyrophosphate; *k13: kelch13*; MaxR: maximum dose response; MIPE: Mechanism Interrogation Plate; NCATS: National Center for Advancing Translational Sciences; *mdr2: multidrug-resistance protein 2*; PfAtg18: *P. falciparum* autophagy-related protein 18; PIP: phosphatidylinositol phosphate; PI3P: phosphatidylinositol 3-phosphate; PAM: protospacer adjacent motif; sgRNA: single guide RNA; SNPs: single nucleotide polymorphisms; TRAC: Tracking Resistance to Artemisinin Collaboration; TEM: transmission electron microscopy; UPR: unfolded protein response; WIPI: WD-repeat protein Interacting with Phosphoinositides; WGS: whole genome sequencing; yDHODH: yeast dihydroorotate dehydrogenase.

Authors' contributions
KFB, RMF, DR, and AKS conceived of the project. KFB, RE, PL, CK-T, CM, and JMS performed the experiments. KFB, SG and DWD performed imaging. RA and RG performed statistical and bioinformatics analyses. KFB wrote the manuscript with significant edits by DR, CT, and AKS. All authors read and approved the final manuscript.

Author details
[1] National Center for Advancing Translational Sciences, National Institutes of Health, Bethesda, MD, USA. [2] Nuffield Department of Medicine, University of Oxford, Oxford, UK. [3] Wellcome Sanger Institute, Wellcome Genome Campus, Hinxton, Cambridge, UK. [4] National Institute of Allergy and Infectious Diseases, National Institutes of Health, Bethesda, MD, USA. [5] Vertex Pharmaceuticals, Boston, MA, USA. [6] Rocky Mountain Laboratories, National Institute of Allergy and Infectious Diseases, National Institutes of Health, Bethesda, MD, USA. [7] Radcliffe Department of Medicine, Medical Sciences Division, University of Oxford, Oxford, UK. [8] Kennedy Institute of Rheumatology and Medical Research Council Human Immunology Unit, Weatherall Institute of Molecular Medicine, University of Oxford, Oxford, UK.

Acknowledgements
We are grateful to study participants and clinical staff that made this study possible. We thank David Ito for advice in the production of mutant parasites and Thomas Wellems and Chanaki Amaratunga for advice and support of this work. We thank David Fidock and Jose Juan Lopez-Rubio for use of materials. Whole genome sequencing was done by the Wellcome Sanger Institute (WSI) as part of the MalariaGEN *Plasmodium falciparum* Community Project, and coordinated by the MalariaGEN Resource Centre. We thank the staff of the WSI Sample Logistics, Sequencing, and Informatics facilities for their contribution.

Competing interests
The authors declare that they have no competing interests.

Funding
This study was funded by the Intramural Research Programs of the National Institute of Allergy and Infectious Diseases and the National Center for Advancing Translational Sciences, the Wellcome Trust, Bill & Melinda Gates Foundation, Medical Research Council, and the NIH OxCam Scholars Program.

References
1. Amaratunga C, Lim P, Suon S, Sreng S, Mao S, Sopha C, et al. Dihydroartemisinin-piperaquine resistance in *Plasmodium falciparum* malaria in Cambodia: a multisite prospective cohort study. Lancet Infect Dis. 2016;16:357–65.
2. Duru V, Khim N, Leang R, Kim S, Domergue A, Kloeung N, et al. *Plasmodium falciparum* dihydroartemisinin-piperaquine failures in Cambodia are associated with mutant K13 parasites presenting high survival rates in novel piperaquine in vitro assays: retrospective and prospective investigations. BMC Med. 2015;13:305.
3. Ashley EA, Dhorda M, Fairhurst RM, Amaratunga C, Lim P, Suon S, et al. Spread of artemisinin resistance in *Plasmodium falciparum* malaria. N Engl J Med. 2014;371:411–23.
4. Ghorbal M, Gorman M, Macpherson CR, Martins RM, Scherf A, Lopez-Rubio JJ. Genome editing in the human malaria parasite *Plasmodium falciparum* using the CRISPR-Cas9 system. Nat Biotechnol. 2014;32:819–21.
5. Straimer J, Gnadig NF, Witkowski B, Amaratunga C, Duru V, Ramadani AP, et al. Drug resistance. K13-propeller mutations confer artemisinin resistance in *Plasmodium falciparum* clinical isolates. Science. 2015;347:428–31.
6. Miotto O, Amato R, Ashley EA, MacInnis B, Almagro-Garcia J, Amaratunga C, et al. Genetic architecture of artemisinin-resistant *Plasmodium falciparum*. Nat Genet. 2015;47:226–34.
7. Taylor SM, Parobek CM, DeConti DK, Kayentao K, Coulibaly SO, Greenwood BM, et al. Absence of putative artemisinin resistance mutations among *Plasmodium falciparum* in Sub-Saharan Africa: a molecular epidemiologic study. J Infect Dis. 2015;211:680–8.
8. Mukherjee A, Bopp S, Magistrado P, Wong W, Daniels R, Demas A, et al. Artemisinin resistance without pfkelch13 mutations in *Plasmodium falciparum* isolates from Cambodia. Malar J. 2017;16:195.
9. Kheang ST, Sovannaroth S, Ek S, Chy S, Chhun P, Mao S, et al. Prevalence of K13 mutation and Day-3 positive parasitaemia in artemisinin-resistant malaria endemic area of Cambodia: a cross-sectional study. Malar J. 2017;16:372.
10. Ouattara A, Kone A, Adams M, Fofana B, Maiga AW, Hampton S, et al. Polymorphisms in the K13-propeller gene in artemisinin-susceptible *Plasmodium falciparum* parasites from Bougoula-Hameau and Bandiagara, Mali. Am J Trop Med Hyg. 2015;92:1202–6.
11. Muwanguzi J, Henriques G, Sawa P, Bousema T, Sutherland CJ, Beshir KB. Lack of K13 mutations in *Plasmodium falciparum* persisting after

artemisinin combination therapy treatment of Kenyan children. Malar J. 2016;15:36.

12. Cooper RA, Conrad MD, Watson QD, Huezo SJ, Ninsiima H, Tumwebaze P, et al. Lack of artemisinin resistance in *Plasmodium falciparum* in Uganda based on parasitological and molecular assays. Antimicrob Agents Chemother. 2015;59:5061–4.

13. Bansal P, Tripathi A, Thakur V, Mohmmed A, Sharma P. Autophagy-related protein ATG18 regulates apicoplast biogenesis in Apicomplexan parasites. MBio. 2017;8:e01468–517.

14. Klionsky DJ, Abdelmohsen K, Abe A, Abedin MJ, Abeliovich H, Acevedo Arozena A, et al. Guidelines for the use and interpretation of assays for monitoring autophagy 3rd ed. Autophagy. 2016;12:1–222.

15. Dogovski C, Xie SC, Burgio G, Bridgford J, Mok S, McCaw JM, et al. Targeting the cell stress response of *Plasmodium falciparum* to overcome artemisinin resistance. PLoS Biol. 2015;13:e1002132.

16. Li J, Zhou B. Biological actions of artemisinin: insights from medicinal chemistry studies. Molecules. 2010;15:1378–97.

17. Thorpe GW, Fong CS, Alic N, Higgins VJ, Dawes IW. Cells have distinct mechanisms to maintain protection against different reactive oxygen species: oxidative-stress-response genes. Proc Natl Acad Sci USA. 2004;101:6564–9.

18. Mbengue A, Bhattacharjee S, Pandharkar T, Liu H, Estiu G, Stahelin RV, et al. A molecular mechanism of artemisinin resistance in *Plasmodium falciparum* malaria. Nature. 2015;520:683–7.

19. Mok S, Ashley EA, Ferreira PE, Zhu L, Lin Z, Yeo T, et al. Population transcriptomics of human malaria parasites reveals the mechanism of artemisinin resistance. Science. 2015;347:431–5.

20. Behrends C, Sowa ME, Gygi SP, Harper JW. Network organization of the human autophagy system. Nature. 2010;466:68–76.

21. Lim P, Dek D, Try V, Eastman RT, Chy S, Sreng S, et al. Ex vivo susceptibility of *Plasmodium falciparum* to antimalarial drugs in western, northern, and eastern Cambodia, 2011-2012: association with molecular markers. Antimicrob Agents Chemother. 2013;57:5277–83.

22. Bacon DJ, Latour C, Lucas C, Colina O, Ringwald P, Picot S. Comparison of a SYBR green I-based assay with a histidine-rich protein II enzyme-linked immunosorbent assay for in vitro antimalarial drug efficacy testing and application to clinical isolates. Antimicrob Agents Chemother. 2007;51:1172–8.

23. Wu Y, Sifri CD, Lei HH, Su XZ, Wellems TE. Transfection of *Plasmodium falciparum* within human red blood cells. Proc Natl Acad Sci USA. 1995;92:973–7.

24. Deitsch KW, Driskill CL, Wellems TE. Transformation of malaria parasites by the spontaneous uptake and expression of DNA from human erythrocytes. Nucleic Acids Res. 2001;29:850–3.

25. Fidock DA, Wellems TE. Transformation with human dihydrofolate reductase renders malaria parasites insensitive to WR99210 but does not affect the intrinsic activity of proguanil. Proc Natl Acad Sci USA. 1997;94:10931–6.

26. Mathews Griner LA, Guha R, Shinn P, Young RM, Keller JM, Liu D, et al. High-throughput combinatorial screening identifies drugs that cooperate with ibrutinib to kill activated B-cell-like diffuse large B-cell lymphoma cells. Proc Natl Acad Sci USA. 2014;111:2349–54.

27. Inglese J, Auld DS, Jadhav A, Johnson RL, Simeonov A, Yasgar A, et al. Quantitative high-throughput screening: a titration-based approach that efficiently identifies biological activities in large chemical libraries. Proc Natl Acad Sci USA. 2006;103:11473–8.

28. Yuan J, Johnson RL, Huang R, Wichterman J, Jiang H, Hayton K, et al. Genetic mapping of targets mediating differential chemical phenotypes in *Plasmodium falciparum*. Nat Chem Biol. 2009;5:765–71.

29. Smilkstein M, Sriwilaijaroen N, Kelly JX, Wilairat P, Riscoe M. Simple and inexpensive fluorescence-based technique for high-throughput antimalarial drug screening. Antimicrob Agents Chemother. 2004;48:1803–6.

30. Bennett TN, Paguio M, Gligorijevic B, Seudieu C, Kosar AD, Davidson E, et al. Novel, rapid, and inexpensive cell-based quantification of antimalarial drug efficacy. Antimicrob Agents Chemother. 2004;48:1807–10.

31. Wang Y, Jadhav A, Southal N, Huang R, Nguyen D-T. A grid algorithm for high throughput fitting of dose-response curve data. Curr Chem Genomics. 2010;4:57–66.

32. Blom N, Gammeltoft S, Brunak S. Sequence and structure-based prediction of eukaryotic protein phosphorylation sites. J Mol Biol. 1999;294:1351–62.

33. Faris R, Moore RA, Ward A, Race B, Dorward DW, Hollister JR, et al. Cellular prion protein is present in mitochondria of healthy mice. Sci Rep. 2017;7:41556.

34. Kite WA, Melendez-Muniz VA, Moraes Barros RR, Wellems TE, Sa JM. Alternative methods for the *Plasmodium falciparum* artemisinin ring-stage survival assay with increased simplicity and parasite stage-specificity. Malar J. 2016;15:94.

35. Proikas-Cezanne T, Waddell S, Gaugel A, Frickey T, Lupas A, Nordheim A. WIPI-1alpha (WIPI49), a member of the novel 7-bladed WIPI protein family, is aberrantly expressed in human cancer and is linked to starvation-induced autophagy. Oncogene. 2004;23:9314–25.

36. Vicinanza M, Korolchuk Viktor I, Ashkenazi A, Puri C, Menzies Fiona M, Clarke Jonathan H, et al. PI(5)P regulates autophagosome biogenesis. Mol Cell. 2015;57:219–34.

37. Mott BT, Eastman RT, Guha R, Sherlach KS, Siriwardana A, Shinn P, et al. High-throughput matrix screening identifies synergistic and antagonistic antimalarial drug combinations. Sci Rep. 2015;5:13891.

38. Proikas-Cezanne T, Ruckerbauer S, Stierhof YD, Berg C, Nordheim A. Human WIPI-1 puncta-formation: a novel assay to assess mammalian autophagy. FEBS Lett. 2007;581:3396–404.

39. Amaratunga C, Neal AT, Fairhurst RM. Flow cytometry-based analysis of artemisinin-resistant *Plasmodium falciparum* in the ring-stage survival assay. Antimicrob Agents Chemother. 2014;58:4938–40.

40. Blackman RK, Cheung-Ong K, Gebbia M, Proia DA, He S, Kepros J, et al. Mitochondrial electron transport is the cellular target of the oncology drug elesclomol. PLoS ONE. 2012;7:e29798.

41. Kirshner JR, He S, Balasubramanyam V, Kepros J, Yang CY, Zhang M, et al. Elesclomol induces cancer cell apoptosis through oxidative stress. Mol Cancer Ther. 2008;7:2319–27.

42. Wang Z, Cabrera M, Yang J, Yuan L, Gupta B, Liang X, et al. Genome-wide association analysis identifies genetic loci associated with resistance to multiple antimalarials in *Plasmodium falciparum* from China-Myanmar border. Sci Rep. 2016;6:33891.

43. Yeh E, DeRisi JL. Chemical rescue of malaria parasites lacking an apicoplast defines organelle function in blood-stage *Plasmodium falciparum*. PLoS Biol. 2011;9:e1001138.

44. Proikas-Cezanne T, Takacs Z, Dönnes P, Kohlbacher O. WIPI proteins: essential PtdIns3P effectors at the nascent autophagosome. J Cell Sci. 2015;128:207–17.

45. Hanahan D, Weinberg RA. The hallmarks of cancer. Cell. 2000;100:57–70.

46. Hanahan D, Weinberg RA. Hallmarks of cancer: the next generation. Cell. 2011;144:646–74.

47. Straimer J, Gnädig NF, Stokes BH, Ehrenberger M, Crane AA, Fidock DA. *Plasmodium falciparum* k13 mutations differentially impact ozonide susceptibility and parasite fitness in vitro. MBio. 2017;8:e00172–1117.

48. Cui L, Wang Z, Miao J, Miao M, Chandra R, Jiang H, et al. Mechanisms of in vitro resistance to dihydroartemisinin in *Plasmodium falciparum*. Mol Microbiol. 2012;86:111–28.

49. Becker K, Tilley L, Vennerstrom JL, Roberts D, Rogerson S, Ginsburg H. Oxidative stress in malaria parasite-infected erythrocytes: host–parasite interactions. Int J Parasitol. 2004;34:163–89.

50. Mejia P, Trevino-Villarreal JH, Hine C, Harputlugil E, Lang S, Calay E, et al. Dietary restriction protects against experimental cerebral malaria via leptin modulation and T-cell mTORC1 suppression. Nat Commun. 2015;6:6050.

51. Hunt NH, Manduci N, Thumwood CM. Amelioration of murine cerebral malaria by dietary restriction. Parasitology. 1993;107(Pt 5):471–6.

52. Murray MJ, Murray NJ, Murray AB, Murray MB. Refeeding-malaria and hyperferraemia. Lancet. 1975;1:653–4.

53. Mancio-Silva L, Slavic K, Grilo Ruivo MT, Grosso AR, Modrzynska KK, Vera IM, et al. Nutrient sensing modulates malaria parasite virulence. Nature. 2017;547:213–6.

54. Kim J, Kundu M, Viollet B, Guan K-L. AMPK and mTOR regulate autophagy through direct phosphorylation of Ulk1. Nat Cell Biol. 2011;13:132.

55. Delves M, Plouffe D, Scheurer C, Meister S, Wittlin S, Winzeler EA, et al. The activities of current antimalarial drugs on the life cycle stages of *Plasmodium*: a comparative study with human and rodent parasites. PLoS Med. 2012;9:e1001169.

56. Groth-Pedersen L, Ostenfeld MS, Høyer-Hansen M, Nylandsted J, Jäättelä M. Vincristine induces dramatic lysosomal changes and sensitizes cancer cells to lysosome-destabilizing Siramesine. Cancer Res. 2007;67:2217–25.

57. Morrison G, Fu X, Shea M, Nanda S, Giuliano M, Wang T, et al. Therapeutic potential of the dual EGFR/HER2 inhibitor AZD8931 in circumventing endocrine resistance. Breast Cancer Res Treat. 2014;144:263–72.

58. Lum JJ, Bauer DE, Kong M, Harris MH, Li C, Lindsten T, et al. Growth factor regulation of autophagy and cell survival in the absence of apoptosis. Cell. 2005;120:237–48.

59. Tan X, Thapa N, Sun Y, Anderson RA. A kinase-independent role for EGF receptor in autophagy initiation. Cell. 2015;160:145–60.

60. Liu JT, Li WC, Gao S, Wang F, Li XQ, Yu HQ, et al. Autophagy inhibition overcomes the antagonistic effect between gefitinib and cisplatin in epidermal growth factor receptor mutant non–small-cell lung cancer cells. Clin Lung Cancer. 2015;16:e55–66.

61. Hambright HG, Ghosh R. Autophagy: in the cROSshairs of cancer. Biochem Pharmacol. 2017;126:13–22.

62. Yu KY, Wang YP, Wang LH, Jian Y, Zhao XD, Chen JW, et al. Mitochondrial KATP channel involvement in angiotensin II-induced autophagy in vascular smooth muscle cells. Basic Res Cardiol. 2014;109:416.

63. Zhu L, Wei W, Zheng YQ, Jia XY. Effects and mechanisms of total glucosides of paeony on joint damage in rat collagen-induced arthritis. Inflamm Res. 2005;54:211–20.

64. Witkowski B, Amaratunga C, Khim N, Sreng S, Chim P, Kim S, et al. Novel phenotypic assays for the detection of artemisinin-resistant Plasmodium falciparum malaria in Cambodia: in vitro and ex vivo drug-response studies. Lancet Infect Dis. 2013;13:1043–9.

65. Witkowski B, Khim N, Chim P, Kim S, Ke S, Kloeung N, et al. Reduced artemisinin susceptibility of Plasmodium falciparum ring stages in western Cambodia. Antimicrob Agents Chemother. 2013;57:914–23.

11

Baseline entomologic data on malaria transmission in prelude to an indoor residual spraying intervention

Albert S. Salako[1,2]*, Idelphonse Ahogni[1,2], Casimir Kpanou[1,2], Arthur Sovi[3], Roseric Azondekon[1,4], André A. Sominahouin[1,5], Filémon Tokponnon[6], Virgile Gnanguenon[7], Fortuné Dagnon[8], Laurent Iyikirenga[9] and Martin C. Akogbeto[1]

Abstract

Background: Despite the success of indoor residual insecticide spraying (IRS) in Africa, particularly in Benin, some gaps of information need to be filled to optimize the effectiveness of this intervention in the perspective of the country's effort to eliminate malaria. In anticipation to the 2018 IRS campaign in two targeted regions of northern Benin, this study aimed, to collect baseline information on vector composition, spatio-temporal variation and peak malaria transmission in the Alibori and Donga, two targeted regions of northern Benin. Information collected will help to better plan the implementation and later on the impact assessment of this IRS campaign.

Methods: The study was carried out in four districts of the two IRS targeted regions of northern Benin. Human landing catches and pyrethrum spray catches protocols were used to assess the biting rate (HBR) and, biting/resting behaviour of malaria vector populations. After morphological identification of collected *Anopheles*, the heads and thoraxes of *Anopheles gambiae* sensu lato (s.l.) were analysed by the ELISA CSP tests to estimate the sporozoite index (SI). The entomological inoculation rate was calculated as the product of mosquito biting rate (HBR) and the SI.

Results: The biting rates of *An. gambiae* s.l., the major vector in this study sites, varied significantly from region to region. It was higher: in rural than in urban areas, in rainy season than in dry season, indoors than outdoors. Overall, SI was comparable between sites. The highest EIRs were observed in the Donga region (16.84 infectious bites/man/month in Djougou district and 17.64 infectious bites/man/month in Copargo district) and the lowest in the Alibori region (10.74 infectious bites/man/month at Kandi district and 11.04 infectious bites/man/month at Gogounou district).

Conclusion: This study showed the heterogeneous and various nature of malaria epidemiology in Northern Benin. Indeed, the epidemiological profile of malaria transmission in the Alibori and Donga regions is made of a single season of transmission interrupted by a dry season. This period of transmission is relatively longer in Donga region than in Alibori. This information can be used to guide the extension of IRS in the Alibori and in the Donga, by primarily targeting areas with short periods of transmission, and easy to cover.

Keywords: Malaria transmission, *Anopheles gambiae* s.l., IRS, Alibori, Donga, Benin

*Correspondence: albertsourousalako@ahoo.fr
[1] Centre de Recherche entomologique de Cotonou (CREC), Cotonou, Benin
Full list of author information is available at the end of the article

Background

Indoor residual spraying (IRS) and insecticide-treated nets (ITNs) are two key and effective strategies designed to interrupt malaria transmission [1–3]. IRS has greatly contributed to reduce or eliminate malaria from many areas of the world, particularly in situations where mosquito vectors feed and rest indoors and where the transmission of malaria is seasonal [4–7]. In Benin, after 6 years of intervention, IRS has proved to be an effective vector control intervention [8]. Started in 2008 in the Oueme region (southern Benin), then relocated to the Atacora region (North Benin) from 2011 to 2015, the intervention was effective in reducing the level of malaria transmission [8–10]. The same trend has been observed in other sub-Saharan countries with this intervention: Swaziland, Botswana, South Africa, Zimbabwe and Mozambique [11], Madagascar [12], Equatorial Guinea (Bioko Island) [13–15], in Uganda [16], Kenya [17] and Tanzania [18]. Unfortunately, IRS effectiveness is being jeopardized by the spread and intensification of insecticide resistance, including to pyrethroids [19–24] and more recently to bendiocarb [25–27]. Density and distribution of *Anopheles,* vectors of malaria vary according to the region and the time of year, and these variations can modify malaria transmission levels [28–31]. Several studies have shown that malaria infection is influenced by environmental factors, such as temperature, precipitation, and relative humidity that vary from region to region [32]. However, in most parts of Africa, there are still gaps in information regarding the dynamics of malaria transmission resulting in the implementation of vector control interventions without sufficient decision-making basis [33–35].

This was the case of Benin where, from 2008 to 2009, a single round of IRS instead of two was implemented in the Oueme region to cover the period of malaria transmission [9]. In 2017, the IRS campaign, with pirimiphos methyl (Actellic 300CS), has targeted all eligible households in the Alibori and Donga regions. These two regions being located in two different eco-geographical areas despite their proximity, it was hypothesized that variations in vectors ecology may affect the micro-epidemiology of malaria. It is in this context that this study was initiated with the aim of obtaining useful information for a better planning and assessment of IRS intervention.

Methods

Study site

Entomological data were collected from two regions with two districts each: Alibori (Gogounou, Kandi) and Donga (Copargo, Djougou) (Fig. 1). The region of Alibori is characterized by a Sudanese climate and the Donga by a Sudano-guinean climate, with a single dry season (December to May) and a single rainy season (June to November). The annual average rainfall varies between 700–1200 mm and 1200–1300 mm, respectively in Alibori and Donga regions. The average monthly temperature varies between 23 and 40 °C. The region of Donga has more rivers than the region of Alibori. The major economic activity is farming of cotton, maize and millet [36, 37].

Malaria prevalence is generally higher in Donga region than in Alibori [38]. Long-lasting insecticide-treated mosquito nets (LLINs) distributed every 3 years throughout the mass campaign distribution are the main tools used to prevent human–vector contact in the four districts. In each district, two sites, one in urban and one in rural setting, were selected for mosquito collections. These sites are:

- In Djougou district:
  Zountori: a urban area of Djougou (09°42′10.1″ N latitude and 01°40′55.4″ E longitude);
  Barienou: a rural village of Djougou (09°42′58.4″ N latitude and 01°46′06.5″ E longitude) (Fig. 1).
- In Copargo district:
  Parakounan: a urban area of Copargo (09°50′19.3″ N latitude and 01°32′39.5″ E longitude);
  Kataban: a rural village of Copargo (09°54′34.3″ N latitude and 01°31′26.9″ E longitude);
- In Kandi district:
  Kossarou: a urban area of Kandi (11°07′29.32″ N latitude and 2°56′9.57″ E longitude);
  Sonsoro: a rural village of Kandi (11°4′58.91″ North latitude and 2°13′37.60″ East longitude);
- In Gogounou district:
  Bantansoue: a urban area of Gogounou (10°50′30.6″ N latitude and 2°50′20.3″ E longitude);
  Gounarou: a rural village of Gogounou (10°52′20.8″ N latitude and 2°50′51.2″ E longitude) (Fig. 1).

Sampling of *Anopheles* vectors of malaria was conducted from May 2016 to February 2017.

Ethical considerations

The protocol of this study has been reviewed and approved by the Institutional Ethics Committee of the Center for the Research in Entomology of Cotonou (IECC). Verbal consent was obtained from local mosquito collectors before being involved in the study. They subsequently received a vaccine against yellow fever as a prophylactic measure. An agreement with health facilities close to sites was also obtained for the free anti-malarial

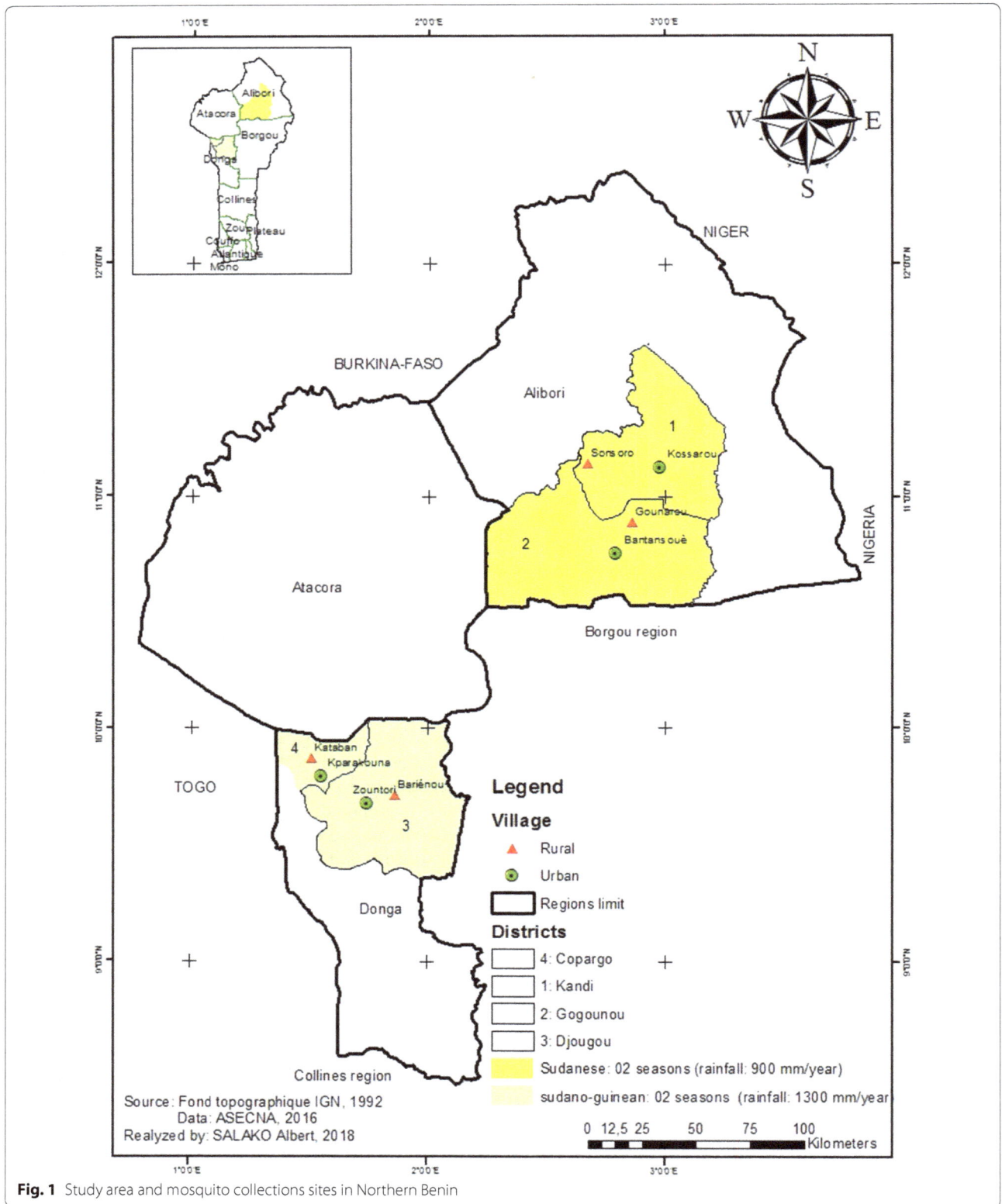

Fig. 1 Study area and mosquito collections sites in Northern Benin

treatment of mosquito collectors who would suffered from malaria.

Anopheles adult collection

Malaria transmission dynamics were assessed in the 08 identified and described sites in the study area. This is why two classical methods were used for the sampling of *Anopheles* mosquitoes. The first sampling method is termed as Human Landing Catch (HLC), and was carried out from 9:00 p.m. to 5:00 a.m. in 2 nights per month per district, enabled the evaluation of the frequency of human–vector contact (human biting rate). For this purpose, four volunteers (02 inside and 02 outside) captured mosquitoes in 02 randomly selected houses per site, making a total of eight collectors per district per night. The collectors are rotated in the different houses to avoid biases related to their ability or their individual attractiveness. The second sampling method is pyrethrum spray catch (PSC) which was carried out through two morning sessions (between 6 a.m. and 8:30 a.m.) per month in 40 houses per district. This method allowed the collection of resting mosquitoes inside houses.

Mosquito processing

These mosquitoes as well as those caught on human bait were examined for *Plasmodium falciparum* infectivity. After each collection, collected mosquitoes were counted and morphologically identified using the taxonomic key of Gillies and De Meillon [39]. Females of *An. gambiae* s.l. (refered to as *An. gambiae* thereafter in the text) caught on human bait were then dissected to assess their physiological age [40]. Each specimen was finally stored in a labelled Eppendorf tube containing silicagel for further laboratory analysis.

The heads and thorax of females of *An. gambiae* collected at each site were analysed by enzyme-linked immunosorbent assay (ELISA) according to the method described by Wirtz et al. [41]. This allows the detection of *P. falciparum* infection and the calculation of infectivity rates.

Estimation of entomological parameters

The *human biting rate* (HBR) for identified vector species was calculated as the number of *An. gambiae* caught per person per night of sampling effort. The *sporozoite index* (SI) is the proportion of *An. gambiae* s.l. with circumsporozoite protein of *P. falciparum*: $SI = (Thorax + / Thorax\ analysed) \times 100$. The *parity rate* is a percentage of *An. gambiae* that have laid eggs at least once (parous) out of the total number of *An. gambiae* dissected for the examination of the physiological status of their ovaries. It indicates the proportion of older mosquitoes within the population during

the survey. The *entomological inoculation rate* (EIR), a key variable expressing the malaria transmission level and which is defined as the number of infective bites received/man/night. It is the product of *An. gambiae* biting rate and SI data acquired from HLCs and the ELISA tests, respectively.

Data analysis

Data were analysed with the R statistics software, version 2.8. The Poisson method was used to estimate the confidence intervals [42] of HBRs and EIRs of *An. gambiae*. The binomial method for calculation of confidence intervals [42] was used to estimate the confidence intervals of parity and infectivity rates of *An. gambiae*. The unconditional maximum likelihood estimation method Wald, or median unbiased estimation (mid-p) of the risk ratio (RR) followed by their confidence intervals obtained using the normal approximation or the exact method p-values obtained by Khi^2 or mid-p.exact [43] was used to compare EIR. Proportion comparison tests were used to compare SI and parity rates. A difference is considered as significant when the p-value is less than 0.05.

Results

Vector species composition

A total of 3876 specimens of *Anopheles* mosquitoes from six different species were collected in the regions of Alibori and Donga. The most abundant species was *An. gambiae*, which accounted for 97.72% (3788/3876) of the collected vectors, followed by *Anopheles funestus* (1.88%, 73/3876). The biting behaviour of these two vector species was generally higher in the Donga compared to the Alibori. It should be noted that *An. funestus* was mainly collected in the district of Djougou which provided about 82.2% (60/73) of the specimens (Table 1). Among *Anopheles* species which were collected, there were only 9 *Anopheles coustani* (0.23%), 3 *Anopheles pharoensis* (0.077%), 2 *Anopheles ziemanni* (0.05%) and 1 *Anopheles paludis* (0.025%) (Table 1).

Variability of human biting rates

The biting rate of *An. gambiae* varied significantly from region to region: 6.55–7.51 bites/man/night (b/m/n) in the Donga against 4.4–4.78 bites/man/night in the Alibori (p < 0.05) (Table 2). The HBR was four times higher in rural areas compared to urban areas (RR = 4.27; p < 0.0001). The data also show that the average biting rate of *An. gambiae* was higher indoors (6.37 bites/man/night) than outdoors (5.25 bites/man/night). In the dry season, it was 2.27 bites/man/night compared to 9.95 bites/man/night in the rainy season, an increase of more than four times (RR = 4.38; p < 0.0001) (Table 2). In both regions, the highest biting rates were observed between

Table 1 Vector species composition in all districts, May 2016–February 2017

Regions	Districts	Anopheles gambiae s.l.	Anopheles funestus	Anopheles pharoensis	Anopheles ziemanni	Anopheles coustani	Anopheles paludis
Donga	Djougou	1086	60	0	0	1	0
	Copargo	1188	8	2	1	8	1
	Sub-total	2274	68	2	1	9	1
Alibori	Kandi	869	4	0	1	0	0
	Gogounou	645	1	1	0	0	0
	Sub-total	1514	5	1	1	0	0
	Total	3788	73	3	2	9	1

Table 2 *An. gambiae* s.l. average monthly biting trends by district, settings and seasons (May 2016 to February 2017)

Variables	Modalities	May	June	July	August	October	January	February	HBR/night	CI-95%	RR and CI-95%	p (Wald)
Donga	Djougou	2	2.88	9.13	13.06	9.06	2.38	5.13	6.55[a]	[6.07–7.06]	1	–
	Copargo	0.75	7.06	10.56	16.63	10.5	1.5	2.25	7.51[b]	[7.00–8.06]	1.15 [1.03–1.27]	0.0089
Alibori	Kandi	0.13	4.19	6.75	8.75	10.81	0.25	0.31	4.78[c]	[4.37–5.22]	0.73 [0.65–0.82]	< 0.001
	Gogounou	0.38	1.31	4.56	9	10.63	2	0.94	4.4[c]	[4–4.83]	0.67 [0.59–0.76]	< 0.001
Settings	Urban area	0.13	0.63	2.78	5.09	4.28	0.72	0.78	2.18[a]	[1.99–2.39]	1	–
	Rural area	1.50	7.09	12.72	18.63	16.22	2.34	3.53	9.42[b]	[9.01–9.85]	4.27 [3.85–4.75]	< 0.0001
Location	Indoor	1.06	3.53	8.50	12.13	11.97	1.97	2.81	6.37[a]	[6.03–6.72]	1	–
	Outdoor	0.56	4.19	7.00	11.59	8.53	1.09	1.50	5.25[b]	[4.95–5.58]	0.83 [0.76–0.89]	< 0.001
Seasonality	Dry season	0.81	–	–	–	–	1.53	2.16	2.27[a]	[2.07–2.47]	1	–
	Rainy season	–	3.86	7.75	11.86	10.25	–	–	9.95[b]	[9.51–10.40]	4.38 [3.97–4.83]	< 0.0001

[a,b,c] The values of the same variable with different letters are statistically different

June and October with a peak in October and August, respectively in Alibori and Donga (Table 2).

Sporozoite index of *Anopheles gambiae*

Overall, out of a total of 3788 head-thoraxes of *An. gambiae* assessed by ELISA, approximately 305 were found to be positive for the circumsporozoitic antigen of *P. falciparum*, which equates to a mean SI of 8.05% [7.20–8.96]. The SI were similar between urban (6.35% [4.63–8.46]) and rural (8.42% [7.6–9.45]) areas (p = 0.086). The highest infection rates were observed in Gounarou (11.65% [8.48–15.46]) and Kossarou (11.36% [5.58–19.90]) and the lowest in Bantansoue (4.44% [2.38–7.46]) (Table 3).

Overall, mosquito infectivity was 7.48% [5.81–9.43], 8.37% [6.35–10.78], 8.56% [6.96–10.38] and 7.82% [6.36–9.50], respectively in the districts of Kandi, Gogounou, Djougou and Copargo (Table 3). By cumulating data by region, SI was also similar (7.86% [6.55–9.33] in the Alibori versus 8.18% [7.08–9.38] in the Donga, p = 0.769) (Table 3).

Cumulative data from both regions show similar average of infectivity rates in the rainy season (8.07% [7.14–9.07]) and in the dry season (7.95% [5.95–10.34]) (p = 0.981). In Kandi, Gogounou and Djougou, mosquito infectivity was respectively 8.89% [3.91–16.76], 4.38%

[1.43–9.93] and 11.26% [7.92–15.37] in the dry season versus 7.32% [5.58–9.37], 9.23% [6.90–12.01] and 7.53% [5.77–9.60] in the rainy season (p > 0.05). Conversely, in Copargo, the SI was significantly higher in the rainy season (8.45% [6.84–10.28]) than in the dry season (2.44% [0.63–7.50]) (p = 0.0297) (Table 3).

Entomological inoculation rate of *Anopheles gambiae*

Tables 4 and 5 show the spatio-temporal variation in entomological inoculation rates (EIR). A variation of the EIR across districts was significantly higher in the rainy season (June, July, August and October) than in the dry season (May, January and February) (p < 0.05) (Table 4).

Overall, the lowest infectivity was observed in Kandi (10.74 infective bites/man/month) and Gogounou (11.04 infective bites/man/month) in Alibori region than in Djougou (16.84 infective bites/man/month) and Copargo (17.64 infectious bites/man/month) in Donga region (Table 4). In the four districts, the infectivity was higher in rural areas than in urban areas (p < 0.05). Cumulative data revealed an average EIR of 23.79 infectious bites/man/month in rural areas versus 4.15 infectious bites/man/month in urban areas (p < 0.0001) (Table 5). In Alibori's districts (Kandi and Gogounou), the period of malaria transmission was relatively shorter than in

Table 3 Sporozoite index of *Anopheles gambiae* s.l.

Districts	Sites	May (DS)	June (RS)	July (RS)	August (RS)	October (RS)	January (DS)	February (DS)	Mean (DS)	Mean (RS)	Mean (7 months)	CI 95%	p-value
Kandi	Sonsoro*												
	Thorax	38	119	175	166	244	10	29	77	704	781		0.212
	Thorax+	6	6	9	4	30	0	0	6	49	55		
	SI	15.79	5.04	5.14	2.41	12.30	0	0	7.79[a]	6.96[a]	7.042	[5.34–9.06]	
	Kossarou												
	Thorax	7	4	6	16	49	2	4	13	75	88		
	Thorax+	1	0	0	0	8	1	0	2	8	10		
	SI	14.29	0	0	0	16.33	50	0	15.38[a]	10.67[a]	11.36	[5.58–19.90]	
	Total												
	Thorax	45	123	181	182	293	12	33	90	779	869		
	Thorax+	7	6	9	4	38	1	0	8	57	65		
	SI	15.56	4.88	4.97	2.20	12.97	8.33	0	8.89[a]	7.32[a]	7.47	[5.81–9.43]	
Gogounou	Gounarou*												
	Thorax	7	8	33	93	167	22	22	51	301	352		0.0016
	Thorax+	0	1	2	10	27	0	1	1	40	41		
	SI	0	12.50	6.06	10.75	16.17	0	4.55	1.96[a]	13.29[b]	11.65	[8.48–15.46]	
	Bantansoue												
	Thorax	0	23	64	72	71	33	30	63	230	293		
	Thorax+	0	1	1	2	5	3	1	4	9	13		
	SI	–	4.35	1.56	2.78	7.04	9.09	3.33	6.35[a]	3.91[a]	4.44	[2.38–7.46]	
	Total												
	Thorax	7	31	97	165	238	55	52	114	531	645		
	Thorax+	0	2	3	12	32	3	2	5	49	54		
	SI	0	6.45	3.09	7.27	13.45	5.45	3.85	4.39[a]	9.23[a]	8.37	[6.35–10.78]	
Total (Alibori region)	Thorax	52	154	278	347	531	67	85	204	1310	1514		
	Thorax+	7	8	12	16	70	4	2	13	106	119		
	SI	13.46	5.19	4.32	4.61	13.18	5.97	2.35	6.37[a]	8.09[a]	7.86	[6.55–9.33]	
Djougou	Barienou*												
	Thorax	56	57	251	198	145	51	171	278	651	929		0.223
	Thorax+	15	4	6	25	16	3	15	33	51	84		
	SI	26.79	7.02	2.39	12.63	11.03	5.88	8.77	11.87[a]	7.83[a]	9.04	[7.27–11.07]	
	Zountori												
	Thorax	0	0	33	59	41	18	6	24	133	157		
	Thorax+	0	0	1	5	2	1	0	1	8	9		
	SI	–	–	3.03	8.47	4.88	5.56	0	4.17[a]	6.02[a]	5.73	[2.65–10.60]	
	Total												
	Thorax	56	57	284	257	186	69	177	302	784	1086		
	Thorax+	15	4	7	30	18	4	15	34	59	93		
	SI	26.79	7.02	2.46	11.67	9.68	5.80	8.47	11.26[a]	7.53[a]	8.56	[6.96–10.38]	

Table 3 (continued)

Districts	Sites	May (DS)	June (RS)	July (RS)	August (RS)	October (RS)	January (DS)	February (DS)	Mean (DS)	Mean (RS)	Mean (7 months)	CI 95%	p-value
Copargo	Kataban*												
	Thorax	13	189	274	284	198	35	56	104	945	1049		1
	Thorax+	0	8	16	34	21	3	0	3	79	82		
	SI	0	4.23	5.84	11.97	10.61	8.57	0	2.88a	8.36a	7.81	[6.26–9.61]	
	Kparakouna												
	Thorax	1	11	27	61	21	4	14	19	120	139		
	Thorax+	0	0	0	6	5	0	0	0	11	11		
	SI	0	0	0	9.84	23.81	0	0	0a	9.16a	7.91	[4.01–13.71]	
	Total												
	Thorax	14	200	301	345	219	39	70	123	1065	1188		
	Thorax+	0	8	16	40	26	3	0	3	90	93		
	SI	0	4	5.32	11.59	11.87	7.69	0	2.44a	8.45b	7.83	[6.36–9.50]	
Total (Donga region)	Thorax	70	257	585	602	405	108	247	425	1849	2274		
	Thorax+	15	12	23	70	44	7	15	37	149	186		
	SI	21.43	4.67	3.93	11.63	10.86	6.48	6.07	8.71a	8.06a	8.18	[7.08–9.38]	
Total (rural areas)	Thorax	114	373	733	741	754	118	278	510	2601	3111		0.086
	Thorax+	21	19	33	73	94	6	16	43	219	262		
	SI	18.42	5.09	4.50	9.85	12.47	5.08	5.76	8.43a	8.42a	8.42	[7.46–9.45]	
Total (urban areas)	Thorax	8	38	130	208	182	57	54	119	558	677		
	Thorax+	1	1	2	13	20	5	1	7	36	43		
	SI	12.50	2.63	1.54	6.25	10.99	8.77	1.85	5.88a	6.45a	6.35	[4.63–8.46]	
Grand total	Thorax	122	411	863	949	936	175	332	629	3159	3788		
	Thorax+	22	20	35	86	114	11	17	50	255	305		
	SI	18.03	4.87	4.06	9.06	12.18	6.29	5.12	7.95a	8.07a	8.05	[7.20–8.96]	

SI: sporozoite index; CI: confidence interval; *: rural area; DS: dry season; RS: rainy season

a,b The SI/season of the same site bearing different letters are statistically different

Donga's districts where it extended from May to February at Djougou and, from June to January at Copargo (Fig. 2). In Alibori region, the peak of transmission was recorded in October at Kandi (42.06 infectious bites/man/month) and Gogounou (42.86 infectious bites/man/month). Conversely, in Donga region, it was observed in August at Djougou (45.6 infectious bites/man/month) and Copargo (57.6 infectious bites/man/month) (Fig. 2 and Table 5).

Seasonal variation of the parity of Anopheles gambiae

Ovaries dissection of 1640 females of *An. gambiae* collected through HLCs were performed to determine parity rates. 1185 (72.3%) were found parous. Vectors' parity rate was 81.90% [73.19–88.73], 91.38% [81.01–97.14] and 89.13% [76.43–96.37] during the dry season against 71.14% [66.39–75.56], 70.59% [65.90–74.96] and 68.58% [62.57–74.16] during the rainy season (p < 0.05), respectively in Djougou, Copargo and Gogounou. In Kandi, no significant difference was observed between parous rates

of both seasons, probably due to the low number of mosquitoes dissected in the dry season (Table 6). Overall, cumulative data showed an average parous rate estimated at 86.70% [81.45–90.90] in the dry season against 70.04% [67.58–72.41] in the rainy season (p < 0.001).

Discussion

The study of the dynamics of malaria transmission is a prerequisite to not only understand the epidemiology of this disease, but also to establish effective and targeted control of mosquito, vectors of diseases [44]. The entomological monitoring that we carried out revealed that *An. gambiae* and *An. funestus* were the main malaria vectors in Alibori and Donga regions, which confirms the results of previous studies conducted in West Africa, and specifically in Benin [45–47]. *Anopheles gambiae* appeared as the major vector (97.72%) in the two regions. This finding corroborates previous data published by Aikpon et al. [48] in Atacora and Gnanguenon et al.

Table 4 Entomological inoculation rates (EIR) per district according to the season

Districts	Parameters	Dry season (May–January–February)	Rainy season (June–October)	Total	RR (95% CI)	p (Wald)
Kandi	HBR/night	0.25	7.625	4.78		
	SI	8.89	7.32	7.48		
	EIR/night	0.022	0.558	0.358		
	EIR/month	0.66[a]	16.74[b]	10.75	1	–
Gogounou	HBR/night	1.25	6.375	4.4		
	SI	4.4	9.2	8.37		
	EIR/night	0.055	0.588	0.368		
	EIR/month	1.645[a]	17.648[b]	11.06	1.03 [1.012–1.046]	0.0006
Djougou	HBR/night	3.4	8.53125	6.55		
	SI	11.3	7.5	8.56		
	EIR/night	0.38	0.64	0.561		
	EIR/month	11.48[a]	19.26[b]	16.85	1.56 [1.54–1.58]	< 0.001
Copargo	HBR/night	1.65	11.1875	7.5		
	SI	2.44	8.45	7.82		
	EIR/night	0.04	0.945	0.588		
	EIR/month	1.21[a]	28.36[b]	17.66	1.64 [1.62–1.66]	< 0.001

EIR: entomological inoculation rate; RR: rate ratio; CI: confidence interval; p-Wald: p-value of the significance of the ratio of entomological inoculation rate between districts

[a,b] The EIR/season of the same district bearing different letters are statistically different

[47] in Kandi and Malanville, two districts of the region of Alibori. According to Akogbéto et al. [49], in Alibori and Donga regions, *An. gambiae* is composed of two sibling species (*An. gambiae* and *Anopheles coluzzii*) whose proportions vary depending on the region. In Alibori region, species composition showed *An. coluzzii* (62.2%) and *An. gambiae* (37.8%). In Donga, *An. gambiae* was the most abundant (64.7%). The two species were present throughout the transmission season [49]. *Anopheles gambiae* showed endophagic tendency. This behaviour of *An. gambiae* which feeds on man, preferentially inside houses, is justified by the fact that *An. gambiae* populations rest exclusively indoors during the rainy season, a period of vector abundance. However, this strong endophagy could also be facilitated by the alteration of the repulsive and lethal properties of the LLINs distributed in 2014 within the communities in both regions. In fact, according to Darriet [50], a new Olyset net reduces the entry rate of *An. gambiae* in the huts by 44% compared to an untreated net, whereas when it is 3 years old, its repellent effect is halved and this effect does no longer exist when it is washed. In addition, the dosage of the amount of insecticide carried out by Azondékon et al. [51] on LLINs fibers surface revealed a decrease in chemical efficacy only 6 months after the distribution of the LLINs Furthermore, the endophagic nature of *An. gambiae* in the study area is an asset for a preventive control based on IRS.

Regarding *An. funestus*, it represents the secondary vector encountered in the study area as it was found in a very low density compared to *An. gambiae*. This very low density has already been reported by Aikpon et al. [48] in the region of Atacora and by Gnanguenon et al. [47] in the Alibori (particularly in Kandi). The low abundance of *An. funestus* in Kandi and Gogounou may be due to the absence of its typical larval habitat (permanent or semi-permanent shaded freshwater streams, swamps, ponds and lakes) in these areas in view of the length of the drought period.

However, Aikpon et al. [52] reported a marked seasonal trend of *An. funestus* in Copargo (Donga region) with high abundance in the dry season. Conversely, the relatively high density of *An. funestus* in Djougou district, compared to other districts, is due to the existence of a small semi-permanent river, with surrounding vegetation, located not far from one of the study sites (Barienou).

The proportion of *An. gambiae* tested positive to circumsporozoitic antigen of *P. falciparum* was very high in the Alibori and in the Donga (SI = 8.05%), which stresses the need for the implementation of an effective malaria vectors control strategy in these two regions. A similar SI was previously reported in the Atacora, a northern region in Benin (SI = 6.63%) [48], in the Ouidah-Kpomasse-Tori region (southern Benin) (SI = 9.63%) [53] and in western Kenya (SI = 8.2%) [54]. This SI is lower than

Table 5 Monthly variation of EIR per site and per district

Districts	Sites		May	June	July	August	October	January	February	EIR/night	EIR/month	EIR/year	RR (95% IC)	P (Wald)
Kandi	Sonsoro[a]													< 0.0001
		HBR/night	0	8.25	13.25	15.75	17.63	0.38	0.38	0.6	18.08	216.96	1	
		EIR/night	0	0.42	0.68	0.38	2.17	0	0					
	Kossarou													
		HBR/night	0.25	0.13	0.25	1.75	4	0.13	0.25	0.12	3.47	41.7	0.19 [0.17–0.21]	
		EIR/night	0.04	0	0	0	0.65	0.06	0					
	Total													
		HBR/night	0.13	4.19	6.75	8.75	10.81	0.25	0.31	0.358	10.75	128.94		
		EIR/night	0.019	0.204	0.336	0.192	1.402	0.021	0					
Gogounou	Gounarou[a]													< 0.0001
		HBR/night	0.75	0.63	3	10.88	14.38	1.75	1	0.57	17.2	206.43	1	
		EIR/night	0	0.08	0.18	1.17	2.32	0	0.05					
	Bantansoue													
		HBR/night	0	2	6.13	7.13	6.88	2.25	0.88	0.17	5.17	62.05	0.30 [0.28–031]	
		EIR/night	0	0.09	0.1	0.2	0.48	0.2	0.03					
	Total													
		HBR/night	0.38	1.31	4.56	9	10.63	2	0.94	0.369	11.06	132.73		
		EIR/night	0	0.08	0.14	0.65	.43	0.11	0.04					
Djougou	Barienou[a]													< 0.0001
		HBR/night	4	5.75	15.88	20	14.38	4.38	9.75	1.003	30.1	361.19	1	
		EIR/night	1.07	0.4	0.38	2.53	1.59	0.26	0.86					
	Zountori													
		HBR/night	0	0	2.38	6.13	3.75	0.38	0.5	0.057	1.72	20.64	0.11 [0.10–0.12]	
		EIR/night	0	0	0.03	0.085	0.049	0.056	0					
	Total													
		HBR/night	2	2.88	9.13	13.06	9.06	2.38	5.13	0.562	16.85	202.17		
		EIR/night	0.54	0.20	0.22	1.52	0.88	0.14	0.43					

Table 5 (continued)

Districts	Sites		May	June	July	August	October	January	February	EIR/night	EIR/month	EIR/year	RR (95% IC)	P (Wald)
Copargo	Kataban[a]													
		HBR/night	1.25	13.75	18.75	27.88	18.5	2.88	3					< 0.0001
		EIR/night	0	0.582	1.095	3.337	1.962	0.246	0	1.027	30.81	369.72	1	
	Kparakouna													
		HBR/night	0.25	0.38	2.38	5.38	2.5	0.13	1.5					
		EIR/night	0	0	0	0.529	0.595	0	0	0.151	4.52	54.24	0.14 [0.13–0.15]	
	Total													
		HBR/night	0.75	7.06	10.56	16.63	10.50	1.50	2.25					
		EIR/night	0	0.28	0.56	1.92	1.24	0.11	0	0.589	17.66	211.91		
Urbanization	Rural areas[a]													
		HBR/night	1.5	7.09	12.72	18.63	16.2	2.34	3.53					< 0.0001
		EIR/night	0.27	0.36	0.57	1.83	2.023	0.119	0.203	0.793	23.79	285.54	1	
	Urban area													
		HBR/night	0.13	0.63	2.78	5.09	4.28	0.72	0.78					
		EIR/night	0.016	0.017	0.043	0.318	0.470	0.063	0.014	0.138	4.15	49.83	0.176 [0.174–0.179]	

EIR: entomological inoculation rate; RR: rate ratio; CI: confidence interval of RR; p-Wald: p-value of the significance of the ratio of entomological inoculation rate between the rural and urban areas

[a] Rural area

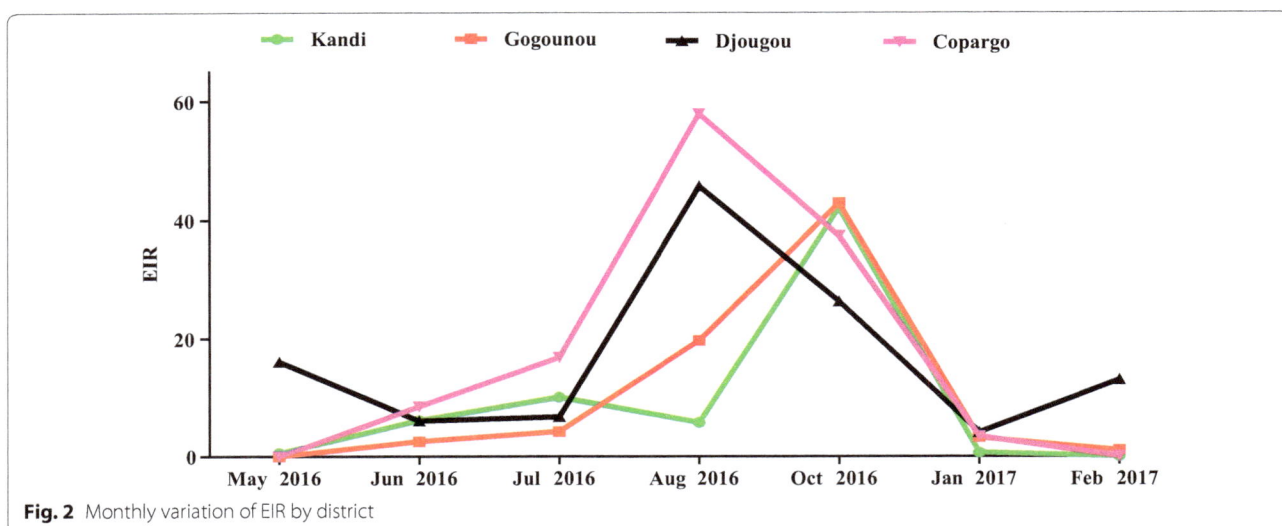

Fig. 2 Monthly variation of EIR by district

Table 6 Parity rates of *Anopheles gambiae* s.l.

Districts	Dry season (May–January–February)			Rainy season (June–October)			p-value
	Number dissected	Parous	Parous rate (%)	Number dissected	Parous	Parous rate (%)	
Djougou	105	86	81.90	395	281	71.14	0.0361
Copargo	58	53	91.38	408	288	70.59	0.0014
Kandi	9	9	100	358	248	69.27	0.1055
Gogounou	46	41	89.13	261	179	68.58	0.0074
Total	218	189	86.70	1422	996	70.04	0.00042

those observed in Eastern Gambia (SI = 17.73%) [55] and in Guinea-Bissau (SI = 12%) [56, 57]. This relatively high infection rate could be due to an increase in human–vector contact facilitated by anthropogenic behaviours (late hours at which people go to bed, non-usage of LLINs and others) and some factors that affect physical integrity (usage of sharp objects and lighted candles) and chemical effectiveness (high washing frequency) of LLINs. Other environmental factors, including high ambient temperature, prompt people to sleep outside without any protection against mosquito bites. This observation underscores the need to support IRS campaign with appropriate information, education and communication campaigns to combat this sleeping are misbehaviour in sprayed areas.

Although the infectivity rate was not the same in the four districts the highest rates were obtained in Djougou (16.84 infectious bites/man/month) and Copargo (17.64 infectious bites/man/month) and the lowest in Kandi (10.74 infectious bites/man/month) and Gogounou (11.04 infectious bites/man/month). These results suggest that the intensity of malaria transmission is higher

in Donga region than in Alibori. Considering that the entomological inoculation rate is calculated using human biting and SI and, on the other hand, the similarity of SI in the two regions, it is legitimate to infer that the biting rate of *An. gambiae* was the main factor causing the difference observed between malaria transmission levels of the two regions. This deduction confirms the findings of Garrett-Jones [58], who reported that vector abundance is an important determinant in the malaria transmission level. In the case of the present study, the highest biting frequency of *An. gambiae* was observed in Donga region compared to Alibori (p < 0.0001), which could be due to some environmental characteristics (rainfall and soil humidity higher in the Donga region than in that of Alibori, thus promoting vector proliferation). Variation in malaria transmission levels between the two investigated regions may also be related to differences in topographies. In Alibori region, Kandi and Gogounou districts are located in areas of sloping plateaus that favour the runoff of water towards the south of the country after the rains. This situation prevents the on-site formation of a large number of breeding sites, resulting in lower vector abundance in Alibori region compared to Donga region. These results are consistent with findings of Omukunda et al. [59] who investigated similar bioecological areas in western Kenya.

The higher infection rates in rural areas compared to urban areas (p = 0) in the four districts confirm the spatial polymorphism in malaria epidemiology as previously observed by Sovi et al. [60] in the region of the Plateau, southeast of Benin. High EIRs obtained in rural areas were likely due to a high biting rate of *An. gambiae* resulting from an exponential proliferation in breeding sites meeting optimum conditions for development, in contrast to urban areas where the larval habitats are generally quite polluted and, therefore, more conducive to the development of *Culicines* [61]. Similar results have been observed in Dar es Salaam, Tanzania [62], in Ouagadougou, Burkina Faso [63], in Tori-bossito, southern Benin [64], in Kandi, northeastern Benin [31] and in the north–south transect of Benin [47]. In the study area, the risk of malaria infection was very high during the rainy season, but too low during the dry season despite the high parity rate in *An. gambiae* during this period compared to the rainy season. The period of malaria transmission is relatively longer in Donga region than in Alibori with a peak, respectively in August and October. These results are typical of tropical facies to which belong the two regions and characterized by a seasonal transmission of malaria interrupted by a dry season covering a non-negligible time in a year. A similar epidemiological facies was found in Zimbabwe, Kenya, Tanzania, northern areas of Nigeria, Benin, Ghana, Côte d'Ivoire and Guinea [65]. This observation should be taken into account to schedule spraying operations for a better impact of the intervention. Indeed, it is more appropriate to start the IRS campaign before the transmission period. In the four district covered by this study, June appeared to be the best period to start the IRS intervention. Since the CS formulation of pirimiphos methyl to be used for the next IRS campaign has a 4-month persistence period in field conditions of Atacora region [8], the short duration of malaria transmission in the Alibori region could be considered as an advantage.

Conclusion

The Alibori and Donga regions are characterized by one transmission season relatively longer in Donga region than in Alibori. Spatio-temporal variation in entomological inoculation rates was also observed with higher rates in rural areas and during the rainy season. Given the duration of persistence of pirimiphos methyl selected for the IRS operations, the month of June would be the ideal period to start the implementation of the intervention. The information collected in this study provides a reference for the monitoring and evaluation of the IRS intervention in four districts of the study area.

Abbreviations
EIR: entomological inoculation rate; HBR: human biting rate; HLC: human landing catch; SI: sporozoite index; IRS: indoor residual spraying; ITN: insecticide treated net; LLIN: long lasting insecticidal nets; PSC: pyrethrum spray catch; CS: micro-encapsulated formulation.

Authors' contributions
ASS, IA, CK, FT and MCA conceived the study. ASS and MCA have participated in the design of the study. ASS, IA, CK, AAS and VG carried out the field activities and the laboratory analysis. ASS and MCA drafted the manuscript. RA, AS, LI, FT, FD and MCA critically revised the manuscript for intellectual content. All authors read and approved the final manuscript.

Author details
[1] Centre de Recherche entomologique de Cotonou (CREC), Cotonou, Benin.
[2] Faculté des Sciences et Techniques de l'Université d'Abomey-Calavi, Abomey-Calavi, Benin. [3] PMI VectorLink Project, Abt Associates, Bamako, Mali.
[4] University of Wisconsin Milwaukee, Milwaukee, WI, USA. [5] Faculté des Sciences Humaines et Sociales de l'Université d'Abomey-Calavi, Abomey-Calavi, Benin. [6] Programme Nationale de Lutte contre le Paludisme, Cotonou, Benin.
[7] PMI VectorLink Project, Abt Associates, Bujumbura, Burundi. [8] US President's Malaria Initiative, US Agency for International Development, Cotonou, Benin.
[9] PMI VectorLink Project, Abt Associates, Cotonou, Benin.

Acknowledgements
We are grateful to the President's Malaria Initiative which supported financially this study. We thank Bruno AKINRO for statistical analysis and also the populations of Sonsoro, Kossarou, Gounarou, Bantansouè, Bariénou, Zountori, Kataban and Kparakouna centre for their collaboration. We acknowledge Monica Patton, Peter Thomas and Raymond Beach of US Centers for Disease Control and Prevention for providing technical assistance and proofreading the manuscript.

Competing interests
The authors declare that they have no competing interests.

Funding
This study was financially supported by the US President's Malaria Initiative (PMI) thru the United States Agency for International Development (USAID) Africa Indoor Residual Spraying Project (AIRS).

References

1. WHO. Global Malaria Programme. Indoor residual spraying: use of indoor residual spraying for scaling up global malaria control and elimination. Geneva: World Health Organization; 2006.
2. WHO. Global Malaria Programme. Insecticide-treated mosquito nets: a position statement. Geneva: World Health Organization; 2007.
3. Roll Back Malaria. The global malaria action plan 2012. 2013. http://www.rollbackmalaria.org/gmap. Accessed 26 Feb 2018.
4. Schiff C. Integrated approach to malaria control. Clin Microbiol Rev. 2002;15:278–93.
5. Lengeler C, Sharp B. Indoor residual spraying and insecticide-treated nets. In: Murphy C, Ringheim K, Woldehanna S, Volmink J, editors. Reducing malaria's burden: evidence of effectiveness for decision makers. Washington, DC: Global Health Council; 2003. p. 17–24.
6. Roberts D, Curtis C, Tren R, Sharp B, Shiff C, Bate R. Malaria control and public health. Emerg Infect Dis. 2004;10:1170–1.
7. WHO. World malaria report 2015. Geneva: World Health Organization; 2015.
8. Akogbeto MC, Aikpon R, Azondekon R, Padonou G, Osse R, Agossa FR, et al. Six years of experience in entomological surveillance of indoor residual spraying against malaria transmission in Benin: lessons learned challenges and outlooks. Malar J. 2015;14:242.
9. Akogbeto M, Padonou GG, Bankole HS, Gazard DK, Gbedjissi GL. Dramatic decrease in malaria transmission after large-scale indoor residual spraying with bendiocarb in Benin, an area of high resistance of Anopheles gambiae to pyrethroids. Am J Trop Med Hyg. 2011;85:586–93.
10. Ossè R, Aikpon R, Padonou GG, Oussou O, Yadouléton A, Akogbéto M. Evaluation of the efficacy of bendiocarb in indoor residual spraying against pyrethroid resistant malaria vectors in Benin: results of the third campaign. Parasit Vectors. 2012;5:163.
11. Mabaso ML, Sharp B, Lengeler C. Historical review of malarial control in southern African with emphasis on the use of indoor residual house-spraying. Trop Med Int Health. 2004;9:846–56.
12. Brutus L, Le Goff G, Rasolomaina LG, Rajaonarivelo V, Raveloson A, Cot M. Lutte contre le paludisme dans le moyen-ouest de Madagascar : Comparaison de l'efficacité de la lambda-cyhalothrine et du DDT en aspersions intradomiciliaires. I. Etude entomologique. Parasite. 2001;8:309–16.
13. Kleinschmidt I, Sharp B, Benevente L, Schwabe C, Torrez M, Kuklinski J, et al. Reduction in infection with Plasmodium falciparum one year after the introduction of malaria control interventions on Bioko Island, Equatorial Guinea. Am J Trop Med Hyg. 2006;74:972–8.
14. Sharp BL, Kleinschmidt I, Streat E, Maharaj R, Barnes KI, Durrheim DN, et al. Seven years of regional malaria control collaboration—Mozambique, South Africa and Swaziland. Am J Trop Med Hyg. 2007;76:42–7.
15. Overgaard HJ, Reddy VP, Abaga S, Matias A, Reddy MR, Kulkarni V, et al. Malaria transmission after five years of vector control on Bioko Island, Equatorial Guinea. Parasit Vectors. 2012;5:253.
16. Kigozi R, Baxi SM, Gasasira A, Sserwanga A, Kakeeto S, Nasr S, et al. Indoor residual spraying of insecticide and malaria morbidity in a high transmission intensity area of Uganda. PLoS ONE. 2012;7:e42857.
17. Gimnig JE, Otieno P, Were V, Marwanga D, Abong'o D, Wiegand R, et al. The effect of indoor residual spraying on the prevalence of malaria parasite infection, clinical malaria and anemia in an area of perennial transmission and moderate coverage of insecticide treated nets in Western Kenya. PLoS ONE. 2016;11:0145282.
18. Protopopoff N, Wright A, West PA, Tigererwa R, Mosha FW, Kisinza W, et al. Combination of insecticide treated nets and indoor residual spraying in Northern Tanzania provides additional reduction in vector population density and malaria transmission rates compared to insecticide treated nets alone: a randomised control trial. PLoS ONE. 2015;10:e0142671.
19. Chandre F, Manguin S, Brengues C, Dossou Yovo J, Darriet F, Diabate A, et al. Current distribution of pyrethroid resistance gene (kdr) in Anopheles gambiae complex from West Africa and further evidence for reproductive isolation of Mopti form. Parassitologia. 1999;41:319–22.
20. Corbel V, N'Guessan R, Brengues C, Chandre F, Djogbenou L, Martin T, et al. Multiple insecticide resistance mechanisms in Anopheles gambiae and Culex quinquefasciatus from Benin, West Africa. Acta Trop. 2007;101:207–16.
21. Yadouleton A, Asidi A, Djouaka R, Braïma J, Agossou C, Akogbeto M. Development of vegetable farming. A cause of the emergence of

22. insecticide resistance in populations of Anopheles gambiae in urban areas of Benin. Malar J. 2009;8:103.
22. Djogbenou L, Pasteur N, Bio-Bangana S, Baldet T, Irish SR, Akogbeto M, et al. Malaria vectors in the Republic of Benin: distribution of species and molecular forms of the Anopheles gambiae complex. Acta Trop. 2010;114:116–22.
23. Djegbe I, Boussari O, Sidick A, Martin T, Ranson H, Chandre F, et al. Dynamics of insecticide resistance in malaria vectors in Benin: first evidence of the presence of L1014S kdr mutation in Anopheles gambiae from West Africa. Malar J. 2011;10:261.
24. Sovi A, Djegbe I, Soumanou L, Tokponnon F, Gnanguenon V, Azondekon R, et al. Microdistribution of the resistance of malaria vectors to deltamethrin in the region of Plateau (southeastern Benin) in preparation for an assessment of the impact of resistance on the effectiveness of long lasting insecticidal nets (LLINs). BMC Infect Dis. 2014;14:103.
25. Aïzoun N, Aïkpon R, Gnanguenon V, Oussou O, Agossa F, Padonou GG, et al. Status of organophosphate and carbamate resistance in Anopheles gambiae sensu lato from the south and north Benin, West Africa. Parasit Vectors. 2013;6:274.
26. Aïkpon R, Agossa F, Ossè R, Oussou O, Aïzoun N, Oké-Agbo F, et al. Bendiocarb resistance in Anopheles gambiae s.l. populations from Atacora department in Benin, West Africa: a threat for malaria vector control. Parasit Vectors. 2013;6:192.
27. Gnanguenon V, Agossa FR, Badirou K, Govoetchan R, Anagonou R, Oke-Agbo F, et al. Malaria vectors resistance to insecticides in Benin: current trends and mechanisms involved. Parasit Vectors. 2015;8:223.
28. Cox J, Craig MH, Le Sueur D, Sharp BL. Mapping malaria risk in the highlands of Africa. Technical report. London/Durban: MARA/HIMAL; 1999.
29. Kleinschmidt I, Sharp B, Mueller I, Vounatsou P. Rise in malaria incidence rates in South Africa: small area spatial analysis of variation in time trends. Am J Epidemiol. 2002;155:257–64.
30. Munga S, Yakob L, Mushinzimana E, Zhou G, Ouna T, Minakawa N, et al. Land use and land cover changes and spatiotemporal dynamics of Anopheline larval habitats during a four-year period in a highland community of Africa. Am J Trop Med Hyg. 2009;81:1079–84.
31. Govoetchan R, Gnanguenon V, Azondékon R, Agossa RF, Sovi A, Oké-Agbo F, et al. Evidence for perennial malaria in rural and urban areas under the Sudanian climate of Kandi, Northeastern Benin. Parasit Vectors. 2014;7:79.
32. Kazembe LN, Kleinschmidt I, Holtz TH. Spatial analysis and mapping of malaria risk in Malawi using point-referenced prevalence of infection data. Int J Health Geograph. 2006;5:41.
33. Le Sueur D, Binka F, Lengeler C, de Savigny D, Snow B, Teuscher T, et al. An atlas of malaria in Africa. Afr Health. 1997;19:23–4.
34. Carter R, Mendis KN, Roberts D. Spatial targeting of interventions against malaria. Bull World Health Organ. 2000;78:1401–11.
35. Killeen GF, Okumu FO, N'Guessan R, Coosemans M, Adeogun A, Awolola S, et al. The importance of considering community-level effects when selecting insecticidal malaria vector products. Parasit Vectors. 2011;4:160.
36. INSAE, RGPH4 2013. Cahiers des villages et quartiers de ville du département de l'Alibori; 2016. http://www.insae-bj.org/recensement-population.html/enquêtes-recensements/rgph/Cahier_village_2013/Alibori.pdf. Accessed 20 Apr 2018.
37. INSAE, RGPH4 2013. Cahiers des villages et quartiers de ville du département de la Donga; 2016. http://www.insae-bj.org/recensement-population.html/enquêtes-recensements/rgph/Cahier_village_2013/Donga.pdf. Accessed 20 Apr 2018.
38. Ministère de la Santé. Annuaire des statistiques sanitaires 2016. Cotonou: Direction de la Programmation et de la Prospective; 2017.
39. Gillies MT, De Meillon B. The Anophelinae of Africa south of the Sahara. South Afri Inst Med Res. 1968;54:1–343.
40. Detinova TS, Gillies MT. Observations on the determination of the Age composition and epidemiological importance of populations of Anopheles gambiae Giles and Anopheles funestus Giles in Tanganyika. Bull World Health Organ. 1964;30:23–8.
41. Wirtz R, Zavala F, Charoenvit Y, Campbell G, Burkot T, Schneider I, et al. Comparative testing of monoclonal antibodies against Plasmodium falciparum sporozoites for ELISA development. Bull World Health Organ. 1987;65:39.
42. Rothman KJ. Epidemiology: an introduction. Oxford: Oxford University Press; 2012.

43. Jewell NP. Statistics for epidemiology. Boca Raton: CRC Press; 2003.
44. Fontenille D, Simard F. Unraveling complexities in human malaria transmission dynamics in Africa through a comprehensive knowledge of vectors populations. Comp Immunol Microbiol Infect Dis. 2004;27:357–75.
45. Akogbeto M, Di Deco M. Distribution of members of the *Anopheles gambiae* complex and their chromosomal variants in Benin and Togo, West Africa. Afr Zool. 1995;109:443–54.
46. Kelly-Hope LA, Mckenzie FE. The multiplicity of malaria transmission: a review of entomological inoculation rate measurements and methods across sub-Saharan Africa. Malar J. 2009;8:19.
47. Gnanguenon V, Govoetchan R, Agossa FR, Osse R, Oke-Agbo F, Azondekon R, et al. Transmission patterns of *Plasmodium falciparum* by *Anopheles gambiae* in Benin. Malar J. 2014;13:444.
48. Aïkpon R, Osse R, Govoetchan R, Sovi A, Oke-Agbo F, Akogbeto MC. Entomological baseline data on malaria transmission and susceptibility of *Anopheles gambiae* to insecticides in preparation for indoor residual spraying (IRS) in Atacora, (Benin). J Parasitol Vector Biol. 2013;5:102–11.
49. Akogbéto MC, Salako SA, Dagnon F, Aïkpon R, Kouletio M, Sovi A, et al. Blood feeding behaviour comparison and contribution of *Anopheles coluzzii* and *Anopheles gambiae*, two sibling species living in sympatry, to malaria transmission in Alibori and Donga region, northern Benin, West Africa. Malar J. 2018;17:307.
50. Darriet F. Moustiquaires imprégnées et résistance des moustiques aux insecticides. Paris: Éditions IRD; 2007.
51. Azondekon R, Gnanguenon V, Oke-Agbo F, Houevoessa S, Green M, Akogbeto M. A tracking tool for long-lasting insecticidal (mosquito) net intervention following a 2011 national distribution in Benin. Parasit Vectors. 2014;7:6.
52. Aïkpon R, Ossè R, Padonou G, Anagonou R, Salako A, Ahogni I, et al. Involvement of both *Anopheles gambiae* and *Anopheles funestus* (Diptera: Culicidae) in the perennial malaria transmission through a seasonal abundance in savannah area in Benin. Int J Mosq Res. 2017;4:107–12.
53. Djènontin A, Bio-Bangana S, Moiroux N, Henry M-C, Bousari O, Chabi J, et al. Culicidae diversity, malaria transmission and insecticide resistance alleles in malaria vectors in Ouidah-Kpomasse-Tori district from Benin (West Africa): a preintervention study. Parasit Vectors. 2010;3:83.
54. Taylor KA, Koros JK, Nduati J, Copeland R, Collins FH, Brandling-Bennett AD. *Plasmodium falciparum* infection rates in *Anopheles gambiae, An.*

arabiensis, and *An. funestus* in Western Kenya. Am J Trop Med Hyg. 1990;43:124–9.
55. Thomson MC, D'Alessandro U, Bennett S, Connor SJ, Langerock P, Jawara M, et al. Malaria prevalence is inversely related to vector density in The Gambia, West Africa. Trans R Soc Trop Med Hyg. 1994;88:638–43.
56. Snounou G, Pinheiro L, Gonçalves A, Fonseca L, Dias F, Brown KN, et al. The importance of sensitive detection of malaria parasites in the human and insect hosts in epidemiological studies, as shown by the analysis of field samples from Guinea Bissau. Trans R Soc Trop Med Hyg. 1993;87:649–53.
57. Jaenson TG, Gomes MJ, Barreto dos Santos RC, Petrarca V, Fortini D, Evora J, et al. Control of endophagic *Anopheles* mosquitoes and human malaria in Guinea Bissau, West Africa by permethrin-treated bed nets. Trans R Soc Trop Med Hyg. 1994;88:620–4.
58. Garrett-Jones C. Prognosis for interruption of malaria transmission through the assessment of mosquito vectorial capacity. Nature. 1964;204:1173–5.
59. Omukunda E, Githeko A, Ndong'a MF, Mushinzimana E, Atieli H, Wamae P. Malaria vector population dynamics in highland and lowland regions of western Kenya. J Vector Borne Dis. 2013;50:85–92.
60. Sovi A, Govoétchan R, Tokponnon F, Hounkonnou H, Aïkpon R, Agossa F, et al. Impact of land-use on malaria transmission in the Plateau region, southeastern Benin. Parasit Vectors. 2013;6:352.
61. Omumbo JA, Guerra CA, Hay SI, Snow RW. The influence of urbanization on measures of *Plasmodium falciparum* infection prevalence in East Africa. Acta Trop. 2005;93:11–21.
62. Wang SJ, Lengeler C, Mtasiwa D, Mshana T, Manane L, Maro G, et al. Rapid urban malaria appraisal (RUMA) II: epidemiology of urban malaria in Dar es Salaam (Tanzania). Malar J. 2006;5:29.
63. Wang SJ, Lengeler C, Smith TA, Vounatsou P, Diadie DA, Pritroipa X, et al. Rapid urban malaria appraisal (RUMA) I: epidemiology of urban malaria in Ouagadougou. Malar J. 2006;4:43.
64. Pierrat C. Des moustiques et des hommes: les territoires du paludisme à Tori-Bossito (sud du Bénin). Thèse de Doctorat de Géographie, Université Paris I Panthéon-Sorbonne; 2010.
65. Mouchet J, Carnevale P, Coosemans M, Fontenille D, Ravaonjanahary C, Richard A, Robert V. Typologie du paludisme en Afrique. Santé: Cahiers d'Etudes et de Recherches Francophones. 1993;3(4):220–38

12

Analysis of erythrocyte dynamics in Rhesus macaque monkeys during infection with *Plasmodium cynomolgi*

Luis L. Fonseca[1,2*], Chester J. Joyner[2,3], Celia L. Saney[2,3], The MaHPIC Consortium[2], Alberto Moreno[2,3], John W. Barnwell[2,4], Mary R. Galinski[2,3] and Eberhard O. Voit[1,2]

Abstract

Background: Malaria is a major mosquito transmitted, blood-borne parasitic disease that afflicts humans. The disease causes anaemia and other clinical complications, which can lead to death. *Plasmodium vivax* is known for its reticulocyte host cell specificity, but many gaps in disease details remain. Much less is known about the closely related species, *Plasmodium cynomolgi*, although it is naturally acquired and causes zoonotic malaria. Here, a computational model is developed based on longitudinal analyses of *P. cynomolgi* infections in nonhuman primates to investigate the erythrocyte dynamics that is pertinent to understanding both *P. cynomolgi* and *P. vivax* malaria in humans.

Methods: A cohort of five *P. cynomolgi* infected Rhesus macaques (*Macaca mulatta*) is studied, with individuals exhibiting a plethora of clinical outcomes, including varying levels of anaemia. A discrete recursive model with age structure is developed to replicate the dynamics of *P. cynomolgi* blood-stage infections. The model allows for parasitic reticulocyte preference and assumes an age preference among the mature RBCs. RBC senescence is modelled using a hazard function, according to which RBCs have a mean lifespan of 98 ± 21 days.

Results: Based on in vivo data from three cohorts of macaques, the computational model is used to characterize the reticulocyte lifespan in circulation as 24 ± 5 h ($n = 15$) and the rate of RBC production as 2727 ± 209 cells/h/µL ($n = 15$). Analysis of the host responses reveals a pre-patency increase in the number of reticulocytes. It also allows the quantification of RBC removal through the bystander effect.

Conclusions: The evident pre-patency increase in reticulocytes is due to a shift towards the release of younger reticulocytes, which could result from a parasite-induced factor meant to increase reticulocyte availability and satisfy the parasite's tropism, which has an average value of 32:1 in this cohort. The number of RBCs lost due to the bystander effect relative to infection-induced RBC losses is 62% for *P. cynomolgi* infections, which is substantially lower than the value of 95% previously determined for another simian species, *Plasmodium coatneyi*.

Keywords: Mathematical model, Host–pathogen interactions, *Macaca mulatta*, *Plasmodium cynomolgi*, *Plasmodium vivax*, Reticulocytes, Anaemia, Zoonosis

*Correspondence: llfonseca@gatech.edu
[2] Malaria Host–Pathogen Interaction Center, Emory Vaccine Center, Yerkes National Primate Research Center, Emory University, Atlanta, GA 30322, USA
Full list of author information is available at the end of the article

Background

Malaria is a major life-threatening disease caused by parasites of the genus *Plasmodium* [1]. The genus *Plasmodium* includes parasites of different species that can infect humans as well as nonhuman primates (NHPs), rodents, bats, reptiles and birds [2]. *Plasmodium vivax* has a wide geographical distribution and is responsible for almost half of the malarial cases outside of Africa, where *Plasmodium falciparum* predominates [1, 3, 4]. Having been responsible for 8.5 million cases globally in 2016, *P. vivax* constitutes a major challenge towards the goals of the World Health Organization and its partners of eliminating malaria from 35 countries and reducing incidence and mortality rates by 90% by 2030 [1]. Its closely related sister species, *Plasmodium cynomolgi*, is a simian malaria parasite that has been an important model for research [5–8] and is now also recognized as a zoonosis [9].

In the vertebrate host, the infection process begins with a blood-meal by a female *Anopheles* mosquito, which typically results in the inoculation of the host with fewer than 100 sporozoites [10, 11]. Successful sporozoites travel from the skin to the liver, where they infect hepatocytes. From each infected hepatocyte, tens of thousands of merozoites may develop and be released into the bloodstream [12, 13]. Several species including *P. vivax* and *P. cynomolgi* have the additional ability to produce hypnozoites during the liver stage, which are dormant forms of the parasite that may be activated and thus able to cause relapse infections weeks to months after the primary infection [14–17].

During the blood stage of the parasite's life cycle, merozoites exclusively infect red blood cells (RBCs). The productivity of an infected RBC is much lower than that of an infected hepatocyte, with an infected RBC only producing up to 30 new merozoites, depending on the *Plasmodium* species. In the case of *P. cynomolgi*, the number of released merozoites per infected RBC is on average 16, with a range of 14–20 [18]. At some point during the blood stage cycle, some merozoites become committed to the production of gametocytes, which, if taken up by a mosquito, begin the arthropod stage of the infection.

Whereas the liver stage of the infection proceeds asymptomatically, the blood stage often presents symptoms that are shared by common viral infections, i.e., headaches, fever, chills, dizziness, myalgia, nausea and vomiting [19, 20]. On the other end of the clinical spectrum is severe malaria, which is most often caused by *P. falciparum*, although *P. vivax* may also cause severe disease [21]. Severe malaria complications can develop very rapidly and progress to death within hours or days [22]. Disease manifestations can include, among others, respiratory distress, pulmonary oedema, acute renal failure, thrombocytopaenia, and severe anaemia [23]. With that said, many infections can be asymptomatic, as also shown recently for relapsing [17] and zoonotic cases [9] of *P. cynomolgi*. Both species exhibit tropism toward reticulocytes, which is nearly strict in the case of *P. vivax* and conditional for *P. cynomolgi* [8, 24, 25]. Also, both species produce caveola vesicle complexes in the infected RBCs, which involves remodelling of the host RBC cytoskeleton, and results in increased membrane deformability [24, 26, 27]. And, as mentioned above, both species produce hypnozoites capable of causing relapses.

To characterize and quantify the RBC dynamics during malaria, various mathematical models have been developed with the particular goal of deconvolving and quantifying the different processes of RBC removal. Models of the malarial host–pathogen interactions have been proposed since the late 1980s [28] (reviewed in [29]). Dynamic models for such a purpose are often formulated as sets of ordinary differential equations (ODEs), and in their simplest form are commonly represented with three compartments, namely, RBCs, infected RBCs, and either merozoites or some marker of the immune response [30–33]. More complex models may contain more than three compartments, especially when they focus on antigenic variation, where many parasite variants are considered, and specific and cross-reactive immune responses are included [29]. Attempts have also been made to model the delays inherent to this system, in which case it was necessary to use delayed differential equations, age-structured ODEs, partial differential equations, or discrete implementations of their continuous analogs. All these approaches have advantages and drawbacks [34] that should be taken into consideration, depending on the ultimate goals of the model, i.e., whether the model was developed as a tool for further analytical investigations, data fitting, hypothesis generation, or other purposes.

Here, a time-dependent discrete recursive equation (DRE) model with age structure is used. The model has four compartments: reticulocytes, mature RBCs, infected RBCs and merozoites, all of which have an age structure, except for the merozoites. Unlike most other models [29], the processes here are quantified time-dependently rather than imposing certain kinetic formulations, such as a mass-action representation. This strategy was used to assess the reticulocyte maturation time in circulation, loss of RBCs, and the impact of the immune response. It also permits the time-dependent quantification of the extent of RBC production and of RBC loss through different processes (random death, senescence, parasitization, or bystander effect), as well as an assessment of the reticulocyte timespan in circulation and of the immune response. The result is in each case a personalized model of each macaque's response to the infection, which is then analysed a posteriori.

The experimental data used in this work were generated from a longitudinal study involving a cohort of Rhesus macaques that were infected with *P. cynomolgi* (B/M strain) sporozoites and followed for 100 days, with sampling of blood and bone marrow at different points in time. Of particular importance for the model, complete blood counts (CBCs) and parasitaemia counts were performed. The data are publicly available [35], and a comprehensive clinical analysis of these infections [17], as well as multi-omic integrated analyses have been reported [36].

Methods

Model formulation

A dynamic mathematical model was developed to characterize the within-host host–pathogen interactions during a malarial (*P. cynomolgi*) infection in Rhesus macaques (*Macaca mulatta*). This model was developed using the same discrete recursive framework previously shown to be well suited for these types of problems [34].

In the model (Fig. 1), the erythropoietic system releases reticulocytes (*Ret*) into the bloodstream, where they remain for a certain period of time before becoming mature RBCs (*RBC*). Mature RBC may be removed by normal physiological processes, invasion by merozoites, or destruction during an infection by the so-called bystander effect. The normal physiological processes of removing RBCs include random death, a process through which about 10% of all produced cells eventually die [37], and senescence. For the latter, a hazard function was

determined [38], based on data obtained through RBC biotinylation of a cohort of macaques [39] kept under the same conditions as the macaques used in the present study. The bystander effect is a process by which RBCs are removed even though they are uninfected [40, 41]; it is modelled here under the assumption that it is age-independent, as suggested previously [38].

Merozoites (*M*) invade not only mature RBCs but actually prefer reticulocytes, with a reported preference of 477:1 over RBCs [25]. The invasion of reticulocytes is assumed to be age-independent, as these cells are short-lived, lasting about 1 day in circulation. Among the mature RBCs, the parasite invasion preference is assumed to follow a decreasing exponential distribution, which is defined in such a way that the relative likelihood of infecting a young RBC, relative to a RBC 11 days older, is twice as large, $\frac{PoI_a}{PoI_{a+264}} = 2$, where PoI_a is the probability

of infecting a RBC of age a and a is the RBC age expressed in hours. The purpose of this function is to approximate the merozoite preference for younger mature RBCs and, thus, allowing the model to represent the effects of an infection on the age distribution of mature RBCs as accurately as possible. Modelling *P. cynomolgi*'s well-documented age preference for younger RBCs, as just described, does not alter the total number of RBCs removed, but allows the model simulations to produce a more realistic representation of the RBC age distribution during and after an infection.

Both, invaded RBCs and reticulocytes become infected RBCs (*iRBC*). Infected RBCs live for 48 h, which is the length of the intraerythrocytic cycle in *P. cynomolgi* [18],

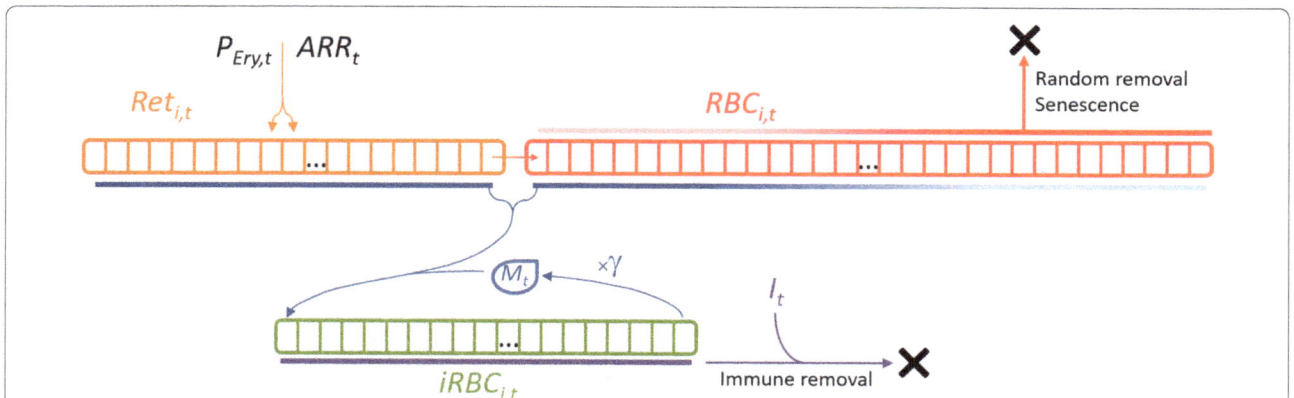

Fig. 1 Scheme of the within-host host–pathogen interaction model. In the proposed model, reticulocytes (*Ret*) are released from the bone marrow at a rate of P_t cells/h/μL and with an age given by $121—ARR_t$ hours, where ARR_t stands for the age class into which reticulocytes are produced. All cells move from one age class to the next (right) at every hourly step. When reticulocytes reach their last age class, they mature into RBCs. In the absence of an infection, RBCs are removed at random or through senescence processes, in which older cells are more likely to be removed than young cells (depicted by the red bar over the RBC age classes). During an infection, merozoites (*M_t*) will, preferentially, invade reticulocytes and young RBCs (blue bars under the reticulocyte and RBCs pools). Upon infection, reticulocytes and RBCs become infected RBCs (*iRBC_{i,t}*), which live for 24 h, after which they burst and release γ new merozoites. The immune response (*I_t*) removes infected RBCs in an age-independent way

after which they burst and release about 16 merozoites [18]. A variable representing the immune-response (I) is used to control infected RBCs.

Assumptions

The structure of the model requires very few mechanistic assumptions. In many other models, the authors assume that the formation of infected RBCs follows a mass action format [29], as it is, for instance, used in most epidemiological SIR models (i.e., $dI/dt = \beta \cdot I \cdot S - \dots$). Here, all merozoites present at time point t infect RBCs or reticulocytes by time point $t+1$, i.e., 1 h later. Similarly, the erythropoietic output does not depend on a hypothetical function of the remaining RBCs, of the missing RBCs, or some other feature of the anaemia. Rather, a time-dependent profile (P_t) is estimated for each macaque, given its health trajectory, which directly quantifies the RBC production at each time-point. A discrete recursive framework with age-classes is chosen, instead of an ODE, as this formulation mimics more accurately the natural physiological process of aging.

The implementation of this discrete model does require some assumptions, which are listed in Table 1.

Variables

The model contains five dependent variables: $Ret_{i,t}$, $RBC_{i,t}$, $iRBC_{i,t}$, $rRBC$ and, M. The definitions of all model variables are given in Table 2.

Equations

The within-host host–pathogen interaction model is set up as a discrete recursive system and solved with a 1-h time step. The next paragraphs describe each compartment and the formulation of all associated processes.

Reticulocyte compartment

In primates, reticulocytes are produced in the bone marrow and released into circulation before maturing into RBCs. The common maturation time in circulation for human reticulocytes is about 24 h, but can change in response to anaemia [42]. To account for this variable maturation time, the reticulocyte pool ($Ret_{i,t}$) is defined as having a total of 120 age classes, which corresponds to a maximum of 5 days or 120 h (Eq. 1). Reticulocytes are produced at a rate of P_t into age class ARR_t (Fig. 1), and then allowed to age until they reach their last age class, 120, at which point the reticulocytes become mature RBCs. In order for the model to respond in a quasi-continuous fashion to ARR_t, newly released reticulocytes are distributed among the two age classes $int(ARR_t)$ and $int(ARR_t)+1$ based on the decimal part of ARR_t (Eqs. 1, 3). *P. cynomolgi*, unlike *P. coatneyi*, has the ability to invade reticulocytes and does so with a 477:1 preference over RBCs, according to [25]. Therefore, reticulocyte removal was introduced using $SfRet_{i,t}$ (Eqs. 1, 13, 24). Modelled this way, a normal 24-h maturation time in circulation for reticulocytes is modelled by these cells being released into age class $ARR_t = 121 - 24 = 97$, which ensures that 24 h later they become mature RBCs. Thus, the equations governing reticulocytes are given as follows:

Table 1 List of model assumptions

#	Description
1	The general scheme shown in Fig. 8 is assumed to represent sufficiently well the real physiological interactions between the host cells and the parasites
2	Reticulocytes are produced and released from the bone marrow at a rate of P_t and with a remaining maturation time of 121 ARR_t, at the end of which they become mature RBCs
2.1	Reticulocytes are not subject to random or senescent death as they become mature RBCs within one to 2 days after entering circulation
2.2	Reticulocytes may be infected by the parasite
3	Mature RBCs are, theoretically, allowed to live for up to 160 days
3.1	Random death removes 10% of all produced RBCs
3.2	Senescent death follows a hazard function that causes RBCs to have a mean lifespan of 98 days
3.3	Mature RBCs can be lost due to invasion by a parasite
3.4	Mature RBCs may be lost due to the bystander effect
4	Free merozoites live only for 1 h, during which time they infect reticulocytes and RBCs
4.1	Merozoites have a reported 477.2:1 preference for reticulocytes over RBCs
4.2	Among mature RBCs, merozoites have an age preference that leads a younger RBC to be two times more likely to be infected than a RBC 11 days older
5	Infected RBCs live for 2 days and then burst, releasing a new brood of merozoites
5.1	Infected RBCs are removed by the immune response

Table 2 Definition of all variables. The first five variables ($Ret_{i,t}$, $RBC_{i,t}$, $iRBC_{i,t}$, $rRBC$ and, M) are the key dependent variables of the model for which time recursions are defined

Variable	Description
$Ret_{i,t}$	Number of circulating reticulocytes of age i at time t
$RBC_{i,t}$	Number of mature red blood cells of age i at time t
$iRBC_{i,t}$	Number of infected red blood cells of age i at time t
$rRBC_t$	Number of RBCs that will die due to random death
M_t	Number of free merozoites at time t
P_t	Hourly production and release of reticulocytes from bone marrow into the bloodstream at time t
ARR_t	Age-class into which reticulocytes are released
$iARR_t$	Integer part of ARR_t
$dARR_t$	Decimal part of ARR_t
$SfRet_{i,t}$	Fraction of reticulocytes in age class i at time point t that survive to time point $t+1$
$SfRBC_{i,t}$	Fraction of RBCs in age class i at time-point t that survive to time point $t+1$
$SfiRBC_{i,t}$	Fraction of infected RBCs in age class i at time point t that survive to time point $t+1$
ToI	Time point at which an infection starts
NoI	Number of infected RBCs that start an infection at time point ToI
RDt	Number of RBCs removed at time point t due to random death
hf_i	Hazard function for RBCs
$RBCInv_{i,t}$	Fraction of RBCs in age class i at time point t lost to merozoite invasion
$RetInv_{i,t}$	Fraction of reticulocytes in age class i at time point t lost to merozoite invasion
UR_t	Number of RBCs removed by bystander effect
$TRBC_t$	Total number of RBCs at time t
$TRet_t$	Total number of reticulocytes at time t
Ret_{Pref}	Reticulocyte preference over mature RBCs
$RBCAPf_i$	Merozoite-RBC age preference function
$PiRet$	Percentage that a merozoite will infect a reticulocyte
$NiRet$	Number of reticulocytes to be infected
$PiRBC_i$	Probability that a merozoite will infect an RBC of age i
$MerLeft$	Number of merozoites left after accounting for invasion of reticulocytes
$NiRBC_f$	Number of RBCs of age class f to be invaded by a merozoite

$$\begin{cases} Ret_{i,t+1} = 0 & i = 1 \\ Ret_{i,t+1} = Ret_{i-1,t} \cdot SfRet_{i-1,t} & i \in \{2, \ldots, iARR_t - 1\} \\ Ret_{i,t+1} = Ret_{i-1,t} \cdot SfRet_{i-1,t} + P_t \cdot dARR_t & i = iARR_t + 1 \\ Ret_{i,t+1} = Ret_{i-1,t} \cdot SfRet_{i-1,t} + P_t \cdot dARR_t & i \in \{iARR_t + 2, \ldots, 120\} \end{cases} \tag{1}$$

$$Ret_{i,0} = \begin{cases} 0 & i \in \{1, \ldots, iARR_0 - 1\} \\ P_0 \cdot (1 - dARR_0) & i = iARR_0 \\ P_0 & i \in \{iARR_0 + 1, \ldots, 120\} \end{cases} \tag{2}$$

Here, $iARR_t$ and $dARR_t$ are the integer and decimal parts of ARR_t (age class into which reticulocytes are released, Table 2):

$$iARR_t = int(ARR_t) \quad \text{and} \quad dARR_t = ARR_t - iARR_t \tag{3}$$

RBC compartment

The RBC compartment ($RBC_{i,t}$) has 3840 ($= 160 \times 24$) age classes (Eq. 4), which allows for a maximum lifespan of 160 days. Although RBCs live on average only for 98 days in Rhesus macaques [38], significant numbers survive to about 120 days and sometimes longer [38]. The remaining 40 age classes ensure that even under conditions where large numbers of RBCs are produced in a short period of time, RBCs never "artificially" disappear due to a lack of age classes. In most simulations, the oldest age classes are empty. RBCs are produced from reticulocytes by maturation, and removal occurs by two sets of processes: physiological and pathophysiological. The two normal, physiological processes are random loss and senescence. Random loss of RBCs is modelled under the assumption that 10% of all RBCs produced will die by this process; this mechanism is modelled with the auxiliary variable $rRBC_t$ [37, 38]. Senescent death is governed by a power-law hazard function, which was previously parameterized for Rhesus macaques [38]. The pathophysiological processes are merozoite invasion and RBC removal by bystander effect. Merozoites are released at the end of the intraerythrocytic developmental cycle and within 1 h re-infect RBCs and reticulocytes (Fig. 1). The bystander effect is an ill-characterized process that is known to occur during some malarial infections and leads to additional, sometimes substantial, losses of RBCs. Fonseca et al. [38] recently suggested that the bystander mechanism removes RBCs in an age-independent manner, and that it does not seem to occur due to an increased rate of RBC senescence. Consequently, the bystander effect is modelled as an age-independent process, namely

$$RBC_{i,t+1} = RBC_{i-1,t} \cdot SfRBC_{i-1,t}, \qquad i \in \{2, 3, \ldots, 3840\} \tag{4}$$

$$RBC_{1,t+1} = Ret_{120,t} \cdot Sfret_{120,t}. \tag{5}$$

The initial state $RBC_{i,0}$ may be analytically deduced, but this deduction is complex. Instead, it was numerically calculated by starting without any RBCs ($RBC_{i,0}=0$) and running the model absent of infection or loss of RBCs by bystander effect for over 1500 days, when it had long reached the steady state. Under these conditions, the model is asymptotically stable at the initial state. This final RBC age distribution ($RBC_{i,\mathrm{end}}$) is saved and used as the initial state for all subsequent simulations.

Merozoite compartment

Merozoites are produced in infected RBCs and released upon completion of the intra-erythrocytic developmental cycle (Fig. 1). Although *P. cynomolgi* is known to produce an average of 16 merozoites, with a range of 14–20 [18], some of the macaques analysed here exhibited higher rates. In view of this fact, this parameter was individually fitted for each parasitaemia peak in each macaque assuming the growth of the parasite population follows an exponential function and calculating the multiplication rate as the increase in numbers (γ) during 48 h. Therefore, the number of merozoites released will be γ times the number of surviving infected RBCs in their last age class.

$$M_{t+1} = \gamma \cdot iRBC_{48,t} \cdot SfiRBC_{48,t} \tag{6}$$

$$M_{t=0} = 0 \tag{7}$$

Note that M_{t+1} does not depend on M_t, because the free merozoites present at time t infect RBCs within 1 h (Eq. 9) since their appearance in blood. The merozoites that will be present at time $t+1$ are those released from infected RBCs that finished their intra-erythrocytic developmental cycle at time t and were not removed by the immune-response (Eq. 6).

Compartment of infected RBCs

Infected RBCs ($iRBC_{i,t}$) are produced from merozoite invasion of RBCs or reticulocytes and destroyed by the immune system (I_t, Fig. 1). All infected RBCs that survive for the entire intra-erythrocytic developmental cycle of 48 h are assumed to burst and release γ merozoites each. It is furthermore assumed that all released merozoites are infectious. Additionally, since *P. cynomolgi* has a 2-day intra-erythrocytic cycle, this compartment is modelled with 48 age classes.

$$iRBC_{i,t+1} = iRBC_{i-1,t} \cdot SfiRBC_{i-1,t}, \quad i \in \{2, 3, \ldots, 48\} \tag{8}$$

$$iRBC_{1,t+1} = M_t \tag{9}$$

$$iRBC_{i,0} = 0, \quad i \in \{1, 2, \ldots, 48\} \tag{10}$$

Infections are initiated in the model (Eq. 11) by stating how many infected RBCs (NoI) exist at the time the infection starts (ToI), close to the time the infection becomes patent. Here, it is assumed that the infection has a uniform age-distribution at the time of patency; i.e., all parasite life stages are equally present at any time point as shown by the experimental data. Therefore:

$$iRBC_{i,t=TOI} = \frac{NoI}{48}, \quad i \in \{1, 2, \ldots, 48\} \tag{11}$$

Destruction of RBCs and reticulocytes

While reticulocytes are assumed to be destroyed only by merozoite invasion, RBCs are assumed to be removed by random death, senescence, merozoite invasion or bystander effect (Fig. 1). Thus, the fractions of surviving RBCs and reticulocytes are:

$$SfRBC_{i,t} = \left(1 - \frac{RD_t}{TRBC_t} - hf_i - RBCInv_{i,t} - \frac{UR_t}{TRBC_t}\right), \quad i \in \{1, 2, \ldots, 3840\} \tag{12}$$

$$SfRet_{i,t} = \left(1 - RetInv_{i,t}\right), \quad i \in \{1, 2, \ldots, 120\} \quad (13)$$

where RD_t is the number of RBCs that are removed by random destruction, hf_i is the RBC hazard function that determines the fraction of RBCs lost due to senescence, $RBCInv_{i,t}$ is the fraction of RBCs lost to invasion, UR_t is the number of RBCs removed by the bystander effect, $RetInv_{i,t}$ is the fraction of reticulocytes lost to invasion, and

$$TRBC_t = \sum_{i=1}^{3840} RBC_{i,t}. \quad (14)$$

Random death is modelled as:

$$rRBC_{t+1} = rRBC_t + 0.1 \cdot P_t - \frac{rRBC_t}{800} \quad (15)$$

$$RD_t = \frac{rRBC_t}{800} \quad (16)$$

$$rRBC_0 = 80 \cdot P_t \quad (17)$$

where RD_t is given by the number of RBCs lost through Eq. (15). This removal process is characterized by a first-order rate of $(800 \text{ h})^{-1}$, which was approximated from the corresponding rate in humans (1024^{-1}) [37, 38] by rescaling to $\approx 4/5$, given the ratio of RBC lifespans in macaques and humans of 100 and 120 days, respectively.

The hazard function used here was obtained elsewhere [38] as

$$hf_i = 8.488 \cdot 10^{-45} \cdot i^{12.25}, \quad i \in \{1, 2, \ldots, 3840\}. \quad (18)$$

The hazard function is defined for the 3840 age classes of RBCs, which corresponds to 160 days and thus the maximum theoretical lifespan. In practice, the average RBC is removed at an age of 98 days. RBC and reticulocyte destruction by merozoite invasion was implemented as described below and is only executed if merozoites are present. Once the presence of merozoites has been ascertained, the algorithm checks if there are more RBCs than merozoites ($T RBC_t + T Ret_t > M_t$). If merozoites outnumber RBCs, the simulation is stopped due a lack of RBCs, which implies that the host has died. The total number of reticulocytes is given by:

$$TRet_t = \sum_{i=1}^{120} Ret_{i,t}. \quad (19)$$

Taking into consideration the reticulocyte-to-RBC preference (Ret_{Pref}) [25] and the RBC age preference ($RBCAPf$), given by

$$Ret_{Pref} = 477.2, \quad (20)$$

$$RBCAPf_i = e^{-\frac{10i}{3840}}, \quad i \in \{1, 2, \ldots, 3840\}, \quad (21)$$

the percentage of merozoites infecting reticulocytes is calculated as:

$$PiRet = \frac{Ret_{Pref} \cdot TRet_t}{Ret_{Pref} \cdot TRet_t + TRBC_t}. \quad (22)$$

Thus, the number of reticulocytes being infected is:

$$NiRet = \begin{cases} M_t \cdot PiRet, & if \ M_t \cdot PiRet < TRet_t \\ TRet_t, & if \ M_t \cdot PiRet \geq TRet_t \end{cases} \quad (23)$$

Equation (23) ensures that even at high reticulocyte/RBC preference rates and low RBC numbers, no more than the actually existing reticulocytes are removed. The fraction of reticulocytes lost to invasion ($RetInv_{i,t}$) is then given by:

$$RetInv_{i,t} = \frac{NiRet}{TRet_t}, \quad i \in \{1, 2, \ldots, 120\}, \quad (24)$$

which guarantees that the same proportion of reticulocytes is removed from every age class. In other words, the invasion of reticulocytes is assumed to be age-independent. At this point, there are still $M_t - N \ iRET$ merozoites available to infect RBCs, and the removal of these RBCs follows the age-preference function ($RBCAPf_i$). This removal is accomplished with the auxiliary function described in supplemental materials (Additional file 1).

Removal of infected RBCs by the immune system

In order to account for the immune system's ability to control the infection, an immune response function is introduced, which leads to the removal of infected RBCs:

$$SfiRBC_{i,t} = (1 - I_t), \quad i \in \{1, 2, \ldots, 48\}. \quad (25)$$

Modelling the healthy state

A healthy macaque is characterized by a steady state in terms reticulocytes and RBCs. For this state, only two time-invariant parameters need to be determined, namely the erythropoietic output, which corresponds to RBC production and release rate, $PO_{MacaqueX}$, and the reticulocyte maturation time in circulation, which is determined as the age of that which reticulocytes are released from the bone marrow; it is given as ARR

$0_{MacaqueX}$. The steady state is achieved by specifying that there is no infection, no immune response, and no bystander effect.

$$\begin{cases} P_t = P0_{MacaqueX} \\ ARR_t = ARR0_{MacaqueX} \\ M_t = 0, \quad \forall t > 0 \\ NoI = 0 \\ ToI = +\infty \\ UR_t = 0, \quad \forall t > 0 \\ I_t = 0, \quad \forall t > 0 \end{cases} \quad (26)$$

The parameters $P0_{MacaqueX}$ and $ARR0_{MacaqueX}$ were obtained by optimization of the model, as defined in Eq. (26), against reticulocyte and RBC data obtained either for healthy macaques (E13 cohort, see below) or for infected macaques (E04 and E03 cohorts, see below). In the case of infected macaques, only the first 5- to 7 days of data are used, as long as these show no changes. The optimizations were performed in MatLab using the (fminsearch) algorithm to solve the nonlinear least-square problem.

Modelling an infected blood profile of a macaque

The modelling of an infected macaque's profile starts by calculating its healthy haematological parameters, as shown above for a non-infected macaque. Next, the infected RBC profile is modelled by optimization of the NoI and ToI parameters, which cause the blood infection to appear at a certain point in time (ToI) and, at a certain level (NoI). The infected RBC profile is fitted by optimization of the immune response (I_t).

The time-dependent characterization of the infection is accomplished by adjusting the remaining physiological responses, namely the erythropoietic output, P_t; reticulocyte maturation time, ARR_t; and bystander effect, UR_t. In order to transform the determination of a temporal profile into a standard parametric estimation problem, these functions are modelled as sums of peak functions (Eqs. 27–30)

$$P_t = P0_{MacaqueX} \cdot \left(1 + \sum_i f\left(t | \alpha_{1,i}, \beta_{1,i}, \gamma_{1,i}, \delta_{1,i}, \varepsilon_{1,i}\right) \right) \quad (27)$$

$$ARR_t = ARR0_{MacaqueX} + \sum_i f\left(t | \alpha_{2,i}, \beta_{2,i}, \gamma_{2,i}, \delta_{2,i}, \varepsilon_{2,i}\right) \quad (28)$$

$$UR_t = \sum_i f\left(t | \alpha_{3,i}, \beta_{3,i}, \gamma_{3,i}, \delta_{3,i}, \varepsilon_{3,i}\right) \quad (29)$$

$$I_t = \sum_i f\left(t | \alpha_{4,i}, \beta_{4,i}, \gamma_{4,i}, \delta_{4,i}, \varepsilon_{4,i}\right) \quad (30)$$

where the following peak function is used due to its flexibility (Eq. 31) in generating symmetrical and asymmetrical peaks and plateaus:

$$f(t|\alpha, \beta, \gamma, \delta, \varepsilon) = \alpha \cdot \frac{1}{1 + \beta^{\gamma-t}} \cdot \left(1 - \frac{1}{1 + \delta^{\varepsilon-t}}\right), \quad \varepsilon > \gamma. \quad (31)$$

This function (Eq. 31) results from the juxtaposition of two logistic functions, where α represents the top of the peak or plateau; β and δ allow the modulation of the rate of ascent and descent, respectively; and γ and ε define the points in time where half of the ascent and of the descent occurs, respectively.

All responses (Eqs. 27–30) are modelled with a sum of a variable number of peak functions. In this way the characterization of the response profile of a macaque is converted into a parameter estimation problem, which was implemented in MatLab using a Levenberg–Marquardt algorithm (lsqnonlin) that solves the nonlinear least-squares problem.

Experimental datasets

Three datasets are used in this work; they have been denoted as 'E04', 'E03', and 'E13' in the malaria host–pathogen interaction consortium (MaHPIC). 'E04' is the main dataset, which is used throughout this work, whereas 'E03' and 'E13' are used only to provide additional data for the characterization of the maturation time of reticulocytes in circulation and the reticulocyte production rate. A summary of each of these cohorts is provided below; more detailed descriptions and data are also publicly available [35].

E04 cohort

The 'E04' experiment was performed to study *P. cynomolgi* infections in Rhesus macaques (*Macaca mulatta*). A detailed clinical analysis of the results of this experiment has been published elsewhere [17]. Briefly, five malaria-naïve male macaques, with designations RFa14, RIc14, RMe14, RSb14, RFv13, born and raised at the Yerkes National Primate Research Center, were infected with *P. cynomolgi* B strain through an intravenous inoculation of 2000 freshly-isolated sporozoites per animal. The animals were followed for 100 days, during which ear-prick blood samples were collected daily and analysed for complete blood counts (CBC) and parasitaemia counts.

Four macaques of the E04 cohort (RFa14, RIc14, RMe14, RSb14) survived the 100-day infection study [17].

Macaque RFv13 had to be euthanized due to acute kidney failure and was excluded from this modelling analysis, as it was never able to mount an effective response to the infection. Two of the remaining macaques, RFa14 and RMe14, had a severe clinical outcome and received sub-curative anti-malaria treatments. RMe14 was also provided with a blood transfusion as a precautionary measure given that its haemoglobin levels approached 6 g/dl.

E13 cohort

The 'E13' experiment was performed as a control for other studies. In this experiment, healthy macaques were treated in the same way as other cohorts, but never infected with malaria. The E13 cohort consisted of five malaria-naïve male Rhesus macaques which were followed for 100 days, without ever being exposed to malaria, and were treated with pyrimethamine on days 26, 57, 58, 59, 95, 96 and 97. Pyrimethamine treatment had no effect on blood cell counts [43], and therefore can be considered a true control experiment.

E03 cohort

The design of experiment 'E03' was very similar to the design of 'E04'. The target was, however, to study the effects of a different malaria parasite species, *P. coatneyi*, on Rhesus macaques. Specifically, five malaria-naïve male Rhesus macaques were infected with *P. coatneyi* sporozoites and followed for 100 days during which many samples were taken for different measurements, including daily CBC and parasitaemia levels [43]. Here, only the first 7 days of RBC and reticulocyte measurements are used.

Experimental validation of the reticulocyte maturation time in circulation

In vitro macaque blood cultures

Venous blood from healthy Rhesus macaques was collected in EDTA. A buffy coat preparation was then performed by centrifuging each sample at $200 \times g$ for 10 min. After centrifugation, the buffy coat was removed and discarded. The remaining red blood cell pellet was washed four times in RPMI by centrifugation at $400 \times g$ for 10 min. After washing, the RBC pellet was resuspended in complete RPMI supplemented with L-glutamine, 0.25% sodium bicarbonate, 50 μg/mL hypoxanthine, 7.2 mg/mL HEPES, 2 mg/mL glucose, and 10–20% Human AB + serum to 10% haematocrit. The 10% haematocrit solution was aliquoted into close-cap culture flasks and incubated at 37 °C under blood gas conditions (5%:5%:90%; O_2:CO_2:N_2). Samples were taken at 0, 4, 20, 25.5, and 48 h after incubation to enumerate reticulocytes by flow cytometry and by new methylene blue staining.

Monitoring reticulocyte maturation by flow cytometry

Twenty microlitres of the RBC culture were taken from each culture flask and washed in PBS by centrifugation at $800 \times g$ for 7 min. After washing, the supernatant was aspirated and discarded. The remaining RBC pellet was then resuspended in a cocktail of fluorescently-conjugated antibodies (Clone D058-1283; Fluorochrome APC-Cy7). After resuspension, the antibodies were incubated for 15 min in the dark at room temperature. The samples were then washed in PBS by centrifugation at $800 \times g$ for 7 min. The supernatant was discarded, and the remaining RBC pellet was resuspended for flow cytometry analysis. Data were acquired immediately without fixation using a BD LSR Fortessa flow cytometer. Raw FCS files were imported into FlowJo and compensated followed by importing the compensated files into the Cytobank platform for analysis.

Reticulocyte enumeration by new methylene blue staining

Ten microlitres of the RBC culture were taken from each culture flask and incubated with ten microlitres of new methylene blue for 20 min at 37 °C. After incubation, a thin blood smear was made and allowed to dry prior to the determination of the number of reticulocytes in the sample. For each sample, the number of reticulocytes out of 1000 RBCs was determined, and the percentage of reticulocytes in each sample was calculated for analysis.

Results

Host-parasite interaction model

The proposed model of the malaria blood-stage dynamics uses a discrete recursive framework with a 1-h time-step and an age-structure for reticulocytes, RBCs and infected RBCs [34]. A simplified diagram of the model structure is shown in Fig. 2. The model assumes that reticulocytes are released from the bone marrow at a given rate and age (Eq. 1). At the end of their maturation time, the reticulocytes become mature RBCs. These RBCs have an average lifespan of 98 days in Rhesus macaques [38] and, under normal conditions, are removed due to either senescence or random death. These processes were mathematically characterized elsewhere [38] and are reused here. Upon infection of the blood, the *Plasmodium cynomolgi* merozoites are able to invade reticulocytes and mature RBCs. *P. cynomolgi* within infected RBCs complete their intra-erythrocytic developmental cycle in 2 days, after which the RBCs burst and release a new brood of merozoites.

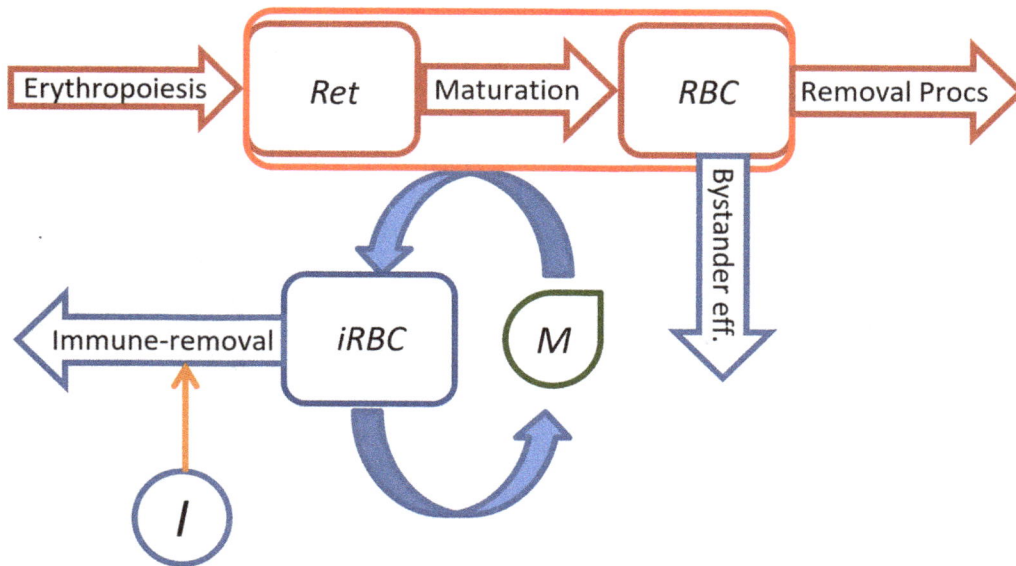

Fig. 2 Simplified diagram of the model. In the absence of an infection, reticulocytes (*Ret*) are produced through *erythropoiesis* and mature into RBCs (*RBC*). These are prone to be removed by the physiological removal processes (*Removal Procs*). In the presence of an infection (processes depicted in blue), merozoites (*M*) invade both reticulocytes and RBCs, thereby generating infected RBCs (*iRBC*). At the end of the parasites' intraerythrocytic development cycle, the infected RBCs burst and release a new brood of merozoites. Up-regulation of the immune-response (*I*) leads to removal of infected RBCs and ideally to control of the parasitaemia. The presence of an infection may also cause loss of RBCs by other means besides parasite invasion (*Bystander eff.*)

During the infection, the increased level of destruction of RBCs is not only attributable to invasion by merozoites but may also be due to a significant bystander effect, which is included in the model. The infection may be controlled either by the host through an up-regulation of the immune response which causes the removal of infected RBCs, or by anti-malarial treatment regimens.

Reticulocyte maturation time in Rhesus macaques

In control animals, RBC and reticulocyte numbers stay essentially constant, absent of any insult [43]. Therefore, model optimization against control macaque data allows the inference of the haematological parameters for reticulocyte release rate and maturation time. In the case of infected macaques, it was assumed that the haematological steady state, observed between the pre-infection period and the first 5 days post-infection, represents reasonably well the non-infected baseline state of each macaque. Using this procedure, the reticulocyte release rate and maturation time were calculated for each macaque in three separate cohorts: E04 [17] (the main cohort modelled in this paper), E03 (Cordy et al. pers. comm.) and E13 [43]. The data for these cohorts are publicly available [35, 43].

Analysis of the results obtained for these three cohorts (Fig. 3) shows only modest inter-cohort differences,

and the overall averages for the reticulocyte maturation time in circulation and the reticulocyte release rate are 24 ± 5 h and 2727 ± 209 cells/h/µL, respectively.

To validate the inferred in vivo reticulocyte maturation time in circulation, freshly drawn RBCs from two different healthy macaques were incubated in vitro, and reticulocytes followed over time (Fig. 4). The reticulocytes were assessed by measuring RBCs staining positive for RNA (Fig. 4). Using the former method, fewer than 20% of the reticulocytes were found after 25 h of incubation in vitro (Fig. 4), which is similar to what was determined in vivo (Fig. 3).

Characterization of responses to malarial infections

The optimization of the model towards reproducing the experimental blood profile of a given macaque leads to inferences regarding the temporal host response to the infection. This characterization includes the profile of the reticulocyte release rate (or erythropoietic output); the reticulocyte maturation time in circulation; the RBC removal due to bystander effect, parasitization, senescence, and random processes; and the immune response.

Modelling RFa14

Applying the model to the data obtained for RFa14 (Fig. 5a, c, f) permits the inference of this macaque's infection response profile (Fig. 5b, d, e, f). During the first

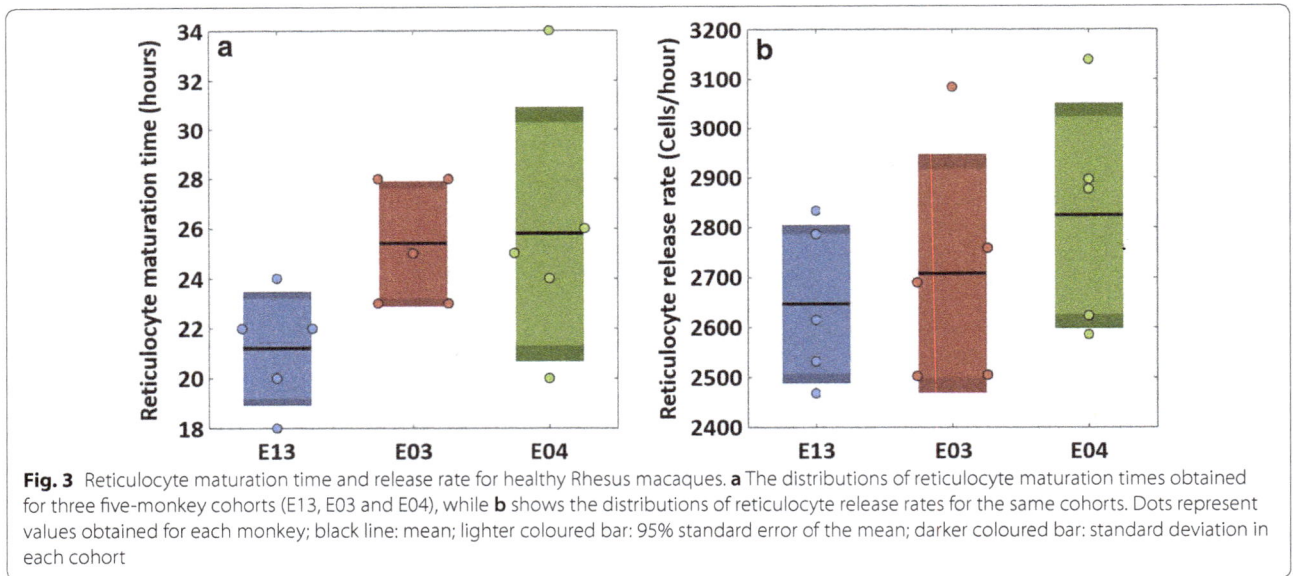

Fig. 3 Reticulocyte maturation time and release rate for healthy Rhesus macaques. **a** The distributions of reticulocyte maturation times obtained for three five-monkey cohorts (E13, E03 and E04), while **b** shows the distributions of reticulocyte release rates for the same cohorts. Dots represent values obtained for each monkey; black line: mean; lighter coloured bar: 95% standard error of the mean; darker coloured bar: standard deviation in each cohort

7 days, this macaque presented with a healthy phenotype (Fig. 5a, c, f), which allowed an assessment of its baseline values. The reticulocyte maturation time in circulation was determined to be 25 h, and the erythropoietic output was 2623 RBCs/h/μL (Fig. 5b). During this same interval, RBCs were mainly removed due to senescence (2361 RBCs/h/μL, Fig. 5e), and considerably fewer cells were lost through random processes (262 RBCs/h/μL).

At days 8 and 9, the maturation time of reticulocytes started to increase, suggesting that these cells started to be released from the bone marrow at a younger stage and giving rise to an increased percentage of reticulocytes (Fig. 5a), without a corresponding change in RBC

numbers (Fig. 5c). This trend slowly became stronger, and on day 11, reticulocytes were being released 25 h younger than normal. Upon release, these cells subsequently spent a total of 50 h in circulation before maturating into RBCs, except if they happened to be infected before completing their maturation.

The observed growth rate of the parasite in this macaque, expressed as the number of merozoites released per infected RBC in a 48 h cycle, was 54.4 and 40.6 for the first and second parasitaemia peaks, respectively (ranges 11–19 and 23–26 days). These values are much larger than what is expected for *P. cynomolgi*, as this parasite is known to release, on average, 16 merozoites per infected RBC, with a range of 14–20. While at first counterintuitive, these results have been shown to be suggestive of concealment of the infected RBCs in tissues, away from the peripheral circulation [44]. In the present model, the assumption of a concealed population of infected RBCs was not used. The model assumes a rate of parasite growth equal to the observed rate. In this way, the observed growth kinetics is modelled, but no assumption or information on the magnitude and kinetics of the concealed population are required.

Infection patency occurred at day 12, and shortly thereafter, RBC death by parasitization became significant, causing the RBC and reticulocyte titers to start tumbling. Accounting for *P. cynomolgi*'s reported 477:1 preference for reticulocytes over mature RBCs [25] leads the model to predict a complete removal of reticulocytes at peak parasitaemia (Days 16–18, Fig. 5a). This result is in stark contrast to the experimental data, which indicate only a modest drop in reticulocytes (Fig. 5a). To explore this

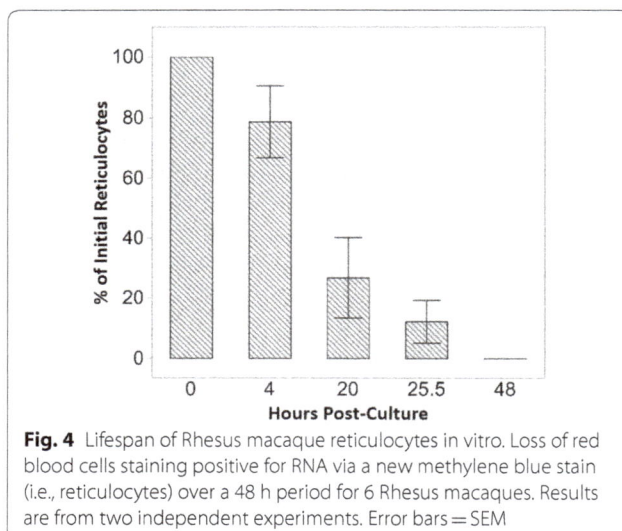

Fig. 4 Lifespan of Rhesus macaque reticulocytes in vitro. Loss of red blood cells staining positive for RNA via a new methylene blue stain (i.e., reticulocytes) over a 48 h period for 6 Rhesus macaques. Results are from two independent experiments. Error bars = SEM

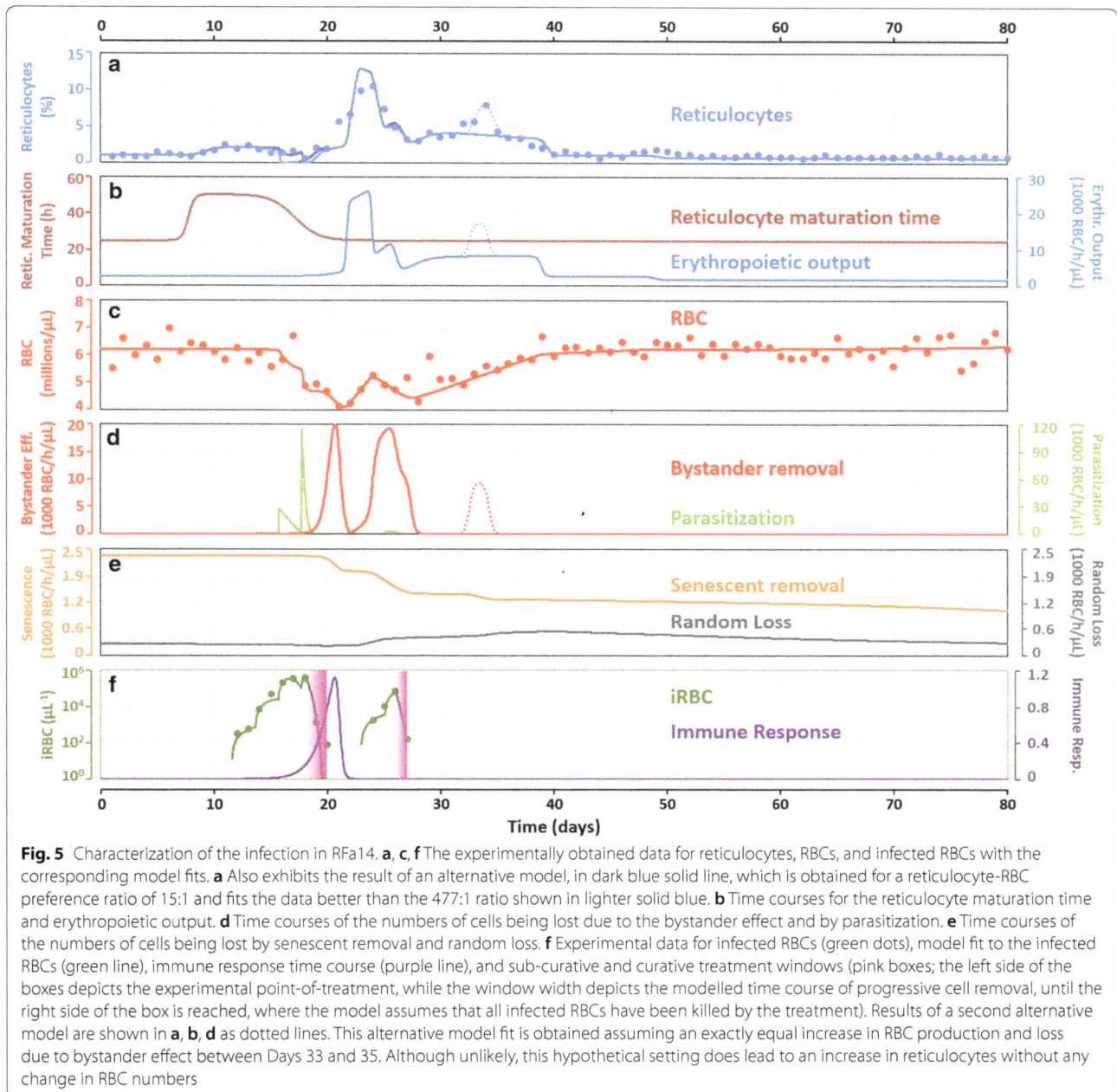

Fig. 5 Characterization of the infection in RFa14. **a**, **c**, **f** The experimentally obtained data for reticulocytes, RBCs, and infected RBCs with the corresponding model fits. **a** Also exhibits the result of an alternative model, in dark blue solid line, which is obtained for a reticulocyte-RBC preference ratio of 15:1 and fits the data better than the 477:1 ratio shown in lighter solid blue. **b** Time courses for the reticulocyte maturation time and erythropoietic output. **d** Time courses of the numbers of cells being lost due to the bystander effect and by parasitization. **e** Time courses of the numbers of cells being lost by senescent removal and random loss. **f** Experimental data for infected RBCs (green dots), model fit to the infected RBCs (green line), immune response time course (purple line), and sub-curative and curative treatment windows (pink boxes; the left side of the boxes depicts the experimental point-of-treatment, while the window width depicts the modelled time course of progressive cell removal, until the right side of the box is reached, where the model assumes that all infected RBCs have been killed by the treatment). Results of a second alternative model are shown in **a**, **b**, **d** as dotted lines. This alternative model fit is obtained assuming an exactly equal increase in RBC production and loss due to bystander effect between Days 33 and 35. Although unlikely, this hypothetical setting does lead to an increase in reticulocytes without any change in RBC numbers

discrepancy further, alternate levels of the reticulocyte/RBC preference were tested, and a ratio of 15:1 emerged to fit the data best. The model predictions with this alternate parameter value are shown in dark blue (Fig. 5a). This new parameter value does not change any other model outputs, since the same numbers of RBCs are still being removed. Apart from the time period between days 16 and 18, the effects of this adjusted parameter value are only noticeable at day 26. During peak parasitaemia, the

release of younger reticulocytes subsides, and the reticulocyte maturation time returns to 25 h.

Interestingly, the model predicts that the bystander effect increases after the sub-curative treatment and peaks just before Day 21. By Day 22, the bystander effect subsides, and RBC production increases (Fig. 5b). This peak of RBC production is responsible for the peak of reticulocytes between Days 22–25 (Fig. 5a) and for the increase in RBC numbers between Days 22 and 24 (Fig. 5c). To reproduce these two observations, the model predicts an erythropoietic output increase from its baseline value of 2623 to 26,080 RBCs/h/μL. This tenfold jump is able to replenish approximately half of the RBCs lost up until Day 20. Between Days 23 and 27, a new smaller peak of parasitaemia develops. This peak is accompanied by RBC losses that are mainly due to the bystander effect (Fig. 5d), given that the relatively low levels of parasites (Fig. 5f) cannot explain the numbers of RBCs lost (Fig. 5b).

At Day 26, this macaque received curative treatment, and the last day of recorded parasitaemia occurred 1 day later. By Day 28, the bystander effect subsides and RBC recovery restarts at a rate of approximately 8100 RBCs/h/μL, which led to full recovery of the RBC numbers by Day 40. Within the period between Days 28 and 40, reticulocytes seem to rise again during Days 33–34. This peak could simply have been an error or noise in the determination, or due to a combination of biological events. In the latter case, since this peak is not accompanied by an increased RBC production, one of two explanations seems most likely: either the reticulocyte maturation time increased and decreased briefly, or a simultaneous increase in RBC production and loss due to bystander effect occurred. Neither one seems likely at this point of the infection, as the macaque had been curatively treated by Day 26 and no parasitaemia was recorded since then. Furthermore, given that the peak is rather short, it is not very likely due to a release of younger reticulocytes.

To explore the situation further, a slightly altered model was created, where it was assumed that a peak of production of RBCs and loss due to bystander effect occurred simultaneously and with the same magnitude (Fig. 5b, d); output from this model is shown in dotted lines in Fig. 5a, b, d. While the results are satisfactory, the explanation of two simultaneous processes with the same magnitude seems unlikely, and this model will, therefore, not be explored further.

During the period between Days 40 and 48, the erythropoietic output returns to its normal value. However, after Day 49 the model predicts a small drop in the erythropoietic output to 1740 RBCs/h/μL. This decrease reflects the decrease in RBC deaths by senescence, relative to the start of the infection. After Day 20, senescent cell death (Fig. 5e) decreases due to a changed age profile of RBCs (Additional file 2). Namely, during the infection large numbers of RBCs of all age classes are killed and subsequently replaced by newly produced RBCs. This replacement means that the older age classes are, after Day 50, notably less populated than under normal conditions (Additional file 2). Thus, until the age class profile is restored to its normal state, fluctuations in the senescent death rate are expected to occur for some time after the infection. Nevertheless, this drop in erythropoietic

output, which is predicted after Day 49, also causes a small drop in reticulocytes and, indeed, the experimental data show a similar drop in reticulocytes numbers (Fig. 5a).

Modelling RMe14, RSb14, and RIc14

The response profiles of the remaining macaques to the infections are documented as supplemental material (Additional file 3).

Pre-patent increase in reticulocyte numbers

All macaques modelled here showed evidence of an increase in reticulocyte numbers early in the infection (Fig. 5, Additional file 3: Figs. S2.1, S2.2, S2.3). Replotting these observations for all cases shows more clearly that the reticulocyte numbers increased before the infection patency (Fig. 6). The increases averaged at $1.7 \pm 0.6\%$, with RFa14 increasing from 1.05 to 2.12% (Fig. 6a), RMe14 from 1.43 to 3.87% (Fig. 6b), RSB14 from 1.0 to 3.1% (Fig. 6c) and RIc14 from 1.1 to 2.44% (Fig. 6d). An analogous increase in reticulocytes was also detected in RIc14 just before the relapse infection peak (Fig. 6e). At the beginning of this time-period, between Days 42 and 66, RIc14 had recovered from the anaemia caused by the primary infection, and the erythropoietic production had been reduced (Additional file 3: Fig. S2.3B) to compensate for the lower rate of senescent RBC removal. The predicted levels of reticulocytes in the absence of an increase in reticulocyte maturation time in circulation are shown in panel E in gray (Fig. 6). This gray line clearly misses all data points, demonstrating that it is, indeed, necessary to assume an increase in the maturation time of reticulocytes in circulation between Days 42 and 58. Accounting for this increased maturation time in circulation leads to an increased percentage of peripheral blood reticulocytes from 0.87% (grey line) to 1.70% (blue line) (Fig. 6e).

If these increases in reticulocyte numbers in peripheral blood are caused by an increase in their maturation time in circulation, then the cause of this increase must precede it. In this model, the age of the reticulocytes released from the bone marrow is given by ARR_t (Eq. 1). It is the decrease of this quantity, representing the decrease in the age of newly released reticulocytes, which ultimately leads to the increase in their maturation time and the accumulation of reticulocytes in circulation. On average, the age of reticulocytes entering circulation starts to decrease 4 days before the detection of the infection by microscopy (7 days post-infection), at which time the parasitic infection is either still restricted to the liver or just beginning to be present in the blood.

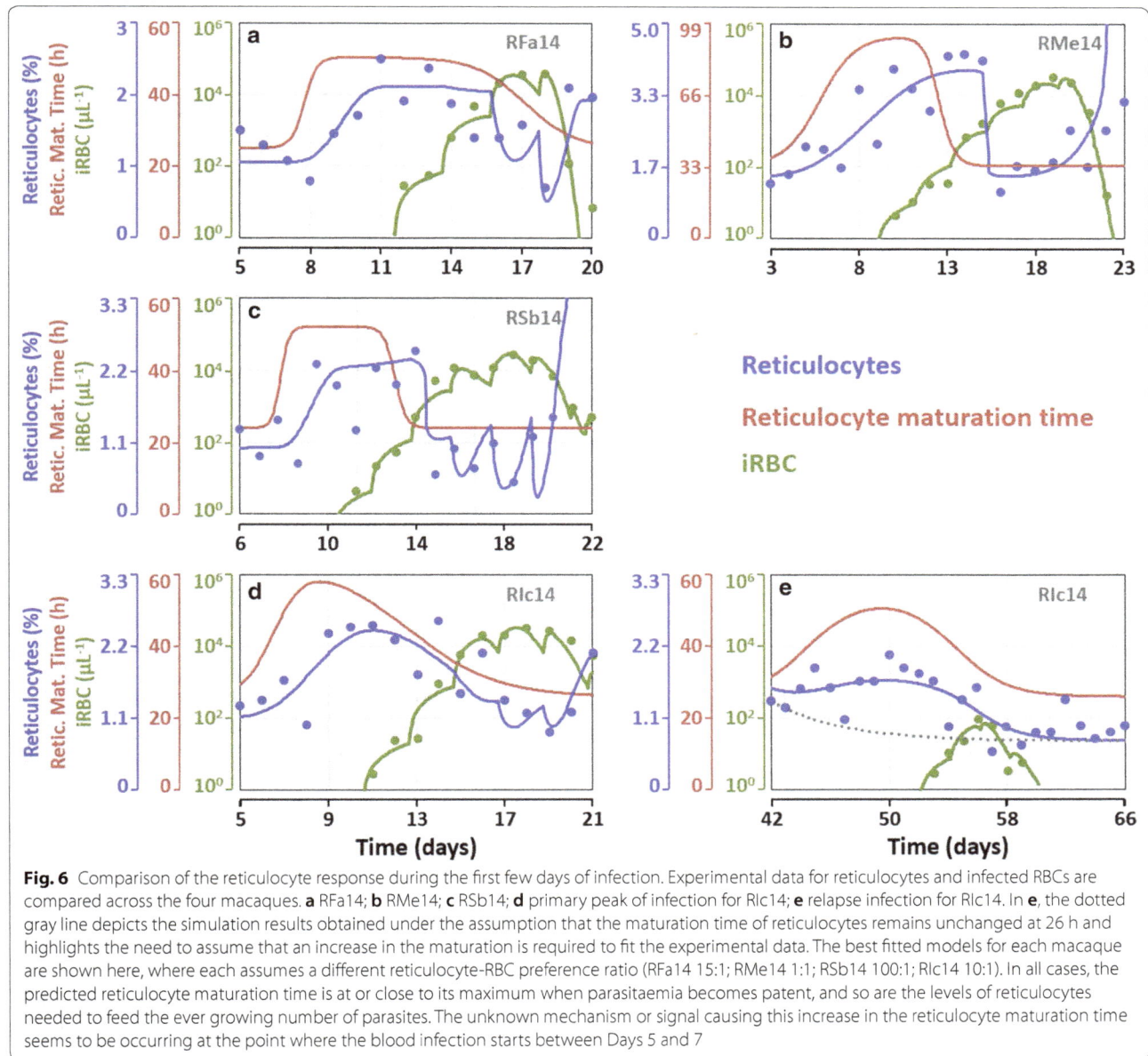

Fig. 6 Comparison of the reticulocyte response during the first few days of infection. Experimental data for reticulocytes and infected RBCs are compared across the four macaques. **a** RFa14; **b** RMe14; **c** RSb14; **d** primary peak of infection for RIc14; **e** relapse infection for RIc14. In **e**, the dotted gray line depicts the simulation results obtained under the assumption that the maturation time of reticulocytes remains unchanged at 26 h and highlights the need to assume that an increase in the maturation is required to fit the experimental data. The best fitted models for each macaque are shown here, where each assumes a different reticulocyte-RBC preference ratio (RFa14 15:1; RMe14 1:1; RSb14 100:1; RIc14 10:1). In all cases, the predicted reticulocyte maturation time is at or close to its maximum when parasitaemia becomes patent, and so are the levels of reticulocytes needed to feed the ever growing number of parasites. The unknown mechanism or signal causing this increase in the reticulocyte maturation time seems to be occurring at the point where the blood infection starts between Days 5 and 7

RBC fate during *P. cynomolgi* infection

The infection response profiles inferred for each macaque (Fig. 5 and Additional file 3: Figs. S2.1, S2.2, S2.3) were analysed for RBC production and removal, and the results are summarized in Fig. 7. Since these profiles are time-dependent and different for each macaque, the number of RBCs removed by each process was summed for the first 50 days of each infection, which in all cases includes the onset of the infection, anaemia, and recovery, but excludes relapses. RMe14 was excluded from the average as he received a blood transfusion, which clearly changed his reticulocyte and RBC profiles (Additional file 3: Fig. S2.1), and consequently would have invalidated

the quantification of the haematological processes. If these macaques had not been infected but remained healthy with the same trajectory shown at their baselines, they would have produced, during these 50 days, an average of 3.5 ± 0.3 million RBCs/µL, of which 10% would have died by random processes and the remaining 90% by senescence. Yet, in every case, these infections resulted in the removal of twice as many RBCs, with an average of 7.6 ± 0.9 million RBCs/µL. Fewer RBCs were lost by the normal physiological processes (random and senescent), since many more were prematurely killed by the infection dependent processes. Interestingly, similar to what has been seen before in *Plasmodium coatneyi* infections

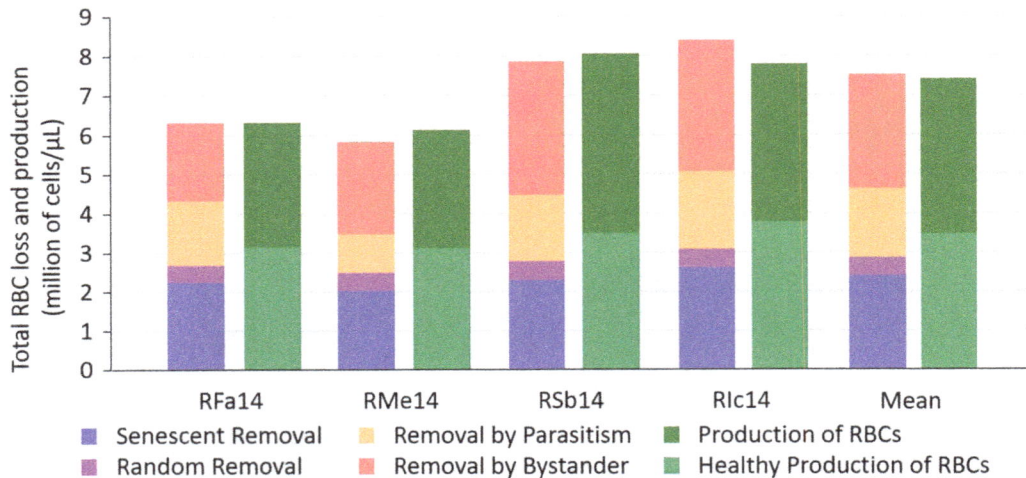

Fig. 7 Comparison of the levels of RBC production and removal among 'E04' macaques. Total extent of RBC production and removal per macaque and for the average of RFa14, Rsb14 and Rlc14 during the first 50 days of infection is shown. RMe14 was excluded from the average as this macaque received a blood transfusion that invalidates the true quantification of RBC production and removal. The extent of RBC production each macaque would have had if it had remained in its healthy state, shown during the first few days is highlighted with a lighter shade of green, out of the total measured RBC production. RBC removal is shown per process. The normal physiological processes are senescence and random loss. Infection-induced pathological processes are parasitism (invasion by the parasite) and bystander effect (loss of uninfected RBCs). Throughout the first 50 days of the infections, which include the primary parasitaemia peak but exclude relapses, 38 ±4% of RBCs were lost by the physiological processes (senescence and random loss), 38 ±6% due to bystander effect, and only 23 ±2% due to invasion by the parasite

[38], of the total number of RBCs removed due to the infection, only 38 ± 6% were actually killed by parasite invasion. The remaining 62 ± 8% were removed by the bystander effect. In contrast, *P. coatneyi* had 5% removed by parasite invasion and 95% by bystander effect [38].

Dependence of the erythropoietic production on the severity of the anaemia

The level of erythropoietic output in the model, i.e., the rate of RBC production, was inferred from each macaque's profile data (Fig. 5, Additional file 3: Figs. S2.1, S2.2, S2.3). Since this property is not being assumed to be explicitly dependent on the severity of the anaemia, nor on the number of RBCs, it becomes possible to test these dependencies and the underlying assumptions. Figure 8 shows the erythropoietic output of each macaque, plotted against the RBC levels (Fig. 8a) and against anaemia (Fig. 8b). Here, anaemia represents the number of missing RBCs relative to the healthy state of each macaque. Therefore, periods where the macaques had very mild or no anaemia (Fig. 8b) correspond to periods with high levels (6–7.5 million) of RBCs (Fig. 8a).

A usual assumption in the field is that the erythropoietic output decreases as the RBC levels approach a healthy value, which is to say that the erythropoietic output is negatively correlated with RBC levels and a negative trend would be visible in panel A. Similarly, a positive correlation would be found in panel B if the

RBC production increased with the severity of the anaemia. Yet, such correlations are not present. One possible explanation for this lack of correlation could be that there is a time lag between the onset of the anaemia and the increase in the RBC production, as it takes time for the kidneys to detect the low levels of oxygen in the blood, produce erythropoietin, allow this hormone to travel to the bone marrow, exert its effect on RBC progenitors, and actually to increase the release of reticulocytes. Different time lags were tested and none resulted in a correlation being detected in either case, which suggests a couple of possible explanations. The response could be highly non-linear, and/or the presence of a malarial infection may interfere with the bone marrow response to such a degree that the correlation disappears. Unsurprisingly, bone marrow dysfunction has been previously reported for this cohort of animals, when infected with *P. cynomolgi* [36].

Discussion

Nonhuman primate model systems hold the greatest potential for understanding malarial host-parasite dynamics and pathogenesis in vivo [14, 45–47]. A new computational model is presented here for the analysis of erythrocyte dynamics during infections with *P. cynomolgi*, a relapsing simian malaria parasite that is a zoonosis and can serve as an experimental model for *P. vivax*. This computational model was parameterized to

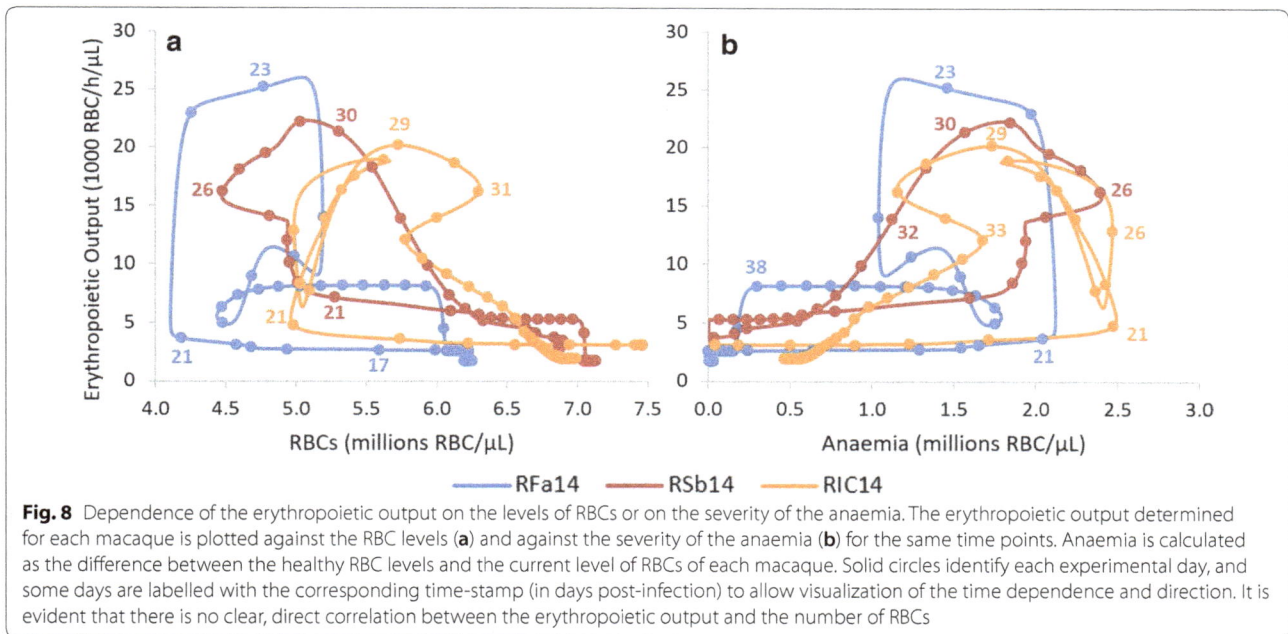

Fig. 8 Dependence of the erythropoietic output on the levels of RBCs or on the severity of the anaemia. The erythropoietic output determined for each macaque is plotted against the RBC levels (**a**) and against the severity of the anaemia (**b**) for the same time points. Anaemia is calculated as the difference between the healthy RBC levels and the current level of RBCs of each macaque. Solid circles identify each experimental day, and some days are labelled with the corresponding time-stamp (in days post-infection) to allow visualization of the time dependence and direction. It is evident that there is no clear, direct correlation between the erythropoietic output and the number of RBCs

reproduce experimental data obtained from *P. cynomolgi* infection of Rhesus macaques [17] and allowed the characterization of the lifespan of reticulocytes in healthy malaria-naïve animals, the interactions between parasite and host, and the host responses during a blood-stage infection.

Process quantification in this model was done by inference of a time-dependent function from the experimental data, rather than assuming that these processes follow a mass-action model in an *ad-hoc* fashion, as it is commonly done in the field [30–33]. By avoiding the assumption of such relationships, it becomes possible to test assumptions and system properties in an unbiased manner. One such property examined was the erythropoietic output, which corresponds to the rate of RBC production and the rate of reticulocyte release from the bone marrow. This property is usually assumed to depend linearly on present or recent anaemia or to be inversely proportional to the present or recent RBC levels [48, 49]. Yet, the results show no correlation between either, which suggests that the true function is more complex and likely includes delays.

In humans, the maturation time of reticulocytes in circulation is about 24 h [50, 51], but this period may be increased to as many as 3 days under erythropoietic stress [52]. Here, the computational model shows that the maturation time of circulating reticulocytes in healthy *Macaca mulatta* is about 24 ± 5 h (n = 15). This value is corroborated by an in vitro analysis of the surviving reticulocytes in fresh RBC cultures from healthy macaques. In these cultures, reticulocytes remained detectable for 25 h, as identified by their RNA content. Overall, these

results point to a similar reticulocyte kinetics between *Macaca mulatta* and humans. From the same analysis, the normal healthy RBC production rate was determined to be 2727 ± 209 cells/h/μL (n = 15) for *Macaca mulatta*.

All macaques exhibited a period of elevated reticulocyte levels 11–13 days after the inoculation with sporozoites, which preceded the detection of patent parasitaemia in the blood and occurred concurrently without any change in RBC numbers. Theoretically, an increase in reticulocyte numbers can only be due to one of two processes, or both: (1) increased RBC production and release from the bone marrow; or (2) a shift towards the release of younger reticulocytes, as it has been observed during erythropoietic stress [52]. The first would lead to increased reticulocyte numbers in circulation, along with an increase in the overall RBC numbers. In the latter, the same total number of RBCs is still being produced, so no increase in RBC numbers would be observed. However, if reticulocytes are released at a younger stage from the bone marrow, these would take a longer time to mature in circulation, thus leading to an increased accumulation of reticulocytes in circulation. Given that an increase in the total number of RBCs was not observed, an increase in the RBC production does not explain the current data. Therefore, the more likely explanation is a shift toward the release of less mature reticulocytes. Under this assumption, this shift would have to occur around days 6–8 to be consistent with the observed changes, which puts this shift at around the time the parasites are coming out of the liver and starting the infection's blood stage. A plausible explanation may be that during the beginning of the blood-stage infection the parasite releases a factor that ultimately results in the release of younger reticulocytes from the bone marrow. This mechanism would ensure an increase of circulating reticulocytes, which are arguably the parasite's preferred host cells, although the preference is not exclusive [8, 24, 25]. The increased number of reticulocytes seems to subside before a subsequent reticulocyte peak occurs due to the host's response to the anaemia. During the high parasitaemia period, the reticulocyte numbers exhibit oscillations. These seem to be due to the cycles of RBC infection. In this period of the infection, it is difficult for the model to distinguish precisely between the high consumption of reticulocytes and the decrease in maturation time of these cells. However, the decrease in maturation time has to happen during this time period, because the model only fits the reticulocyte peak in response to the anaemia if the reticulocyte maturation time has returned to normal. These observations are interesting as they suggest that P. cynomolgi parasites may be capable of causing a shift in the age at which reticulocytes are released from the bone marrow. This shift may be advantageous for the parasite as it happens in anticipation of the parasite's high demand for reticulocytes and, secondarily, red blood cells, and occurs a week after the release from the liver, when the parasite numbers reach their maximum.

It has long been recognized that certain *Plasmodium* species show preferences for invading mature RBCs or reticulocytes [25, 53]. Species like *Plasmodium ovale* and *P. vivax* have almost strict reticulocyte tropism, whereas *P. coatneyi*, *Plasmodium knowlesi* and *Plasmodium malariae* have mature RBC tropism [24]. By contrast, *P. falciparum* invades both mature and immature RBCs. *P. cynomolgi* resembles *P. vivax*, which has an almost strict reticulocyte tropism [24], whereas the tropism appears to be conditional in the case of *P. cynomolgi* [25, 54], thus exhibiting a preference for reticulocytes while maintaining the ability to infect both RBC maturation stages. Using the computational model developed here, the reticulocyte preference calculated for each macaque is about 15, 1, 100 and 10 (RFa14, RMe14, RSb14 and RIc14, respectively), which gives an average of 32 ± 46 (n = 4) or a median of 13 for this cohort. These results are rough estimates, as they depend highly on the level of reticulocytes during peak parasitaemia, a short time span with just about six time points for each macaque. Additionally, the reticulocyte preference parameter also suffers from structural correlation with the reticulocyte maturation time. The model results show that the reticulocyte maturation and release timing returns to normalcy by the time high parasitaemias are observed, which allows averting the issue of structural non-identifiability. The value determined here for the reticulocyte preference is lower than what was measured for *Plasmodium berghei*, 153 [55],

and closer to what was recently obtained for *P. berghei* ANKA strain, 74 [56]. Additionally, a recent in vitro study showed that *P. cynomolgi* B strain has strict tropism towards human reticulocytes, but this was not evident when testing *Macaca mulatta* RBCs [8]. Unfortunately, this study did not address possible host cell preferences using co-cultures of reticulocytes and RBCs, thus preventing the quantification of *P. cynomolgi* preference for *Macaca mulatta* reticulocytes. Overall it appears that the reticulocyte preference is an important parameter for the infection dynamics, as it has been shown that the preference may be correlated with parasitaemia levels and ultimately with disease severity [33, 48, 49].

Analysis of the parasite growth rates within each macaque revealed that the parasite population grew at unexpectedly fast rates, mostly with values in the range of 30–54 merozoites per infected RBC. In the case of the *P. cynomolgi* infected macaque RFv13, the computed value actually reached 110 merozoites per infected RBC, which is likewise unrealistic. This monkey had a particularly high peak parasitaemia (19.5%), suffered severe manifestations of the disease and ultimately needed to be euthanized [7, 17]. A likely explanation of the apparently high growth rates is that not all parasite forms circulate freely but may rather become concealed in venules or tissues [44], such that parasitaemia readings from peripheral blood smears may not reflect the total parasite load in the blood. If indeed a substantial number of infected RBCs go into concealment for some of their 48-h life cycle, then the parasite population based on blood smear readings may at times appear to grow at a faster rate than what is biologically possible. This hypothesis has been analysed for *P. cynomolgi*, where the analysis of in vivo data suggested the existence of a population of non-circulating concealed parasites [44]. The model here did not consider concealment and accounted only for parasites observed on blood smears. However, as compensation, the parasitaemias were allowed to grow at the observed, seemingly inflated, growth rates, even though these are higher than what would be biologically possible. In this way, the growth of the parasitaemias does take into consideration any non-visible, and thus concealed, parasites, without requiring any assumption regarding possible concealment probabilities, kinetics, or sites.

Analysis of the infection profiles of RFa14 and RIc14 points to a temporal segregation of RBC production and removal (Fig. 5 and Additional file 3: Fig. S2.3), and similar results were found for *P. coatneyi* [38]. Interestingly, RSb14 (Additional file 3: Fig. S2.2) does not fit this pattern, as it shows an increased level of RBC production that lasts 15 days with its maximum at Day 30, during which time losses due to bystander effect and parasite invasion are recorded. Given the limited sample size, all cases are being reported here. In addition to the deconvolution of loss and production of RBCs in RFa14 and RIc14, RBC losses by parasite invasion and bystander effect tend not to occur simultaneously. This observation gives confidence that loss due to bystander effect is real and not due to a miss-calculation of parasite invasion. Additionally, removal by bystander effect is also detected in periods where parasitaemia is low, which further strengthens this point. Yet, the fact that these two losses tend to be segregated from RBC production does suggest that something involved with the RBC losses prevents up-regulation of the erythropoietic system even during periods of anaemia.

For example, the profile of RIc14 contains a period (Days 23–28) where the main parasitaemia peak had subsided, and the erythropoietic production is high. Suddenly, parasitaemia increases again, and the model measures an increase in RBC death, due to both invasion and bystander effect, which is accompanied by a decrease in RBC production. The decrease in production is inferred by the model as a result of the decrease in reticulocyte counts. What the mediator of this effect could be is not known, but the unknown factor could be mediated by the immune system, as suggested by the analysis of the bone marrow transcriptome of this macaque cohort [36]. Additionally, it is possible that some aspect of the immune response may be the culprit for the bystander effect, which would simultaneously explain uninfected and infected RBC losses and the failure to up-regulate RBC production.

However, the analysis never shows a reduction of the erythropoietic flux during the infection and recovery periods. The healthy baseline RBC production is determined from the RBC status of each macaque during the first 5–7 days of the experiment, and across all infections, the RBC production is never inferred to dip below this healthy level. Thus, anaemia cannot be due to decreased RBC production, but is more likely due to increased RBC destruction, either by parasite invasion and a bystander effect, and to suppression of the erythropoietin-dependent up-regulation of erythropoiesis in response to anaemia, despite elevated levels of erythropoietin in this macaque cohort between Days 20 and 30 [36]. By contrast, decreased RBC production is observed only after full recovery of the macaques, but that is due to a shift in the age distribution of RBCs which becomes skewed toward a younger than normal population (see Additional file 1). This younger population of RBCs is, therefore, subject to fewer losses due to old age, and the erythropoietic system of these macaques transiently adjusts the production to meet these reduced losses at normal haematocrit levels.

The bystander effect was estimated from all RBCs produced and lost throughout the first 50 days of the infection. This period of 50 days post-inoculation includes the main parasitaemia peak, anaemia, treatment if needed, and recovery, but excludes relapses. As a consequence of the infections, RBC production and removal doubled to 217% (from 3.5 ± 0.3 to 7.6 ± 0.9 million RBCs/µL). During this same period, RBC removal occurred due to normal physiological processes of senescence and random loss ($38 \pm 4\%$), invasion by the parasite ($23 \pm 2\%$), and the bystander effect ($38 \pm 6\%$). These results suggest that the bystander effect accounts for $62 \pm 8\%$ of all infection-induced RBC losses.

Bystander removal of RBCs during malaria has been documented in humans [41, 57, 58], yet accurate measurements are difficult to obtain [41]. Using a mathematical model similar to the one used here, the bystander removal of RBCs was inferred for *Macaca mulatta* during *P. coatneyi* infections as 95% [38], which is similar to values estimated for humans with falciparum malaria (90–92%) [41, 58]. Bystander loss of RBCs has also been documented in vivax malaria [58] and may be due to changes in membrane rigidity, although other mechanisms are under investigation [59, 60]. The present data do not allow inferences regarding the possible underlying causes of the bystander effect, but they do show that proportionally fewer RBCs are removed by the bystander effect in *P. cynomolgi* (62%) infections than in *P. coatneyi* (95%) [44]. Whether this difference is indicative of the difference between the human counterparts of these infections (vivax and falciparum, respectively) is yet to be determined.

Conclusions

Nonhuman primate models of malaria are as close to human malaria as possible, and much can be inferred regarding the disease progression in humans from NHP models. Here, the dynamics of reticulocytes and RBCs was investigated with a new mathematical model. This model uses a discrete recursive framework with age-structure, which allows the estimation of the healthy maturation time of reticulocytes in circulation and of normal RBC production in Rhesus macaques. The maturation time was determined as 24 ± 5 h ($n = 15$), and RBC production as 2727 ± 209 cells/h/µL ($n = 15$). The reticulocyte maturation time in circulation was validated in ex vivo experiments and is similar to that in humans. Analysis of the responses of Rhesus macaques to *P. cynomolgi* infections revealed a period during the early blood-stage of the infection when the numbers of reticulocytes in the peripheral blood increase. The model analysis suggests that this short period comprising the early rise in blood-stage parasitaemia may be associated with reticulocyte tropism of this *Plasmodium* species, which would be consistent with previous indications of host cell preferences by *P. cynomolgi* [25]. The results also suggest a temporal segregation between RBC producing and RBC removing processes, which points towards the existence of some unidentified factor, which may prevent up-regulation of erythropoiesis during anaemia and while RBCs are being destroyed either by invasion or due to the bystander effect. The main infection peak and subsequent recovery resulted in an overall doubling (214%) of the number of RBCs produced relative to what would be expected in the absence of infection. Of the total number of RBCs lost due to these infections, 62% were lost by processes other than parasitic invasion, here designated as the bystander effect. This value is significantly lower than the value of 95% that was obtained previously for *P. coatneyi* infections in rhesus macaques [38].

Authors' contributions
Conceived and designed the model: LLF and EOV. Performed simulations and optimizations: LLF. Managed and deposited the data and metadata: members of the MaHPIC consortium. Performed data analysis: LLF, CJJ. Generated the figures: LLF, CJJ. Interpreted the results: LLF, EOV, AM, CJJ, MRG, and JWB. Wrote the paper: LLF and EOV. Executed validations experiments and analysis: CS and CJJ. Provided expert knowledge, viewpoints and manuscript contributions: MRG, AM, JWB and members of the MaHPIC consortium. All authors read and approved the final manuscript.

Author details
[1] The Wallace H. Coulter Department of Biomedical Engineering, Georgia Institute of Technology and Emory University, Atlanta, GA 30332-2000, USA. [2] Malaria Host–Pathogen Interaction Center, Emory Vaccine Center, Yerkes National Primate Research Center, Emory University, Atlanta, GA 30322, USA. [3] Division of Infectious Diseases, Department of Medicine, Emory University, Atlanta, GA 30322, USA. [4] Malaria Branch, Division of Parasitic Diseases and Malaria, Centers for Disease Control and Prevention, Atlanta, GA 30322, USA.

Acknowledgements
The authors would like to thank Anuj Gupta, James Wade, and Nathan Chiappa for fruitful discussions. The authors would also like to thank Daniel Olivença for proof-reading the methods section and for all the discussions.

Competing interests
The authors declare that they have no competing interests.

Funding
This project was funded in part by Federal funds from the US National Institute of Allergy and Infectious Diseases, National Institutes of Health, Department

of Health and Human Services under contract # HHSN272201200031C (PI: Mary R. Galinski), which supports the Malaria Host–Pathogen Interaction Center (MaHPIC), as well as the Office of Research Infrastructure Programs/OD P51OD011132 (formerly National Center for Research Resources P51RR000165).

References
1. WHO. Control and elimination of *Plasmodium vivax* malaria—a technical brief. Geneva: World Health Organization; 2015.
2. Borner J, Pick C, Thiede J, Kolawole OM, Kingsley MT, Schulze J, et al. Phylogeny of haemosporidian blood parasites revealed by a multigene approach. Mol Phylogenet Evol. 2016;94:221–31.
3. Baird JK. Evidence and implications of mortality associated with acute *Plasmodium vivax* malaria. Clin Microbiol Rev. 2013;26:36–57.
4. Howes RE, Battle KE, Mendis KN, Smith DL, Cibulskis RE, Baird JK, et al. Global epidemiology of *Plasmodium vivax*. Am J Trop Med Hyg. 2016;95:15–34.
5. Pacheco MA, Battistuzzi FU, Junge RE, Cornejo OE, Williams CV, Landau I, et al. Timing the origin of human malarias: the lemur puzzle. BMC Evol Biol. 2011;11:299.
6. Pasini EM, Bohme U, Rutledge GG, Voorberg-Vander Wel A, Sanders M, Berriman M, et al. An improved *Plasmodium cynomolgi* genome assembly reveals an unexpected methyltransferase gene expansion. Wellcome Open Res. 2017;2:42.
7. Joyner C, Consortium TM, Wood JS, Moreno A, Garcia A, Galinski MR. Severe and complicated cynomolgi malaria in a Rhesus macaque resulted in similar histopathological changes as those seen in human malaria. Am J Trop Med Hyg. 2017;97:548–55.
8. Kosaisavee V, Suwanarusk R, Chua ACY, Kyle DE, Malleret B, Zhang R, et al. Strict tropism for cd71(+)/cd234(+) human reticulocytes limits the zoonotic potential of *Plasmodium cynomolgi*. Blood. 2017;130:1357–63.
9. Imwong M, Madmanee W, Suwannasin K, Kunasol C, Peto TJ, Tripura R, et al. Asymptomatic natural human infections with the simian malaria parasites *Plasmodium cynomolgi* and *Plasmodium knowlesi*. J Infect Dis. 2018;1:1. https://doi.org/10.1093/infdis/jiy519 **(Epub ahead of print)**.
10. Medica DL, Sinnis P. Quantitative dynamics of *Plasmodium yoelii* sporozoite transmission by infected anopheline mosquitoes. Infect Immun. 2005;73:4363–9.
11. Ponnudurai T, Lensen AH, van Gemert GJ, Bolmer MG, Meuwissen JH. Feeding behaviour and sporozoite ejection by infected *Anopheles stephensi*. Trans R Soc Trop Med Hyg. 1991;85:175–80.
12. Prudencio M, Rodriguez A, Mota MM. The silent path to thousands of merozoites: the *Plasmodium* liver stage. Nat Rev Microbiol. 2006;4:849–56.
13. Vaughan AM, Aly AS, Kappe SH. Malaria parasite pre-erythrocytic stage infection: gliding and hiding. Cell Host Microbe. 2008;4:209–18.
14. Joyner C, Barnwell JW, Galinski MR. No more monkeying around: primate malaria model systems are key to understanding *Plasmodium vivax* liverstage biology, hypnozoites, and relapses. Front Microbiol. 2015;6:145.
15. Krotoski WA, Collins WE, Bray RS, Garnham PC, Cogswell FB, Gwadz RW, et al. Demonstration of hypnozoites in sporozoite-transmitted *Plasmodium vivax* infection. Am J Trop Med Hyg. 1982;31:1291–3.
16. White NJ. Determinants of relapse periodicity in *Plasmodium vivax* malaria. Malar J. 2011;10:297.
17. Joyner C, Moreno A, Meyer EV, Cabrera-Mora M, Ma HC, Kissinger JC, et al. *Plasmodium cynomolgi* infections in Rhesus macaques display clinical and parasitological features pertinent to modelling *vivax* malaria pathology and relapse infections. Malar J. 2016;15:451.
18. Coatney GR, Allergy NIO. Diseases I: the primate malarias. Washington: U.S. National Institute of Allergy and Infectious Diseases; 1971.
19. Murphy GS, Oldfield EC. Falciparum malaria. Infect Dis Clin North Am. 1996;10:747–75.
20. Genton B, D'Acremont V. Clinical features of malaria in returning travelers and migrants. Decker: Travelers' malaria Hamilton; 2001. p. 371–92.
21. Rahimi BA, Thakkinstian A, White NJ, Sirivichayakul C, Dondorp AM, Chokejindachai W. Severe vivax malaria: a systematic review and meta-analysis of clinical studies since 1900. Malar J. 2014;13:481.
22. WHO. Severe falciparum malaria. Trans R Soc Trop Med Hyg. 2000;94:S190.

23. WHO. Severe malaria. Trop Med Int Health. 2014;19:7–131.
24. Russell BM, Cooke BM. The rheopathobiology of *Plasmodium vivax* and other important primate malaria parasites. Trends Parasitol. 2017;33:321–34.
25. Warren M, Skinner JC, Guinn E. Biology of the simian malarias of southeast Asia. I. Host cell preferences of young trophozoites of four species of *Plasmodium*. J Parasitol. 1966;52:14–6.
26. Akinyi S, Hanssen E, Meyer EVS, Jiang J, Korir CC, Singh B, et al. A 95 kDa protein of *Plasmodium vivax* and *P. cynomolgi* visualized by three-dimensional tomography in the caveola vesicle complexes (Schüffner's dots) of infected erythrocytes is a member of the phist family. Mol Microbiol. 2012;84:816–31.
27. Aikawa M, Miller LH, Rabbege J. Caveola–vesicle complexes in the plasmalemma of erythrocytes infected by *Plasmodium vivax* and *P. cynomolgi*. Unique structures related to Schüffner's dots. Am J Pathol. 1975;79:285–300.
28. Mideo N, Day T, Read AF. Modelling malaria pathogenesis. Cell Microbiol. 2008;10:1947–55.
29. Khoury DS, Aogo R, Randriafanomezantsoa-Radohery G, McCaw JM, Simpson JA, McCarthy JS, et al. Within-host modeling of blood-stage malaria. Immunol Rev. 2018;285:168–93.
30. Anderson RM, May RM, Gupta S. Non-linear phenomena in host—parasite interactions. Parasitology. 1989;99:S59–79.
31. Hetzel C, Anderson RM. The within-host cellular dynamics of blood-stage malaria: theoretical and experimental studies. Parasitology. 1996;113:25–38.
32. Johnson PLF, Kochin BF, Ahmed R, Antia R. How do antigenically varying pathogens avoid cross-reactive responses to invariant antigens? Proc R Soc Lond B Biol Sci. 2012;279:2777–85.
33. Mcqueen PG, Mckenzie FE. Competition for red blood cells can enhance *Plasmodium vivax* parasitemia in mixed-species malaria infections. Am J Trop Med Hyg. 2006;75:112–25.
34. Fonseca LL, Voit EO. Comparison of mathematical frameworks for modeling erythropoiesis in the context of malaria infection. Math Biosci. 2015;270:224–36.
35. Access data from mahpic—the malaria host-pathogen interaction center. http://plasmodb.org/plasmo/mahpic.jsp.
36. Tang Y, Joyner CJ, Cabrera-Mora M, Saney CL, Lapp SA, Nural MV, et al. Integrative analysis associates monocytes with insufficient erythropoiesis during acute *Plasmodium cynomolgi* malaria in Rhesus macaques. Malar J. 2017;16:384.
37. Schirm S, Engel C, Loeffler M, Scholz M. A biomathematical model of human erythropoiesis under erythropoietin and chemotherapy administration. PLoS ONE. 2013;8:1–17.
38. Fonseca LL, Alezi HS, Moreno A, Barnwell JW, Galinski MR, Voit EO. Quantifying the removal of red blood cells in *Plasmodium coatneyi* infection. Malar J. 2016;15:1.
39. Moreno A, Cabrera-Mora M, Garcia A, Orkin J, Strobert E, Barnwell JW, et al. *Plasmodium coatneyi* in Rhesus macaques replicates the multisystemic dysfunction of severe malaria in humans. Infect Immun. 2013;81:1889–904.
40. Dasari P, Fries A, Heber SD, Salama A, Blau I-W, Lingelbach K, et al. Malarial anemia: digestive vacuole of *Plasmodium falciparum* mediates complement deposition on bystander cells to provoke hemophagocytosis. Med Microbiol Immunol. 2014;203:383–93.

41. Jakeman GN, Saul A, Hogarth WL, Collins WE. Anaemia of acute malaria infections in non-immune patients primarily results from destruction of uninfected erythrocytes. Parasitology. 1999;119:127–33.
42. Lichtman M, Beutler E, Kipps T, Seligsohn U, Kaushansky K, Prchal J. Williams hematology. 8th ed. New York: McGraw-Hill Education; 2010.
43. Lee KJ, Yin W, Arafat D, Tang Y, Uppal K, Tran V, et al. Comparative transcriptomics and metabolomics in a Rhesus macaque drug administration study. Front Cell Dev Biol. 2014;2:54.
44. Fonseca LL, Joyner CJ, Consortium M, Galinski MR, Voit EO. A model of *Plasmodium vivax* concealment based on *Plasmodium cynomolgi* infections in *Macaca mulatta*. Malar J. 2017;16:375.
45. Langhorne J, Buffet P, Galinski M, Good M, Harty J, Leroy D, et al. The relevance of non-human primate and rodent malaria models for humans. Malar J. 2011;10:23.
46. Ng S, March S, Galstian A, Gural N, Stevens KR, Mota MM, et al. Towards a humanized mouse model of liver stage malaria using ectopic artificial livers. Sci Rep. 2017;7:45424.
47. Vallender EJ, Miller GM. Nonhuman primate models in the genomic era: a paradigm shift. ILAR J. 2013;54:154–65.
48. Antia R, Yates A, Roode JCD. The dynamics of acute malaria infections. I. Effect of the parasite's red blood cell preference. Proc R Soc Lond B Biol Sci. 2008;275:1449–58.
49. Mcqueen PG, Mckenzie FE. Age-structured red blood cell susceptibility and the dynamics of malaria infections. Proc Natl Acad Sci USA. 2004;101:9161–6.
50. Kaushansky K, Lichtman MA, Beutler E, Kipps TJ, Seligsohn U, Prchal JT. Williams hematology. 4th ed. New York: McGraw-Hill Medical; 2011.
51. Skadberg O, Brun A, Sandberg S. Human reticulocytes isolated from peripheral blood: maturation time and hemoglobin synthesis. Lab Hematol. 2003;9:198–206.
52. Brugnara C. Use of reticulocyte cellular indices in the diagnosis and treatment of hematological disorders. Int J Clin Lab Res. 1998;28:1–11.
53. Craik R. The erythrocytes in malaria. Lancet. 1920;198:1110.
54. Sutton PL, Luo Z, Divis PCS, Friedrich VK, Conway DJ, Singh B, et al. Characterizing the genetic diversity of the monkey malaria parasite *Plasmodium cynomolgi*. Infect Genet Evol. 2016;40:243–52.
55. Cromer D, Evans KJ, Schofield L, Davenport MP. Preferential invasion of reticulocytes during late-stage *Plasmodium berghei* infection accounts for reduced circulating reticulocyte levels. Int J Parasitol. 2006;36:1389–97.
56. Thakre N, Fernandes P, Mueller A-K, Graw F. Characterizing malaria blood-stage infection patterns of two *Plasmodium* parasite strains. Front Microbiol. 2017;00:00.
57. Collins WE, Jeffery GM, Roberts JM. A retrospective examination of anemia during infection of humans with *Plasmodium vivax*. Am J Trop Med Hyg. 2003;68:410–2.
58. Price RN, Simpson JA, Nosten F, Luxemburger C, Hkirjaroen L, ter Kuile F, et al. Factors contributing to anemia after uncomplicated falciparum malaria. Am J Trop Med Hyg. 2001;65:614–22.
59. Handayani S, Chiu DT, Tjitra E, Kuo JS, Lampah D, Kenangalem E, et al. High deformability of *Plasmodium vivax*-infected red blood cells under microfluidic conditions. J Infect Dis. 2009;199:445–50.
60. Paul A, Padmapriya P, Natarajan V. Diagnosis of malarial infection using change in properties of optically trapped red blood cells. Biomed J. 2017;40:101–5.

13

Detection of foci of residual malaria transmission through reactive case detection

Endalew Zemene[1]*, Cristian Koepfli[2], Abebaw Tiruneh[1], Asnakew K. Yeshiwondim[3], Dinberu Seyoum[4], Ming-Chieh Lee[2], Guiyun Yan[2†] and Delenasaw Yewhalaw[1,5†]

Abstract

Background: Sub-microscopic and asymptomatic infections could be bottlenecks to malaria elimination efforts in Ethiopia. This study determined the prevalence of malaria, and individual and household-level factors associated with *Plasmodium* infections obtained following detection of index cases in health facilities in Jimma Zone.

Methods: Index malaria cases were passively detected and tracked in health facilities from June to November 2016. Moreover, family members of the index houses and neighbours located within approximately 200 m from the index houses were also screened for malaria.

Results: A total of 39 index cases initiated the reactive case detection of 726 individuals in 116 households. Overall, the prevalence of malaria using microscopy and PCR was 4.0% and 8.96%, respectively. Seventeen (43.6%) of the index cases were from Doyo Yaya *kebele*, where parasite prevalence was higher. The majority of the malaria cases (90.74%) were asymptomatic. Fever (AOR = 12.68, 95% CI 3.34–48.18) and history of malaria in the preceding 1 year (AOR = 3.62, 95% CI 1.77–7.38) were significant individual-level factors associated with detection of *Plasmodium* infection. Moreover, living in index house (AOR = 2.22, 95% CI 1.16–4.27), house with eave (AOR = 2.28, 95% CI 1.14–4.55), area of residence (AOR = 6.81, 95% CI 2.49–18.63) and family size (AOR = 3.35, 95% CI 1.53–7.33) were main household-level predictors for residual malaria transmission.

Conclusion: The number of index cases per *kebele* may enhance RACD efforts to detect additional malaria cases in low transmission settings. Asymptomatic and sub-microscopic infections were high in the study area, which need new or improved surveillance tools for malaria elimination efforts.

Keywords: Reactive case detection, Malaria, Residual malaria transmission, Low-transmission setting, Ethiopia

Background

The global pattern of malaria epidemiology has changed remarkably over the last decade. Between 2010 and 2015, malaria mortality rates declined by 35% among children under 5 years of age, with 21% fall in incidence among the population at risk [1]. Implementation of key malaria prevention and control measures have played a pivotal role in decreasing morbidity and mortality due to malaria [2, 3]. Furthermore, concerted control and elimination efforts of malaria in some countries, such as the United Arab Emirates and Sri Lanka, have resulted in malaria-free status in recent years [4, 5]. Despite the achievements gained in the control of malaria, the disease still remains a significant public health problem in many sub-Saharan African countries, including Ethiopia.

The epidemiology of malaria in Ethiopia appears unique, compared to other countries in sub-Saharan Africa, in that both *Plasmodium falciparum* and *Plasmodium vivax* coexist. While almost all cases of malaria are due to the two species, there is high spatiotemporal heterogeneity in the distribution of these parasite species.

*Correspondence: endalew2005@yahoo.com
†Guiyun Yan and Delenasaw Yewhalaw contributed equally to this work
[1] School of Medical Laboratory Sciences, Faculty of Health Sciences, Jimma University, Jimma, Ethiopia
Full list of author information is available at the end of the article

According to the 2015 National Health Sector Development Plan report [6], out of the total microscopy or rapid diagnostic test (RDT) confirmed malaria cases, 63.7% and 36.3% were due to *P. falciparum* and *P. vivax*, respectively. In a recent study done in Jimma in south-western Ethiopia, however, more than three-quarters of the cases were due to *P. vivax* [7]. *Plasmodium ovale* plays a minor role in Ethiopia, and appears to be often misdiagnosed [8].

Over the last decade, during which malaria elimination was put back on the global health agenda, morbidity and mortality due to malaria has remarkably declined in Ethiopia [9, 10]. Besides the sharp decline of malaria including from some of the historically malarious areas of the country [11], no major malaria epidemics, which usually recur every 5- to 8 years, have been reported since 2005 [12]. Implementation and scale-up of the powerful vector control interventions, including indoor residual spraying (IRS) and long-lasting insecticidal nets (LLINs) appear to have played key roles [13]. More than 17 million LLINs have been distributed in 2014/2015 alone, with cumulative number of the nets distributed since 2009 being scaled up to more than 75 million [6]. Access to malaria diagnostics and treatment has also remarkably improved over the last decade, mainly via the innovative health extension programme [14] that operates at community level.

Based on the malaria control achievements gained, and with the help of international partners, Ethiopia has set goals to eliminate malaria by 2030. However, substantial portions of human *Plasmodium* infections are asymptomatic, often remaining undetected by microscopic examination [15]. Asymptomatic infections can serve as reservoirs of infection to the vector mosquitoes [16], potentially sustaining transmission.

To further sustain control of malaria and move towards elimination, adequate detection and prompt treatment of both symptomatic and asymptomatic cases in the community is critical [17]. One of the strategies of addressing malaria cases not presenting to the health care facilities is reactive case detection (RACD) with focal test and treatment methods. Reactive case detection makes use of the spatial clustering trend of malaria carriers particularly in low endemic settings [18, 19]. Hence, in RACD, following passive case detection, household members of the index case and neighbours located at certain distance from the index household are screened. This method has been utilized in several low malaria transmission settings [20, 21], despite lack of established standard approach to the spatial range of neighbouring households to be within the screening radius.

Reactive case detection also allows detection of asymptomatic malaria infections, which play a major role in sustaining malaria transmission in low-transmission settings [22]. However, active case detection of malaria is not yet fully implemented in the routine health care system in Ethiopia. Thus, this study is aimed at detecting malaria cases using RACD in two health centres in Jimma Zone, south-western Ethiopia.

Methods

Study setting

The study was conducted in catchment *kebeles* (smallest government administrative units in Ethiopia) of Kishe and Nada health centres, located in Shebe Sambo and Omo Nada districts of Jimma Zone, respectively (Fig. 1). Shebe Sambo and Omo Nada districts are located at 415 and 285 kms south west of the capital, Addis Ababa, respectively. The geographical coordinates of Shebe Sambo and Omo Nada are approximately 7°30′14″N, 36°30′44″E and 7°38′00″N, 37°15′05″E, respectively. The inhabitants in both areas mainly depend on subsistence farming, cultivating mainly maize and *teff*. Moreover, in Kishe area rice is cultivated in small scale.

Historically, the catchment areas of both health centres have been malarious [23–25]. As in most parts of Ethiopia, the transmission of malaria in these areas is seasonal. The transmission usually peaks from September to October, following the major rains from June to September, and minor transmission occurs in April and May, following the short rains of February to March. According to the information obtained from both health centres, malaria cases detected in the health facilities have remarkably declined in recent years. A total 43 malaria cases have been registered in Kishe Health Centre in 2016. Of these, 62.8% were due to *P. falciparum*. Kishe Health Centre has been serving a total of 26,843 population in 2016. In the same year, a total of 51 malaria cases were recorded at Nada Health Centre, 49% of which were due to *P. falciparum*. The health centre has been serving a total of 32,264 population in 2016.

Population and sampling

A prospective observational study was conducted for 6 months (June to November 2016) in two health centres and their catchment *kebeles*. Index malaria cases residing within the catchment *kebeles* of the two health centres who did not travel within 2 weeks prior to presenting to the health centres, and diagnosed with malaria at the health centres during the study period were included in the study. The index cases were identified in the health centres based on the routine blood film microscopy by the laboratory staff at each health facility. Following detection of the index cases, household members of the index houses and neighbours within 200 m radius were included in the study.

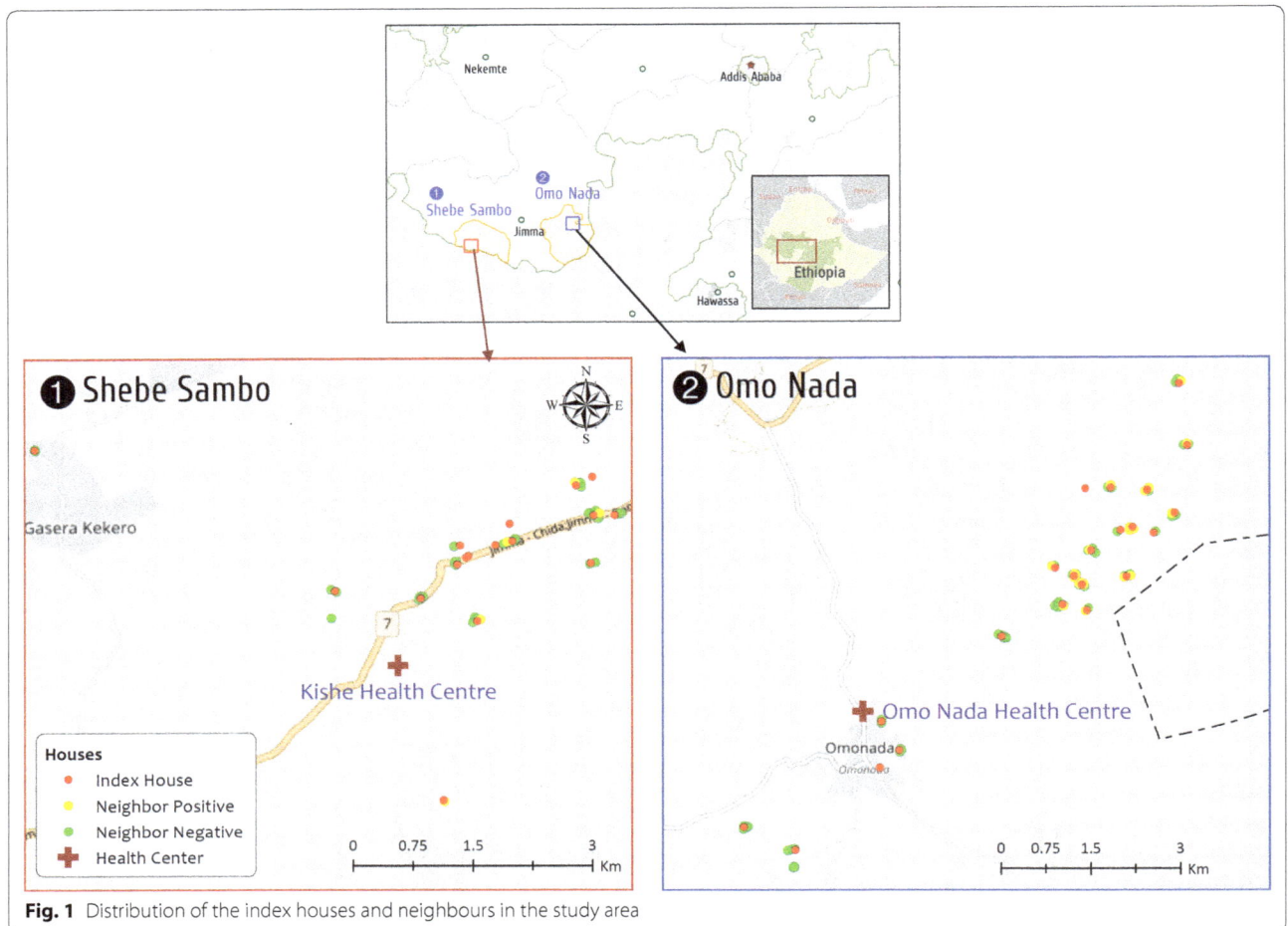

Fig. 1 Distribution of the index houses and neighbours in the study area

Data collection

Passive case detection

Febrile patients who sought treatment at Kishe and Nada Health Centres from June 1 to November 31, 2016, were screened for malaria using microscopy by the resident laboratory personnel as a routine practice. Consenting index cases that were microscopy-positive and who agreed that a research team will visit them within 1 week provided their home address. To locate the index household easily, names of three nearby household heads were also recorded.

Reactive case detection

Presence of index cases was communicated to the research team on the same day of presentation to the health centres. The index houses and neighbours were visited within 1 week of detecting the index cases, in most cases, within 3 days. After obtaining consent, family members of the index houses and neighbours within 200 m radius from the index houses were screened for *Plasmodium* infection using RDT. Moreover,

demographic information and some individual and household-level risk factors of malaria were collected using a semi-structured questionnaire. The field data was collected by experienced laboratory technologists.

The individual-level factors assessed included demographic characteristics (age, sex, educational status and occupation), recent travel history, history of malaria infection in the last 1 year, LLIN usage the previous night before the survey and axillary body temperature. Fever was defined in this study as having axillary temperature of ≥ 37.5 °C, which was measured during the survey. The household-level factors assessed included housing conditions such as roof structure, presence of visible hole on the wall, presence of eave and presence of window(s), and presence of animals within the house, family size, total number of LLINs owned during the survey and whether the house was sprayed with insecticide during the last 1 year. In Ethiopia, indoor residual spraying is performed once in a year, usually around July to September (before malaria cases peak) as transmission is mainly seasonal. Apart from the household-level characteristics, an approximate distance of each house from the index house was estimated, and coordinates of each house was taken using hand-held global positioning system unit (GPS).

All consenting members of the index houses and neighbours were enrolled in this study. Infants less than 6 months of age were not included, with the assumption that they are likely protected from malaria due to passively acquired maternal antibody, and presence of foetal haemoglobin. The household members available during the visit and those found in the nearby farming sites were included in the study. The samples were collected by a team of two laboratory technologists deployed at a time. The data collection team spent, in most cases, all the day around the index houses to maximize coverage of the screened population. However, few individuals who were not available on the day of screening around their houses were not captured, as there was no follow-up to the community members.

Specimen collection and laboratory processing

Finger-prick blood samples were collected from consenting study participants for blood examination by RDT and microscopy. The RDT was done for rapid diagnosis and treatment; hence, RDT-positive individuals were referred to the health centres for confirmation and treatment. Moreover, thick and thin blood smears were prepared for each study participant in the field. After air drying, the thin films were fixed with absolute methanol, and Giemsa stained at Jimma University Medical Parasitology Laboratory on the same day of collection. The slides were examined by two experienced laboratory technologists independently. Approximately 200 high-power fields of the thick blood smears were examined before declaring a microscopy-negative result. The personnel reading the slides were also blinded of the RDT results. Apart from the blood smears, three to four drops of blood were spotted on Whatman 3MM filter paper for further molecular analysis. The blood spots were air-dried and kept individually in air-tight plastic bags and stored at − 20 °C until DNA extraction.

DNA was extracted from approximately 20 μL whole blood using the QiaCube DNA extraction system as per standard protocols. DNA was eluted in 100 μL buffer, and 4 μL DNA was screened using a multiplex *P. falciparum/P. vivax* qPCR with limit of detection of 1 DNA copy per reaction [26]. Thus, the limit of detection of the qPCR was 1–2 parasites/μL blood.

Data management and analysis

Household was defined in this study as group of human subjects residing in the same house as family members. Household access to LLINs was considered "sufficient" when the ratio of the total LLINs owned by a household

to the family members is at least 0.5 (assuming that one LLIN covers two individuals), and "not sufficient" when the ratio is less than 0.5 [27]. While a total of 726 individuals participated in this study providing samples for microscopic examination, sufficient DBS sample for PCR was obtained from 603 individuals. Specimens of sufficient quantity could not be obtained from the remaining individuals for PCR following blood film preparation and RDT testing, the results of which were used for immediate care. Hence, the data analysis was based on the PCR-run samples. Asymptomatic malaria infection was considered when an individual who did not experience fever at the time of the survey (axillary body temperature is less than 37.5 °C) and no malaria-related symptoms was positive for *Plasmodium* species by PCR.

The collected data were coded, entered into Excel (Microsoft Office 2010) and cleaned. The data were analysed using a statistical software package STATA 12 (StataCorp., TX, USA). Descriptive statistics including frequency, percentages and median were calculated to summarize demographic profile of the study participants. Univariate and multivariate logistic regressions were employed to determine individual and household-level factors associated with malaria infection. Multi-level regression model (mixed-effects logistic regression) was utilized to determine predictors of malaria infection among individual and household-level variables. Variables with significant association with malaria infection by the univariate analysis and those with *p* values less than 0.2 were candidates for the multivariate analyses. Odds ratio and the corresponding 95% confidence intervals were calculated to show the strength of the association. Statistical significance was set at $p < 0.05$ during the analysis.

Results

Socio-demographic characteristics

Thirty-nine passively detected microscopy-positive malaria cases (index cases) initiated the RACD. Most of the index cases (56.4%, n = 22) were from Nada Health Centre, with the remaining 17 (43.6%) being from Kishe Health Centre. Twenty-four (61.5%) and 15 (38.5%) of the index cases were due to *P. falciparum* and *P. vivax* infections, respectively. Following detection of the index cases, a total of 726 individuals residing in 116 households were screened for *Plasmodium* infection. Most of them were female (55.6%, n = 404), and the median age was 16 years (range 1 to 80 years). Demographic characteristics of the study participants are presented in Table 1.

Table 1 Demographic characteristics of the study participants

Characteristics	Frequency, n (%)
Age group in years	
<5	144 (19.8)
5–15	221 (30.4)
>15	361 (49.7)
Sex	
Male	322 (44.4)
Female	404 (55.6)
Site	
Kishe	220 (30.30)
Nada	506 (69.69)
Educational status	
Illiterate	235 (42.6)
Literate	316 (57.4)
Occupation	
Farmers	155 (21.4)
Housewives	143 (19.7)
Students	214 (29.5)
Others	38 (5.2)
House structure	
Iron sheet	496 (68.3)
Thatched	230 (31.7)
Spray status of the house	
Not sprayed	417 (57.4)
Sprayed	309 (42.6)

Prevalence of malaria

The overall prevalence of malaria from the RACD by microscopy and PCR was 4.0% (29/726) and 8.96% (54/603), respectively. Majority of the PCR-detected cases (92.59%, n = 50) were *P. falciparum*, the remaining 4 (7.41%) being *P. vivax*. The prevalence of malaria among individuals residing in the index houses and neighbours was 17.5% and 6.83%, respectively. The majority (90.74%, n = 49) of malaria cases detected in the RACD were asymptomatic. A relatively larger number of the malaria cases were detected in Doyo Yaya *kebele* (Table 2).

Factors associated with *Plasmodium* infection

Bivariate analysis of individual and household-level factors associated with malaria positivity is shown in Table 3. The analysis revealed that several individual-level factors were significantly associated with *Plasmodium* infection, including age (COR = 1.99, 95% CI 1.06–3.74), self-reported history of malaria infection in the last 1 year before the survey (COR = 3.71, 95% CI 1.94–7.07) and fever (COR = 6.12, 95% CI 1.97–18.98). The study participants were asked if they travelled to other villages in the preceding 2 weeks before the survey. Only 3 (0.5%) reported travel and none of them were positive.

Among the household-level factors assessed in this study, IRS (COR = 6.86, 95% CI 2.69–17.48), living within index house (COR = 2.89, 95% CI 1.60–5.21), area of residence (COR = 6.70, 95% CI 2.63–17.08) and family size (COR = 3.73, 95% CI 1.88–7.38) were significant risk factors of malaria.

Long-lasting insecticidal nets ownership (proportion of households who reported to have at least one LLIN) was 90.9%, but 56.82% of the households having insufficient LLINs. Bivariate analysis showed that individuals living in households with insufficient access to LLINs were at higher risk of *Plasmodium* infection (COR = 2.35, 95% CI 1.18–4.65).

Table 4 shows predictors of *Plasmodium* infection. After adjusting for other variables, fever (AOR = 10.13, 95% CI 2.76–37.16) and history of malaria (AOR = 3.97, 95% CI 1.96–8.04) were the main individual-level predictors of *Plasmodium* infection. Moreover, household-level

Table 2 Residence of the index cases and frequency of individuals screened following the index cases, Jimma, southwestern Ethiopia

Health facility	Kebele	Index cases, n (%)	Examined by PCR, n (%)	Ratio of # screened to index cases	Additional RACD cases, n (%)
Kishe Health Centre	Kishe	7 (17.9)	59 (9.8)	8.4	1 (1.7)
	Halo Sebaka	7 (17.9)	91 (15.1)	13.0	4 (4.1)
	Gasera Kekero	1 (2.6)	6 (1.0)	6.0	0 (0)
	Wala Kela	1 (2.6)	7 (1.2)	7.0	0 (0)
Omo Nada Health Centre	Doyo Yaya	17 (43.6)	375 (62.2)	22.1	49 (13.1)
	Nada	4 (10.3)	18 (3.0)	4.5	0 (0)
	Nada Chala	1 (2.6)	24 (4.0)	24.0	0 (0)
	Nada Sekote	1 (2.6)	23 (3.8)	23.0	0 (0)
Total		39 (100)	603 (100)	15.5	54 (8.96)

Table 3 Bivariate analysis results showing individual and household-level factors associated with *Plasmodium* infection among the study participants, Jimma, south-western Ethiopia

Variables	Examined by PCR, n (%)	Positive, n (%)	p-value	COR (95% CI)
Age (years)				
<5	117 (19.40)	11 (9.40)	0.336	1.46 (0.68–3.14)
5–15	185 (30.68)	23 (12.43)	0.032	1.99 (1.06–3.74)*
>15	301 (49.92)	20 (6.64)	Ref	
Sex				
Male	270 (44.78)	24 (8.89)	Ref	
Female	333 (55.22)	30 (9.01)	0.959	1.01 (0.58–1.78)
Malaria in the preceding 1 year				
Yes	72 (11.94)	16 (22.22)	0.001	3.71 (1.94–7.07)*
No	531 (88.06)	38 (7.16)	Ref	
Fever at the time of survey				
Yes	14 (2.32)	5 (35.71)	0.002	6.12 (1.97–18.98)*
No	589 (97.68)	49 (8.32)	Ref	
ITN usage the preceding night				
Yes	243 (40.30)	18 (7.41)	Ref	
No	360 (59.70)	36 (10.00)	0.276	1.39 (0.77–2.51)
Roof structure				
Iron sheet	398 (66.00)	32 (8.04)	Ref	
Thatched	205 (34.00)	22 (10.73)	0.274	1.38 (0.78–2.43)
Visible hole on house wall				
No	418 (69.32)	36 (8.61)	Ref	
Yes	185 (30.68)	18 (9.73)	0.658	1.14 (0.63–2.07)
Presence of window				
No	210 (34.83)	16 (7.62)	Ref	
Yes	393 (65.17)	38 (9.67)	0.402	1.30 (0.71–2.39)
Eave gap				
Absent	450 (74.63)	37 (8.22)	Ref	
Present	153 (25.37)	17 (11.11)	0.281	1.40 (0.76–2.56)
Area of residence				
Doyo Yaya	375 (62.19)	49 (13.07)	0.001	6.70 (2.63–17.08)*
Others**	228 (37.81)	5 (2.19)	Ref	
Spray status of the structure				
Not sprayed	372 (61.69)	49 (13.17)	0.001	6.86 (2.69–17.48)*
Sprayed	231 (38.31)	5 (2.16)	Ref	
Animals sleeping in the house				
No	291 (48.26)	25 (8.59)	Ref	
Yes	312 (51.74)	29 (9.29)	0.762	1.09 (0.62–1.91)
Individual residing in				
Index house	120 (19.90)	21 (17.50)	0.001	2.89 (1.60–5.21)*
Neighbour	483 (80.10)	33 (6.83)	Ref	

Table 3 (continued)

Variables	Examined by PCR, n (%)	Positive, n (%)	p-value	COR (95% CI)
Plasmodium species of the index house				
P. vivax	197 (32.67)	9 (4.57)	Ref	
P. falciparum	406 (67.33)	45 (11.08)	0.011	2.60 (1.25–5.44)*
Family size				
Less than five	279 (46.27)	11 (3.94)	Ref	
Five or more	324 (53.73)	43 (13.27)	0.001	3.73 (1.88–7.38)*
Access to ITN				
Sufficient	217 (35.99)	11 (5.07)	Ref	
Not sufficient	386 (64.01)	43 (11.14)	0.015	2.35 (1.18–4.65)*

COR crude odds ratio, *ref* reference

* Significant at p < 0.05, ** includes all the remaining catchment *kebeles* of the selected health centres

Table 4 Results of mixed-effects logistic regression analysis of individual and household-level factors showing main predictors of *Plasmodium* infection, Jimma, south-western Ethiopia

Characteristics	Examined by PCR, n (%)	Positive, n (%)	AOR (95% CI)	p-value
Fever at the time of survey				
Yes	14 (2.32)	5 (35.71)	12.68 (3.34–48.18)	0.001*
No	589 (97.68)	49 (8.32)	Ref	
Malaria history in the preceding 1 year				
Yes	72 (11.94)	16 (22.22)	3.62 (1.77–7.38)	0.001*
No	531 (88.06)	38 (7.16)	Ref	
Area of residence				
Doyo Yaya	375 (62.19)	49 (13.07)	6.81 (2.49–18.63)	0.001*
Others**	228 (37.81)	5 (2.19)		
Individual residing in				
Index house	120 (19.90)	21 (17.50)	2.22 (1.16–4.27)	0.016*
Neighbour	483 (80.10)	33 (6.83)	Ref	
Family size				
<5	279 (46.27)	11 (3.94)	Ref	
≥5	324 (53.73)	43 (13.27)	3.35 (1.53–7.33)	0.003*
Eave				
Absent	450 (74.63)	37 (8.22)	Ref	
Present	153 (25.37)	17 (11.11)	2.28 (1.14–4.55)	0.020*

AOR adjusted odds ratio

* Significant at p < 0.05 ** includes all the remaining catchment *kebeles* of the selected health centres

predictors of *Plasmodium* infection include area of residence (AOR = 6.81, 95% CI 2.49–18.63), living in index house (AOR = 2.22, 95% CI 1.16–4.27), eaves (AOR = 2.28, 95% CI 1.14–4.55) and family size (AOR = 3.35, 95% CI 1.53–7.33).

Discussion

This study revealed that index cases presenting to health facilities enabled detection of good number of additional asymptomatic malaria in the community. Thus, screening of individuals using PCR following index malaria cases presenting to health facilities is a valuable method for detecting additional malaria cases in low transmission settings. However, it should be noted that PCR-based malaria detection techniques are largely restricted to research settings, and not currently in use by the National Malaria Control Programme in Ethiopia. This calls for evaluation of affordable alternative test methods with better sensitivity compared to microscopy to be utilised in elimination settings.

The overall prevalence of malaria detected using the RACD was 8.96%, more than 90% of the cases being due to *P. falciparum*. This is in contrast to the recent report from Jimma, in which less than a third of the malaria cases were due to *P. falciparum* [7], and the national report (63.7% of the documented malaria cases being caused by *P. falciparum*) [6]. There might be high spatio-temporal variation of *Plasmodium* species in a country, and even among villages within the same district, mainly due to difference in ecological, climatic and socio-economic factors, and interventions carried out to control malaria [28, 29]. Significant clustering of *Plasmodium* infection between *kebeles*, and households was observed in this study. The vast majority of cases were found in one of the eight *kebeles* included in this study, and individuals residing within the index house were at twofold higher risk of *Plasmodium* infections as compared to their neighbours. This has an important implication in prioritizing resources for targeted malaria control and elimination efforts in low transmission setting.

Apart from household-level clustering of the malaria cases, significantly higher prevalence of malaria was documented in Doyo Yaya *kebele* compared to other *kebeles*. Heterogeneity in transmission of malaria is a well-known feature [30]. It appears that the clustering of malaria in this *kebele* is likely due to presence of a village not covered in the preceding IRS operation. Indeed, most of the houses which did not receive IRS within the preceding 12 months of the survey were located in this *kebele*. Malaria control interventions in resource-limited areas should, therefore, target such hotspots that may contribute to sustained transmission, and possibly fuel epidemics in such settings. It is worth noting that screening of

malaria was limited to approximately 200 m from index houses in this study, and thus the overall prevalence in the population was not known. Several studies utilized different screening radii around the index houses, often detecting more cases within the index household and among those residing closer to the index houses [20, 31]. However, the optimum screening radius from the index house that should be included during RACD still remains unclear. It appears that the screening radius is mainly influenced by the local epidemiology of malaria and available resources to implement RACD [32].

Improved housing structure is essential in deterring endophagic/endophilic mosquitoes from reaching the occupants [33], thus possibly reducing vector-human contact. In this study, individuals residing in houses with open eaves were significantly more likely to succumb to malaria compared to those living in houses with closed eaves. Significantly higher odds of malaria in houses with open eaves was also reported previously [34, 35]. Earlier reports around the study area indicate that *Anopheles gambiae* sensu lato (presumably *Anopheles arabiensis*), the primary malaria vector in Ethiopia, to be predominantly endophagic [36], which may explain the observed higher prevalence of malaria in those living in houses with open eaves. Significantly higher number of indoor-resting malaria vectors were also observed in houses with open eaves in a previous study from central Ethiopia [37].

The vast majority of the malaria cases detected in this study were asymptomatic, most of which were sub-microscopic. Reports also show that in low-transmission settings, asymptomatic infections are common and most of the asymptomatic infections are sub-microscopic [22, 38]. As asymptomatic malaria carriers apparently do not seek treatment, they may serve as reservoirs of infection [39], jeopardizing elimination efforts. The challenges asymptomatic malaria infections pose to the malaria elimination efforts is also exacerbated by the diagnostic limitations in detecting the infections [40]. In very low transmission settings, sub-microscopic carriers may contribute up to 50% of human-to-mosquito transmissions [41]. Apart from the possible contribution to onward transmission, persistent asymptomatic infections may be associated with other deleterious health outcomes, such as anaemia [42].

In the current study, it was also found that self-reported history of malaria in the preceding 1 year before the survey was significantly associated with *Plasmodium* infection, after adjusting for the other variables. Individuals with history of malaria were more than three times likely to have *Plasmodium* infection. Relapse with vivax malaria is well known, hence, vivax cases could be due to relapse, even if small number of *P. vivax* cases were detected. It could also be attributed to persistent *P. falciparum* asymptomatic infections. The duration of persistence of asymptomatic *P. falciparum* parasitaemia is debatable. A recent report from Cambodia shows limited duration of asymptomatic *P. falciparum* parasitaemia in low transmission setting [43], while cases of asymptomatic falciparum malaria persisting more than a decade have been documented elsewhere [44].

In this study, PCR detected 2.2-fold higher *Plasmodium* infection as compared to microscopy. This difference is comparable with other previous studies [22, 45]. As the current routine malaria diagnostic protocol in health facilities in Ethiopia involve blood film microscopy, it is inevitable that sub-microscopic infections remain a huge challenge to the envisaged malaria elimination efforts. Thus, alternative field-friendly and more sensitive diagnostic tools such as highly sensitive RDTs (HS-RDTs) or loop-mediated isothermal amplification (LAMP) need to be evaluated and used for detection of sub-microscopic/asymptomatic malaria.

The difference in the prevalence of malaria was not significantly different among different age groups and between sexes. However, family size was a one of the main predictors. In households with five or more occupants, the risk of infection was threefold, compared to those living in families with fewer than five family members. This could be due to higher number of anopheline mosquitoes related with increased number of household occupants [46].

Long-lasting insecticidal nets were the only personal protection tools utilized by the study participants. However, the difference in prevalence of malaria among households with sufficient number of LLINs was not significant. Similarly, there was no significant difference in LLIN usage the preceding night on malaria risk. These could perhaps be due to poor integrity of the LLINs, rendering only partial protection from mosquito bite, and/or possibly inaccurate information provided on the number of nets owned and their usage. The apparent lack of association of sufficient ownership or usage of the LLINs and *Plasmodium* infection could also be related with biting activity of the anopheline mosquitoes in the area. It was reported in a neighbouring district that the peak biting time of *An. gambiae* s.l. was at the early part of the night, before 21:00 h [47], during which most of the inhabitants likely do not sleep. As the LLIN coverage was high in this study, it may have 'herd effect', in that, those not utilizing the nets may be protected as a result of usage of the rest [48].

Sustained residual transmission of malaria in the areas necessitates assessing vector behavioural characteristics and human activities that may contribute to the on-going transmission. As LLINs and IRS interventions target vectors which feed and rest indoors, malaria elimination using these interventions alone may not be achieved [49]. Outdoor biting by the vectors as a result of long-term use of the vector control tools, and resistance to insecticides used in IRS and treating the LLINs may contribute to sustained low transmission of malaria [50, 51]. Moreover, night-time human activities may increase malaria risk [52].

The study has the following limitations: First, due to limitation of resources, the RACD was limited to catchment *kebeles* of the two health centres. Hence, passively detected malaria cases which resided out of the catchment of the two selected health centres were not included. Second, this study did not include index cases who might have visited private clinics. However, the areas being predominantly rural, it is expected that most of the residents visit the two public health facilities for treatment of fever. Finally, while this study allowed to identify high number of *Plasmodium* infections around the index cases from one site, no individuals living > 200 m from index case houses were screened for infection. Thus, it was not known how large this cluster of transmission was.

Conclusions

The study revealed that substantial number of malaria cases, largely asymptomatic, were detected using RACD. Reactive case detection strategies utilizing malaria diagnostic tools of high sensitivity, therefore, complement the routine passive case detection in low malaria transmission areas, and may be used in malaria elimination programme. Significant household and *kebele* level clustering of the malaria cases were observed. Moreover, history of malaria, houses with eaves and family size were risk factors to *Plasmodium* infection. Further studies incorporating greater distance from index households, and including environmental factors affecting risk of malaria infection are recommended.

Abbreviations
DBS: dried blood spot; DNA: deoxyribonucleic acid; ITNs: insecticide-treated nets; LLINs: long-lasting insecticide-treated nets; PCR: polymerase chain reaction; RACD: reactive case detection; RDT: rapid diagnostic test.

Authors' contributions
EZ and DY: Conceived and designed the study. AT and EZ involved in data collection. CK, AT, AKY, DS and ML involved in data analysis. EZ, CK, DY and GY drafted the manuscript. DY and GY critically reviewed the manuscript. All authors read and approved the final manuscript.

Author details
[1] School of Medical Laboratory Sciences, Faculty of Health Sciences, Jimma University, Jimma, Ethiopia. [2] Program in Public Health, College of Health Sciences, University of California at Irvine, Irvine, CA 92697, USA. [3] PATH/MACEPA, Addis Ababa, Ethiopia. [4] Department of Statistics, College of Natural Sciences, Jimma University, Jimma, Ethiopia. [5] Tropical and Infectious Diseases Research Centre, Jimma University, Jimma, Ethiopia.

Acknowledgements
We thank the study participants for taking part in the study, administration of the study *kebeles*, the two health centres and Jimma University for their support. We are also grateful to the laboratory staff of the health centres and Tropical and Infectious Diseases Research Center (TIDRC), Jimma University, who gave technical support in slide readings.

Competing interests
The authors declare that they have no competing interests.

Ethics approval and consent to participate
The study protocol was reviewed and approved by the Ethical Review Board (IRB) of College of Health Sciences, Jimma University (Ref No. RPGC/486/06). Permission was obtained from administration of the health facilities prior to data collection. The study participants were provided with full information about the purpose of the study, the specimens to be provided and the procedures followed, before enrolment into the study. Written consent was obtained from each study participant, and from parents/guardians in case of minors. Study participants found RDT-positive for malaria during the field work, and those with fever, regardless of the RDT results, were referred to either health centres for confirmation and treatment.

Funding
The study was supported by Grants from the National Institutes of Health (R01 AI050243, U19 AI129326 and D43 TW001505) and Jimma University. The funders had no role in the design of the study and collection, analysis, and interpretation of data and in writing the manuscript or decision to publish.

References
1. WHO. World Malaria Report 2016. Geneva: World Health Organization; 2016. http://www.who.int/malaria/media/world-malaria-report-2016/en/.
2. Cibulskis RE, Alonso P, Aponte J, Aregawi M, Barrette A, Bergeron L, et al. Malaria: global progress 2000–2015 and future challenges. Infect Dis Poverty. 2016;5:61.
3. Brown G, Rogerson S. Malaria: global challenges for malaria eradication. Microbiol Aust. 2016;37:34–8.
4. Meleigy M. The quest to be free of malaria. Bull World Health Organ. 2007;85:507–8.
5. Lucas G. Malaria-free Sri Lanka. Sri Lanka J Child Health. 2017;46:1–2.
6. FMOH. Health Sector Development Programme Annual Performance Report EFY 2007 (2014/15). Version 1. Addis Ababa: FMOH; 2015.
7. Zhou G, Yewhalaw D, Lo E, Zhong D, Wang X, Degefa T, et al. Analysis of asymptomatic and clinical malaria in urban and suburban settings of southwestern Ethiopia in the context of sustaining malaria control and approaching elimination. Malar J. 2016;15:250.
8. Alemu A, Fuehrer H-P, Getnet G, Tessema B, Noedl H. *Plasmodium ovale curtisi* and *Plasmodium ovale wallikeri* in North-West Ethiopia. Malar J. 2013;12:346.
9. Otten M, Aregawi M, Were W, Karema C, Medin A, Jima D, et al. Initial evidence of reduction of malaria cases and deaths in Rwanda and Ethiopia due to rapid scale-up of malaria prevention and treatment. Malar J. 2009;8:14.
10. Yimer F, Animut A, Erko B, Mamo H. Past five-year trend, current prevalence and household knowledge, attitude and practice of malaria in Abeshge, south-central Ethiopia. Malar J. 2015;14:230.
11. Toyama Y, Ota M, Molla G, Beyene BB. Sharp decline of malaria cases in the Burie Zuria, Dembia, and Mecha districts, Amhara Region, Ethiopia, 2012–2014: descriptive analysis of surveillance data. Malar J. 2016;15:104.
12. FMOH. Health Sector Transformation Plan 2015/16–2019/20. Addis Ababa: FMOH; 2015.
13. Abeku TA, Helinski ME, Kirby MJ, Kefyalew T, Awano T, Batisso E, et al. Monitoring changes in malaria epidemiology and effectiveness of interventions in Ethiopia and Uganda: beyond Garki Project baseline survey. Malar J. 2015;14:337.
14. PMI. Malaria operational plan FY 2017. Addis Ababa: PMI; 2017.
15. Golassa L, Enweji N, Erko B, Aseffa A, Swedberg G. Detection of a substantial number of sub-microscopic *Plasmodium falciparum* infections by polymerase chain reaction: a potential threat to malaria control and diagnosis in Ethiopia. Malar J. 2013;12:352.
16. Kiattibutr K, Roobsoong W, Sriwichai P, Saeseu T, Rachaphaew N, Suansomjit C, et al. Infectivity of symptomatic and asymptomatic *Plasmodium vivax* infections to a Southeast Asian vector, *Anopheles dirus*. Int J Parasitol. 2017;47:163–70.
17. Moonen B, Cohen JM, Snow RW, Slutsker L, Drakeley C, Smith DL, et al. Operational strategies to achieve and maintain malaria elimination. Lancet. 2010;376:1592–603.
18. Sluydts V, Heng S, Coosemans M, Van Roey K, Gryseels C, Canier L, et al. Spatial clustering and risk factors of malaria infections in Ratanakiri Province, Cambodia. Malar J. 2014;13:387.
19. Rulisa S, Kateera F, Bizimana JP, Agaba S, Dukuzumuremyi J, Baas L, et al. Malaria prevalence, spatial clustering and risk factors in a low endemic area of Eastern Rwanda: a cross sectional study. PLoS ONE. 2013;8:e69443.
20. Littrell M, Sow G, Ngom A, Ba M, Mboup B, Dieye Y, et al. Case investigation and reactive case detection for malaria elimination in northern Senegal. Malar J. 2013;12:331.
21. Smith Gueye C, Sanders KC, Galappaththy GN, Rundi C, Tobgay T, Sovannaroth S, et al. Active case detection for malaria elimination: a survey among Asia Pacific countries. Malar J. 2013;12:358.
22. Harris I, Sharrock WW, Bain LM, Gray K-A, Bobogare A, Boaz L, et al. A large proportion of asymptomatic Plasmodium infections with low and sub-microscopic parasite densities in the low transmission setting of Temotu Province, Solomon Islands: challenges for malaria diagnostics in an elimination setting. Malar J. 2010;9:254.
23. Yewhalaw D, Legesse W, Van Bortel W, Gebre-Selassie S, Kloos H, Duchateau L, et al. Malaria and water resource development: the case of Gilgel–Gibe hydroelectric dam in Ethiopia. Malar J. 2009;8:21.
24. Mekonnen SK, Medhin G, Berhe N, Clouse RM, Aseffa A. Efficacy of artemether–lumefantrine therapy for the treatment of uncomplicated *Plasmodium falciparum* malaria in Southwestern Ethiopia. Malar J. 2015;14:317.
25. Adera TD. Beliefs and traditional treatment of malaria in Kishe settlement area, southwest Ethiopia. Ethiop Med J. 2003;41:25–34.
26. Rosanas-Urgell A, Mueller D, Betuela I, Barnadas C, Iga J, Zimmerman PA, et al. Comparison of diagnostic methods for the detection and quantification of the four sympatric Plasmodium species in field samples from Papua New Guinea. Malar J. 2010;9:361.
27. WHO. Methods for maintaining coverage with long-lasting insecticidal nets (LLINs). Geneva: World Health Organization; 2013.
28. Kumar D, Andimuthu R, Rajan R, Venkatesan M. Spatial trend, environmental and socioeconomic factors associated with malaria prevalence in Chennai. Malar J. 2014;13:14.
29. Dhimal M, O'Hara RB, Karki R, Thakur GD, Kuch U, Ahrens B. Spatio-temporal distribution of malaria and its association with climatic factors and vector-control interventions in two high-risk districts of Nepal. Malar J. 2014;13:457.
30. Mogeni P, Omedo I, Nyundo C, Kamau A, Noor A, Bejon P, et al. Effect of transmission intensity on hotspots and micro-epidemiology of malaria in sub-Saharan Africa. BMC Med. 2017;15:121.
31. Sturrock HJW, Novotny JM, Kunene S, Dlamini S, Zulu Z, Cohen JM, et al. Reactive case detection for malaria elimination: real-life experience from an ongoing program in Swaziland. PLoS ONE. 2013;8:e63830.
32. WHO. Disease surveillance for malaria elimination: an operational manual. Geneva: World Health Organization; 2012.

33. Konradsen F, Amerasinghe P, van der Hoek W, Amerasinghe F, Perera D, Piyaratne M. Strong association between house characteristics and malaria vectors in Sri Lanka. Am J Trop Med Hyg. 2003;68:177–81.

34. Kirby MJ, Green C, Milligan PM, Sismanidis C, Jasseh M, Conway DJ, et al. Risk factors for house-entry by malaria vectors in a rural town and satellite villages in The Gambia. Malar J. 2008;7:2.

35. Ghebreyesus TA, Haile M, Witten KH, Getachew A, Yohannes M, Lindsay SW, et al. Household risk factors for malaria among children in the Ethiopian highlands. Trans R Soc Trop Med Hyg. 2000;94:17–21.

36. Lelisa K, Asale A, Taye B, Emana D, Yewhalaw D. Anopheline mosquitoes behaviour and entomological monitoring in southwestern Ethiopia. J Vector Borne Dis. 2017;54:240.

37. Animut A, Balkew M, Lindtjørn B. Impact of housing condition on indoor-biting and indoor-resting Anopheles arabiensis density in a highland area, central Ethiopia. Malar J. 2013;12:393.

38. Tadesse FG, Pett H, Baidjoe A, Lanke K, Grignard L, Sutherland C, et al. Submicroscopic carriage of Plasmodium falciparum and Plasmodium vivax in a low endemic area in Ethiopia where no parasitaemia was detected by microscopy or rapid diagnostic test. Malar J. 2015;14:303.

39. Ganguly S, Saha P, Guha SK, Biswas A, Das S, Kundu PK, et al. High prevalence of asymptomatic malaria in a tribal population in Eastern India. J Clin Microbiol. 2013;51:1439–44.

40. Okell LC, Ghani AC, Lyons E, Drakeley CJ. Submicroscopic infection in Plasmodium falciparum—endemic populations: a systematic review and meta-analysis. J Infect Dis. 2009;200:1509–17.

41. Okell LC, Bousema T, Griffin JT, Ouédraogo AL, Ghani AC, Drakeley CJ. Factors determining the occurrence of submicroscopic malaria infections and their relevance for control. Nat Commun. 2012;3:1237.

42. Chen I, Clarke SE, Gosling R, Hamainza B, Killeen G, Magill A, et al. "Asymptomatic" malaria: a chronic and debilitating infection that should be treated. PLoS Med. 2016;13:e1001942.

43. Tripura R, Peto TJ, Chalk J, Lee SJ, Sirithiranont P, Nguon C, et al. Persistent Plasmodium falciparum and Plasmodium vivax infections in a western Cambodian population: implications for prevention, treatment and elimination strategies. Malar J. 2016;15:181.

44. Ashley EA, White NJ. The duration of Plasmodium falciparum infections. Malar J. 2014;13:500.

45. Manjurano A, Okell L, Lukindo T, Reyburn H, Olomi R, Roper C, et al. Association of sub-microscopic malaria parasite carriage with transmission intensity in north-eastern Tanzania. Malar J. 2011;10:370.

46. Kateera F, Mens PF, Hakizimana E, Ingabire CM, Muragijemariya L, Karinda P, et al. Malaria parasite carriage and risk determinants in a rural population: a malariometric survey in Rwanda. Malar J. 2015;14:16.

47. Taye B, Lelisa K, Emana D, Asale A, Yewhalaw D. Seasonal dynamics, longevity, and biting activity of Anopheline mosquitoes in southwestern Ethiopia. J Insect Sci. 2016;16:6.

48. Howard SC, Omumbo J, Nevill C, Some ES, Donnelly CA, Snow RW. Evidence for a mass community effect of insecticide-treated bednets on the incidence of malaria on the Kenyan coast. Trans R Soc Trop Med Hyg. 2000;94:357–60.

49. Govella NJ, Ferguson H. Why use of interventions targeting outdoor biting mosquitoes will be necessary to achieve malaria elimination. Front Physiol. 2012;3:199.

50. Reddy MR, Overgaard HJ, Abaga S, Reddy VP, Caccone A, Kiszewski AE, et al. Outdoor host seeking behaviour of Anopheles gambiae mosquitoes following initiation of malaria vector control on Bioko Island, Equatorial Guinea. Malar J. 2011;10:184.

51. Haji KA, Khatib BO, Smith S, Ali AS, Devine GJ, Coetzee M, et al. Challenges for malaria elimination in Zanzibar: pyrethroid resistance in malaria vectors and poor performance of long-lasting insecticide nets. Parasit Vectors. 2013;6:82.

52. Monroe A, Asamoah O, Lam Y, Koenker H, Psychas P, Lynch M, et al. Outdoor-sleeping and other night-time activities in northern Ghana: implications for residual transmission and malaria prevention. Malar J. 2015;14:35.

14

Screening and field performance of powder-formulated insecticides on eave tube inserts against pyrethroid resistant *Anopheles gambiae* s.l.

Welbeck A. Oumbouke[1,2]*, Innocent Z. Tia[2], Antoine M. G. Barreaux[3], Alphonsine A. Koffi[2], Eleanore D. Sternberg[3], Matthew B. Thomas[3] and Raphael N'Guessan[1,2]

Abstract

Background: The widespread emergence of insecticide resistance in African malaria vectors remains one of the main challenges facing control programmes. Electrostatic coating that uses polarity to bind insecticide particles is a new way of delivering insecticides to mosquitoes. Although previous tests demonstrated the resistance breaking potential of this application method, studies screening and investigating the residual efficacy of a broader range of insecticides are necessary.

Methods: Eleven insecticide powder formulations belonging to six insecticide classes (pyrethroid, carbamate, organophosphate, neonicotinoid, entomopathogenic fungus and boric acid) were initially screened for residual activity over 4 weeks against pyrethroid resistant *Anopheles gambiae* sensu lato (s.l.) from the M'bé valley, central Côte d'Ivoire. Tests were performed using the eave tube assay that simulates the behavioural interaction between mosquitoes and insecticide-treated inserts. With the best performing insecticide, persistence was monitored over 12 months and the actual contact time lethal to mosquitoes was explored, using a range of transient exposure time (5 s, 30 s, 1 min up to 2 min) in the tube assays in laboratory. The mortality data were calibrated against overnight release-recapture data from enclosure around experimental huts incorporating treated inserts at the M'bé site. The natural recruitment rate of mosquitoes to the tube without insecticide treatment was assessed using fluorescent dust particles.

Results: Although most insecticides assayed during the initial screening induced significant mortality (45–100%) of pyrethroid resistant *An. gambiae* during the first 2 weeks, only 10% beta-cyfluthrin retained high residual efficacy, killing 100% of *An. gambiae* during the first month and >80% over 8 subsequent months. Transient exposure for 5 s of mosquitoes to 10% beta-cyfluthrin produced 56% mortality, with an increase to 98% when contact time was extended to 2 min (P = 0.001). In the experimental hut enclosures, mortality of *An. gambiae* with 10% beta-cyfluthrin treated inserts was 55% compared to similar rate (44%) of mosquitoes that contacted the inserts treated with fluorescent dusts. This suggests that all host-seeking female mosquitoes that contacted beta-cyfluthrin treated inserts during host-seeking were killed.

Conclusion: The eave tube technology is a novel malaria control approach which combines house proofing and targeted control of anopheline mosquitoes using insecticide treated inserts. Beta-cyfluthrin showed great promise for

---

*Correspondence: oumbouke.welbeck@gmail.com
[2] Institut Pierre Richet (IPR)/Institut National de Santé Publique (INSP), Bouaké, Côte d'Ivoire
Full list of author information is available at the end of the article

providing prolonged control of pyrethroid resistant *An. gambiae* and has potential to be deployed year-round in areas where malaria parasites are transmitted by highly pyrethroid resistant *An. gambiae* across sub-Saharan Africa.

Keywords: Insecticide resistance, Resistance breaking, Electrostatic coating, Powder-formulated insecticide, Residual efficacy, Eave tubes

Background

Wide-scale use of insecticide-based interventions such as indoor residual sprays (IRS) and long-lasting insecticide-treated nets (LLINs) has contributed to a substantial reduction in the global malaria burden in recent years [1, 2]. However, the sustainability of these approaches is now being threatened by the evolution of insecticide resistance [3, 4], creating a need for more diverse vector control tools [5].

The eave tube is a recent innovation that offers a novel approach for delivering insecticides to malaria mosquitoes [6]. The approach involves blocking the eaves of houses (if open) and inserting pieces of PVC pipe to act as 'chimneys' to channel the human odours mosquitoes use as cues to locate hosts for blood feeding, out of the house. When host-seeking mosquitoes enter a tube, they encounter an insert treated with an insecticide. The current version of the eave tube inserts uses electrostatic netting to hold powder formulations of insecticides. Mosquito contact with the netting results in very efficient transfer of powder particles such that even highly pyrethroid resistant mosquitoes can be killed with pyrethroid insecticides due to the overwhelming dose [7]. When eave tubes are combined with screening of windows and doors to reduce mosquito entry via other routes, the approach provides both physical protection and a killing effect, much like an insecticide treated net but at the level of the household.

Semi-field and modelling studies indicate that screening plus eave tubes (SET) could reduce transmission of malaria at community level above and beyond universal coverage of LLINs [8–10]. Based on these promising results, a cluster randomized controlled trial (CRT) is now being conducted in central Côte d'Ivoire [11] to evaluate epidemiological impact at village level. The current paper reports on a series of initial studies to screen a range of candidate insecticides for use in this trial, together with an evaluation of potential residual activity of a smaller number of promising insecticides to select a final product and inform likely retreatment frequency for the CRT.

Methods

Mosquitoes and insecticides

Experiments were performed with *Anopheles gambiae* mosquitoes collected from a rice growing area adjacent to the M'bé experimental hut station in central Côte d'Ivoire, approximately 40 km north of the city of Bouaké. These rice fields provide mosquito-breeding habitat year-round. A comprehensive characterization of the local mosquito population showed that the M variant of the *An. gambiae* complex, now referred to as *Anopheles coluzzii*, is predominant in the area and exhibits high levels of resistance to pyrethroid and carbamate insecticides [12, 13]. Recently, over 1700 fold resistance against deltamethrin was detected in the M'bé population of *An. gambiae* compared to the Kisumu laboratory strain, using adapted CDC bottle assays [14]. The high resistance intensity exhibited by this vector population makes it a good strain for testing potential resistance breaking chemistry or novel insecticide delivery systems, such as the electrostatic coating technology. In the experiments described below, mosquitoes were collected as larvae and pupae from breeding sites around M'bé and reared to adult in the insectary of the Institut Pierre Richet (IPR) in Bouaké, under ambient climatic conditions. Five-day-old sugar-fed only female mosquitoes were used in all laboratory and semi-field assays.

The list of insecticides initially screened for residual performance is given in Table 1. Overall, 11 products belonging to six insecticide classes (pyrethroid, carbamate, organophosphate, neonicotinoid, entomopathogenic fungus and boric acid) were tested. The products were selected for testing based on, commercial availability as pest control products, however a handful of experimental formulations were also tested. All the insecticides evaluated were powder formulations.

Application of insecticide powders on eave tube inserts

Eave tube inserts that fit into locally produced PVC tubes have been designed with electrostatic netting attached to a polyethylene frame consisting of a plastic circle with six spokes and a central protruding node (see [9] for images of the insert design). The frame provides physical support to the netting and allows easy insertion inside eave tubes. This prototype was used in the present study to investigate the persistence of insecticide applied on eave tube insert.

Candidate active ingredients were applied on eave tube inserts manually; 5 g of each '*active*' (powder-formulated insecticide) was weighed and poured evenly onto an eave tube insert placed in the middle of a 20 cm long PVC tube. To prevent active from falling through the tube,

Table 1 **List of insecticides initially screened for residual performance against pyrethroid resistant *Anopheles gambiae* M'bé strain**

Commercial name (supplier)	Active ingredients (dose)	Chemical classes
Actellic (Syngenta, Switzerland)	Pyrimiphos methyl (1.6%); thiamethoxam (0.36%)	Organophosphate; neonicotinoid
NA	Azamethiphos (10%)	Organophosphate
NA	*Beauveria bassiana* (10%)	Fungus
Ficam D (Bayer, Germany)	Bendiocarb (1.25%)	Carbamate
BISTAR 10 WP (FMC India)	Bifenthrin (10%)	Pyrethroid
BorActin (Rockwell labs Ltd, USA)	Orthoboric acid (99%)	Boric acid
Tempo Ultra (Bayer, Germany)	Beta-cyfluthrin WP (10%)	Pyrethroid
Spritex (Denka International BV, Barneveld, The Netherlands)	Deltamethrin (0.25%)	Pyrethroid
Drione (Bayer, Germany)	Pyrethrin (1%); Piperonyl Butoxide (10%)	Pyrethroid; synergist
NA	Permethrin (25%)	Pyrethroid
Sevin (TechPac LLC, Atlanta)	Carbaryl (5%)	Carbamate

Commercial names are provided for insecticides that are available on the market; NA indicates that the insecticide was an experimental formulation and not a commercially available product

both ends of the pipe was sealed off with a plastic lid and the tube was then shaken by hand for 1 min. To allow for adequate distribution of the insecticide on the two sides of the insert, the tube was turned every 10 s. The tube was then put on a table for 2 min to allow the dust to settle and adhere to the insert, and then the treated insert was moved to a clean tube and shaken for 15 s to remove any excess of powder. After treatment, the insert was placed in a third, clean tube. Four to six inserts were treated for each insecticide; approximately 4 g of powder were collected after treatment, leaving approximately 1 g of powder on the insert. An excess of powder was used during treatment to ensure thorough saturation of the inserts with the powders. Inserts were tested 1 day post-treatment (T0), then kept for subsequent monitoring of residual efficacy at regular intervals. To better approximate decay rates under realistic conditions, the inserts were kept individually in eave tubes inserted in holes drilled at eave level in an experimental house on the IPR campus. The inserts were stored in these tubes throughout the testing period and removed only for persistence monitoring.

The "eave tube" bioassay

This bioassay method uses a 20 cm long piece of PVC tube with an insecticide-treated insert placed in the tube such that it is flush with one end of the pipe (Fig. 1a). The opposite end of the tube is fitted with untreated netting to keep mosquitoes inside of the tube, and mosquitoes are introduced into the tube on this clean end using mouth aspirators. A host cue is placed behind the treated insert and the mosquitoes are allowed to recruit freely to the insert over a fixed period of time. This experimental

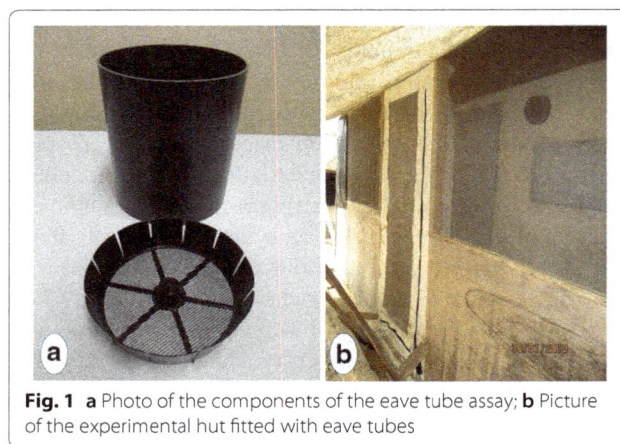

Fig. 1 **a** Photo of the components of the eave tube assay; **b** Picture of the experimental hut fitted with eave tubes

set up was designed to simulate the interaction between mosquitoes and eave tube inserts in the field, where heat and odour cues draw host-seeking female mosquitoes into the tube where they then make contact with the insecticide-laden insert (see [15] for a similar methodology).

Initial screening of powder insecticides

The aim of this set of experiments was to identify chemicals that retained efficacy against pyrethroid resistant mosquitoes for at least 4 weeks post-treatment. Persistence assays were performed on a fortnightly basis, and insecticides with significant decline in residual activity over the testing period were dropped from further testing. A total of ~60 unfed female mosquitoes aged 4–5 days were exposed in batch of 15 to each insert for

3 min using the eave tube bioassay. A hand was used as the attractive cue behind the treated insert. To eliminate any potential biases from differential attractiveness of volunteers, hand from the same individual was used in all assays. Exposure to an untreated insert served as the control. At the end of the exposure period, mosquitoes were released in netted cages with access to a 10% sugar solution on cotton pads. Mortality was scored after a 24 h holding period, except for the fungus-exposed group, which was scored 7 days later.

Persistence monitoring

The only insecticide that persisted for 1 month during the initial screening was 10% beta-cyfluthrin. New inserts were treated with 10% beta-cyfluthrin and residual activity was monitored at approximately monthly intervals for 12 months using the same eave tube bioassays, but with some refinement of the protocol. The three modifications were: (1) the host cue was changed from a hand to a bottle filled up with boiling water and wrapped in a worn sock (worn over night), to allow for more assays to be run in parallel, (2) female mosquitoes were deprived of sugar 6 h prior to the bioassay to maximize host-seeking behaviour, and (3) the duration of the bioassay was extended from 3 min to 1 h. Although mosquitoes remained inside the tube for 1 h, it is important to note that the actual contact time was still determined by the host-seeking response of each individual mosquito. Approximately 60 mosquitoes (four replicates of 15 mosquitoes per tube) were tested. At the end of the 1 h behavioural assay, mosquitoes were transferred to observation cages, supplied with 10% sugar water solution, and mortality scored 24 h.

Supplementary experiments

Results from residual efficacy assays show that 10% beta-cyfluthrin was the longest lasting chemical when applied on eave tube inserts. To further explore the vector control potential of this insecticide formulation, additional experiments were performed in a semi-field setting and in the laboratory using reduced contact times.

Field performance of insecticide-treated insert

Experiments were conducted at the M'bé phase II experimental hut station between June and September 2017 using experimental huts constructed to the West African design [16]. The huts are 3.25 m long, 1.76 m wide and 2 m high. The interior walls of the huts are made of concrete brick, with a corrugated iron roof. A plastic cover was affixed onto the roofing as ceiling. Each hut was built on a concrete base with a water-filled moat, to protect against invertebrate predators. The huts were customized to allow evaluation of eave tube inserts; namely, six holes were drilled at eave level (1.7 m from the ground)

on three sides of the hut (two holes on each side). Eave tubes were fitted into the holes and inserts freshly treated with 10% beta-cyfluthrin were placed in the tubes. To allow for the recapture of mosquitoes after contact with the eave tube inserts, the huts had to be in an enclosed structure (Fig. 1b). A wooden frame was erected on the concrete base, 50 cm from the exterior wall of the hut. Plastic sheeting was used as a roof on the enclosure, and extended beyond the edge of the enclosure as an awning, to protect against rain entering the enclosure. The bottom half of the frame was made out of wooden panels and the top half was screened with polyethylene netting. White plastic sheeting was installed on the floor of the enclosure to facilitate the collection of dead mosquitoes. The door of the enclosure was positioned on the front side of the hut and closed with a zipper to prevent mosquitoes escaping.

Overnight release-recapture experiments were conducted in two modified experimental huts, situated 50 m apart. In the first experiment, six inserts treated with beta-cyfluthrin were installed in one experimental hut and six untreated inserts were placed in tubes in the second experimental house. Two adult volunteers were recruited from nearby villages to sleep in the huts. During the experiment, sleepers were rotated between the two huts. Before the start of the experiment, study participants slept in the experimental huts for a week to build up human odours and maximize mosquito host-seeking response. At 20:00, volunteers entered the huts to sleep under intact, untreated net. A total of 100, 5 day-old female *An. gambiae* (M'bé strain) were released into each enclosure 15 min after volunteers retired to their respective huts. Mosquitoes were sugar-starved for 6 h prior to the release, but still provided tap water to prevent desiccation. In the following morning, at 05:00, mosquitoes were recaptured both inside the experimental huts and within the enclosures using flashlights and aspirators. Live recaptured mosquitoes were subsequently held in netted plastic cups and supplied with 10% sugar solution. Survival was monitored for 24 h.

Measurement of mosquito host-seeking response in the enclosure

To assess how many mosquitoes actually enter the eave tubes and came into contact with the inserts over the course of a night, a second experiment was conducted using fluorescent powder. The procedure for the experiment was similar to that described above, except that the inserts were treated with a non-toxic fluorescent dust instead of beta-cyfluthrin. The procedure for applying the fluorescent dust was similar to that used for hand-treating insert with powder insecticide as described in an earlier section. Again, the experimental huts were fitted with 6 eave tube inserts and 100 sugar-starved *An. gambiae* M'bé mosquitoes were released in each enclosure each study night. To prevent cross-contamination with the fluorescent powder, mosquitoes were caught individually using clean haemolysis tubes. Recaptured mosquitoes were killed with chloroform and their bodies subsequently checked for fluorescent particles, indicative of contact with treated inserts, using a UV light microscope (Dino Lite Premier, USA). A third experiment was also conducted where eave tubes were simply left open overnight to estimate how many mosquitoes passed through the tubes. The following morning at 05:00, the volunteers blocked the eave tubes using untreated inserts and mosquitoes inside and outside the hut were collected and counted.

Short contact assays

Unlike house walls, where a mosquito might rest for a longer period of time, the time that vectors spend in contact with an eave tube insert could be relatively transient [17, 18]. Overnight survival in the enclosures with insecticide-treated inserts could indicate either that the mosquito did not come into contact with a treated insert or that it did not stay in contact long enough to pick up a lethal dose.

Likewise, while the presence of coloured particles on a recaptured mosquito does indicate contact with the eave tube insert, the absence of fluorescent particles could indicate either no contact, or that the mosquito did not stay in contact long enough to be contaminated with a visible amount of particles.

To evaluate whether beta-cyfluthrin can kill even with brief contact, individual mosquitoes were exposed to freshly treated inserts using the same modified eave tube bioassay. A range of exposure time (5 s, 30 s, 1 min and 2 min) was tested on 6 h sugar-starved 5-day-old female *An. gambiae* M'bé. A transparent tube was used instead of a standard PVC tube, to enable direct observation of mosquito behaviour within the tube and to allow measurement of contact duration using a stopwatch. A total of 52 mosquitoes was tested individually for each time period. Following exposure, mosquitoes were removed from the eave tube and housed in 150 mL plastic cups and provided with sugar solution. Mortality was scored 24 h post-exposure.

To test whether a contact time of only 5 s is sufficient for fluorescent particles to transfer from the insert to the mosquito, 50 female *An. gambiae* mosquitoes were exposed individually to inserts treated with fluorescent powder using the same modified eave tube assay. After 5 s of contact, the mosquito was removed and the body examined under UV light for the presence of coloured particles.

Statistical analysis

Data were entered into an excel spreadsheet and transferred into the R statistical software version 3.4.0 for analysis. The decline in efficacy over time across insecticides was analysed using Bayesian generalized linear models (BGLMs) with the "arm" package. Insecticide treatments were included in the model as explanatory variable and mosquito mortality as the outcome. Interactions between insecticides and persistence testing intervals (time since treatment) were also included in the models. Pairwise comparisons were performed with the final model using the "multcomp" package in R. For the release-recapture experiments, generalized linear mixed models (GLMMs) with a binomial distribution and a logit link function was fitted to the data using the "lme4" package for R. Treatment and enclosure were included as fixed effects and sleepers were included as a random effect. Data from the short contact eave tube assays were analysed using Bayesian generalized linear models with a binomial distribution.

Results
Initial screening of powder insecticides

Figure 2 shows the results of the eave tube bioassay tests with the 11 initial candidate powder insecticides, tested at T0, 2 weeks and 1 month post-treatment against the pyrethroid resistant *An. gambiae* M'bé strain. Comparing the 11 insecticides at T0 and 2 weeks post-treatment, most killed a significant proportion (45–100%) of *An. gambiae* mosquitoes. However, there was a significant ($P < 0.05$) decline in activity 4 weeks after treatment, with mortality dropping below 25% for almost all of the insecticides. In contrast, beta-cyfluthrin retained full residual activity (100% mortality) over the screening period of 1 month.

Persistence monitoring

Based on the initial screening, beta-cyfluthrin was selected for its persistence on inserts over 12 months; the results are summarized in Fig. 3. Beta-cyfluthrin was highly effective, continuing to kill > 80% of *An. gambiae* up to 9 months post-treatment. Mortality of *An. gambiae* declined steadily over time down to 67% by month 11 and 20% by month 12.

Experimental hut evaluations

The proportions of *An. gambiae* mosquitoes recaptured in the experimental hut enclosures are presented in Table 2, both for the experiment using insecticide-treated inserts and for the one using inserts treated with fluorescent dust. Table 2 also presents the proportions of

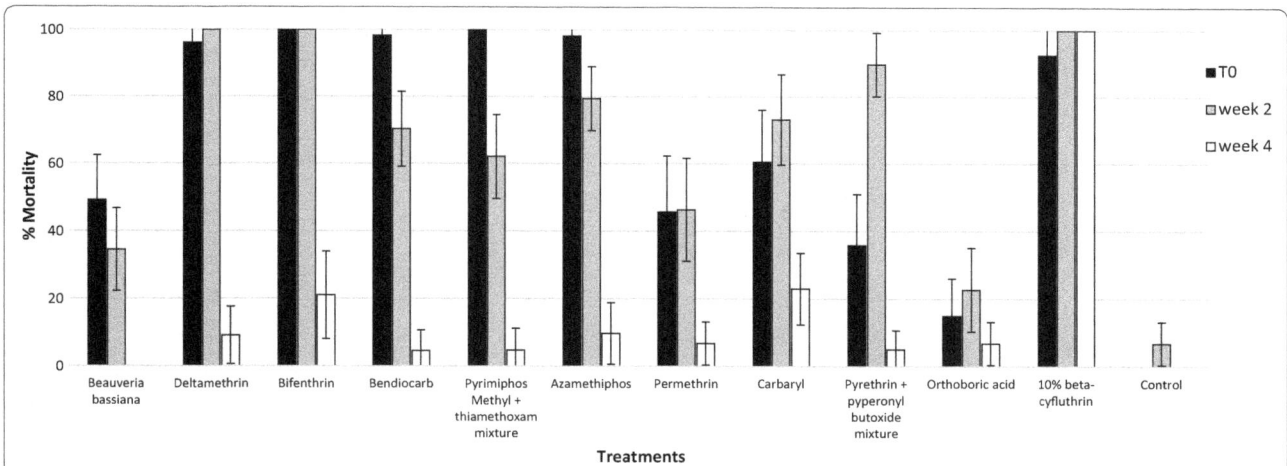

Fig. 2 Weekly mortality rates of pyrethroid resistant *Anopheles gambiae* M'bé strain after exposure to insecticide treated insert using 3 min eave tube assay. Error bars indicate the confidence intervals for the different proportions on the graphs

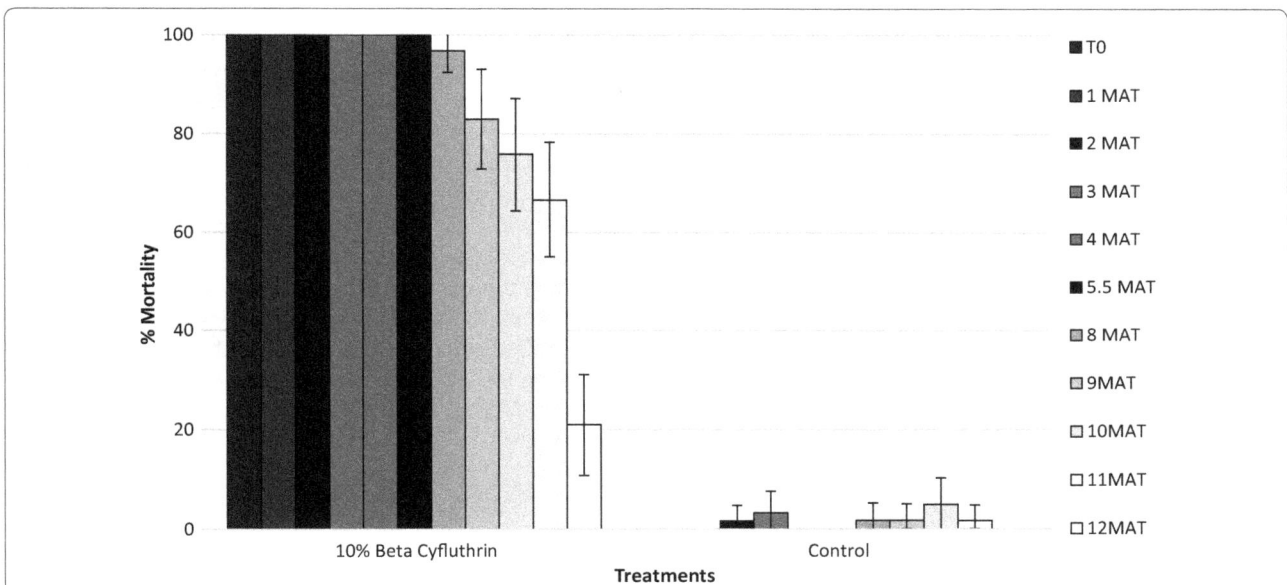

Fig. 3 Residual activity over 12 months of 10% beta-cyfluthrin (selected from initial screening) on insert against pyrethroid resistant *Anopheles gambiae* from M'bé. Error bars indicate the confidence intervals for the different proportions on the graphs (*MAT* months after treatment)

mosquitoes found dead (insecticide treatment) or recaptured with fluorescent dust particles.

Mosquito recapture rate was consistently high in all experiments (more than 80%). It is possible that a few mosquitoes escaped through the door of the enclosure during release, thus accounting for the small difference in number between mosquitoes released and that recaptured.

Mortality with the untreated control inserts was < 5%. When inserts treated with beta-cyfluthrin were used, about half of the mosquitoes tested died by the morning of collection (55% immediate mortality) and this

increased to 64% by 24 h post-exposure, but the difference between immediate mortality and 24 h mortality was not significant (P > 0.05).

Results from the experiment using the fluorescent powder showed that, on average 44% of mosquitoes released in the enclosure had coloured particles on their body after recapture. This suggests that slightly less than half of the released mosquitoes made contact with the inserts overnight. Given that this is similar to the mortality observed when beta-cyfluthrin was used in the experimental huts (44% with coloured particles versus 55% immediate mortality with beta-cyfluthrin), this suggests

Table 2 Release-recapture of pyrethroid resistant *An. gambiae* within enclosure at M'bé, Côte d'Ivoire

Treatment	Total released	% recaptured (95% CI)	% immediate mortality (95% CI)	% 24 h mortality (95% CI)	% with fluorescent dust (95% CI)
Untreated insert	395	90.38 [87.5–93.3]	1.12[a] [0.03–2.21]	2.8[a] [1.1–4.5]	–
10% beta-cyfluthrin treated insert	389	84.31 [80.7–87.9]	55[b] [49.6–60.4]	64[b] [58.8–69.2]	–
Fluorescent dust-treated insert	790	87.6 [85.5–89.7]	–	–	44.4 [40.7 – 48.1]

*Values in the same column not sharing a letter superscript differ significantly (P < 0.05, GLMMs)

that all of the mosquitoes encountering the insecticide-treated inserts were killed. When eave tubes were left open, > 75% of mosquitoes were caught inside the experimental hut. This indicates that, in the absence of the inserts, the majority of mosquitoes will pass through the tubes overnight.

Short contact assay

Figure 4 shows the 24 h mortality of *An. gambiae* mosquitoes after 5 s, 30 s, 1 min or 2 min exposure to inserts freshly treated with beta-cyfluthrin. There was a positive relationship between exposure duration and mortality, i.e. the longer the exposure time the higher the mortality rate. Percent mortality was 56% with the shortest exposure time (5 s), and increased significantly to 88.5% when contact time was increased to 1 min (P = 0.003). A 2-min contact with a freshly treated insert was sufficient to produce almost 100% mortality in a pyrethroid resistant *An. gambiae* strain, but the difference in mortality between 1 min and 2 min exposure was not significant (P > 0.05). There was no mortality in the control group. When mosquitoes were exposed for just 5 s on inserts treated with fluorescent dust, 100% of mosquitoes were contaminated with the coloured particles.

Discussion

Malaria elimination will require innovative vector control tools that are not compromised by insecticide resistance. The eave tube is part of a new mosquito control strategy that involves screening windows, closing eaves, and the targeted delivery of insecticide on eave tube inserts. The intervention will be trialed in Côte d'Ivoire to test whether it can impact malaria incidence. The study presented here was designed, in part, to identify a suitable insecticide for use in the trial, and to explore a diversity of insecticides that could potentially be used in the eave tubes for prolonged control of insecticide resistant anopheline mosquito populations.

Results from residual efficacy bioassays show that the majority of insecticides tested in the present study produced significant mortality (45–100%) in the local M'bé strain of *An. gambiae* mosquitoes, when freshly applied on eave tube insert. This confirms that a wide range of actives from diverse insecticide classes could be successfully applied on electrostatic netting for effective control of insecticide resistant malaria vectors and provides further evidence of the resistance breaking potential of the technology [7].

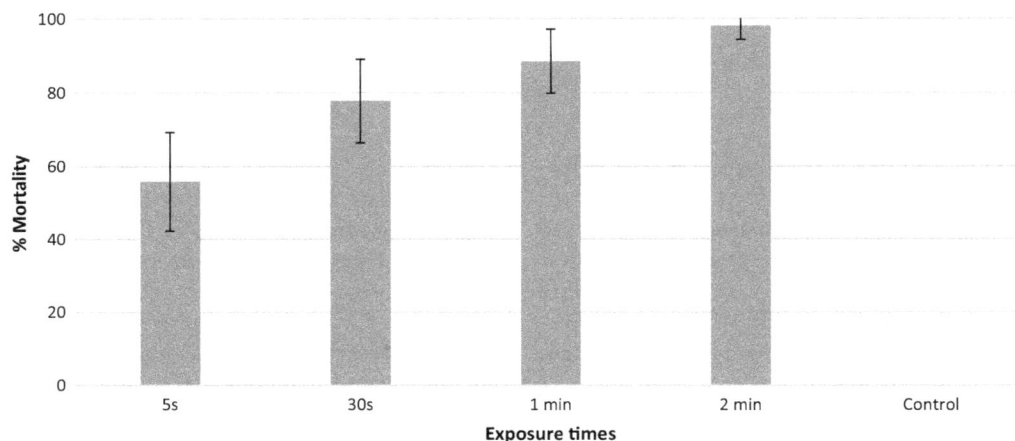

Fig. 4 Exposure time and induced mortality of individual pyrethroid resistant *Anopheles gambiae* from M'bé with 10% beta-cyfluthrin treated insert. Error bars indicate the confidence intervals for the different proportions on the graphs

While most candidate actives were highly effective at killing mosquitoes immediately following treatment, only one (10% beta-cyfluthrin) retained efficacy beyond 1 month. Previous studies with some of the same insecticides have reported longer residual activity than what was observed in the present study but this could be due to the difference in the nature of the substrate (electrostatic netting versus walls). The rapid loss in efficacy observed with some actives could also be due to factors that are known to degrade insecticides used during indoor residual spraying campaign, including temperature, humidity and UV-light [19]. The underlying mechanism for the rapid decay that was observed with some actives should be evaluated in further studies. However, different formulations could help mitigate some of these factors. For example, the use of UV protection additive could prevent insecticide breakdown due to photolysis and prolong the effective lifespan of chemicals. Although candidate actives were exposed to environmental conditions similar to those in local villages, persistence could still differ for a number of reasons when the insecticides are deployed in the field. For example, exposure to smoke from cooking in real houses could impact the long-term insecticidal efficacy of chemicals deployed in the eave tube. This issue has also been reported with insecticide-treated durable wall lining, where the efficacy can be undermined by dirt accumulation [20]. This emphasizes the need for continued monitoring of persistence and timely re-treatment of inserts once efficacy starts to decline.

Although the focus of this study was on readily available formulations of insecticides, there is clearly an opportunity for reformulating or repurposing a number of active ingredients for use in eave tubes. This could be useful, for example, in resistance mitigation and management where one of the recommended strategy is the use of unrelated insecticidal compounds in rotations or mosaics to delay the spread of insecticide resistant genes [21, 22]. Additionally, a diversity of active ingredients suited for deployment in eave tubes could be useful for addressing constraints on IRS. The relatively high cost of non-pyrethroid insecticide formulations coupled with a proposed reduction in IRS funding will result in much fewer houses being sprayed across sub-Saharan Africa [23], but only a small amount of insecticide is needed to protect a house with eave tubes. Moreover, most insecticides are short-lived when applied on mud wall, which is common in most rural endemic areas across sub-Saharan Africa. This may be less of a problem with the eave tube technology given that insecticides are deployed on substrate with standard characteristics.

In the experimental huts, beta-cyfluthrin produced 55% mortality of pyrethroid resistant *An. gambiae* mosquitoes. Although the mortality observed in the experimental huts is consistent with findings from previous studies [8, 9], mortality was much higher in laboratory bioassays. This could be either due to a percentage of mosquitoes not entering the tubes over the course of the night or that contact with the treated inserts was too transient for the mosquito to pick up a lethal dose of insecticide. When inserts were treated with fluorescent powder and placed in the experimental huts, the proportion of mosquitoes that contacted the fluorescent dust (44%) was similar to the mortality (55%) induced by beta-cyfluthrin treated inserts. This suggests that not all female mosquitoes came into contact with the treated inserts but those females that contacted the tube died, and this would have happened within the first 2 min of exposure. In other words, overnight mortality is likely determined by the probability a mosquito will come into contact with the treated insert rather than the probability the mosquito will die given it has contacted a treated insert (if the inserts are freshly treated with insecticides). Interestingly, the proportion of mosquitoes entering through open tubes (> 75%) was higher than the contact rates estimate with beta-cyfluthrin and fluorescent powder. This difference in mosquito behaviour could be due to a change in the flow of human odours emanating from volunteer-occupied hut, which might be attenuated when tubes are screened with the inserts.

Overall, on the basis of its performance and residual activity, as well as commercial availability and existing regulatory approval in Côte d'Ivoire, beta-cyfluthrin was selected for the eave tube CRT. While having a pyrethroid insecticide in the eave tube might not seem an ideal option in an area of pyrethroid resistance, the resistance breaking properties of the electrostatic netting still enables use of a pyrethroid. Nonetheless, it will be important to monitor the potential for further selection for pyrethroid resistance. Moreover, screening for other active ingredients should be considered a priority to develop more sustainable resistance management strategies [24].

Abbreviations
SET: Screening plus eave tubes; PVC: Polyvinyl chloride; CDC: Centers for Disease Control and Prevention; UV: Ultra-violet; BGLMs: Bayesian generalized linear models; GLMMs: Generalized linear mixed models.

Authors' contributions
WAO participated in the study design, analysed the data and drafted the manuscript. WAO, IZT and AMGB performed the experiments. RN, AAK, MBT and EDS contributed to the study design. RN, MBT and EDS edited the manuscript. All authors read and approved the final manuscript.

Author details
[1] Department of Disease Control, London School of Hygiene and Tropical Medicine, London, UK. [2] Institut Pierre Richet (IPR)/Institut National de Santé Publique (INSP), Bouaké, Côte d'Ivoire. [3] Department of Entomology, Center

for Infectious Disease Dynamics, The Pennsylvania State University, University Park, PA 16802, USA.

Acknowledgements

We would like to thank all technicians at IPR for their assistance. The authors also thank the volunteer sleepers for their participation in the experimental hut study.

Competing interests

The authors declare that they have no competing interests.

Funding

This research is supported by a grant to the Pennsylvania State University from the Bill and Melinda Gates foundation. Grant Number: OPP1131603.

References

1. Bhatt S, Weiss DJ, Cameron E, Bisanzio D, Mappin B, Dalrymple U, et al. The effect of malaria control on Plasmodium falciparum in Africa between 2000 and 2015. Nature. 2015;526:207–11.
2. WHO. World malaria report 2016. Geneva: World Health Organization; 2016.
3. Toe KH, Jones CM, N'Fale S, Ismail HM, Dabire RKRH. Increased pyrethroid resistance in malaria vectors and decreased bed net effectiveness, Burkina Faso. Emerg Infect Dis. 2014;20:1691.
4. Hemingway J, Ranson H, Magill A, Kolaczinski J, Fornadel C, Gimnig J, et al. Averting a malaria disaster: will insecticide resistance derail malaria control? Lancet. 2016;387:1785–8.
5. Barreaux P, Barreaux AMG, Sternberg ED, Suh E, Waite JL, Whitehead SA, et al. Priorities for broadening the malaria vector control tool kit. Trends Parasitol. 2017;33:763–74.
6. Knols BGJ, Farenhorst M, Andriessen R, Snetselaar J, Suer RA, Osinga AJ, et al. Eave tubes for malaria control in Africa: an introduction. Malar J. 2016;15:404.
7. Andriessen R, Snetselaar J, Suer RA, Osinga AJ, Deschietere J, Lyimo IN, et al. Electrostatic coating enhances bioavailability of insecticides and breaks pyrethroid resistance in mosquitoes. Proc Natl Acad Sci USA. 2015;112:12081–6.
8. Sternberg ED, Ng'habi KR, Lyimo IN, Kessy ST, Farenhorst M, Thomas MB, et al. Eave tubes for malaria control in Africa: initial development and semi-field evaluations in Tanzania. Malar J. 2016;15:447.
9. Snetselaar J, Njiru BN, Gachie B, Owigo P, Andriessen R, Glunt K, et al. Eave tubes for malaria control in Africa: prototyping and evaluation against Anopheles gambiae s.s. and Anopheles arabiensis under semi-field conditions in western Kenya. Malar J. 2017;16:276.
10. Waite JL, Lynch PA, Thomas MB. Eave tubes for malaria control in Africa: a modelling assessment of potential impact on transmission. Malar J. 2016;15:449.
11. Sternberg ED, Cook J, Ahoua Alou LP, Aoura CJ, Assi SB, Doudou DT, et al. Evaluating the impact of screening plus eave tubes on malaria transmission compared to current best practice in central Côte d'Ivoire: a two armed cluster randomized controlled trial. BMC Public Health. 2018;18:894.
12. Koffi AA, Ahoua Alou LP, Adja MA, Chandre F, Pennetier C. Insecticide resistance status of Anopheles gambiae s.s. population from M'Be: a WHOPES-labelled experimental hut station, 10 years after the political crisis in Côte d'Ivoire. Malar J. 2013;12:151.
13. Camara S, Koffi AA, Ahoua Alou LP, Koffi K, Kabran J-PK, Koné A, et al. Mapping insecticide resistance in Anopheles gambiae (s.l.) from Côte d'Ivoire. Parasit Vectors. 2018;11:19.
14. Glunt KD, Coetzee M, Huijben S, Alphonsine Koffi A, Lynch PA, N'Guessan R, et al. Empirical and theoretical investigation into the potential impacts of insecticide resistance on the effectiveness of insecticide-treated bed nets. Evol Appl. 2017;11(4):431–41.
15. Sternberg ED, Waite JL, Thomas MB. Evaluating the efficacy of biological and conventional insecticides with the new "MCD bottle" bioassay. Malar J. 2014;13:499.
16. WHO. Guidelines for laboratory and field-testing of long-lasting insecticidal nets. Geneva: World Health Organization; 2013.
17. Spitzen J, Koelewijn T, Mukabana WR, Takken W. Visualization of house-entry behaviour of malaria mosquitoes. Malar J. 2016;15:233.
18. Sperling S, Cordel M, Gordon S, Knols BGJ, Rose A. Research: Eave tubes for malaria control in Africa: videographic observations of mosquito behaviour in Tanzania with a simple and rugged video surveillance system. MalariaWorld. 2017;8:9.
19. Sibanda MM, Focke WW, Labuschagne FJWJ, Moyo L, Nhlapo NS, Maity A, et al. Degradation of insecticides used for indoor spraying in malaria control and possible solutions. Malar J. 2011;10:307.
20. Kruger T, Sibanda MM, Focke WW, Bornman MS, de Jager C. Acceptability and effectiveness of a monofilament, polyethylene insecticide-treated wall lining for malaria control after six months in dwellings in Vhembe District, Limpopo Province, South Africa. Malar J. 2015;14:485.
21. malERA Refresh Consultative Panel on Insecticide and Drug Resistance. malERA: An updated research agenda for insecticide and drug resistance in malaria elimination and eradication. PLoS Med. 2017;14:e1002450.
22. WHO. Global plan for insecticide resistance management in malaria vectors. Geneva: World Health Organization; 2012.
23. Winskill P, Slater HC, Griffin JT, Ghani AC, Walker PGT. The US President's Malaria Initiative, Plasmodium falciparum transmission and mortality: a modelling study. PLoS Med. 2017;14:e1002448.
24. Sternberg ED, Thomas MB. Insights from agriculture for the management of insecticide resistance in disease vectors. Evol Appl. 2018;11:404–14.

15

Outdoor malaria transmission risks and social life: a qualitative study in South-Eastern Tanzania

Irene R. Moshi[1,2]*, Lenore Manderson[2], Halfan S. Ngowo[1], Yeromin P. Mlacha[1,3,4,5], Fredros O. Okumu[1,2,6,7] and Ladislaus L. Mnyone[1,2,5]

Abstract

Background: Behaviour changes in mosquitoes from indoor to outdoor biting result in continuing risk of malaria from outdoor activities, including routine household activities and occasional social and cultural practices and gatherings. This study aimed to identify the range of social and cultural gatherings conducted outdoors and their associated risks for mosquito bites.

Methods: A cross-sectional study was conducted in four villages in the Kilombero Valley from November 2015 to March 2016. Observations, focus group discussions, and key informant interviews were conducted. The recorded data were transcribed and translated from Swahili to English. Thematic content analysis was used to identify perspectives on the importance of various social and cultural gatherings that incidentally expose people to mosquito bites and malaria infection.

Results: Religious, cultural and social gatherings involving the wider community are conducted outdoors at night till dawn. Celebrations include life course events, religious and cultural ceremonies, such as Holy Communion, weddings, gatherings at Easter and Christmas, male circumcision, and rituals conducted to please the gods and to remember the dead. These celebrations, at which there is minimal use of interventions to prevent bites, contribute to individual satisfaction and social capital, helping to maintain a cohesive society. Bed net use while sleeping outdoors during mourning is unacceptable, and there is minimal use of other interventions, such as topical repellents. Long sleeve clothes are used for protection from mosquito bites but provide less protection.

Conclusion: Gatherings and celebrations expose people to mosquito bites. Approaches to prevent risks of mosquito bites and disease management need to take into account social, cultural and environmental factors. Area specific interventions may be expensive, yet may be the best approach to reduce risk of infection as endemic countries work towards elimination. Focusing on single interventions will not yield the best outcomes for malaria prevention as social contexts and vector behaviour vary.

Keywords: Community gatherings, Life course events, Kilombero Valley, Outdoor-mosquito bites, Malaria transmission, Vector control, Tanzania

*Correspondence: imoshi@ihi.or.tz
[1] Environmental Health and Ecological Sciences Department, Ifakara Health Institute, Kiko Avenue, Mikocheni, PO Box 78373, Dar es Salaam, United Republic of Tanzania
Full list of author information is available at the end of the article

Background

Between 2000 and 2015, global malaria morbidity and mortality declined by 41% and 62%, respectively [1, 2]. This reduction has largely been associated with the high coverage of frontline vector control measures, such as long-lasting insecticide-treated nets (LLINs) and indoor residual spraying (IRS) [2], and the widespread use of the malaria rapid diagnostic test (RDT) for prompt diagnosis and increased access to treatment [3–5]. Social marketing programmes and substantial global investment have improved universal coverage of bed nets and in turn increased personal and community protection [6–9]. Despite these achievements, the burden of malaria remains unacceptably high, with an estimated 216 million cases in 2016 worldwide, 4 million cases above that of from 212 million cases in 2015 [10].

In sub-Saharan Africa (SSA), which suffers the largest malaria burden, malaria prevalence decreased from 17% in 2010 to 13% in 2015 [1]. Tanzania recorded reduction in under-five mortality from 112 deaths to 67 deaths per 1000 live births between 2004 and 2010 [11], and in Muheza district in Tanga region, malaria incidences decreased by 75% between 2000 and 2015 [12–15]. Continued malaria cases and deaths, despite the wide coverage of LLINs and IRS, is associated with insecticide resistance [16–18], decrease in bed net use [19], and changes in mosquito biting behaviour and patterns from indoor biting to early outdoor biting, therefore reducing their contact with insecticide treated surfaces [20–23]. However, other factors that contribute to increasing outdoor feeding includes climate change [24], human behaviour and land use [25], environmental change [26], ecology and increasing zoophagic vectors may all contribute to continued transmission [27–30]. Previously outdoor biting was not considered as important for allocation of interventions because of its low impact on malaria transmission [31, 32], but the current increasingly outdoor biting by *Anopheles arabiensis* and *Anopheles funestus* [33–35] is contributing to continued malaria rates, frequent infections and inhibiting global malaria elimination efforts [33, 36, 37]. Studies have identified the need to address the risks of outdoor malaria transmission [38, 39]. Despite the reported changes in vector's biting and resting behaviours [40–45], in Tanzania, control efforts have neither attended the outdoor transmission segment nor consider the role of social and cultural factors in malaria transmission [46–50].

Malaria prevalence in Kilombero Valley is about 14% from a study done in 2011 [51]. The major malaria vectors includes *An. arabiensis*, *An. funestus* and *Anopheles gambiae* sensu stricto [34] whereby *An. arabiensis* is the dominant vector for the outdoor settings. The prevalence in this valley might be a result of not only indoor but also outdoor transmission risks, therefore other factors including host-seeking behaviour needs to be well understood to prevent malaria rebound. While behavioural factors are important for individual and household level prevention, a range of social and cultural factors are implicated in malaria transmission and effective interventions use outside human dwellings, that may impact health and well-being of the communities. A study by Dunn et al. [52] has indicated that, minimal bednet use among children in Kilombero Valley is a result of sleeping arrangements within the households thus continue to put this vulnerable group at risks of malaria infection. So, human behaviour and practices that contribute to outdoor malaria transmission risks needs to be well understood for identification and allocation of appropriate intervention to prevent mosquito bites and control malaria. These factors include; local knowledge and perceptions, cultural beliefs and norms, behaviours and practices [53]. This study aimed to identify and explore the significance of social and cultural and practices, and their contributions to exposure and existing outdoor malaria transmission, biting experiences and intervention use in Kilombero Valley.

Methods

Study area

This study was conducted from November 2015 to March 2016 in Kilombero Valley, Morogoro region, South-Eastern Tanzania. The valley is approximately 300 metres above sea level, and experiences a short rainy season from late November to January and a long rainy season from mid-February to May. Annual rainfall ranges from 1000 to 1400 mm; annual temperature ranges from 16 to 32 °C [54]. The study was conducted in Lipangalala and Ifakara Town, Kilombero district, and Minepa and Mavimba, Ulanga district (Fig. 1). The main economic activities of people in the area are rice farming and fishing, and in the semi-urban settings of Lipangalala and Ifakara Town, also small-scale businesses. The majority of houses are made with mud bricks walls, with corrugated iron or thatched roofs and small windows that are rarely covered with insect screens [55].

Study design

A descriptive cross-sectional study was conducted using focus group discussions (FGDs), key informant interviews (KIIs) and direct observations. The FGDs stimulated recall and encouraged people to share experiences and opinions, which helped to understand the existing interactions, practices, and opinions on social and cultural practices within the study communities. To complement the FGDs data, KII were conducted to further probe into community practices, the meanings attached

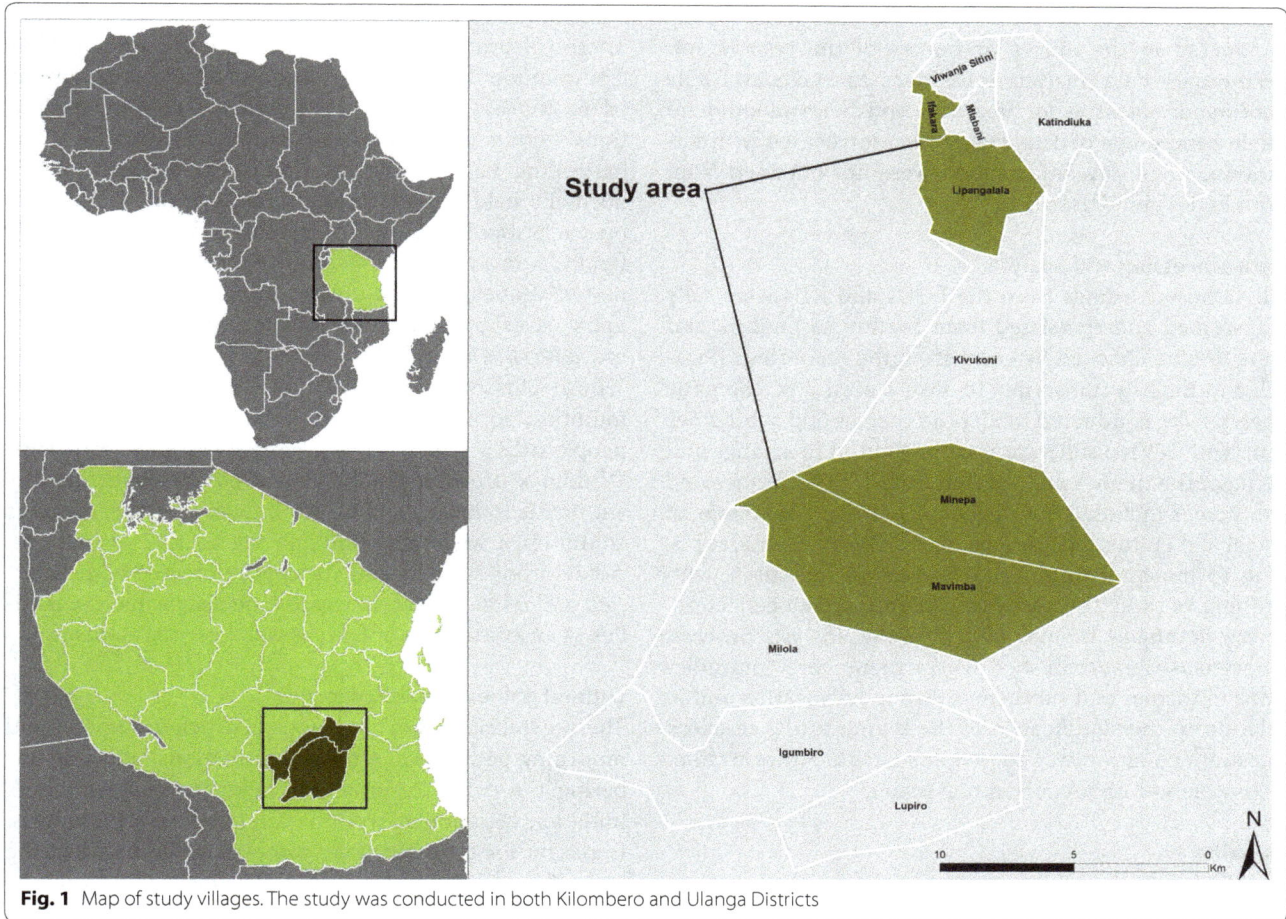

Fig. 1 Map of study villages. The study was conducted in both Kilombero and Ulanga Districts

to them and their importance to the communities. Participants for both FGDs and KIIs were also provided an opportunity to provide recommendations for malaria control. Grounded theory principles guided the study, with theories developing from collected data to generate explanations of relationships and events [56, 57]. In the final stages, thematic analysis was adopted.

Study participants

Purposive sampling was used to select all study participants. FGD participants were selected from community members, with the following inclusion criteria: 18 years or older; either a caregiver or another adult from a household with at least one child below 5 years of age; voluntary agreement to participate in the study. Eight FGDs (two from each study village) were conducted, with 9–11 people per group (total 45 men, 43 women). All groups included both men and women from two ethnic groups such as Ndamba and Pogolo. The similarity to the ethnic groups adhere to the suggested similar characteristics of the FGD participants [58] as among the factors but the

groups were mixed with both sex to stimulate discussion, improve the quality of the discussion, gain comprehensive information on local cultural and social practices within the community and the meanings attached to them [59]. For the KIIs, eight participants (four men, four women) were selected from among village leaders in the four study villages, who were born in the Kilombero Valley or lived in the study villages for at least 10 years.

Data collection

For both FGDs and KIIs, collected data included demographic variables and information on social and cultural gatherings, exposure to mosquitoes, and malaria prevention. All FGDs and KIIs were conducted by the first author in Swahili, the official and widely spoken language. Voluntary informed consent was obtained from each study participants before data collection, including consents for audio recording and note-taking. Venues for the FGDs and KIIs were selected from the study villages according to accessibility and availability. The venues were mostly the primary school classrooms within the study villages for FGDs while for KII were mostly conducted in the offices or homes of the respondent. Preliminary data analysis took place as FGDs and KIIs continued, allowing for iteration and determination of quality and range of data. Data collection ceased with saturation, when new information were not obtained from both FGDs and KIIs.

Data processing and analysis

All audio recordings from the FGDs and KIIs were fully transcribed and translated from Swahili to English, and were double checked by comparing the recordings, Swahili and English transcripts to ensure accuracy. Thematic analysis was conducted to identify themes and subthemes [60], with NVIvo software version 13 used to arrange and connect the themes and subthemes [61]. The themes and subthemes included the range, purpose and meanings of social and cultural gatherings, the timing of events, exposure to mosquito bites, and preventive measures, with probing as these themes emerged during data collection. These dominant themes informed the analysis process. Consensus was established where there were contradictions in themes and subthemes through discussion and in relation to the significance of the theme to the research question, community, and people's health. No contradictions emerged about conceptual issues.

Results

A total of 96 people participated in the study (88 in FGDs; eight KII respondents). Their distribution is provided in Table 1.

Socio-cultural gatherings

Gatherings and celebrations conducted in the study area fell into three primary categories: religious gatherings, cultural celebrations, and other social celebrations.

Religious celebrations

These celebrations were associated with baptism, Holy Communion, confirmation and weddings, and among Islam, Mawlid (the birth of Muhammad). These celebrations were generally planned to coincide with the post-harvesting period. The relevant religious ceremony is normally held indoors in a church, but this is followed by celebrations outdoors at the home of the responsible family. A few celebrations were reported to take place in rented venues, but these are relatively scarce, and have open eaves providing minimal or no protection from mosquito bites.

Both Christianity and Islam are practiced in this communities, so adhering to religious ceremonies provides people with a strong sense of identity among Christians. Weddings provide newly married couples with identity within their local community but also in the religious community, while also fulfilling the social expectations. Adults from 20 years and above are expected to get married and religious weddings are especially valued in families as an affirmation of faith as well as social status.

Cultural gatherings and practices

These gatherings, life course events include funeral and mourning gatherings, children's initiations, and remembering the dead. Respondents indicated that children's initiation ceremonies were held for both boys and girls. Initiation for boys may take place any time between the ages of 7 and 17, and involved circumcision and teaching conducted by the *Ngariba* (the person who conducts circumcision/circumciser). At the time of the research, two types of boys' initiations were conducted, the traditional circumcision and initiation that is mostly practiced in rural Ulanga district, and hospital-based circumcision in urban Kilombero district. Boys' traditional circumcision (*Jando*) is normally conducted in the forest

Table 1 Distribution of FGD and KII respondents by age and sex

Village name

Distribution of respondents for FGDs

Age group	Lipangalala		Ifakara town		Mavimba		Minepa	
	Male	Female	Male	Female	Male	Female	Male	Female
20–29	5	3	3	2	2	3	2	4
30–39	2	1	4	2	4	2	6	4
40–49	3	4	0	5	2	4	3	2
50–59	2	3	3	0	3	2	1	0
Total	12	11	10	11	11	11	12	10
Age distribution of respondents for the KIIs								
All	50	45	72	65	52	49	39	47

without anaesthesia. *Jando* not only base on circumcision, but also involves teachings on how to behave well and the responsibilities of the man in the society [62, 63]. Their stay in the forest is often extending over a period of 2 weeks or more and while in the forest, boys are exposed to mosquito bites, and in most cases, no protection against mosquitoes is used. As one KII then explained, "after coming from *jando*, people prepare for a celebration known as *mtoto katoka sunna*, so people such as family members and neighbours, cook, eat and celebrate" (KII respondent). In contrast, in semi-urban settings of Kilombero district, hospital-based circumcision is increasingly practiced, after which the boys are kept inside their homes to heal. Since they do not participate in forest initiation ceremonies, their risk of exposure to mosquito bites is reduced. However, the hospital-based circumcision is undertaken when children are still young from 6 months to 5 years of age, so the teachings may not be provided and if provided my not be of the level of what is taught at traditional initiations.

For girls, initiation involved teaching only, which is undertaken by a respected senior woman in the family or community such as an aunt who is known as *kungwi (*whose main tasks is to teach girls responsibilities of a woman, how to take care of the house and a man as they are then considered to be old enough to start a family, i.e. soon after first menstruation). The initiation of girls signifies that they have reached adulthood, usually after their first menses and normally kept secret. During such occasions, a group of girls stay in the same household for several days and taught about hygiene, self-care, and sexual behaviour with men, especially after marriage.

The initiations of both boys and girls are followed by commemorative celebrations (*kumtoa sunna* which means "Sunnah" to this society means is the celebration after cleansing the child, which involves prayers and taking the child out of the house after the initiation to celebrate with others [64]) organized by parents and guardians and usually conducted outdoors from day through night and until dawn. The congregation may sometimes consist of more than a hundred people who sit outside celebrating. People recognize the possibility of mosquito bites at such occasions, as one FGD participant noted:

In Ifakara, people have adopted traditions from the *Zaramo* people from the coastal areas. "*Ooh. My daughter has grown, ooh, I have circumcised my child, so I will prepare a sunna (Sunnah) a huge celebration. There are other normal celebrations such as wedding receptions (and) child baptism ... in all these celebrations, mosquitoes get a chance to bite you/people.*" (Respondent, FGD).

Death provides another occasion for communal gathering. As elsewhere in Tanzania, respondents believed

that burying people in their homeland is important to ensure they rest in peace where they belong, and this is portrayed as a way of respecting the deceased and fulfilling their wishes. Death can occur any time, regardless of season and people are expected to provide social support to the bereaved family. As one participant in an FGD reflected, "*the importance of funerals is that there is "God's will," so "kumsitiri mwenzetu" (helping each other during the tough times and do the things as the deceased wishes) is among the ways that we can help our fellow to rest in peace.*" (Respondent, FGD).

Since funerals are rarely timed to the post-harvest period, families of the deceased receive financial assistance from relatives, friends and other community members. Most mourners are women, offering their condolences to the relatives of deceased and performing other activities such as cooking, singing religious songs (*zikiri*) throughout the night, and dancing to please the Gods. Although the deaths of infants or stillbirths are not accompanied by extended celebrations, a simple burial will be attended by the mother and close relatives.

Although respondents had different opinions on the importance and significance of conducting various gatherings and ceremonies, their presence at funerals was seen as maintaining a sense of unity and support among each other; and failure to attend would lead the bereaved to feel isolated from others within the village. For funerals, people also felt it was important to stay overnight at or outside the house of the bereaved family as an expression of support. During these gatherings, the mourners who can be relatives, friends, and neighbors sit outdoors, where they exchange stories, chat and reminisce, sing and pray rather than sleep. While they are outdoors, they are frequently bitten by mosquitoes. There is very minimal use of interventions, although occasionally people use repellents or wear long sleeve clothes to prevent bites. Respondents indicated that use of bed net in an outdoor setting was difficult, but also that it would be considered disrespectful, suggesting lack of compassion to those who had lost their loved one:

"*You cannot come with a net into the house when people are mourning. It suggests you think you are better than the rest of the people who are there*" (Respondent, FGD).

Ceremonies for remembering and pleasing the dead are normally conducted 1 year after a death. These are believed to have cultural significance and are considered to be of great importance. These ceremonies are well prepared, and community members believe that such events are necessary to enable the dead to rest in peace and to prevent misfortune. The ceremonies involve visiting and cleaning the grave, creating a tombstone, and rituals such as particular prayers and chants. Afterwards, people spend time with the bereaved family, providing food to eat, drink and talk. These celebrations are always conducted in the post-harvest period, when people have sufficient food and money from selling their harvest and they are conducted outdoors from day time till dawn, often extended for several days depending on the financial capability of the host. During the post-harvest periods people have less farm work, so ensuring that attendance at such events is optimal. Again respondents reflected on exposure to mosquito bites, as one key informant explained:

"There are these rituals when people gather to celebrate for two days, they cook food, make a local brew, eat and drink together and celebrate. They also pour some local brew on the ground in the belief that they are giving it to their ancestors. These celebrations cannot be done in one day and finished, so most of the time people celebrate for two days. The first day they gather, eat and drink, celebrate the whole night, then in the morning they finalize the celebrations, then celebrate for the second day and finish the following day, and people do not use any prevention from mosquito bites" (Respondent, KII).

"These gatherings are mostly in the dry season because it is the time when people are idle or do not have much to do because they are back from harvest; they are just at home and do not go to the farm anymore, so they may just come up with an idea to do a ceremony. Except for gatherings like funerals and mourning, they can happen anytime" (Respondent, FGD).

In rare cases too, members of the study communities may meet for a certain length of time for family or community issues that require extended discussion and collective decision-making. These discussions too are conducted outdoors in the evening, and mostly preceded by having drinks and foods. Such issues may relate to security and safety, or important government communications, and may be held at any time in the year.

Local economics

The majority of respondents emphasized that the ceremonies were dictated by various personal interests or motivations. Although such gatherings varied in time, place and duration according to the event celebrated, individual interests such as prestige, material, and financial gains were important reasons that motivated hosting or participating in a gathering. Most women in the study communities belonged to various Village Community Bank Groups (VICOBA), to which they contributed a set amount of money on a monthly basis. Group members supported each other in good and hard times, so when a member hosts a ceremony or gathering, other group members attend and provide gifts to the host. As a result, the hosts gain materially from a ceremony such as; clothing and African print cloth *(vitenge)*; household utensils like glassware and dinner sets; and money. During these celebrations (mostly religious events), the majority of supporters and attendees are women and children, but in mourning and funerals children are less comparing to other events.

Agriculture is the main economic activity of people living in Kilombero Valley, with most people engaged in small-scale agriculture for subsistence and small cash returns. Many people depend on their capacity to borrow both personally or from financial institutions to maintain and cultivate their farms then repay after harvest. Most farmers use traditional methods of cultivation, with timing tied to the rainy season. Farming allows people to get by few months after harvest, therefore, purchasing mosquito repellents is less a priority than food and paying school fees. People weigh what is important to them based on the circumstances, and poverty impacts on the use of intervention for malaria prevention in these settings.

"Farmers do not have the ability to buy all the agricultural inputs. As a result one has to borrow them from suppliers/shop owners where they return with interest. Then, yes they got the produce like 50 bags of rice, but they borrowed money for farm preparation and weeding so, after returning all these money, they remain with very little and sometimes remain with five bags for consumption. Still, this person expects to farm the following year, and they do not have any other source of income, so they depend on selling the remaining bags to solve all their problems and meet their needs, such as school fees and medications. It reaches a point that someone does not have any money, so he cannot buy repellent instead of food." (Respondent, KII)

Respondents had mixed views about the overnight celebrations. Some supported their continuation due to the importance of these celebrations in bringing community members together to enhance social bonds. Others did not appreciate their importance and felt they contributed to the risks of being infected by diseases:

"Mosquitoes bite people when they are in gatherings like in places of worship, such as mosques and churches, because they bite people when they are settled and not on the move like dancing or the like. They also bite people who are mourning because

when people get there, they mostly sit down and sleep without protection, hence providing the best opportunity for mosquitoes to bite." (Respondent, FGD).

Most respondents were aware of interventions that repelled mosquitoes when they were outdoors, such as topical repellents and mosquito coils, which they suggest should be freely provided to the communities by the government, but they rarely use them, primarily because of their cost. The most common means of protection that people use are fanning and slapping themselves. A few respondents suggested that some people protected themselves from mosquito bites by wearing heavy pants and long-sleeved tops, but as they pointed out, mosquitoes bite anywhere on the body, mosquitoes could bite through light cloth, protection depended on the thickness of the fabric, and in high temperatures, is was uncomfortable to wear heavy clothing.

Respondents held diverse views about the feasibility of interventions during social and cultural gatherings and ceremonies. Although they acknowledged the need for interventions that could be used to minimize outdoor mosquito bites and possible infection, they also emphasized the need to educate women on the risks of malaria while outdoors, likely associated with women's predominance in various ceremonies, their exposure to bites on an everyday basis when preparing evening meals, and assumptions about their responsibility for infants and children. Further, probably influenced by the association of the first author with the research institute in Ifakara, people emphasized that government should work hand in hand with Malariologists and research organizations to regularly update the community on disease transmission trends and vector behaviour. One FGD participant stated that:

"I'd put more emphasis on organizations, because you as an organization, you mainly focus on this sector. I would advise you to go back and speed up the research on this disease to get the solution. That is my main suggestion because we have been struggling for a very long time." (Respondent, FGD)

Respondents also reiterated their ability to purchase repellents depending on relative poverty and priorities, and several factors hindered the introduction and sustainability of interventions:

"I suggest that wadau (stakeholders) for malaria, like organizations and government, should provide interventions such as repellents at affordable rates or even free of charge so that people can use them during gatherings. It is obvious that people will rate (accept) the need to buy this repellent lotion, but

when comparing the price of buying it with food and salt, due to uchumi (economic situation), they buy food and not repellent, but if they are provided free then people would use them." (Respondent, FGD).

Discussion

Community gatherings and celebrations are viewed as important, reflecting social norms and local traditions, and providing participants with mutual support, opportunities for socialization and community engagement. Life cycle events, including traditional initiation ceremonies, baptisms and weddings, are vital moments in the socialization of young people, providing sexual education, guidelines regarding gender norms, and norms and expectations as adult members of kinship networks and the community. The support that people provide each other over time at funerals and through an extended period of mourning, and at celebrations such as baptisms, weddings and the prophet's birthday, are given high priority. In addition, sleeping at the houses of bereaved villagers, helping each other financially and during preparation of events help build and maintain social capital and inclusion. The beliefs that sustain these events reflect strong understandings of what is the "right way" to do things, and the value of reciprocity and collective action.

The life cycle events, celebrations and gatherings around death, and intermittent community gatherings related to government policy and local politics and economics, provide personal satisfaction as well as benefitting the group [65]. There is, as noted above, both tangible benefits and prestige value to hosts when they initiate a celebration, and those who host an event for a long period than others, extending for more than 2 or 3 days, are evidently wealthier and able. People compare and contrast themselves and others in terms of largesse and power, and in this context, are likely to spend money to host a party while they cannot afford to purchase repellents, which might protect them from mosquito bites. At the same time, the amount of money spent on ceremonies and celebratory gatherings is reciprocated over time. Celebrations that are conducted outdoors were reported as associated with mosquito bites, but the social significance and consequences of participating in such events outweigh the importance of using interventions while outdoors. However, similar findings on the importance of community social norms against intervention use was also observed in Uganda where net use during community gatherings outdoors was observed to indicates ones feel proud [66].

Malaria prevention is viewed within the study community as a shared responsibility of the government and researchers. However, malaria prevention, control and elimination need a collective approach that includes the sustained used of vector control to prevent human-mosquito contact, treatment, and surveillance. In the study villages, increasing outdoor feeding by malaria vectors has been documented [34, 35, 44, 67, 68], but emphasis is still placed on the distribution and use of bed nets only which primarily prevent individual infection while sleeping indoors [69]. In order to move closer to elimination, however, there is a need to change the approaches to designing, implementing and evaluating interventions for malaria in Tanzania by taking into consideration the social and ecological aspects of continued and residual transmission. Policy-makers need to consider social, cultural and behavioural factors associated with risk of infection when designing malaria prevention strategies. One approach is to adapt the model developed by Bronfenbrenner [70], which was used in a study by Panter-Brick et al. [53], which contributed to identification of both social and cultural factors for risks in malaria, intervention use, community participation as well as reduction of malaria impact to the communty (Fig. 2). This explains that individual behaviour is influenced by environmental factors, including people's social, institutional and cultural contexts and the beliefs and attitudes that

influence and shape the social, political and economic conditions of a given society. The model helps to explain the importance of different parts of the system in a given society, and how its members relate and influence each other.

Conclusion

People do not use interventions in the evening when outdoors during social and cultural practices and celebrations. Spending time outdoors to participate in social events, in accordance with cultural norms, expose people to mosquito bites and increase the risk of malaria infection. During such gatherings, the use of interventions to prevent bites is rare. Such gatherings not only provide opportunities for collaboration and contribute to cohesion, but also personal satisfaction and personal identity.

The increasing rate of outdoor feeding of the primary vectors of malaria in the study area, coincident with the use of outdoor areas for everyday activities and for ceremonial and social purposes, point to the need for effective interventions. There is over dependency on current interventions, primarily long lasting insecticide-impregnated bed nets, and single interventions should not be used as "one size fits all," since transmission risks and

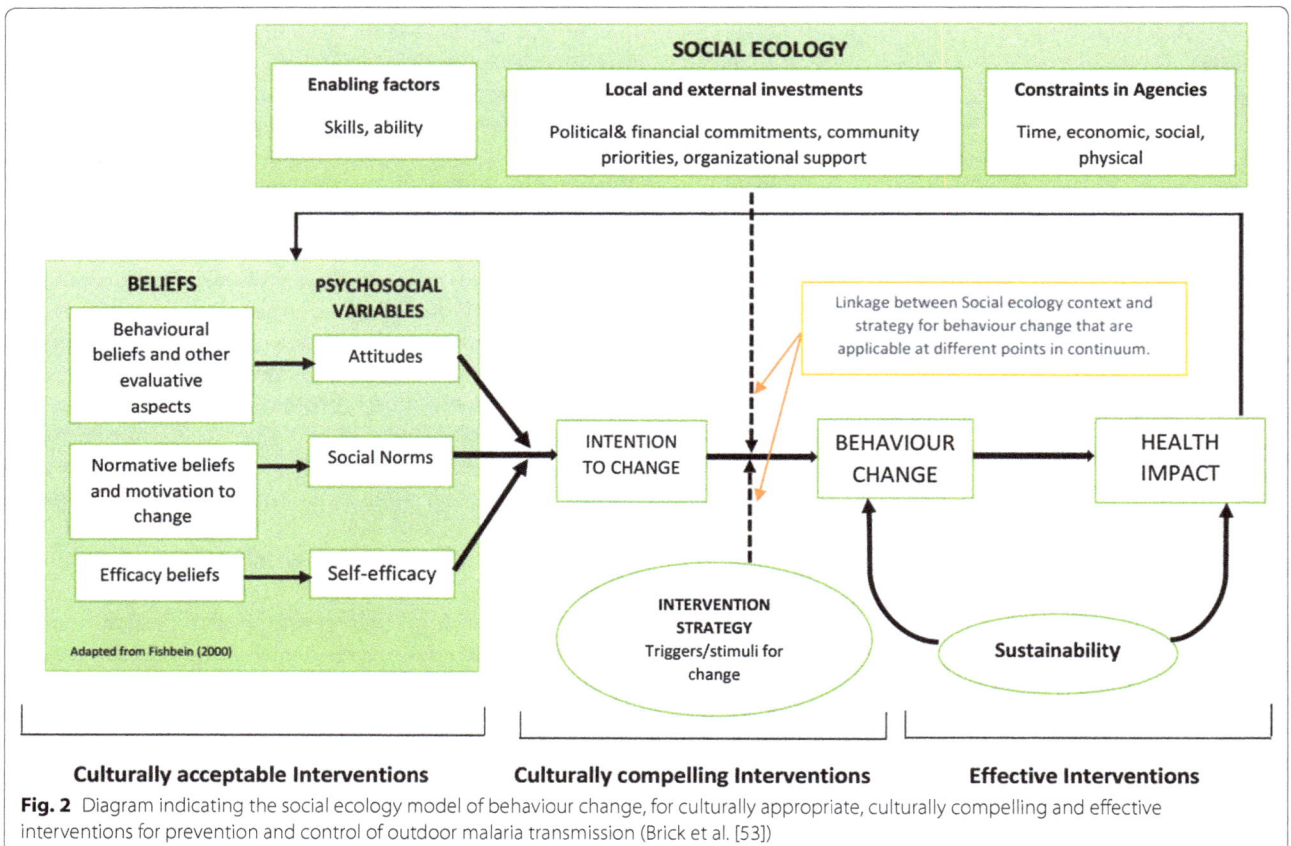

Fig. 2 Diagram indicating the social ecology model of behaviour change, for culturally appropriate, culturally compelling and effective interventions for prevention and control of outdoor malaria transmission (Brick et al. [53])

intensity differ among areas [39]. Although respondents were aware of the risks of infection, further community education on the risks of outdoor malaria and the use of repellents may reduce negative perceptions on the interventions, such as repellents which is perceived to cause skin cancer [71] and increase the uptake of their use. The approach for malaria prevention needs to be culturally compelling [53], despite that area specific interventions, using a social-ecological model that incorporates social, cultural and environment factors, may appear to be expensive but will become inevitable as a strategy for malaria elimination [39]. Interventions are needed that are affordable and can be used during ceremonies and for general protection outdoors, complementing existing methods to prevent indoor transmission.

Abbreviations
FGD: focus group discussion; IRS: insecticide residual spray; KII: key informant interview; LLINs: long-lasting insecticide nets; RDT: rapid diagnostic test; SSA: sub-Sahara Africa.

Authors' contributions
IRM and FOO conceived and designed the research study. LLM and LM supervised the study and were involved in reviewing the study protocol, data analysis, and all drafts of the manuscript. YPM also contributed in preparation and drawing of a map of the study site, HSN has highly contributed to the data collection procedures and actual data collection. All authors read and approved the final manuscript.

Author details
[1] Environmental Health and Ecological Sciences Department, Ifakara Health Institute, Kiko Avenue, Mikocheni, PO Box 78373, Dar es Salaam, United Republic of Tanzania. [2] School of Public Health, Faculty of Health Sciences, University of the Witwatersrand, Parktown, Johannesburg, South Africa. [3] Swiss Tropical and Public Health Institute (Swiss TPH), Basel, Switzerland. [4] University of Basel, Basel, Switzerland. [5] Sokoine University of Agriculture, Pest Management Centre, P.O. Box 3110, Morogoro, Tanzania. [6] Institut de Recherche en Sciences de la Santé, Bobo-Dioulasso, Burkina Faso. [7] Institute of Biodiversity, Animal Health and Comparative Medicine, University of Glasgow, Glasgow G12 8QQ, UK.

Acknowledgements
This research was supported by the Consortium for Advanced Research Training in Africa (CARTA). CARTA is jointly led by the African Population and Health Research Center and the University of the Witwatersrand. We are thankful for the support from and participation in the study by the community members from Kilombero Valley as well as volunteers, technicians, Shraddha Bajaria for assistance in English grammar check and Sara Mtali for assistance during fieldwork (who are all IHI staff). We also, thank CARTA and University of Witwatersrand for both financial assistance and guidance throughout the study,

Competing interests
The authors declare that they have no competing interests.

Funding
This work was funded by the Consortium for Advanced Research Training in Africa (CARTA). CARTA is jointly led by the African Population and Health Research Center and the University of the Witwatersrand. This Consortium is jointly funded by the Carnegie Corporation of New York (Grant No–B 8606.R02), Sida (Grant No: 54100029), the DELTAS Africa Initiative (Grant No: 107768/Z/15/Z). The DELTAS Africa Initiative is an Independent funding scheme of the African Academy of Science (AAS)'s Alliance for Accelerating Excellence in Science in Africa (AESA) and supported by the New Partnership for Africa's Development Planning and Coordinating Agency (NEPAD Agency) with funding from the Wellcome Trust (UK) and the UK government. This research was also supported by a Welcome Trust Post-Doctoral Fellowship and Bill and Melinda Gates Foundation, Grand Challenges Canada.

References
1. WHO. World Malaria Report. Geneva: World Health Organization; 2016.
2. Bhatt S, Weiss D, Cameron E, Bisanzio D, Mappin B, Dalrymple U, et al. The effect of malaria control on *Plasmodium falciparum* in Africa between 2000 and 2015. Nature. 2015;526:207–11.
3. O'Meara WP, Mangeni JN, Steketee R, Greenwood B. Changes in the burden of malaria in sub-Saharan Africa. Lancet Infect Dis. 2010;10:545–55.
4. Ossè RA, Aïkpon R, Gbédjissi GL, Gnanguenon V, Sèzonlin M, Govoétchan R, et al. A shift from Indoor Residual Spraying (IRS) with bendiocarb to Long-Lasting Insecticidal (mosquito) Nets (LLINs) associated with changes in malaria transmission indicators in pyrethroid resistance areas in Benin. Parasit Vectors. 2013;6:73.
5. Steketee RW, Campbell CC. Impact of national malaria control scale-up programmes in Africa: magnitude and attribution of effects. Malar J. 2010;9:299.
6. Hawley WA, Phillips-Howard PA, ter Kuile FO, Terlouw DJ, Vulule JM, Ombok M, et al. Community-wide effects of permethrin-treated bed nets on child mortality and malaria morbidity in western Kenya. Am J Trop Med Hyg. 2003;68:121–7.
7. Killeen GF, Kihonda J, Lyimo E, Oketch FR, Kotas ME, Mathenge E, et al. Quantifying behavioural interactions between humans and mosquitoes: evaluating the protective efficacy of insecticidal nets against malaria transmission in rural Tanzania. BMC Infect Dis. 2006;6:161.
8. Killeen GF, Smith TA, Ferguson HM, Mshinda H, Abdulla S, Lengeler C, et al. Preventing childhood malaria in Africa by protecting adults from mosquitoes with insecticide-treated nets. PLoS Med. 2007;4:e229.
9. Schellenberg J, Abdulla S, Nathan R, Mukasa O, Marchant TJ, Kikumbih N, et al. Effect of large-scale social marketing of insecticide-treated nets on child survival in rural Tanzania. Lancet. 2001;357:1241–7.
10. WHO. World Malaria Report. Geneva: World Health Organization; 2017.
11. President Malaria Initiative. Fighting malaria and saving lives. Dar es Salaam: USAID-PMI; 2018.
12. Ishengoma DS, Mmbando BP, Alifrangis M, Lemnge MM, Bygbjerg IC. Declining burden of malaria over two decades in a rural community of Muheza district, north-eastern Tanzania. Malar J. 2013;12:338.

13. Mmbando BP, Vestergaard LS, Kitua AY, Lemnge MM, Theander TG, Lusingu JP. A progressive declining in the burden of malaria in north-eastern Tanzania. Malar J. 2010;9:216.

14. Mtove G, Amos B, Nadjm B, Hendriksen IC, Dondorp AM, Mwambuli A, et al. Decreasing incidence of severe malaria and community-acquired bacteraemia among hospitalized children in Muheza, north-eastern Tanzania, 2006–2010. Malar J. 2011;10:320.

15. Rutta AS, Francis F, Mmbando BP, Ishengoma DS, Sembuche SH, Malecela EK, et al. Using community-owned resource persons to provide early diagnosis and treatment and estimate malaria burden at community level in north-eastern Tanzania. Malar J. 2012;11:152.

16. Prapanthadara L, Hemingway J, Ketterman AJ. DDT-resistance in Anopheles gambiae (Diptera: Culicidae) from Zanzibar, Tanzania, based on increased DDT-dehydrochlorinase activity of glutathione S-transferases. Bull Entomol Res. 1995;85:267–74.

17. Ranson H, N'Guessan R, Lines J, Moiroux N, Nkuni Z, Corbel V. Pyrethroid resistance in African anopheline mosquitoes: what are the implications for malaria control? Trends Parasitol. 2011;27:91–8.

18. Trape J-F, Tall A, Diagne N, Ndiath O, Ly AB, Faye J, et al. Malaria morbidity and pyrethroid resistance after the introduction of insecticide-treated bednets and artemisinin-based combination therapies: a longitudinal study. Lancet Infect Dis. 2011;11:925–32.

19. United Republic of Tanzania. Tanzania demographic and health survey and malaria indicator survey 2015–2016. Dar es Salaam, 2016.

20. Kitau J, Oxborough RM, Tungu PK, Matowo J, Malima RC, Magesa SM, et al. Species shifts in the Anopheles gambiae complex: do LLINs successfully control Anopheles arabiensis? PLoS ONE. 2012;7:e31481.

21. Kouznetsov R. Malaria control by application of indoor spraying of residual insecticides in tropical Africa and its impact on community health. Trop Doctor. 1977;7:81–91.

22. Muirhead-Thomson R. The significance of irritability, behaviouristic avoidance and allied phenomena in malaria eradication. Bull World Health Organ. 1960;22:721.

23. Okumu FO, Kiware SS, Moore SJ, Killeen GF. Mathematical evaluation of community level impact of combining bed nets and indoor residual spraying upon malaria transmission in areas where the main vectors are Anopheles arabiensis mosquitoes. Parasit Vectors. 2013;6:17.

24. Martens W, Niessen LW, Rotmans J, Jetten TH, McMichael AJ. Potential impact of global climate change on malaria risk. Environ Health Perspect. 1995;103:458–64.

25. Lindblade KA, Walker ED, Onapa AW, Katungu J, Wilson ML. Land use change alters malaria transmission parameters by modifying temperature in a highland area of Uganda. Trop Med Int Health. 2000;5:263–74.

26. Patz JA, Graczyk TK, Geller N, Vittor AY. Effects of environmental change on emerging parasitic diseases. Int J Parasitol. 2000;30:1395–405.

27. Kiware SS, Chitnis N, Moore SJ, Devine GJ, Majambere S, Merrill S, et al. Simplified models of vector control impact upon malaria transmission by zoophagic mosquitoes. PLoS ONE. 2012;7:e37661.

28. Nkya TE, Akhouayri I, Poupardin R, Batengana B, Mosha F, Magesa S, et al. Insecticide resistance mechanisms associated with different environments in the malaria vector Anopheles gambiae: a case study in Tanzania. Malar J. 2014;13:28.

29. Ranson H, Abdallah H, Badolo A, Guelbeogo WM, Kerah-Hinzoumbé C, Yangalbé-Kalnoné E, et al. Insecticide resistance in Anopheles gambiae: data from the first year of a multi-country study highlight the extent of the problem. Malar J. 2009;8:299.

30. Ranson H, Lissenden N. Insecticide resistance in African Anopheles mosquitoes: a worsening situation that needs urgent action to maintain malaria control. Trends Parasitol. 2016;32:187–96.

31. Ferguson HM, Dornhaus A, Beeche A, Borgemeister C, Gottlieb M, Mulla MS, et al. Ecology: a prerequisite for malaria elimination and eradication. PLoS Med. 2010;7:e1000303.

32. Killeen GF. A second chance to tackle African malaria vector mosquitoes that avoid houses and don't take drugs. Am J Trop Med Hyg. 2013;88:809–16.

33. Govella NJ, Chaki PP, Killeen GF. Entomological surveillance of behavioural resilience and resistance in residual malaria vector populations. Malar J. 2013;12:124.

34. Kaindoa EW, Matowo NS, Ngowo HS, Mkandawile G, Mmbando A, Finda M, et al. Interventions that effectively target Anopheles funestus mosquitoes could significantly improve control of persistent malaria transmission in south–eastern Tanzania. PLoS ONE. 2017;12:e0177807.

35. Lwetoijera DW, Harris C, Kiware SS, Dongus S, Devine GJ, McCall PJ, et al. Increasing role of Anopheles funestus and Anopheles arabiensis in malaria transmission in the Kilombero Valley, Tanzania. Malar J. 2014;13:331.

36. Durnez L, Coosemans M. Residual transmission of malaria: an old issue for new approaches. In: Anopheles mosquitoes—New insights into malaria vectors (S. Manguin, Ed). Intech; 2013.

37. Russell TL, Beebe NW, Cooper RD, Lobo NF, Burkot TR. Successful malaria elimination strategies require interventions that target changing vector behaviours. Malar J. 2013;12:56.

38. Zhu L, Müller GC, Marshall JM, Arheart KL, Qualls WA, Hlaing WM, et al. Is outdoor vector control needed for malaria elimination? An individual-based modelling study. Malar J. 2017;16:266.

39. WHO. A framework for malaria elimination. Geneva: World Health Organization; 2017.

40. Bayoh MN, Mathias DK, Odiere MR, Mutuku FM, Kamau L, Gimnig JE, et al. Anopheles gambiae: historical population decline associated with regional distribution of insecticide-treated bed nets in western Nyanza Province, Kenya. Malar J. 2010;9:1.

41. Gillies MT, Furlong M. An investigation into the behaviour of Anopheles parensis Gillies at Malindi on the Kenya coast. Bull Entomol Res. 1964;55:1–16.

42. Reddy MR, Overgaard HJ, Abaga S, Reddy VP, Caccone A, Kiszewski AE, et al. Outdoor host seeking behaviour of Anopheles gambiae mosquitoes following initiation of malaria vector control on Bioko Island, Equatorial Guinea. Malar J. 2011;10:184.

43. Renggli S, Mandike R, Kramer K, Patrick F, Brown NJ, McElroy PD, et al. Design, implementation and evaluation of a national campaign to deliver 18 million free long-lasting insecticidal nets to uncovered sleeping spaces in Tanzania. Malar J. 2013;12:85.

44. Russell TL, Govella NJ, Azizi S, Drakeley CJ, Kachur SP, Killeen GF. Increased proportions of outdoor feeding among residual malaria vector populations following increased use of insecticide-treated nets in rural Tanzania. Malar J. 2011;10:80.

45. Russell TL, Lwetoijera DW, Maliti D, Chipwaza B, Kihonda J, Charlwood JD, et al. Impact of promoting longer-lasting insecticide treatment of bed nets upon malaria transmission in a rural Tanzanian setting with pre-existing high coverage of untreated nets. Malar J. 2010;9:187.

46. Dunn CE, Le Mare A, Makungu C. Malaria risk behaviours, socio-cultural practices and rural livelihoods in southern Tanzania: implications for bednet usage. Soc Sci Med. 2011;72:408–17.

47. Adongo PB, Kirkwood B, Kendall C. How local community knowledge about malaria affects insecticide-treated net use in northern Ghana. Trop Med Int Health. 2005;10:366–78.

48. Atkinson JM, Fitzgerald L, Toaliu H, Taleo G, Tynan A, Whittaker M, et al. Community participation for malaria elimination in Tafea Province, Vanuatu: Part I Maintaining motivation for prevention practices in the context of disappearing disease. Malar J. 2010;9:93.

49. Mazigo HD, Obasy E, Mauka W, Manyiri P, Zinga M, Kweka EJ, et al. Knowledge, attitudes, and practices about malaria and its control in rural northwest Tanzania. Malar Res Treatment. 2010;2010.

50. Nieto T, Méndez F, Carrasquilla G. Knowledge, beliefs and practices relevant for malaria control in an endemic urban area of the Colombian Pacific. Soc Sci Med. 1999;49:601–9.

51. Harchut K, Standley C, Dobson A, Klaassen B, Rambaud-Althaus C, Althaus F, et al. Over-diagnosis of malaria by microscopy in the Kilombero Valley, Southern Tanzania: an evaluation of the utility and cost-effectiveness of rapid diagnostic tests. Malar J. 2013;12:159.

52. Dunn CE, Le Mare A, Makungu C. Malaria risk behaviours, socio-cultural practices and rural livelihoods in southern Tanzania: implications for bednet usage. Soc Sci Med. 2010;72:408–17.

53. Panter-Brick C, Clarke SE, Lomas H, Pinder M, Lindsay SW. Culturally compelling strategies for behaviour change: a social ecology model and case study in malaria prevention. Soc Sci Med. 2006;62:2810–25.

54. Bekker C, Rance W, Monteuuis O. Teak in Tanzania. II. The Kilombero Valley Teak Company. Bois et forêts des Tropiques. 2004;279:1.

55. Ogoma SB, Lwetoijera DW, Ngonyani H, Furer B, Russell TL, Mukabana WR, et al. Screening mosquito house entry points as a potential method for integrated control of endophagic filariasis, arbovirus and malaria vectors. PLoS Negl Trop Dis. 2010;4:e773.

56. Strauss A, Corbin J. Basics of qualitative research: Techniques and procedures for developing grounded theory. Sage Publications, Inc; 1998.

57. Strauss A, Corbin JM. Grounded theory in practice. Thousand Oaks: Sage Publications, Inc; 1997.

58. Krueger RA. Focus groups: a practical guide for applied research. Thousand Oaks: Sage Publications, Inc; 2014.

59. Freitas H, Oliveira M, Jenkins M, Popjoy O. The Focus Group, a qualitative research method. JISRC Working Paper. 1998;010298.

60. Weber RP. Basic content analysis. Thousand Oaks: Sage Publications, Inc; 1990.

61. Bringer JD, Johnston LH, Brackenridge CH. Using computer-assisted qualitative data analysis software to develop a grounded theory project. Field Methods. 2006;18:245–66.

62. Jens F. Traditional Music and Cultures of Kenya: Kikuyu- Circumcision. 2000–2003.

63. A Culture of Circumcision in the Kurya Tribe of Tanzania. https://blog.compassion.com/circumcision-in-africa-a-culture-of-circumcision-in-the-kurya-tribe-of-tanzania/.

64. 3 Meanings of Sunnah. http://aboutislam.net/shariah/hadith/hadith-faqs/3-meanings-sunnah/.

65. Azar OH. What sustains social norms and how they evolve? The case of tipping. J Econ Behav Organ. 2004;54:49–64.

66. Monroe A, Harvey SA, Lam Y, Muhangi D, Loll D, Kabali AT, et al. "People will say that I am proud": a qualitative study of barriers to bed net use away from home in four Ugandan districts. Malar J. 2014;13:82.

67. Matowo NS, Moore J, Mapua S, Madumla EP, Moshi IR, Kaindoa EW, et al. Using a new odour-baited device to explore options for luring and killing outdoor-biting malaria vectors: a report on design and field evaluation of the Mosquito Landing Box. Parasit Vectors. 2013;6:137.

68. Okumu FO, Sumaye RD, Matowo NS, Mwangungulu SP, Kaindoa EW, Moshi IR, et al. Outdoor mosquito control using odour-baited devices: development and evaluation of a potential new strategy to complement indoor malaria prevention methods. Malar World J. 2013;4:8.

69. Programme National Malaria Control. National malaria strategic plan 2014–2020. Dar es Salaam: The United Republic of Tanzania; 2014.

70. Bronfenbrenner U. International encyclopedia of education. Oxford: Elsevier; 1994.

71. Moshi IR, Ngowo H, Dillip A, Msellemu D, Madumla EP, Okumu FO, et al. Community perceptions on outdoor malaria transmission in Kilombero Valley, Southern Tanzania. Malar J. 2017;16:274.

16

Combination of PURE-DNA extraction and LAMP-DNA amplification methods for accurate malaria diagnosis on dried blood spots

Jeanne Perpétue Vincent[1,2], Kanako Komaki-Yasuda[1], Moritoshi Iwagami[1,4], Satoru Kawai[3,4] and Shigeyuki Kano[1,2,4*] (iD)

Abstract

Background: Malaria is one of the most important parasitic infectious diseases for which almost half of the world's population is at risk. Although several diagnostic methods are now available to detect the infection, more sensitive and applicable tests are still required in the field. The loop-mediated isothermal amplification (LAMP) method is a DNA amplification tool in which the DNA amplification can be achieved by incubation at a stable temperature. A malaria detection kit based on this methodology has already been commercialized and is being used in some countries. The kit includes two reaction tubes: one targeting the common *Plasmodium* genus (Pan tube) and the other specifically targeting *Plasmodium falciparum* (Pf tube). In parallel, a simple DNA extraction method, the procedure for ultra rapid extraction (PURE), which can produce a DNA solution suitable for the LAMP reaction without the use of a centrifuge, has also become available. In this study, the sensitivity of the combination of the PURE and LAMP methods (PURE–LAMP) was evaluated with archived dried clinical blood samples of imported malaria cases, including *P. falciparum*, *Plasmodium vivax*, *Plasmodium ovale*, and *Plasmodium malariae*.

Results: Using a nested PCR as the reference, 117 samples including 46 *P. falciparum*, 7 *P. vivax*, 9 *P. ovale*, 4 *P. malariae*, and 51 negative cases were tested. The PURE–LAMP Pan correctly identified 64 of the 66 positives and the 51 negatives. Among the Pan-positive samples 45 *P. falciparum* were also detected with the PURE–LAMP Pf. The PURE–LAMP Pan and PURE–LAMP Pf had respective sensitivities of 96.96% (95% CI 89.47–99.63) and 97.82% (95% CI 88.47–99.94) and common specificity of 1.

Conclusion: The PURE–LAMP system is accurate when used with dried blood spots and extendable to the field.

Keywords: Malaria diagnosis, Procedure for ultra rapid extraction (PURE), Loop-mediated isothermal amplification (LAMP), Dried blood spots (DBS), Nested PCR

*Correspondence: kano@ri.ncgm.go.jp
[1] Department of Tropical Medicine and Malaria, Research Institute, National Center for Global Health and Medicine, Tokyo 162-8655, Japan
Full list of author information is available at the end of the article

Background

As one of the world's major infectious diseases, malaria totaled around 216 million cases in 2016 [1]. Since the discovery of the parasites in human erythrocytes by Laveran in 1880, the capacity for malaria diagnosis has been paired with the development of biomedical techniques [2–4]. However, the observation of Giemsa-stained parasites under light microscopy remains the gold standard diagnostic technique. It presents various advantages such as allowing estimation of parasitaemia, evaluation of parasite morphology, differentiation between *Plasmodium* species or sometimes with other causes of fever, and economic affordability. Nevertheless, it can only diagnose parasitaemia with about 10–100 parasites/μL, and its sensitivity varies depending on the microscopist's skill and the quality of the smear [5]. Rapid diagnostic tests (RDT) based on immunochromatography are also commonly used for malaria diagnosis. They are an extremely convenient point-of-care diagnostic method as they require no electrical power, no special skills, and results can be easily obtained within 15 min. Although they perform with high sensitivity on *Plasmodium falciparum* infections of ≥ 100 parasites/μL, they are less accurate for other species. Furthermore, false-positive results are not rare; HRP-2 Pf-specific antigen detection by RDT is useless for the evaluation of recent treatment due to its persistence in the blood for weeks after treatment [6, 7].

In endemic fields, differential diagnosis with other tropical diseases is of great importance; confirmation of the diagnosis before treatment prevents unnecessary exposure to drugs, which can facilitate the rise of drug-resistant parasites. This is also important from the point of view of preventing unnecessary risk of adverse drug reactions and wastefulness. This optimizes treatment, and even ruling out malaria will help to shift the focus to other possible causes.

Parasitological diagnosis by microscopy or RDT is recommended by the World Health Organization on all suspected malaria cases whenever either method is accessible [8]. Polymerase chain reaction (PCR) offers a lower limit of detection. Nested PCR limits of 0.4 and 0.05 parasites/μL have been reported, but it is barely applicable for routine diagnosis in endemic malaria fields due to its technical and economical requirements [9–11]. While these three methods are useful and bear different advantages to fit varied settings, none combines the accuracy of the nested PCR and field friendliness of the RDT.

In 2000, loop-mediated isothermal amplification (LAMP) became available as a novel DNA amplification and detection tool that was reported to operate at a sensitivity similar to that of PCR [12]. This amplification method uses four primers specifically designed to allow formation of a loop-structured complement of the target DNA by strand displacement. Such loop-structured DNA are later amplified at a stable temperature (~ 65 °C) and detected by the presence of magnesium pyrophosphate (by-product of DNA amplification) using a turbidimeter or calcein (released from its quenched state during amplification) fluorescence under ultraviolet light excitation.

Efforts to produce more accurate and field-friendly malaria diagnostic methods has given birth to several assays based on the LAMP [13–17]. Among them, the Loopamp™ Malaria Pan/Pf Detection Kit (Eiken Chemical, Tokyo, Japan) is the first LAMP kit for the detection of malaria parasites to be commercialized in field-friendly packaging containing tubes filled with reagents stable at room temperature. The Loopamp kit includes two types of reaction tubes: one with primers targeting the DNA sequence of the common *Plasmodium* genus (Pan tube), and the other specifically targeting that of *P. falciparum* (Pf tube). Thus, it allows the diagnosis of malaria and detects whether the causal agent(s) involve *P. falciparum* or other *Plasmodium* species. In parallel, a simple DNA extraction method, the procedure for ultra rapid extraction (PURE, Eiken Chemical), which produces DNA solution suitable for the LAMP reaction without the use of a centrifuge, has also been supplied. A study previously reported the Loopamp kit to be accurate for the detection of plasmodial DNA from dried blood samples on filter paper coupled with a conventional DNA extraction method [18]. In the present study, the accuracy of Loopamp malaria detection using DNA extracted from dried blood samples by the PURE method was evaluated in comparison to standard diagnosis by nested PCR, microscopy, and RDT. Hereafter, the term PURE–LAMP is used to refer to the combination of the PURE and Loopamp methods.

Methods

Blood samples

The samples included in this study were collected by venipuncture from patients who consulted the Center Hospital of the National Center for Global Health and Medicine (NCGM, Tokyo). The diagnosis of malaria was achieved with a combination of microscopic observation, RDT and nested PCR with these patients' blood samples. To conduct PURE–LAMP, dried blood samples stored at room temperature on paper of a single-well preservation plate (WATSON, Tokyo, Japan) were used, and the results were retrospectively compared. One hundred and seventeen samples diagnosed in the period from July 2011 through December 2016 were included. The storage length before performing PURE–LAMP varied between the samples: roughly, the shortest period was 2 weeks and the longest was 5 years (Additional file 1).

Microscopic diagnosis

The microscopic diagnosis was conducted by expert microscopists on light microscopes with Giemsa-stained thin blood smears. Malaria-negative samples were declared after counting ≥ 200,000 erythrocytes.

RDT

RDT were conducted using BinaxNow® Malaria (Alere Inc., Waltham, MA, USA). The test includes T1 and T2 bands. The T1 band contains the antibody for detection of a *P. falciparum*-specific HRP2 antigen, whereas the T2 band contains the antibody for detection of a *Plasmodium* common aldolase antigen. Pale bands were counted as positive.

DNA extraction from patient blood samples

To obtain the template DNA used in the PCR reactions, several methods indicated below were utilized. In many cases, DNA was extracted from 200 µL of fresh blood or 100 µL of frozen RBC concentrate using a QIAamp® DNA Mini Kit (QIAGEN, Hilden, Germany). An automated DNA extraction system, the Maxwell RSC Instrument (Promega, Madison, WI, USA), was also used. With this instrument, DNA samples were extracted from 200 µL of fresh blood or 100 µL of frozen RBC concentrate with a Maxwell RSC Blood DNA Kit (Promega), and after purification steps, DNA samples were eluted in 50 or 100 µL of elution buffer. In other cases, DNA were extracted from 3 dried blood spots (DBS) of φ 3 mm using a Maxwell RSC DNA FFPE Kit (Promega) with the automated Maxwell RSC Instrument, and DNA was eluted in 50 µL of buffer.

Nested PCR

Two protocols were used for the nested PCR [19, 20]. In both protocols, the first PCR was conducted with primers targeting the universal partial sequences of the 18S ribosomal RNA (rRNA) gene of the *Plasmodium* genus. For the second PCR, dilutions of the first PCR products were used as templates along with a species-specific primer for each human Plasmodium species per tube.

Sequencing analysis

Samples diagnosed as *Plasmodium ovale* were further defined into subspecies by sequencing of 365 nucleotides of the 18S rRNA gene. A nested PCR was designed for amplification of *P. ovale*-specific sequences. For the first PCR, 2 µL of template DNA eluted from the patient's blood was added into 25 µL of reaction mix; a forward primer, F1 (5′-CTGGTGCCAGCAGCCGCGGTA-3′)

and a reverse primer, R1 (5′-ATGAGAAATCAAAGT CTTTGGGTTC-3′), which are targeting a segment of ~ 660 bp of the *P. ovale* universal 18S rRNA gene, were used. After 1000-fold dilution of the first PCR product, 2 µL was added as template in 20 µL of the second PCR reaction mix with an inner forward primer, F2 (5′-CTG CGTTTGAATACTACAGCATGGA-3′), and the same reverse primer, R1. PrimeSTAR GXL DNA Polymerase (TaKaRa Bio Inc., Kusatsu, Japan) was used for both PCR reactions. After sequencing of the secondary amplicons, the subspecies were determined by sequence homology with the same genes of *P. ovale* subspecies registered in the GenBank sequence database (accession numbers AB182489 and AB182490 for *P. o. curtisi* and AB182491, AB182492, and AB182493 for *P. o. wallikeri*).

PURE DNA extraction and LAMP reaction

DNA was extracted using the Loopamp™ PURE DNA Extraction Kit (Eiken Chemical) according to the manufacturer's supplied protocol. Briefly, 3 DBS of φ 3 mm were punched into the heating tube containing extraction buffer, mixed by shaking and placed in a heating block (Loopamp™ LF-160, Eiken Chemical) at 75 °C for 5 min. After a rough powder purification of the lysate, the DNA-containing solution was eluted through an injection cap.

The LAMP reactions with the Loopamp™ MALARIA Pan/Pf Detection Kit were performed using 30 µL of the PURE-extracted DNA placed on a Loopamp™ LF-160 reaction block at 65 °C for 40 min followed by 5 min of incubation at 80 °C for enzyme inactivation. Each run was loaded with negative and positive controls, which were supplied in the kit. The results were evaluated by observation of fluorescence under excitation with an ultraviolet lamp incorporated into the same apparatus.

Limit of detection

The PURE–LAMP limit of detection was analysed using infected human blood of known parasitaemia. Cultured *P. falciparum* strain FCR3 were synchronized with 5% D-sorbitol, and 40-h post-synchronization ring stage-infected RBCs were harvested, observed under 1000× light microscopy to determine parasitaemia, and dissolved in human whole blood to reach a concentration of 1000 parasites/µL. Series of 10× dilutions were prepared until the concentration reached 10^{-3} parasites/µL. A part of these blood samples was seeded on filter paper on the same day, and 30 µL was used to conduct the PURE–LAMP. After 3 months of storage at room temperature, the PURE–LAMP was repeated using 3 DBS of φ 3 mm. The PURE–LAMP could sometimes detect up to 0.1 parasite/µL in fresh blood but always 1 parasite/µL. The limit of detection of 1 parasite/µL was sustained with the DBS.

Statistical analysis

Sensitivity [true positive/(true positive + false negative)] and specificity [true negative/(true negative + false positive)] with their exact 95% confidence interval were estimated using nested PCR as the gold-standard reference. Stata ver. 14.2 (StataCorp, College Station, TX, USA) was used for statistical analysis.

Results

Overview of the clinical samples used in this study

One hundred and seventeen samples were retrospectively analysed. A range of 7–19 positive cases was diagnosed per year (Additional file 1). The places of travel included countries in Africa, South America, Asia, and the West-Pacific region. Africa (66.66%) was the most prevalent region of provenance reported among the subjects, with

histories of travel from Uganda (8 cases/10 samples) on top for number of positives. India was the most common country of provenance (2 cases/11 samples).

There were 46 (39.32%) cases of *P. falciparum*, 9 (7.69%) of *P. ovale*, 7 (5.98%) of *Plasmodium vivax*, 4 (3.42%) of *Plasmodium malariae* and 51 (43.59%) negative samples included in this study (Fig. 1). Two *P. ovale* cases classified as *P. o. wallikeri* and 6 cases classified as *P. o. curtisi*. One *P. ovale* sample could not be sequenced due to an extremely low amount of DNA.

Comparison of PURE–LAMP and nested PCR

The results of the PURE–LAMP and the nested PCR were considerably correlated. The Pan tubes of the PURE–LAMP correctly identified 64 [Pan(+)] of 66

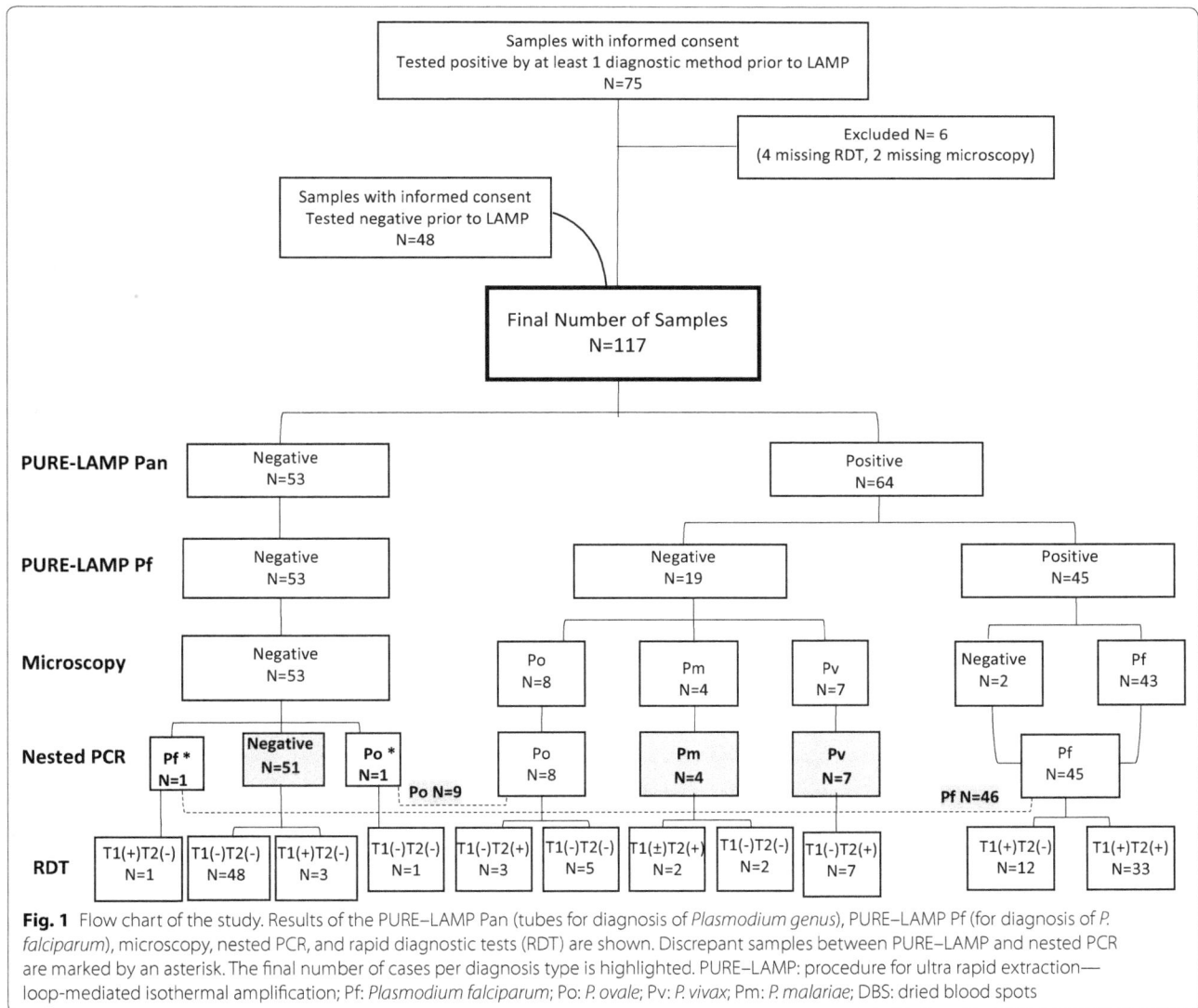

Fig. 1 Flow chart of the study. Results of the PURE–LAMP Pan (tubes for diagnosis of *Plasmodium genus*), PURE–LAMP Pf (for diagnosis of *P. falciparum*), microscopy, nested PCR, and rapid diagnostic tests (RDT) are shown. Discrepant samples between PURE–LAMP and nested PCR are marked by an asterisk. The final number of cases per diagnosis type is highlighted. PURE–LAMP: procedure for ultra rapid extraction—loop-mediated isothermal amplification; Pf: *Plasmodium falciparum*; Po: *P. ovale*; Pv: *P. vivax*; Pm: *P. malariae*; DBS: dried blood spots

positive samples and all 51 [Pan(−)] negative samples. Among the 64 Pan(+) samples, 45 were also positive by the *P. falciparum*-specific tubes [Pf(+)]; these were 45 of 46 *P. falciparum* samples. No samples showed a result of Pan(−)Pf(+) (Fig. 1; Tables 1, 2).

Comparison of PURE–LAMP and microscopic observations
All negatives by PURE–LAMP were also negative by microscopy. Only 2 positive samples by PURE–LAMP [Pan(+)Pf(+)], which were in conformity with the *P. falciparum* diagnosis by the nested PCR, were misdiagnosed by microscopy as negative. Parasitaemia by microscopy varied within a countable range from 0.001 to 21.7% and at uncountable level when 1 gametocyte is observed for over 200,000 erythrocytes (Additional file 1).

Comparison of PURE–LAMP and RDT
The HRP2 band (T1) correctly detected all *P. falciparum* samples. Three of the PURE–LAMP negatives showed false positive [T1(+), PCR(−)]. All 7 *P. vivax* samples were detected by the T2 band, also were 3 of 9 *P. ovale* cases, 2 of 4 *P. malariae* cases and 33 of the 46 *P. falciparum* cases. The 2 *P. malariae* single infections were detected by the RDT indicating *P. falciparum* or mixed infection [T1(+)T2(+)]; and by the PURE–LAMP as Pan(+)Pf(−). In general, 8 positives non-*P. falciparum*

samples were missed by the RDT while PURE–LAMP missed 1 *P. falciparum* and 1 *P. ovale* samples only.

Discussion
This study examined the sensitivity of PURE–LAMP with archived clinical blood samples stored on dried filter paper in comparison to other standard methods. The results suggested a sensitivity higher than that of microscopy, around 97% of the nested PCR and a specificity of 1. Such sensitivity was expected based on previous evaluations of the Loopamp kit with other DNA extraction methods [16–18, 21, 22]. The 2 false-negative samples by PURE–LAMP in this study came from patients with negative microscopic observation and a history of recent anti-malarial drug use. Previous investigations showed the PURE–LAMP limit of detection to range between 0.33 and 3.33 parasites/µL using dried materials in which cultured *P. falciparum* parasites were mixed into healthy human blood [22], whereas Aydin-Schmidt et al. [18] reported a limit of ≤2 parasites/µL for the Loopamp kit using DNA extracted with Chelex (Bio-Rad, Hercules, CA, USA) from dried blood spots. As a limit of 1 parasite/µL was found with the method studied in this paper, it seems that both discrepant samples had parasitaemia under the Loopamp kit limit of detection or remaining DNA of dead parasites. The study by Aydin-Schmidt et al. [18] showed the accuracy of the Loopamp kit to detect malaria parasites at low density from dried samples on filter paper. The present study supported this finding and revealed that the use of the new PURE DNA extraction method reached similar results. Although the present PURE–LAMP analysis was conducted retrospectively, it also corroborates the usefulness of the method for the diagnosis of imported malaria in travellers as reported previously [16]. As exposed earlier, microscopy allows us more than dichotomous characterization of samples. However, the difference observed in sensitivity between PURE–LAMP and microscopy in the present study is expected to be wider in the field, where the PURE–LAMP sensitivity should be maintained, but the sensitivity of microscopy is expected to be lower at times [17, 21, 23].

Table 1 Sensitivity and specificity of PURE–LAMP, microscopy observation, and RDT compared to nested PCR

Test	Sensitivity [95% CI]	Specificity [95% CI]
PURE–LAMP Pan	96.96% [89.47–99.63]	100%
PURE–LAMP Pf	97.82% [88.47–99.94]	100%
Microscopy	93.93% [85.20–98.32]	100%
RDT	T1: 100% T2: 68.18% [55.56–79.11]	T1: 92.95% [84.32–97.67] T2: 100%

PURE–LAMP procedure for ultra rapid extraction-loop-mediated isothermal amplification, *RDT* rapid diagnostic test, *PCR* polymerase chain reaction, *CI* confidence interval, *Pan Plasmodium* genus, *Pf P. falciparum*, *T1* band of the rapid test containing the antibody for detection of a *Plasmodium falciparum*-specific HRP2 antigen, *T2* band containing the antibody for detection of a *Plasmodium* common aldolase antigen

Table 2 Detailed information of samples with discrepant results between PURE–LAMP and nested PCR

Sample no.[a]	RDT	Microscopy	PURE–LAMP Pan	PURE–LAMP Pf	Nested PCR
12	Negative T1(−)T2(−)	Negative	Negative	Negative	Po
78	PfT1(+)T2(−)	Negative	Negative	Negative	Pf

PURE–LAMP procedure for ultra rapid extraction-loop-mediated isothermal amplification, *Pan Plasmodium* genus, *Pf P. falciparum*, *PCR* polymerase chain reaction, *RDT* rapid diagnostic test, *T1* band of the rapid test containing the antibody for detection of a *Plasmodium falciparum*-specific HRP2 antigen, *T2* band containing the antibody for detection of a *Plasmodium* common aldolase antigen

[a] Sample numbering is according to the list of all samples in the Additional file 1

This study included parasites of multiple provenances, with all 4 human transmissible species including both *P. ovale* subspecies that could be seen as an advantage however the modest sample size constituted a limitation (Additional file 1). No case of *Plasmodium knowlesi* was included: however, it can also be detected by PURE–LAMP (Kawai, unpublished data).

The LAMP technique has been adapted for use in the diagnosis of different infectious diseases with notoriously high burdens, including tuberculosis and malaria, for which high sensitivity, specificity, affordability, and applicability to the tropical field are desired [24]. Among the advantages of this kit compared to PCR are that it requires less investment, staff training, and operating time. Results can be ready within 1.5 h from punching DBS through DNA extraction and recording the results. A common disadvantage is the need for power during heating and reaction time.

Conclusion

Filter paper is already a well-known field support method as it allows the collection, transfer, and storage of samples without a cold chamber. Considering the designed-in field-friendliness of this PURE–LAMP combination method, use of this system with dried blood samples will allow maximum exploitation of this characteristic while still performing accurately.

Cost-effectiveness is beyond the scope of this paper, but technically this system is predicted to be extendable to the field, while it is effective for malaria diagnosis in travellers.

Additional file

Additional file 1. List of samples analysed: Combination of PURE-DNA extraction and LAMP-DNA amplification methods for accurate malaria diagnosis on dried blood spots. PURE-LAMP: Procedure for ultra rapid extraction–loop-mediated isothermal amplification; Pan: *Plasmodium* genus; Pf: *Plasmodium falciparum*; Pv: *P. vivax*; Pm: *P. malariae*; Po: *P. ovale*; Poc: *P. o. curtisi*; Pow: *P. o. wallikeri*; RBC: red blood cells; T1: band of the rapid test containing the antibody for detection of a *Plasmodium falciparum*-specific HRP2 antigen; T2: band containing the antibody for detection of a *Plasmodium* common aldolase antigen. +: positive; −: negative; ±: positive (pale band). *DNA extracted from 200 µL of fresh blood or 100 µL of frozen RBC concentrate, nested PCR method 1 [19]. **DNA extracted from 200 µL of fresh blood or 100 µL of frozen RBC concentrate, nested PCR method 2 [20]. ***DNA extracted from 3 dried blood spots of φ 3 mm, nested PCR method 2 [20].

Abbreviations
LAMP: loop-mediated isothermal amplification; PCR: polymerase chain reaction; Pf: *P. falciparum*; Pm: *P. malariae*; Po: *P. ovale*; PURE: procedure for ultra rapid extraction; Pv: *P. vivax*; RDT: rapid diagnostic tests; rRNA: small subunit ribosomal RNA; DBS: dried blood spot; RBC: red blood cells.

Authors' contributions
JPV, KKY, S Kawai and S Kano conceived and designed this study. JPV, MI and KKY performed the experiments. JPV, KKY and S Kano wrote the manuscript. All authors read and approved the final manuscript.

Author details
[1] Department of Tropical Medicine and Malaria, Research Institute, National Center for Global Health and Medicine, Tokyo 162-8655, Japan. [2] Graduate School of Comprehensive Human Sciences, University of Tsukuba, Ibaraki 305-8575, Japan. [3] Department of Tropical Medicine and Parasitology, Dokkyo Medical University, Tochigi 321-0293, Japan. [4] SATREPS Project for Parasitic Diseases, Vientiane, Lao People's Democratic Republic.

Acknowledgements
We sincerely acknowledge Dr. Kazuhiko YANO (NCGM, Tokyo, Japan) for his support with microscopic observation and Dr. Masami NAKATSU (NCGM, Tokyo, Japan) for advice on DNA extraction. Technical advices on LAMP were received from Eiken Chemical Co. Ltd.

Competing interests
The authors declare that they have no competing interests.

Funding
This study was partly supported by an AMED grant of the SATREPS project for the "Development of innovative research technique in genetic epidemiology of malaria and other parasitic diseases in the Lao PDR for containing their expanding endemicity".

References
1. WHO. World malaria report 2017. Geneva: World Health Organization; 2017.
2. Gilles HM, Warrell DA. Bruce-Chwatt's essential malariology. 3rd ed. London: Edward Arnold; 1993.
3. Hänscheid T. Diagnosis of malaria: a review of alternatives to conventional microscopy. Clin Lab Haematol. 1999;21:235–45.
4. Abdul-Ghani R, Al-Mekhlafi AM, Karanis P. Loop-mediated isothermal amplification (LAMP) for malarial parasites of humans: would it come to clinical reality as a point-of-care test? Acta Trop. 2012;122:233–40.
5. Wongsrichanalai C, Barcus MJ, Muth S, Sutamihardja A, Wernsdorfer WH. A review of malaria diagnostic tools: microscopy and rapid diagnostic test (RDT). Am J Trop Med Hyg. 2007;77(Suppl 6):119–27.
6. McMorrow ML, Aidoo M, Kachur SP. Malaria rapid diagnostic tests in elimination settings—can they find the last parasite? Clin Microbiol Infect. 2011;17:1624–31.
7. Moody A. Rapid diagnostic tests for malaria parasites. Clin Microbiol Rev. 2002;15:66–78.
8. WHO. Guidelines for the treatment of malaria. 2nd ed. Geneva: World Health Organization; 2010.
9. Hänscheid T, Grobusch MP. How useful is PCR in the diagnosis of malaria? Trends Parasitol. 2002;18:395–8.
10. Mixson-Hayden T, Lucchi NW, Udhayakumar V. Evaluation of three PCR-based diagnostic assays for detecting mixed *Plasmodium* infection. BMC Res Notes. 2010;3:88.

11. Polley SD, Sutherland CJ, Regan F, Hassan M, Chiodini PL. Increased sensitivity for detecting malaria parasites in human umbilical cord blood using scaled-up DNA preparation. Malar J. 2012;11:62.

12. Notomi T, Okayama H, Masubuchi H, Yonekawa T, Watanabe K, Amino N, et al. Loop-mediated isothermal amplification of DNA. Nucleic Acids Res. 2000;28:E63.

13. Lucchi NW, Demas A, Narayanan J, Sumari D, Kabanywanyi A, Kachur SP, et al. Real-time fluorescence loop mediated isothermal amplification for the diagnosis of malaria. PLoS ONE. 2010;5:e13733.

14. Mohon AN, Lee LD, Bayih AG, Folefoc A, Guelig D, Burton RA, et al. NINA–LAMP compared to microscopy, RDT, and nested PCR for the detection of imported malaria. Diagn Microbiol Infect Dis. 2016;85:149–53.

15. Britton S, Cheng Q, Sutherland CJ, McCarthy JS. A simple, high-throughput, colourimetric, field applicable loop-mediated isothermal amplification (HtLAMP) assay for malaria elimination. Malar J. 2015;14:335.

16. Polley SD, González IJ, Mohamed D, Daly R, Bowers K, Watson J, et al. Clinical evaluation of a loop-mediated amplification kit for diagnosis of imported malaria. J Infect Dis. 2013;208:637–44.

17. Hopkins H, González IJ, Polley SD, Angutoko P, Ategeka J, Asiimwe C, et al. Highly sensitive detection of malaria parasitemia in a malaria-endemic setting: performance of a new loop-mediated isothermal amplification kit in a remote clinic in Uganda. J Infect Dis. 2013;208:645–52.

18. Aydin-Schmidt B, Xu W, González IJ, Polley SD, Bell D, Shakely D, et al. Loop mediated isothermal amplification (LAMP) accurately detects malaria DNA from filter paper blood samples of low density parasitaemias. PLoS ONE. 2014;9:e103905.

19. Kimura M, Kaneko O, Liu Q, Zhou M, Kawamoto F, Wataya Y, et al. Identification of the four species of human malaria parasites by nested PCR that targets variant sequences in the small subunit rRNA gene. Parasitol Int. 1997;46:91–5.

20. Komaki-Yasuda K, Vincent JP, Nakatsu M, Kato Y, Ohmagari N, Kano S. A novel PCR-based system for the detection of four species of human malaria parasites and Plasmodium knowlesi. PLoS ONE. 2018;13:e0191886.

21. Vallejo AF, Martínez NL, González IJ, Arévalo-Herrera M, Herrera S. Evaluation of the loop mediated isothermal DNA amplification (LAMP) kit for malaria diagnosis in P. vivax endemic settings of Colombia. PLoS Negl Trop Dis. 2015;9:e3453.

22. Komaki-Yasuda K, Matsumoto-Takahashi ELA, Kawai S, Kano S. Application of PURE/LAMP method for malaria diagnosis. Clin Parasitol. 2015;26:83–5.

23. Ayalew F, Tilahun B, Taye B. Performance evaluation of laboratory professionals on malaria microscopy in Hawassa Town, Southern Ethiopia. BMC Res Notes. 2014;7:839.

24. Kaku T, Minamoto F, D'Meza R, Morose W, Boncy J, Bijou J, et al. Accuracy of LAMP–TB method for diagnosing tuberculosis in Haiti. Jpn J Infect Dis. 2016;69:488–92.

17

Insecticide resistance in *Anopheles gambiae* from the northern Democratic Republic of Congo, with extreme knockdown resistance (*kdr*) mutation frequencies revealed by a new diagnostic assay

Amy Lynd[1*] , Ambrose Oruni[1], Arjen E. van't Hof[1], John C. Morgan[1], Leon Bwazumo Naego[2], Dimitra Pipini[1], Kevin A. O'Kines[1], Thierry L. Bobanga[3], Martin J. Donnelly[1] and David Weetman[1]

Abstract

Background: Mutations in the voltage-gated sodium channel at codon 1014 confer knock-down resistance (*kdr*) to pyrethroids in a wide range of insects. *Anopheles gambiae* exhibits two mutant alleles at codon 1014, serine and phenylalanine; and both are now widespread across Africa. Existing screening methods only allow for one resistant allele to be detected per assay. A new locked nucleic acid (LNA) qPCR assay was developed for the simultaneous detection of both mutant alleles and the wild type allele in a single assay. This tri-allelic detection assay was assessed as part of a study of the insecticide resistance in *An. gambiae* sensu stricto (s.s.) in the previously un-sampled area of Nord Ubangi, Democratic Republic of the Congo.

Methods: Samples from three sites were tested for insecticide susceptibility using WHO bioassays, with and without the synergist PBO preceding pyrethroid exposures, and were subsequently analysed for frequency and resistance-association of the *Vgsc*-1014 and *Vgsc*-N1575Y mutations. Results from the LNA-*kdr* 1014 assay were compared to results from standard TaqMan-*kdr* assays.

Results: *Anopheles gambiae* sensu lato (s.l.) was by far the predominant vector captured (84%), with only low frequencies of *Anopheles funestus* s.l. (9%) detected in Nord Ubangi. Molecular identification found *An. gambiae* s.s. to be the principal vector (99%) although *Anopheles coluzzii* was detected at very low frequency. *Anopheles gambiae* were susceptible to the carbamate insecticide bendiocarb, but resistant to DDT and to the pyrethroids permethrin and deltamethrin. Susceptibility to both pyrethroids was partially restored with prior exposure to PBO suggesting likely involvement of metabolic resistance. *Anopheles gambiae* s.s. was homozygous for *kdr* resistant alleles with both the L1014F and L1014S mutations present, and the N1575Y polymorphism was present at low frequency. The LNA-*kdr* assay simultaneously detected both resistant alleles and gave results entirely consistent with those from the two TaqMan-*kdr* assays.

Conclusion: This study provides rare data on insecticide resistance and mechanisms in *Anopheles* from the centre of Africa, with the first detection of N1575Y. Nord Ubangi populations of *An. gambiae* s.s. show insecticide resistance mediated by both metabolic mechanisms and *Vgsc* mutations. The LNA-*kdr* assay is particularly suitable for use in

*Correspondence: amy.lynd@lstmed.ac.uk
[1] Liverpool School of Tropical Medicine, Liverpool, UK
Full list of author information is available at the end of the article

populations in which both 1014S and 1014F *kdr* alleles co-occur and provides robust results, with higher throughput and at a quarter of the cost of TaqMan assays.

Background

Malaria is a major cause of mortality and morbidity in The Democratic Republic of the Congo (DRC), with over 40,000 deaths per year [1]. It is estimated that 60% of the country's population live in areas with an average *Plasmodium falciparum* prevalence above 50% (hyperendemic to holoendemic transmission), making the DRC one of the countries with the most intense transmission [2]. Efforts to reduce the malaria burden are focusing on case management and treatment, and on vector control via the distribution of long-lasting insecticide-treated nets (LLINs) [2]. Successful implementation of a vector control programme is reliant on knowledge of vector species and their resistance to insecticides. Few recent studies have been published on the vector species of the DRC or their insecticide resistance and those that exist are principally concerned with locations to the South and East of the country. Over 60 species of *Anopheles* have been described in the DRC, with *Anopheles gambiae* sensu lato (s.l.) and *Anopheles funestus* thought to be the main malaria vectors, but other species, such as *Anopheles pharoensis*, *Anopheles moucheti*, and *Anopheles coustani* are potentially important for transmission (reviewed in [2]). In the *An. gambiae* s.l. species group, *An. gambiae* sensu stricto (s.s.) was found to be the predominant vector in eastern DRC, whereas *Anopheles coluzzii* was the main species found in Bandundu in the West. Both species were found in sympatry in several locations including Kinshasa, as well as Kisangani and Lodja (central West) and Kalemie (East). Only *An. gambiae* s.s. was found in Equateur Province (North West) [1, 3–5].

Contemporary data on insecticide resistance status in malaria vectors is improving but remains sparse for DRC and central Africa generally [6]. A study in 2009 of four locations, Kingasani and Kimpese in the South West, Bolenge, in the West, and Katana located in the East demonstrated that all *An. gambiae* s.s. populations were resistant to DDT, three were resistant to the pyrethroids deltamethrin, permethrin, lambda-cyhalothrin, and a single population was resistant to the organophosphate malathion [3]. In 2012, *An. gambiae* s.s. in the North East were found to be resistant to deltamethrin, DDT and bendiocarb. Pre-exposure to PBO (piperonyl butoxide), a synergist that inhibits the activity of cytochrome P450 enzymes and some esterases which may be involved in the detoxification of pyrethroids, significantly increased mortality in bioassays suggesting that metabolic enzymes were at least partly responsible for

the resistance phenotype [7]. A study in 2013 of two sites near Kinshasa found that *An. coluzzii* were resistant to DDT and permethrin but fully susceptible to propoxur, bendiocarb and deltamethrin. Pre-exposure to PBO did not restore susceptibility in this population [8]. A recent study carried out from 2013 to 2016 found *An. gambiae* s.l. populations were resistant to permethrin in five of seven provinces studied in 2016 (Lodja and Kabondo located centrally, Mikalayi in the South, Kingasani in the West, and Kalemie in the East). A significant impact of PBO showed that metabolic resistance was involved in four of these sites. Resistance to deltamethrin was observed in Mikalayi and Kabondo, whilst resistance to DDT was observed in all six provinces where monitoring was carried out [5]. A study in Kinshasa in 2015, found that *An. gambiae* s.l. were resistant to DDT, four types of pyrethroid, dieldrin and bendiocarb, and that whilst P450 enzymes were involved, they were only partly responsible for the resistance observed [4].

Point mutations in the voltage gated sodium channel (VGSC), the target for pyrethroids, at the L1014 locus (L995 using *An. gambiae* codon nomenclature [9]) typically cause knock down resistance (*kdr*) to pyrethroids (and DDT), and are widespread in *An. gambiae* s.l. [10]. Two resistance alleles are found at this locus, resulting from the replacement of the wild type leucine allele with phenylalanine, L1014F [11], or alternatively serine, L1014S [12]. Both alleles can occur in the same population [7, 13] and the frequency of both alleles appears to be increasing [14–18].

In DRC the *Vgsc*-1014F mutation was found at four locations in *An. gambiae* s.s. specimens collected in 2009 with allele frequencies ranging from 0.13 to 0.95 [3]. The L1014F *kdr* mutation was also detected in *An. coluzzii* at frequencies of 0.33 and 0.38 in two study sites near Kinshasa [8]. The L1014F mutation was found in *An. gambiae* s.l. in all five provinces studied in 2014 with extremely variable frequencies ranging from near fixation to near absence [5]. The *Vgsc*-1014S mutation has only been detected in one location in the North East where it occurred at high frequencies and co-occurred with both the *Vgsc*-1014F mutation and the wild type allele [7]. A study in Kinshasa, 2015, found both L1014S and L1014F, whilst the wild type allele was almost entirely absent [4].

Detection of the *kdr* mutations, which act as useful partial resistance diagnostics for pyrethroid resistance [10], is important for monitoring the spread of resistance in areas were vector control is principally carried out using pyrethroid treated nets. A number of different assays exist for the detection of *kdr* including allele specific PCR (AS-PCR) [11, 12], Heated Oligonucleotide Ligation Assay (HOLA), [19] Sequence Specific Oligonucleotide Probe Enzyme-Linked ImmunoSorbent Assay (SSOP-ELISA) [20], PCR-Dot Blot [21], and the widely-used real-time TaqMan qPCR probe assay [22]. However, all of these methods are reliant on performing two assays in order to detect both the *Vgsc*-1014F and *Vgsc*-1014S mutations. With the spread of both mutations across Africa [9] there is a growing need for an assay that can detect both resistant alleles and the wild type allele in a single assay to aid interpretation, increase throughput, and reduce the cost per specimen. A newly-developed assay utilizing Locked Nucleic Acid (LNA) probes to simultaneously detect all three alleles whilst utilizing the same quantitative PCR platform used for TaqMan assays is presented. LNA probes incorporate modified RNA nucleotides that significantly increase target affinity and the melting temperature (Tm) of an allele-specific probe. This allows very short allele specific oligonucleotides to be produced that have a high difference in Tm between the target sequence and any mis-match sequence. Utilizing this technology, it was possible to design probes to detect all three alleles reliably in a single qPCR reaction and this assay was used to explore *kdr* frequencies in samples from Nord Ubangi, DRC.

Methods

Mosquito collections and bioassays

As part of baseline entomological monitoring for a LLIN distribution campaign in Nord Ubangi, Equateur province in March–April 2016, three rural collection sites (Pambwa, 3.937433, 20.7726; Fiwa, 4.318532, 20.77830; Bassa, 4.267017, 21.283383) were selected in the area surrounding the major town of Gbadolite, near the border with the Central African Republic (Additional file 1).

Anopheles larvae were collected from roadside breeding sites in the proximity of Fiwa and Pambwa, but none were detected around Bassa. Adult mosquito collections were carried out in all three villages using both manual and mechanical ('Prokopack') aspirators [23]. Blood-fed female *Anopheles* were maintained in a field insectary in Gbadolite until egg-laying. Larvae collected directly, and those raised from eggs, were reared until the adult stage and 3–5 day old females were used for insecticide susceptibility testing.

All mosquitoes were identified to species group using phenotypic keys [24] and insecticide testing was carried out on *An. gambiae* s.l. to assess the prevalence of resistance to permethrin (0.75%) and deltamethrin (0.05%) with and without PBO (4%) using standard World Health Organization (WHO) protocols [25]. A limited number

of tests were also performed with DDT (4%) and the carbamate insecticide, bendiocarb (0.1%). Negative controls were carried for all insecticide assays. Mosquitoes were pre-exposed to PBO for one hour before exposure to the control paper in synergist assays. Abbotts correction was carried according to WHO criteria. All mosquitoes were stored on silica gel in 0.2 ml tubes for later DNA analyses.

DNA extraction and molecular species identification

DNA was extracted from individual mosquitoes using Nexttec Biotechnologie GmbH extraction plates according to manufacturer's instructions; or from legs using the following method. Two mosquito legs were removed and placed in 20 µl of 1 × STE buffer in a 0.2 ml PCR tube. Samples were incubated for 30 min at 95 °C. The supernatant was used as template for subsequent PCR reactions.

Mosquitoes from insecticide bioassays previously identified as *An. gambiae* s.l. were identified to species level by SINE [26], using 1 µl of DNA in a 25 µl reaction, with bands visualised on a 2% TAE agarose gel.

TaqMan assays for resistance mutations

Vgsc-L1014F and *Vgsc*-L1014S mutations were screened using the TaqMan assay [22]. Results were analysed using AriaMX software V1.5 and the fluorescence (ΔR) threshold adjusted manually for each dye, if necessary, to enable the correct scoring of positive controls. Results for ΔR last, the final baseline-corrected fluorescence reading as measured in the last cycle, were then exported into Microsoft Excel for analysis and the genotype at locus 1014 determined by combining results from the two assays. Specimens were also screened for the presence of the *Vgsc*-N1575Y and *Ace-1*-G119S resistance mutations using TaqMan assays [27, 28].

LNA-*kdr* assay for locus 1014

Primers were designed to amplify a single 141 bp region surrounding the *Vgsc*-1014 codon. LNA probes were designed according to suggested parameters [29]. The three probes were optimized utilizing the online IDT Biophysics software [30] to give an off-target Tm difference of at least 10 °C whilst keeping the exact match target Tm within 3 °C to allow target binding but preventing non-target binding of each probe within a single assay. All primers and probes were synthesised by IDT; sequence details are given in Table 1.

Each assay contained a final concentration of 1× PrimeTime Master Mix (IDT) or 1× Luna Universal qPCR Master Mix (NEB), 0.1 µM for each of the three probes (LNAkdr-Ser:Cy5, LNAkdr-Phe:Fam, LNAkdr-Leu:Hex), 0.2 µM of primers (VGSC-F, VGSC-R) in a total reaction volume of 10 µl with 1 µl of DNA template.

Table 1 Sequences of primers and probes used in the LNA kdr assay with 5′ and 3′ modifications indicated

Name	5′ Fluorescence modification	Sequence	3′ Quencher modification
VGSC-F		CGTGTGCTATGCGGAGAATG	
VGSC-R		CGATCTTGGTCCATGTTAATT TGC	
Kdr-Leu	HEX	A+CGA+C+T+AAAT+TTC+C	IBFQ
Kdr-Phe	6-FAM	A+CGA+C+A+AAAT+TTC+C	IBFQ
Kdr-Ser	Cy5	+CGA+C+T+GAAT+TTC+C	IBRQ

+, preceding a base indicates it is a LNA nucleotide

Reactions were set up in optical PCR tubes and run on an AriaMX qPCR cycler with Fam, Hex and Cy5 filters. Reaction conditions were 95 °C for 3 min, followed by 40 cycles of 95 °C for 5 s and 60 °C for 30 s, giving a total run time of 52 min. Results were analysed using the AriaMX software V1.5 and the endpoint fluorescence (ΔR Last) threshold adjusted manually for each dye if necessary to enable the correct scoring of controls. Due to current software limitations automated analysis is restricted to bi-allelic genotype calling. Therefore, values for ΔR Last and genotype calling thresholds were exported to Microsoft Excel; ΔR Last values exceeding the threshold were counted as a positive call for each allele. The *kdr* genotype at locus 1014 was then determined for each sample. The R package Plotly [31] was used to produce a 3D scatterplot for all genotypes. To verify the method, final genotype calls were then compared to those produced in the TaqMan *kdr* assays from endpoint fluorescent data. To provide additional testing of the LNA-*kdr* assay for suitability across Africa, 172 *An. gambiae* s.s. samples, collected from four districts in Eastern Uganda in 2017 were also included.

Allele frequencies were calculated from the genotypes observed in the LNA assay. Association of genotype and susceptibility phenotype were analysed using X^2 tests, and odds ratios were calculated using Poptools 3.2. The R package Genetics [32] was used to carry out an Exact test of Hardy–Weinberg Equilibrium.

Results
Species and phenotypic resistance in Nord Ubangi
Over 250 female mosquitoes were obtained from house collections in Fiwa, Pambwa and Bassa (Nord Ubangi), the majority of which (84%) were identified morphologically as *An. gambiae* s.l. *Anopheles funestus* was found in significant numbers (28%) from house collections in Pambwa. Larval collections from sites around Fiwa and Pambwa yielded only *An. gambiae* s.l.

Molecular species identification of *An. gambiae* s.l. showed that the predominant vector collected in all sampling areas was *An. gambiae* s.s. *Anopheles coluzzii* was found in larval collections from only one site (Fiwa) at low frequency, 12.5% (N = 4 of 32). This species was not detected in any other site.

Adults reared from larval collections from Fiwa and Pambwa, and from F1 adults reared from eggs obtained from females in house collections from all three study sites, were exposed to permethrin and deltamethrin with and without prior PBO exposure, and the insecticides bendiocarb and DDT according to the WHO protocol [25]. Control assays yielded low mortality (mean = 3%) and results were corrected using Abbott's formula when mortality in the control assays was between 5 and 20%. Prior exposure to PBO in the control assays also yielded low mortality (mean = 4%), and was no higher than controls without PBO ($\chi^2 = 0.52$, P = 0.47). Bioassay test results are shown in Fig. 1.

Resistance to permethrin and deltamethrin was detected in each study site although susceptibility was partially restored when PBO was used in conjunction with permethrin, and nearly completely restored when used in conjunction with deltamethrin. Despite the relatively small geographical scale (sites are < 100 km apart) significant variation in pyrethroid resistance was detected between the sample areas (Additional file 1). Data from Fiwa and Bassa study sites suggest the populations are fully susceptible to bendiocarb but show very high resistance to DDT.

Molecular resistance diagnostics
Anopheles gambiae s.s. control specimens of known genotype were screened using the newly-developed LNA *kdr* detection method. The assay gave distinct genotypes and clear cut-offs between wildtype, heterozygous and homozygous genotypes for all three alleles (Fig. 2). The assay was successful utilizing two different qPCR master mixes (IDT PrimeTime Master Mix or NEB Luna Universal qPCR Master Mix) suggesting other commercial qPCR mixes may also be suitable thus allowing both greater flexibility and potential for reductions in cost.

LNA *kdr* detection versus TaqMan method
In total 356 *An. gambiae* from DRC and 172 specimens from Uganda (Additional file 2) were analysed for the *Vgsc*-1014 mutations using both the traditional TaqMan assays and the new LNA probe-based method in a blind assay. All samples analysed gave a result in both the TaqMan and LNA kdr assays. The LNA-*kdr* assay gave identical results to the TaqMan assays for all samples, which included homozygotes and heterozygotes for all three alleles. The Ugandan specimens provided a

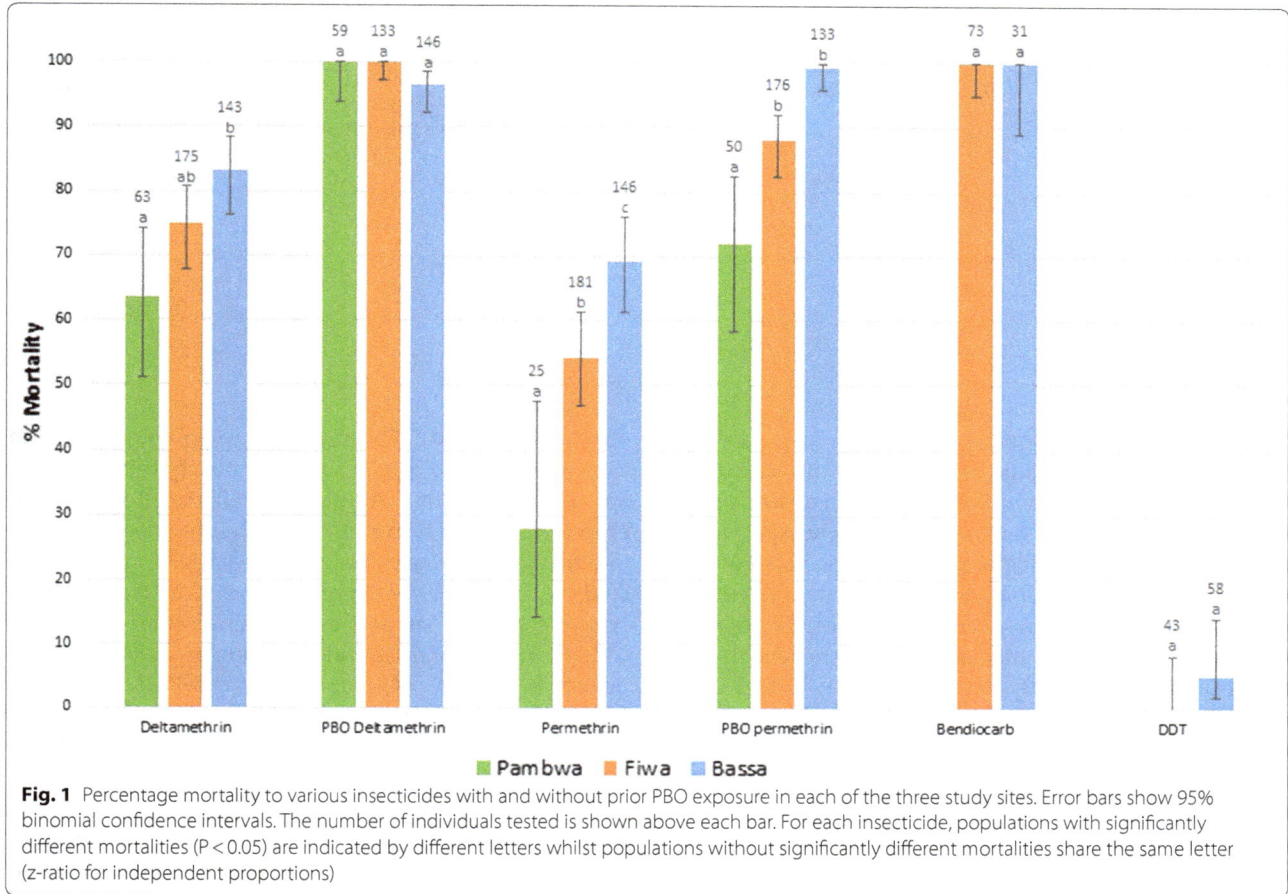

Fig. 1 Percentage mortality to various insecticides with and without prior PBO exposure in each of the three study sites. Error bars show 95% binomial confidence intervals. The number of individuals tested is shown above each bar. For each insecticide, populations with significantly different mortalities (P < 0.05) are indicated by different letters whilst populations without significantly different mortalities share the same letter (z-ratio for independent proportions)

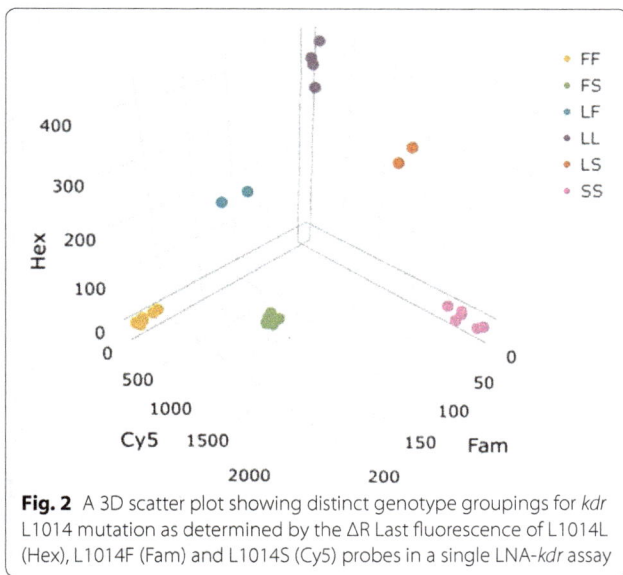

Fig. 2 A 3D scatter plot showing distinct genotype groupings for *kdr* L1014 mutation as determined by the ΔR Last fluorescence of L1014L (Hex), L1014F (Fam) and L1014S (Cy5) probes in a single LNA-*kdr* assay

contrasting genotypic profile to those from DRC, with 1014S dominant, which allowed a more robust test of the LNA-*kdr* assay (Additional file 2).

The L1014F and L1014S mutations were discovered in *An. gambiae* s.s. specimens assayed from the three Nord Ubangi sample locations (Additional file 1) with the predominant genotype being *Vgsc*-1014F homozygotes in each area (Table 2). Wild type alleles were found only in two of the four *An. coluzzii* specimens collected from the village of Fiwa; both occurred as heterozygotes with the L1014F mutation. Population genotype frequencies conformed to Hardy–Weinberg expectations (Table 2). Association studies of genotype and susceptibility phenotype showed that the 1014F was significantly associated with survival to permethrin ($\chi^2 = 10.43$, P < 0.01; odds ratio = 3.7), deltamethrin ($\chi^2 = 6.86$, P < 0.05; odds ratio = 3.8) and with permethrin with prior PBO exposure ($\chi^2 = 6.71$, P < 0.05; odds ratio = 2.9). Note that in each case the tests involve comparison of to 1014S, rather than 1014L, which was absent.

Table 2 Genotype frequencies for the L1014 kdr mutation in *Anopheles gambiae* s.l. specimens from DRC. Tests of Hardy–Weinberg equilibrium (χ^2) with corresponding P-values are shown

L1014 genotype	*Anopheles gambiae* s.s.			*Anopheles coluzzii*
	Bassa (N = 100)	Pambwa (N = 92)	Fiwa (N = 161)	Fiwa (N = 4)
FF	0.79	0.82	0.64	0.5
FS	0.20	0.17	0.29	0.00
SS	0.01	0.01	0.07	0.00
LF	0.00	0.00	0.00	0.5
χ^2	0.05	0.02	2.85	0.44
P value	1.00	1.00	0.10	1.00

The LNA-*kdr* assay was not subject to false positives resulting from non-specific binding of the mutant alleles to wild type probe as occurs in the TaqMan assays, resulting in more robust determination of genotype (Additional file 3). Non-specific binding can lead to a 1014F/S heterozygote sample being initially scored as having all three alleles meaning manual evaluation of the data and correction of the combined genotype is needed (Additional file 3). Importantly, in such cases, failure to carry out both Taqman-*kdr* assays may result in the reporting of false positives for the wild-type allele.

Molecular analysis of the third known *An. gambiae* resistance mutation N1575Y (N1570Y using *An. gambiae* codon numbering) in the voltage-gated sodium channel found the mutation was present in both *An. gambiae* s.s. and *An. coluzzii* populations albeit at very low frequency, 0.011 (N = 364) and 0.25 (N = 4) respectively. The N1575Y mutation was only found in conjunction with L1014F homozygote (Additional file 4). The important carbamate and organophosphate resistance mutation *Ace-1*-G119S was not found in any of the 368 specimens analysed.

Discussion

The primary malaria vector species in the three study sites in Nord Ubangi was found to be *An. gambiae* s.s., although *An. coluzzii* was also found in low numbers. Data for this region of DRC are lacking, but previous studies in southern Equateur Province found only *An. gambiae* s.s. [1, 3]. The presence of *An. coluzzii* in Nord Ubangi further extends the known range of this species.

Molecular analysis revealed the *kdr* L1014F resistance mutation to be present at high frequency (over 0.79–0.90), and the *kdr* L1014S mutation found to be present at moderate frequency (0.1–0.21) across all three study sites (Table 2). The wild-type susceptible allele was not detected in *An. gambiae* s.s. but was found in the few *An. coluzzii* specimens analysed. The N1575Y mutation, also located in the VGSC, has a synergistic effect

on pyrethroid and DDT resistance when combined with the L1014F mutation [27, 33]. Previously this mutation has been found in Burkina Faso, Ghana, Benin, Cameroon and Côte d'Ivoire [27, 34–36]. It has been detected in both *An. gambiae* s.s. and *An. coluzzii* [27, 34]. In this study the N1575Y was found at very low frequency in two of the three survey sites (Pambwa, 0.01 and Fiwa, 0.02) in *An. gambiae* s.s. The mutation was found at a frequency of 0.25 (N = 4) in *An. coluzzii* from Fiwa. This is first report of this mutation in DRC.

This study detected confirmed phenotypic resistance to deltamethrin, permethrin and DDT; the presence of both L1014 *kdr* resistance alleles at high frequency, the absence of the wild type L1014L mutation and the first detection of N1575Y. Such a resistance profile, mediated by both target site and metabolic mechanisms (indicated by PBO results) may provide challenges for LLIN-based vector control programmes in this region of DRC. However, susceptibility to bendiocarb and the absence of the Ace-1 G119S mutant suggest that indoor residual spraying (IRS) using non-pyrethroid formulations may not be compromised. Interestingly, the effect of PBO was not consistent across the two pyrethroids tested, with near-full susceptibility restored with deltamethrin, but not permethrin, suggesting a different balance in the contribution of different resistance mechanisms, with the latter perhaps more dependent upon target site resistance.

The LNA-kdr assay was found to perform as well as the TaqMan kdr assay in all populations of *An. gambiae* s.s. analysed, but with substantial time savings (67% reduction in run time) and since it utilizes non-proprietary probes also permits large cost savings (75%), which may be reduced further by use of different amplification master mixes. In addition, this single assay detection method may reduce the reporting of false positive wild-type alleles and permit the discovery of resistance alleles in places where they are not yet being screened for in single mutant detection assays. The development of a single assay for detection of both *kdr* alleles will allow rapid, reliable and low-cost screening of these important resistance mutations facilitating the monitoring of resistance across Africa.

Conclusion

Anopheles gambiae s.s. populations in Nord Ubangi show insecticide resistance mediated by both metabolic mechanisms and target site mutations. The LNA-*kdr* assay developed was able to simultaneously detect all three *kdr* alleles in Nord Ubangi and has proved a reliable diagnostic tool for *An. gambiae* s.s. populations in which both 1014S and 1014F *kdr* alleles co-occur.

Additional files

Additional file 1. Collection sites in the Gbadolite region of DRC. (A) Location of Gbadolite in DRC (shown in red) within Equateur province and the capital city, Kinshasa ★. (B) Fine-scale map of collection sites.

Additional file 2. Genotype frequencies for the VGSC L1014 mutations in *Anopheles gambiae* s.s. specimens from Uganda.

Additional file 3. Taqman genotype plots demonstrating mis-calling of genotype due non-specific binding of the mutant alleles. Mis-called genotypes are circled in black and the actual genotype indicated. A: Taqman kdr for L1014F detection. B: Taqman kdr for L1014S detection.

Additional file 4. Genotype frequencies for the VGSC N1575Y mutation *in Anopheles gambiae* s.l. specimens from DRC.

Authors' contributions

AL and DW conceived and designed the experiments. AO, AVN and DP made substantial contributions to the design and optimization of the LNA-*kdr* assay. AI, JM, KK and LBN were responsible for collecting mosquitoes and performing the experiments. TB provided resources and made contributions to conception and discussion of the study. AL, DW and MD conducted data analysis and wrote the manuscript. All authors read and approved the final manuscript.

Author details

[1] Liverpool School of Tropical Medicine, Liverpool, UK. [2] Avenue de l'infirmerie, Quartier Yola Bokonzo, Gemena, Sud Ubangi, Democratic Republic of Congo. [3] University of Kinshasa, Kinshasa, Democratic Republic of Congo.

Acknowledgements

Additional funding was provided by Award Number R01AI116811 from the National Institute of Allergy and Infectious Diseases (NIAID) and a Wellcome Trust MSc Fellowship in Public Health and Tropical Medicine (Oruni-203511/Z/16/Z). The content of the manuscript is solely the responsibility of the authors. The authors are grateful to Dr. Seth Irish, Centers for Disease Control, Atlanta, USA, for advice during manuscript preparation. The authors would also like to gratefully acknowledge the staff at PNLP, World Vision and IMA World Health for their support with this project, in particular Dr Charlotte Ndolerire for her tireless efforts in the field, and Crystal Stafford and Dr. Larry Sthreshley for their assistance and advice. The authors would also like to thank Alexandre Loya for his help collecting mosquitoes.

Competing interests

The authors declare that they have no competing interests.

Funding

This research was funded by the Against Malaria Foundation (AMF) as part of a baseline study prior to a bednet distribution campaign in Nord Ubangi, DRC.

References

1. Bobanga T, Umesumbu SE, Mandoko AS, Nsibu CN, Dotson EB, Beach RF, et al. Presence of species within the *Anopheles gambiae* complex in the Democratic Republic of Congo. Trans R Soc Trop Med Hyg. 2016;110:373–5.
2. PNLP KSPH, Swiss KSPH, INRB, INFORM. An epidemiological profile of malaria in the Democratic Republic of Congo. 2014.
3. Basilua Kanza JP, El Fahime E, Alaoui S, Essassi EM, Brooke B, Nkebolo Malafu A, et al. Pyrethroid, DDT and malathion resistance in the malaria vector *Anopheles gambiae* from the Democratic Republic of Congo. Trans R Soc Trop Med Hyg. 2013;107:8–14.
4. Riveron JM, Watsenga F, Irving H, Irish SR, Wondji CS. High *Plasmodium* infection rate and reduced bed net efficacy in multiple insecticide-resistant malaria vectors in Kinshasa, Democratic Republic of Congo. J Infect Dis. 2018;217:320–8.
5. Wat'senga F, Manzambi EZ, Lunkula A, Mulumbu R, Mampangulu T, Lobo N, et al. Nationwide insecticide resistance status and biting behaviour of malaria vector species in the Democratic Republic of Congo. Malar J. 2018;17:129.
6. Knox TB, Juma EO, Ochomo EO, Pates Jamet H, Ndungo L, Chege P, et al. An online tool for mapping insecticide resistance in major *Anopheles* vectors of human malaria parasites and review of resistance status for the Afrotropical region. Parasit Vectors. 2014;7:76.
7. Nardini L, Hunt RH, Dahan-Moss YL, Christie N, Christian RN, Coetzee M, et al. Malaria vectors in the Democratic Republic of the Congo: the mechanisms that confer insecticide resistance in *Anopheles gambiae* and *Anopheles funestus*. Malar J. 2017;16:448.
8. Bobanga T, Ayieko W, Zanga M, Umesumbu S, Landela A, Fataki O, et al. Field efficacy and acceptability of PermaNet3.0® and OlysetNet® in Kinshasa, Democratic Republic of the Congo. J Infect Dis. 2013;50:206–14.
9. The Anopheles gambiae Genomes Consortium. Genetic diversity of the African malaria vector *Anopheles gambiae*. Nature. 2017;552:96.
10. Donnelly MJ, Isaacs AT, Weetman D. Identification, validation, and application of molecular diagnostics for insecticide resistance in malaria vectors. Trends Parasitol. 2016;32:197–206.
11. Martinez-Torres D, Chandre F, Williamson MS, Darriet F, Berge JB, Devonshire AL, et al. Molecular characterization of pyrethroid knockdown resistance (*kdr*) in the major malaria vector *Anopheles gambiae* s.s. Insect Mol Biol. 1998;7:179–84.
12. Ranson H, Jensen B, Vulule JM, Wang X, Hemingway J, Collins FH. Identification of a point mutation in the voltage-gated sodium channel gene of Kenyan *Anopheles gambiae* associated with resistance to DDT and pyrethroids. Insect Mol Biol. 2000;9:491–7.
13. Pinto J, Lynd A, Vicente JL, Santolamazza F, Randle NP, Gentile G, et al. Multiple origins of knockdown resistance mutations in the Afrotropical mosquito vector *Anopheles gambiae*. PLoS ONE. 2007;2:e1243.
14. Lynd A, Weetman D, Barbosa S, Egyir Yawson A, Mitchell S, Pinto J, et al. Field, genetic, and modeling approaches show strong positive selection acting upon an insecticide resistance mutation in *Anopheles gambiae* s.s. Mol Biol Evol. 2010;27:1117–25.
15. Mathias DK, Ochomo E, Atieli F, Ombok M, Nabie Bayoh M, Olang G, et al. Spatial and temporal variation in the *kdr* allele L1014S in *Anopheles gambiae* s.s. and phenotypic variability in susceptibility to insecticides in Western Kenya. Malar J. 2011;10:10.

16. Dabiré KR, Diabaté A, Namountougou M, Toé KH, Ouari A, Kengne P, et al. Distribution of pyrethroid and DDT resistance and the L1014F *kdr* mutation in *Anopheles gambiae* s.l. from Burkina Faso (West Africa). Trans R Soc Trop Med Hyg. 2009;103:1113–20.

17. Aïzoun N, Aïkpon R, Akogbéto M. Evidence of increasing L1014F *kdr* mutation frequency in *Anopheles gambiae* s.l. pyrethroid resistant following a nationwide distribution of LLINs by the Beninese National Malaria Control Programme. Asian Pac J Trop Biomed. 2014;4:239–43.

18. Dabiré RK, Namountougou M, Diabaté A, Soma DD, Bado J, Toé HK, et al. Distribution and frequency of *kdr* Mutations within *Anopheles gambiae* s.l. populations and first report of the ace.1G119S mutation in *Anopheles arabiensis* from Burkina Faso (West Africa). PLoS One. 2014;9:e101484.

19. Lynd A, Ranson H, McCall PJ, Randle NP, Black WC, Walker ED, et al. A simplified high-throughput method for pyrethroid knock-down resistance (*kdr*) detection in *Anopheles gambiae*. Malar J. 2005;4:16.

20. Kulkarni MA, Rowland M, Alifrangis M, Mosha FW, Matowo J, Malima R, et al. Occurrence of the leucine-to-phenylalanine knockdown resistance (*kdr*) mutation in *Anopheles arabiensis* populations in Tanzania, detected by a simplified high-throughput SSOP-ELISA method. Malar J. 2006;5:56.

21. Kolaczinski JH, Fanello C, Herve JP, Conway DJ, Carnevale P, Curtis CF. Experimental and molecular genetic analysis of the impact of pyrethroid and non-pyrethroid insecticide impregnated bednets for mosquito control in an area of pyrethroid resistance. Bull Entomol Res. 2000;90:125–32.

22. Bass C, Nikou D, Donnelly MJ, Williamson MS, Ranson H, Ball A, et al. Detection of knockdown resistance (*kdr*) mutations in *Anopheles gambiae*: a comparison of two new high-throughput assays with existing methods. Malar J. 2007;6:111.

23. Vazquez-Prokopec GM, Galvin WA, Kelly R, Kitron U. A new, cost-effective, battery-powered aspirator for adult mosquito collections. J Med Entomol. 2009;46:1256–9.

24. Gillies MT, Coetzee M. A supplement to the Anophelinae of Africa south of the Sahara (Afrotropical region). Publications of the South African Institute for Medical Research. 1987.

25. WHO. Test procedures for insecticide resistance monitoring in malaria vector mosquitoes. 2nd Ed. Geneva: World Health Organization; 2016.

26. Santolamazza F, Mancini E, Simard F, Qi Y, Tu Z, della Torre A. Insertion polymorphisms of SINE200 retrotransposons within speciation islands of *Anopheles gambiae* molecular forms. Malar J. 2008;7:163.

27. Jones CM, Liyanapathirana M, Agossa FR, Weetman D, Ranson H, Donnelly MJ, et al. Footprints of positive selection associated with a mutation (N1575Y) in the voltage-gated sodium channel of *Anopheles gambiae*. Proc Natl Acad Sci USA. 2012;109:6614–9.

28. Bass C, Nikou D, Vontas J, Williamson MS, Field LM. Development of high-throughput real-time PCR assays for the identification of insensitive acetylcholinesterase (ace-1R) in *Anopheles gambiae*. Pestic Biochem Physiol. 2010;96:80–5.

29. Rose SD. Genotyping with locked nucleic acid fluorescent probes: Intergrated DNA Technologies; 2011.

30. IDT. Biophysics. Software version 1.02.

31. Plotly Technologies Inc. Collaborative data science, 2015.

32. R Genetics package. Warnes G, Gorjanc G, Leisch F, Man M. Software version 1.3.8.1.

33. Wang L, Nomura Y, Du Y, Liu N, Zhorov BS, Dong K. A mutation in the intracellular loop III/IV of mosquito sodium channel synergizes the effect of mutations in helix IIS6 on pyrethroid resistance. Mol Pharmacol. 2015;87:421–9.

34. Edi A, N'Dri B, Chouaibou M, Kouadio F, Pignatelli P, Raso G, et al. First detection of N1575Y mutation in pyrethroid resistant *Anopheles gambiae* in Southern Côte d'Ivoire. Wellcome Open Res. 2017;2:71.

35. Fossog Tene B, Poupardin R, Costantini C, Awono-Ambene P, Wondji CS, Ranson H, et al. Resistance to DDT in an urban setting: common mechanisms implicated in both M and S forms of *Anopheles gambiae* in the city of Yaoundé, Cameroon. PLoS One. 2013;8:e61408.

36. Djègbè I, Agossa FR, Jones CM, Poupardin R, Cornelie S, Akogbéto M, et al. Molecular characterization of DDT resistance in *Anopheles gambiae* from Benin. Parasit Vectors. 2014;7:409.

18

Age and gender trends in insecticide-treated net use in sub-Saharan Africa: a multi-country analysis

Bolanle Olapeju[1], Ifta Choiriyyah[2], Matthew Lynch[1], Angela Acosta[1], Sean Blaufuss[1], Eric Filemyr[1], Hunter Harig[1], April Monroe[1], Richmond Ato Selby[1], Albert Kilian[3] and Hannah Koenker[1*]

Abstract

Background: The degree to which insecticide-treated net (ITN) supply accounts for age and gender disparities in ITN use among household members is unknown. This study explores the role of household ITN supply in the variation in ITN use among household members in sub-Saharan Africa.

Methods: Data was from Malaria Indicator Surveys or Demographic and Health Surveys collected between 2011 and 2016 from 29 countries in sub-Saharan Africa. The main outcome was ITN use the previous night. Other key variables included ITN supply (nets/household members), age and gender of household members. Analytical methods included logistic regressions and meta-regression.

Results: Across countries, the median (range) of the percentage of households with enough ITNs was 30.7% (8.5–62.0%). Crude analysis showed a sinusoidal pattern in ITN use across age groups of household members, peaking at 0–4 years and again around 30–40 years and dipping among people between 5–14 and 50+ years. This sinusoidal pattern was more pronounced in households with not enough ITNs compared to those with enough ITNs. ITN use tended to be higher in females than males in households with not enough ITNs while use was comparable among females and males in households with enough ITNs. After adjusting for wealth quintile, residence and region, among households with not enough ITNs in all countries, the odds of ITN use were consistently higher among children under 5 years and non-pregnant women 15–49 years. Meta-regressions showed that across all countries, the mean adjusted odds ratio (aOR) of ITN use among children under 5 years, pregnant and non-pregnant women aged 15–49 years and people 50 years and above was significantly higher than among men aged 15–49 years. Among these household members, the relationship was attenuated when there were enough ITNs in the household (dropping 0.26–0.59 points) after adjusting for geographical zone, household ITN supply, population ITN access, and ITN use:access ratio. There was no significant difference in mean aOR of ITN use among school-aged children compared to men aged 15–49 years, regardless of household ITN supply.

Conclusions: This study demonstrated that having enough ITNs in the household increases level of use and decreases existing disparities between age and gender groups. ITN distribution via mass campaigns and continuous distribution channels should be enhanced as needed to ensure that households have enough ITNs for all members, including men and school-aged children.

Keywords: Insecticide-treated nets, Use, Household supply, Age, Gender, Household members, Sub-Saharan Africa

*Correspondence: hkoenker@jhu.edu
[1] PMI VectorWorks Project, Johns Hopkins Center for Communication Programs, School of Public Health, 111 Marketplace, Baltimore, MD 21202, USA
Full list of author information is available at the end of the article

Background

According to the World Malaria Report, there were an estimated 216 million cases of malaria globally in 2016 while the estimated number of malaria deaths was 445,000 in 2016 [1]. Africa continues to carry a disproportionately higher share of the global malaria burden as 90% of malaria cases and deaths occur in this continent with 15 countries in sub-Saharan Africa accounting for 80% of the global malaria burden [1]. The World Health Organization (WHO) recommends the use of insecticide-treated nets (ITNs) as a key element of vector control by all individuals at risk of malaria, and distribution of free ITNs is a core intervention in national malaria control strategies of all sub-Saharan Africa countries [2]. In an effort to achieve universal coverage, i.e., universal access to and use of ITNs by populations at risk of malaria [3], over 800 million nets have been delivered in sub-Saharan Africa between 2011 and 2016, mostly under universal coverage campaigns [1]. This investment has resulted in an increased proportion of Africans in malaria-endemic areas who slept under an ITN, from 2010 30%, to 2016 54% [1]. The concept of universal access and indicators used to measure it are based on the assumption that each ITN protects two people [1]. To further improve ITN coverage in Africa, gaps in ITN access as well as ITN use need to be explored and addressed [4].

Recent studies have shown that the major driver of ITN use is access, as one cannot use an ITN unless there is one available for use [5–8]. After ITN access has been addressed, individual level factors, including age and gender of household members, have also been associated with ITN use. Studies across Africa demonstrate that ITN use is typically higher among females compared to males [9]. ITN use is also correlated with age [10] and has been shown to be higher in certain age groups, e.g., infants [11] or children under 5 years of age [12] compared to older children aged 5–14 years and adolescents and young adults aged 15–24 [13, 14]. The association of age with ITN use also seems to be moderated by gender, such that men, older children and teenagers were less likely to sleep under an ITN compared to women and children under 5 years old [15]. It is unclear whether certain household members are prioritized only because the number of nets in the household is not enough. Thus, the supply of nets in the household might be the reason for the age/gender disparities in ITN use.

This paper explores to what extent ITN supply (having enough nets for household members) accounts for age and gender disparities in IT N use among household members in sub-Saharan Africa. ITN use has been shown to increase dramatically in all age groups and gender following mass free distribution of ITN [13, 16] suggesting that certain household members are prioritized for ITN use when there are not enough ITNs in the household. The relationships between ITN supply, household members and ITN use are worth exploring to understand whether improving supply of ITNs in a household might reduce age and gender disparities in ITN use.

Methods

This study analyses secondary data from recent national surveys in sub-Saharan Africa.

Data from recent (conducted between 2011 and 2016) Malaria Indicator Surveys (MIS) or Demographic and Health Surveys (DHS) among countries in sub-Saharan Africa, were included in the analysis. Recent surveys were defined as those conducted between 2011 and 2016. The most recent publicly available MIS or DHS data from a total of 29 malaria endemic countries (Namibia was excluded given its limited malaria risk [1]) were downloaded with permission from the DHS Programme website, http://www.dhsprogram.com.

The countries were categorized into 3 geographical zones, Central, East and West Africa, based on the United Nations geoscheme for Africa [17]. East Africa region included 10 countries (34.5%), Central Africa, 7 countries (24.1%) and West Africa, 12 countries (41.4%).

The main outcome of the study is use of an ITN the previous night and this was calculated for each de facto member of the household, i.e., all those present in the house the previous night, as recommended by WHO's Roll Back Malaria Monitoring and Evaluation Reference Group (MERG) [7, 18]. A main predictor variable was household ITN supply and this was defined as the number of ITNs present in the household divided by the *de jure* household members and was further dichotomized into 'not enough' (ITN: person ratio of less than 0.5) *versus* 'enough' (ITN: person ratio of 0.5 or more equivalent to one ITN for every 2 people). The other main predictor variables of interest included gender (male *versus* female) and age (categorized in 5–10 year increments (0–4, 5–9, 10–14, 15–19, 20–29, 30–39, 40–49, 50–59, and 60+ years) of de facto household members. In addition, a composite variable called 'demographic group' variable was created based on age, gender and pregnancy status of the de facto household members. The following demographic groups were defined: children under 5 years old, school-aged children 5–14 years, women aged 15–49 years who were currently pregnant, women aged 15–49 years who were not currently pregnant, men aged 15–49 years (reference group) and adults aged 50 years or more.

Other socio-demographic variables included household wealth quintile based on the standard DHS wealth index determined by principal component analysis on household assets, residence (urban/rural), and region (sub-national administrative divisions for each country). Two contextual variables included in the analysis include population level ITN access, and use given access (use:access ratio). The population ITN access indicator for each country was calculated according to MERG guidance by dividing the potential ITN users (number of ITNs in the household multiplied by 2) by the number of de facto members for each household, setting the result to 1 if there were more potential users than de facto members, and determining the overall sample mean of that fraction [7]. To assess whether people who have ITNs actually use them, the ratio of population ITN use to population ITN access was calculated.

All analysis was limited to households with at least one ITN. First, plots of ITN use by age and gender of de facto household members, stratified by household ITN supply were constructed for each country separately. Then, multivariable logistic regressions were conducted for each country, stratified by household ITN supply, to explore differences in ITN use among demographic groups, controlling for household wealth quintile, residence and region. Next, to synthesize the findings across all countries, a meta-regression was conducted to explore the mean adjusted odds ratio (aOR) of ITN use across demographic groups across all 29 countries. Each country was stratified by household ITN supply for a total sample size of 58. Plots of the mean aOR and 95% confidence interval (CI) of ITN use among demographic groups stratified by ITN supply were constructed over all countries and also by the 3 geographic zones (Central, East and West Africa). The model included the following country-level covariates: geographical zone, household ITN supply, population ITN access and ITN use:access ratio. To account for different sample size of each country, the number of de facto populations in households with at least one ITN was used as a probability weight.

Data management and analysis was done using Stata version 14 (Stata Corporation, College Station, TX, USA) and Excel 2016 (Microsoft Corp, Seattle, WA, USA). All country-level analyses used sample weights to adjust for DHS sample design and individual response rate [19].

Results

Table 1 presents the proportion of households with enough ITNs and population-level ITN access and use:access ratio for each survey. Across countries, the median (range) of the percentage of households with enough ITNs was 30.7% (8.5–62.0%). The median (range) of the percentage of households with enough ITNs was 14.5% (8.5–24.3%) in Central; 38.4% (22.7–62.0%) in East Africa; and, 30.7% (9.3–56.7%) in West Africa. In only 3 countries did more than 50% of households own enough ITNs: Uganda (62.0%), Senegal (56.7%) and

Ghana (50.3%). Similarly, the median (range) of the percentage of the de facto population with access to an ITN in their household was 26.9% (19.7–61.2%) in Central; 55.9% (37.2–78.8%) in East; and, 49.0% (25.3–75.7%) in West Africa. Overall, the proportion of the population that used an ITN the previous night was greater than 50% in only 8 countries (Madagascar, Rwanda, Uganda, Democratic Republic of Congo, Benin, Burkina Faso, Mali, Senegal). ITN use:access ratio varied widely across the countries from 0.23 in Zimbabwe to 1.15 in Congo-Brazzaville.

Figures 1, 2, 3 highlight country-level population ITN use stratified by ITN supply, age and gender in Central (Fig. 1), East (Fig. 2) and West (Fig. 3) Africa. In all countries, regardless of age and gender, ITN use was higher among people in households with enough ITNs compared to those in households with not enough ITNs. For people from households with not enough ITNs, ITN use showed a sinusoidal pattern, peaking at 0–4 years and again around 30–40 years and dipping among people between 5–14 and 50+ years. This sinusoidal pattern was less pronounced in households with enough ITNs. In households with not enough ITNs, ITN use was higher in females compared to males in many age groups. Among people living in households with enough ITNs, use was more comparable among males and females in all age groups.

Table 2 presents the aOR of ITN use the previous night among demographic groups (reference group: men 15–49 years) stratified by household ITN supply and controlling for household wealth index, household residence and region.

Among households with not enough ITNs, two demographic groups: children under 5 years and non-pregnant women had consistent significantly higher odds of ITN use compared to men aged 15–49 years in all countries. The median (range) aOR of ITN use among children under 5 years old in all 29 countries was 1.86 (1.22–3.81). Non-pregnant women in all 29 countries had a median (range) aOR of 1.76 (1.22–3.36). In addition, pregnant women in all 27 countries with available data had a median (range) aOR of 2.26 (1.48–4.27), although the aOR was not statistically significant in Zimbabwe, Ivory Coast, Madagascar, and Congo-Brazzaville. Children aged 5–14 years had a median (range) aOR of 0.94 (0.55–1.58); the aOR was significantly lower in 11 countries, significantly higher in 10 countries and not statistically significant in 8 out of 29 countries.

Among households with enough ITNs, the disparities in ITN use across demographic groups was attenuated. There was no demographic group with significantly higher odds of ITN use across all countries. The median (range) aOR of ITN use among children under 5 years old

Table 1 List of countries and key insecticide-treated net indicators

Country	Survey	Year	% of households with enough ITNs[a]	% of *de facto* population with ITN access	% of *de facto* population that used an ITN the previous night	Use:access ratio
Central Africa						
Angola	DHS	2015–16	10.9	19.7	17.6	0.89
Burundi	MIS	2012	23.9	46.0	48.6	1.06
Cameroon	DHS	2011	8.5	20.9	14.8	0.71
Chad	DHS	2014–15	40.8	61.2	33.3	0.54
Congo Brazzaville	DHS	2011–12	10.4	22.6	26.0	1.15
Democratic Republic of Congo	DHS	2013–14	24.3	46.5	50.2	1.08
Gabon	DHS	2012	14.5	26.9	26.7	0.99
East Africa						
Kenya	MIS	2015	40.1	52.5	47.6	0.91
Madagascar	MIS	2016	43.1	62.1	68.2	1.10
Malawi	DHS	2015–16	22.7	38.8	33.9	0.87
Mozambique	DHS	2015	38.4	53.8	45.4	0.84
Rwanda	DHS	2014–15	42.2	63.8	61.4	0.96
Tanzania	DHS	2015–16	37.2	55.9	49.0	0.88
Uganda	MIS	2014–15	62.0	78.8	68.6	0.87
Zambia	DHS	2013–14	25.0	65.0	56.9	0.88
Zimbabwe	DHS	2015	26.1	37.2	8.5	0.23
West Africa						
Benin	DHS	2011–12	43.3	64.0	62.6	0.98
Burkina Faso	MIS	2014	47.4	71.2	67.0	0.94
Cote D'Ivoire	DHS	2011	30.7	49.0	33.2	0.68
Gambia	DHS	2013	20.1	45.3	36.9	0.82
Ghana	MIS	2016	50.3	65.8	41.7	0.63
Guinea	DHS	2012	9.3	25.3	18.9	0.75
Liberia	MIS	2016	23.5	41.5	39.2	0.94
Mali	MIS	2015	37.6	69.5	63.8	0.92
Niger	DHS	2012	14.4	37.3	13.8	0.37
Nigeria	MIS	2015	34.4	54.7	37.3	0.68
Senegal	cDHS	2016	56.7	75.7	63.1	0.83
Sierra Leone	MIS	2016	14.6	37.1	38.6	1.04
Togo	DHS	2013–14	32.5	48.8	33.6	0.69

DHS Demographic Health Survey, *ITN* insecticide-treated nets, *MIS* Malaria Indicator Survey

[a] A household supply of at least 0.5 net per person

was 1.48 (0.93–2.80) although the aOR was not statistically significant in 8 and significantly higher in 21 of the 29 countries. Pregnant women had a median (range) aOR of ITN use of 1.29 (0.90–2.59). Similarly, the aOR was not statistically significant in eight countries and significantly higher in 21 countries of the 29 countries. Among pregnant women, the median (range) aOR of ITN use was 1.75 (0.46–4.36) although the aOR was significantly lower in Zimbabwe, not statistically significant in 14 countries and significantly higher in 12 of the 27 countries with available data. Children aged 5–14 years had

a median (range) aOR of 0.98 (0.60–2.40), the aOR was significantly lower in 9 countries, significantly higher in 5 countries and not statistically significant in 15 countries.

Figure 4 presents results of the meta-regression of the aORs of ITN use among demographic groups, stratified by ITN supply across all 29 countries, and in addition, for each geographic zone. Overall, the mean aOR of ITN use was significantly higher among children under 5 years, pregnant and non-pregnant women aged 15–49 years and people 50 years and above compared to the reference group of men aged 15–49 years. Also, the differences

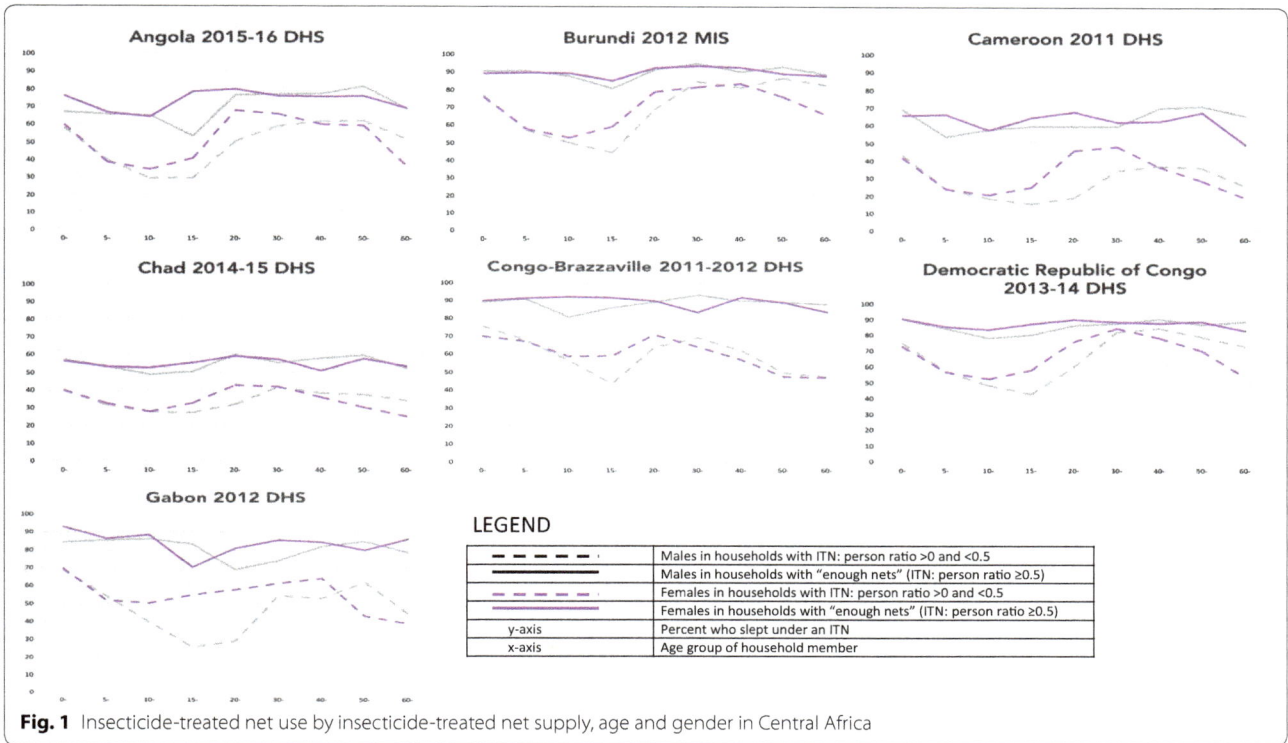

Fig. 1 Insecticide-treated net use by insecticide-treated net supply, age and gender in Central Africa

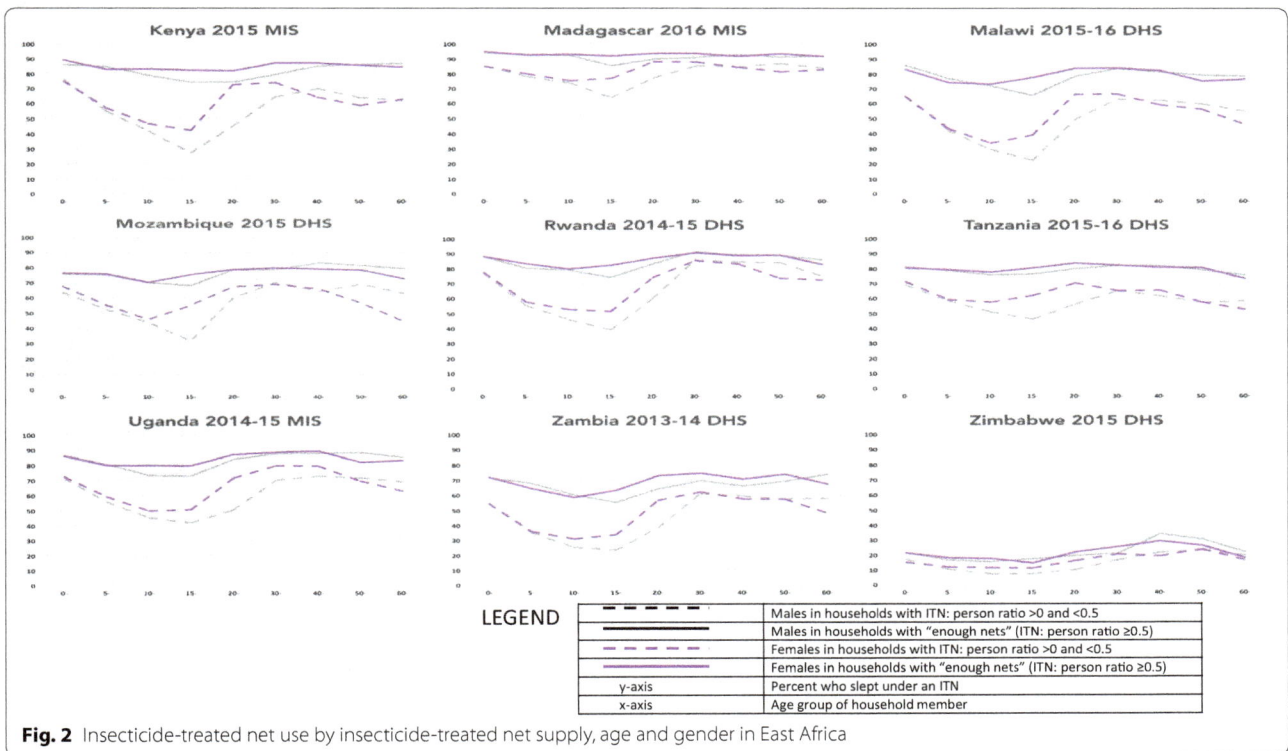

Fig. 2 Insecticide-treated net use by insecticide-treated net supply, age and gender in East Africa

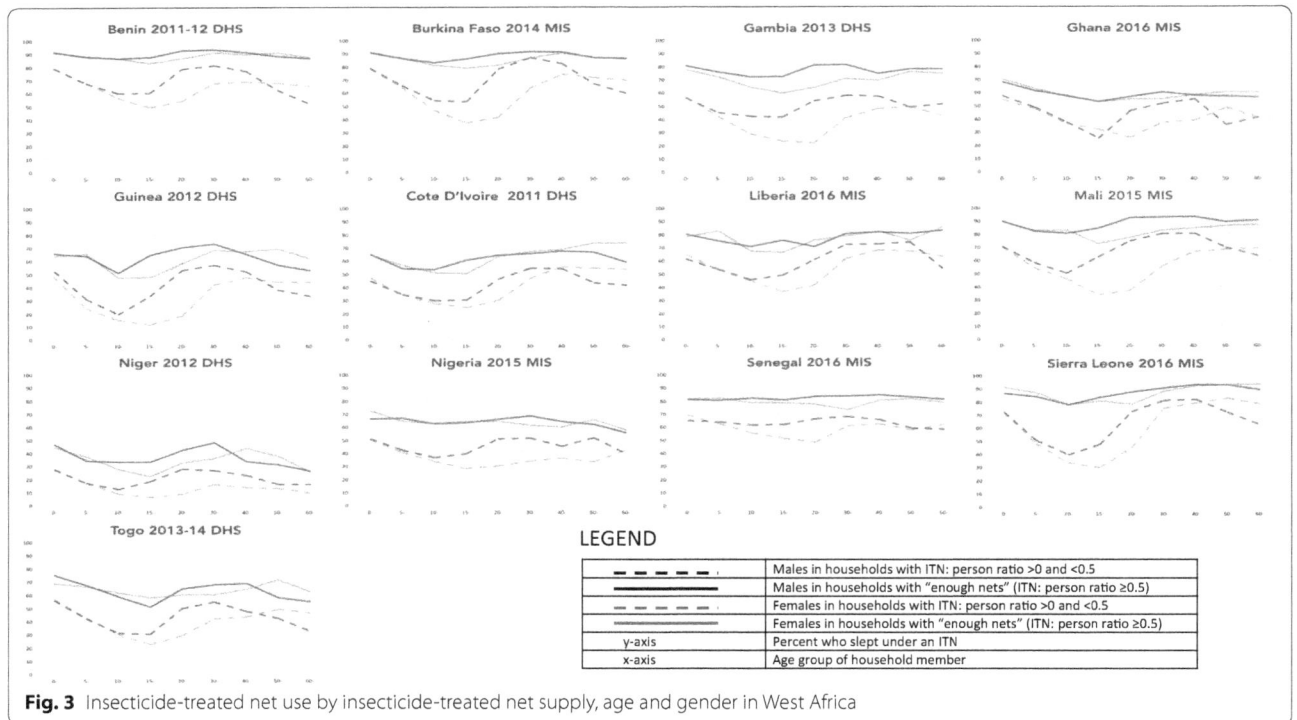

Fig. 3 Insecticide-treated net use by insecticide-treated net supply, age and gender in West Africa

in ITN use across demographic groups tended to be reduced when there were enough ITNs. In addition, for children under 5 years, pregnant and non-pregnant women aged 15–49 years and people 50 years and above, the aORs of ITN use were higher in households with enough ITNs compared to households with not enough ITNs. There was no significant difference in mean aOR of ITN use among school-aged children compared to men aged 15–49 years, regardless of household ITN supply. This trend was seen over all countries and across the 3 geographic zones. Of note, the variation in mean aOR of ITN use across household members was most pronounced in West compared to East or Central Africa.

The meta-regression results in Table 3 highlight the influence of country-level ITN supply, population ITN access, ITN use:access ratio and geographic region on the mean aOR of ITN use for demographic groups across all 29 countries. The effect sizes shown in the Table represent the change in mean aOR per unit change of each covariate, holding others constant. Thus, the mean aOR is treated as a continuous variable in this analysis. For example, the mean aOR of ITN use among children under 5 years reduces by 0.59 points in households with not enough compared to enough ITN supply while each per cent increase in population ITN access has minimal effect on the mean aOR of ITN use. In general, the results confirm earlier findings, as the mean aORs of ITN use decreased (dropping by 0.26–0.59 points) among

almost all demographic groups compared to men age 15–49 years when there are enough ITNs in the household compared to households with not enough ITNs. The only exception was the group children 5–14 years for whom the mean aOR did not change with household ITN supply. The level of population access to ITNs at the time of the survey (as shown in Table 1) did not have any impact on the mean aOR of ITN use among household members, again with the exception of children 5–14 years for whom the mean aOR increased by 0.06 for each 10% increase in population access. Changes in use-to-access ratio did not significantly contribute to differentials in the mean aOR of ITN use across demographic groups. As was suggested in Fig. 4, the mean aOR of ITN use for household members, except the 50 years and over, was significantly higher in West compared to the East Africa.

Discussion

This study demonstrated that regardless of setting and across a large number of countries, the groups most vulnerable to malaria are preferentially being covered, per WHO recommendations that pregnant women and infants in malaria-endemic areas use ITNs. It also suggests that ITNs are not hoarded by heads of households but used among household members, depending on household supply. The study showed that having enough ITNs in the household increases level of use and

Table 2 Logistic regression of insecticide-treated net use among demographic groups (reference: men aged 15–49 years) stratified by insecticide-treated net supply, adjusted for wealth index, residence (urban/rural), and region

Country	aORᵃof ITN use among household members by household ITN supply											
	Households with not enough ITNs (ref: male 15–49 years)					Households with enough ITNs (ref: male 15–49 years)					
	Children under 5 years	School-aged (5–14 years)	Female 15–49 years		50+ years	Children under 5 years	School-aged (5–14 years)	Female 15–49 years		50+ years		
			Not pregnant	Currently pregnant				Not pregnant	Currently pregnant			
East Africa												
Madagascar	1.63*	0.93	1.76*	1.23	1.53*	1.82*	1.46*	1.41*	1.99*	1.21		
Mozambique	1.48*	0.71*	1.48*	1.76*	1.12	0.99	0.80*	1.12	2.42*	1.12		
Zimbabwe	1.22*	0.71*	1.33*	1.07	1.65*	0.97	0.73*	1.10	0.46*	1.08		
Zambia	1.42*	0.56*	1.41*	1.48*	1.51*	1.37*	0.89	1.31*	2.03*	1.33*		
Malawi	2.01*	0.66*	1.65*	1.51*	1.31*	1.73*	0.88*	1.43*	1.05	1.07		
Rwanda	1.68*	0.58*	1.43*	3.55*	1.69*	1.48*	0.85*	1.29*	2.31*	1.38*		
Tanzania	1.83*	1.02	1.60*	1.66*	1.08	1.21*	0.98	1.20*	1.08	0.98		
Uganda	1.98*	0.85	1.80*	2.37*	1.70*	1.27*	0.76*	1.28*	1.61*	1.10		
Kenya	3.2*	1.01	1.9*	3.57*	1.64*	2.04*	1.28*	1.59*	1.54	1.71*		
Central Africa												
Angola	1.45*	0.57*	1.61*	2.26*	1.24	1.13	0.78*	1.41*	2.56*	1.23		
Burundi	1.43*	0.55*	1.30*	2.64*	1.72*	1.08	1.07	1.13	2.74	1.14		
Cameroon	2.34*	0.89	1.94*	2.89*	1.10	1.52*	0.98	1.21	0.76	0.98		
Chad	1.56*	0.94	1.47*	[ ]	1.08	1.22*	0.92	1.14*	[ ]	1.14		
Congo-Brazzaville	1.70*	1.1	1.22*	1.36	0.62*	0.93	0.90	0.90	1.50	0.77		
DRC	1.45*	0.60*	1.57*	1.78*	1.26*	1.5*	0.79*	1.28*	1.70	1.13		
Gabon	3.4*	1.49*	2.24*	2.28*	1.38*	2.8*	2.40*	1.45*	1.75	1.48		
West Africa												
Benin	2.52*	1.20*	2.11*	4.27*	1.13*	1.54*	1.04	1.57*	2.00*	1.06		
Burkina Faso	3.2*	1.22*	2.94*	4.24*	1.87*	1.82*	1.05	1.72*	1.97*	1.26*		
Gambia	3.18*	1.58*	2.65*	3.21*	2.18*	2.25*	1.37*	1.89*	4.36*	1.94*		
Ghana	2.60*	1.46*	1.80*	2.16*	1.35	1.82*	1.16	1.17	1.79*	1.01		
Guinea	2.74*	0.77*	2.72*	3.45*	1.92*	1.49*	1.12	1.80*	1.37	1.38*		
Cote D'Ivoire	1.27*	0.69*	1.47*	1.18	1.46*	0.94	0.60*	1.06	1.51*	1.00		
Liberia	1.60*	0.94	1.72*	1.86*	1.72*	1.05	0.84	1.07	1.23	1.17		
Mali	2.65*	1.24*	3.36*	3.66*	2.37*	2.20*	1.15	2.59*	2.65*	1.87*		
Niger	3.81*	1.57*	3.18*	3.00*	1.43*	2.03*	1.09	1.52*	1.59	0.94		
Nigeria	2.20*	1.30*	2.04*	2.72*	1.54*	1.28*	1.02	1.19*	1.25	0.99		
Senegal	1.66*	1.20*	1.66*	[ ]	1.19	1.47*	1.33*	1.52*	[ ]	1.30*		

Table 2 (continued)

Country	Households with not enough ITNs (ref: male 15–49 years)					Households with enough ITNs (ref: male 15–49 years)				
	Children under 5 years	School-aged (5–14 years)	Female 15–49 years		50 + years	Children under 5 years	School-aged (5–14 years)	Female 15–49 years		50+ years
			Not pregnant	Currently pregnant				Not pregnant	Currently pregnant	
Sierra Leone	1.86*	0.56*	1.90*	2.05*	2.03*	1.08	0.71*	1.37*	2.03	1.80*
Togo	2.56*	1.13*	1.84*	1.93*	1.39*	1.63*	1.13	1.17*	1.37	0.99

Data not available

aOR adjusted odds ratio, *ITN* insecticide-treated net

[a] Adjusted for wealth index, residence (urban/rural), and region

* Significant at *p* value < 0.05

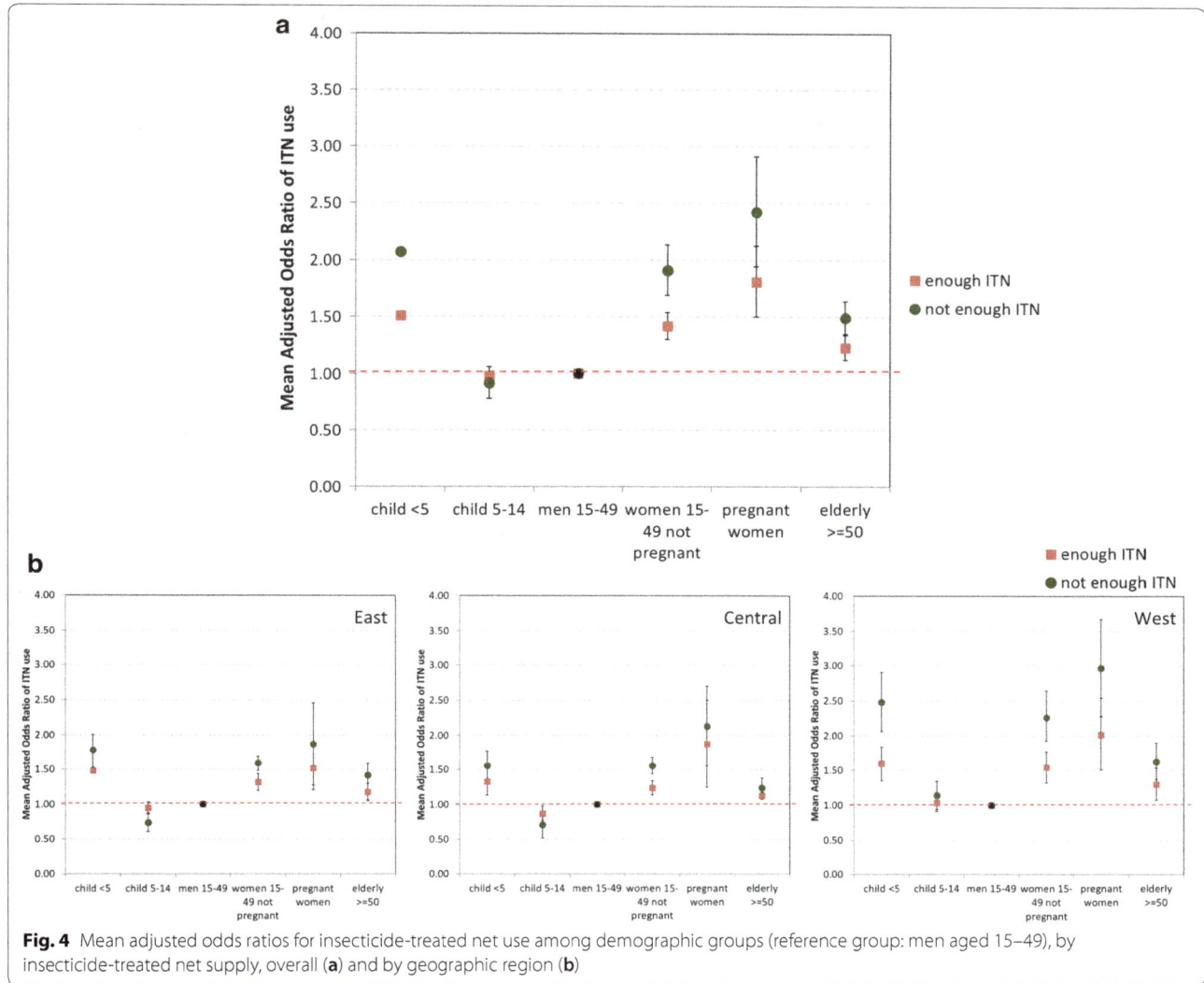

Fig. 4 Mean adjusted odds ratios for insecticide-treated net use among demographic groups (reference group: men aged 15–49), by insecticide-treated net supply, overall (**a**) and by geographic region (**b**)

decreases existing disparities between age and gender groups. ITN use was consistently higher among people in households with enough compared to not enough nets. The role of ITN supply on use is important given the WHO target of 85% coverage of key malaria interventions, including ITN use by all people at risk of malaria, and the WHO recommendation of one ITN for every two people at risk of malaria [1]. Many countries struggle to meet this target among all households but have been able to achieve the target among households with enough ITNs. This suggests that people are typically willing to use ITNs but need to have enough ITNs to increase and sustain ITN use. Thus, increasing the household supply of ITNs improves use among members. These findings provide further evidence that the main barrier to ITN

use is perhaps insufficient access and to a lesser degree unwillingness to use ITNs [5, 7, 8].

Our findings highlight existing disparities in ITN use among household members, corroborating previous research [10–13, 15]. In most of sub-Saharan Africa, households rightfully prioritize children under 5 years as well as pregnant women, especially when there is not enough ITN supply. Children under 5 years and pregnant women of reproductive age may be more likely to sleep under an ITN because, in many settings, those children share sleeping spaces with their mothers or adolescent female siblings [20]. It may also be due to the ITN interventions of the last few decades targeting pregnant women and children under 5 years old [9]. While pregnant women and young children are biologically vulnerable to malaria, there are negative

Table 3 Adjusted linear regression coefficients for mean adjusted odds ratios of insecticide-treated net use

Independent variable	Adjusted linear regression coefficients by demographic group[a]				
	Children under 5 years	School-aged (5–14 years)	Female 15–49 years		50+ years
			Not pregnant	Pregnant	
Household ITN supply enough vs not enough	− 0.568*	0.524	− 0.497*	− 0.591*	− 0.258*
Population access in %[b]	− 0.0001	0.006*	− 0.000	0.013	− 0.005
Use:access ratio[b]	− 0.195	− 0.399	0.221	1.072	0.680
Central Africa vs East	− 0.168	0.036	− 0.040	0.389	− 0.195
West Africa vs East	0.424*	0.231*	0.479*	0.779*	0.179
R squared	0.384	0.332	0.463	0.337	0.328

ITN insecticide-treated net

[a] Covariates included in the model: household ITN supply, population ITN access and geographic zone

[b] Variable shown in Table 1

* Significant at p-value < 0.05

side effects with only prioritizing them for ITN use. Contraction of malaria by other household members still has unwelcome health, social and financial consequences for the family, hence the emphasis on universal coverage [9].

The role of ITN supply on disparities in ITN use among household members is a novel addition of this study to the existing literature. Pregnant women, children under 5 years old, women aged 15–49 years, and those over 50 years were still more likely to have used an ITN the previous night than men but having enough ITNs within the household reduced the gaps in ITN use across these groups. However, school-children aged 5–14 years were among the least prioritized in households, regardless of household ITN supply. Studies have found that school-aged children had the highest prevalence of malaria infection but were most likely to have asymptomatic infection, thus serving as an under recognized reservoir of malaria infection [21, 22]. Protecting this age group with ITNs would reduce adverse health outcomes, such as anaemia and mortality, and educational outcomes such as school absenteeism and lower cognitive function [23]. In addition, protecting this age group with ITNs could protect the rest of the population from malaria transmission. As recommendations shift from covering vulnerable populations to universal coverage, there is a need to ensure that households have enough nets to eliminate disparities in ITN use among members. Mass distribution campaigns have been a major source of ITN supply in households, however, gaps in ITN coverage have been demonstrated between mass campaign cycles. Continuous distribution of ITNs through antenatal care, immunization services, communities, and schools has been recommended by WHO to complement mass campaigns and ensure universal coverage of ITNs, particularly antenatal care

clinic and expanded programmes on vaccination distribution [3]. Continuous community-based [24, 25] and school-based ITN distribution [24, 26] has been shown to improve ITN ownership and access. However, although continuous antenatal care (ANC) and expanded programme on immunization (EPI) distribution systems targeting biologically vulnerable groups, such as children under 5 years and pregnant women, are supposed to be in place in almost every country, these are often low functioning, contributing to gaps in net access [25]. Efforts to improve the quality of existing distribution channels may involve ensuring complete household registration, enhancing data and communication campaigns to promote acceptability and uptake of distribution channels.

There are some limitations within this study. The analysis assumes that all ITNs included in the indicator of ITN supply in the household are all hung or usable. The study also uses slightly different denominators for the ITN indicators. Specifically, ITN supply is calculated from the *de jure* household members while ITN use is calculated from de facto members. This may be important in instances where the de facto and *de jure* members are markedly different. Seasonality of ITN use [27] is one of most important factors of ITN use but was not accounted for in this analysis. Research has shown seasonal variations in ITN use in sub-Saharan Africa, which may explain some of the differences in ITN use across countries as MIS and DHS surveys are usually conducted in different seasons. Typically, MIS is conducted during/at the end of rainy season while the DHS can be done any season. Given that ITN use is higher in the rainy season and immediately thereafter when malaria transmission is at a peak [28, 29], ITN use is higher in MIS survey countries than in DHS countries. Also, the timing of the most recent ITN mass campaigns was not accounted for in the analysis. Mass campaigns that are closely followed by household surveys generally show higher levels of population ITN access, which in turn makes high levels of ITN use feasible [13, 16]. In addition, the data analysed are cross-sectional in nature and thus do not permit causal inferences.

Finally, the study found some differences in ITN use among household members across the geographic zones explored. However due to the country eligibility criteria, not all countries within the three geographic regions are explored. Thus, regional differences in ITN use should be interpreted with caution. Also, malaria control research and programmatic efforts are also needed to understand the specific country level contextual factors that may explain trends in ITN access and use. For example, Zimbabwe has low levels of ITN use even among people in households with enough ITNs, and this may be related to national level indoor residual spraying interventions, resulting in a lower net use culture [30].

Conclusion

This study explored the role of ITN supply on ITN use among household members. The findings suggest that having enough ITNs in the household increases level of use and decreases existing disparities between age and gender groups. School-aged children were also consistently the least prioritized, regardless of a household's ITN supply. ITN distribution via mass campaigns, ANC and EPI, school and community channels should be enhanced as needed in order to ensure that households have enough ITNs for all members, including men and school-aged children.

Abbreviations

aOR: adjusted odds ratio; ANC: antenatal care; CI: confidence interval; DHS: Demographic Health Survey; EPI: expanded programme on immunization; ITN: insecticide-treated nets; MERG: Monitoring and Evaluation Reference Group; MIS: Malaria Indicator Survey; WHO: World Health Organization.

Authors' contributions

HK conceived the study. AA, AK, AM, BO, EF, HH, HK, IC, RAS, and SB managed the datasets and analysed the data. BO and IC drafted the paper with revisions from AA, AK, HK, ML, EF, HH, AM, SB, and RAS. All authors read and approved the final manuscript.

Author details
[1] PMI VectorWorks Project, Johns Hopkins Center for Communication Programs, School of Public Health, 111 Marketplace, Baltimore, MD 21202, USA. [2] Department of Population, Family and Reproductive Health, Johns Hopkins University Bloomberg School of Public Health, Baltimore, USA. [3] PMI VectorWorks Project, Tropical Health LLP, Montagut, Spain.

Acknowledgements
The authors are grateful to Lilia Gerberg, Lia Florey and Anna Bowen for their comments on earlier drafts.

Competing interests

The authors have the following interests: co-author Albert Kilian is employed by Tropical Health LLP.

Funding
This study was made possible by the generous support of the American people through the United States Agency for International Development (USAID) under the terms of USAID/JHU Cooperative Agreement No: AID-OAA-A-14-00057 for the VectorWorks Project. The contents are the responsibility of the authors and do not necessarily reflect the views of USAID or the United States Government. The funders had no role in study design, data collection and analysis, decision to publish, or preparation of the manuscript.

References
1. WHO. World malaria report 2017. Geneva: World Health Organization; 2017.
2. Sexton AR. Best practices for an insecticide-treated bed net distribution programme in sub-Saharan eastern Africa. Malar J. 2011;10:157.
3. WHO. Achieving and maintaining universal coverage with long-lasting insecticidal nets for malaria control. Geneva: World Health Organization; 2017.
4. van Eijk AM, Hill J, Alegana VA, Kirui V, Gething PW, ter Kuile FO, et al. Coverage of malaria protection in pregnant women in sub-Saharan Africa: a synthesis and analysis of national survey data. Lancet Infect Dis. 2011;11:190–207.
5. Eisele TP, Keating J, Littrell M, Larsen D, Macintyre K. Assessment of insecticide-treated bednet use among children and pregnant women across 15 countries using standardized national surveys. Am J Trop Med Hyg. 2009;80:209–14.
6. Graves PM, Ngondi JM, Hwang J, Getachew A, Gebre T, Mosher AW, et al. Factors associated with mosquito net use by individuals in households owning nets in Ethiopia. Malar J. 2011;10:354.
7. Koenker H, Kilian A. Recalculating the net use gap: a multi-country comparison of ITN use versus ITN access. PLoS ONE. 2014;9:e97496.
8. Bhatt S, Weiss DJ, Mappin B, Dalrymple U, Cameron E, Bisanzio D, et al. Coverage and system efficiencies of insecticide-treated nets in Africa from 2000 to 2017. eLife. 2015;4:e09672.
9. Garley AE, Ivanovich E, Eckert E, Negroustoueva S, Ye Y. Gender differences in the use of insecticide-treated nets after a universal free distribution campaign in Kano State, Nigeria: post-campaign survey results. Malar J. 2013;12:119.
10. Ng'ang'a PN, Jayasinghe G, Kimani V, Shililu J, Kabutha C, Kabuage L, et al. Bed net use and associated factors in a rice farming community in Central Kenya. Malar J. 2009;8:64.
11. Larson PS, Minakawa N, Dida GO, Njenga SM, Ionides EL, Wilson ML. Insecticide-treated net use before and after mass distribution in a fishing community along Lake Victoria, Kenya: successes and unavoidable pitfalls. Malar J. 2014;13:466.
12. Fokam EB, Kindzeka GF, Ngimuh L, Dzi KT, Wanji S. Determination of the predictive factors of long-lasting insecticide-treated net ownership and utilisation in the Bamenda Health District of Cameroon. BMC Public Health. 2017;17:263.
13. Loha E, Tefera K, Lindtjorn B. Freely distributed bed-net use among Chano Mille residents, south Ethiopia: a longitudinal study. Malar J. 2013;12:23.

14. Noor AM, Kirui VC, Brooker SJ, Snow RW. The use of insecticide treated nets by age: implications for universal coverage in Africa. BMC Public Health. 2009;9:369.

15. Babalola S, Ricotta E, Awantang G, Lewicky N, Koenker H, Toso M. Correlates of intra-household ITN use in Liberia: a multilevel analysis of household survey data. PLoS ONE. 2016;11:e0158331.

16. Finlay AM, Butts J, Ranaivoharimina H, Cotte AH, Ramarosandratana B, Rabarijaona H, et al. Free mass distribution of long lasting insecticidal nets lead to high levels of LLIN access and use in Madagascar, 2010: a cross-sectional observational study. PLoS ONE. 2017;12:e0183936.

17. Statistics Division UN. Standard country or area codes for statistics use. New York: United Nations, Division S; 1999.

18. MEASURE Evaluation, MEASURE DHS, President's Malaria Initiative, Roll Back Malaria Partnership, UNICEF, WHO. Household survey indicators for malaria control. Chapel Hill: MEASURE Evaluation; 2013.

19. Rutstein SO, Rojas G. Guide to DHS statistics. Calverton: ORC Macro; 2006.

20. Toé LP, Skovmand O, Dabiré KR, Diabaté A, Diallo Y, Guiguemdé TR, et al. Decreased motivation in the use of insecticide-treated nets in a malaria endemic area in Burkina Faso. Malar J. 2009;8:175.

21. Walldorf JA, Cohee LM, Coalson JE, Bauleni A, Nkanaunena K, Kapito-Tembo A, et al. School-age children are a reservoir of malaria infection in Malawi. PLoS ONE. 2015;10:e0134061.

22. Pullan RL, Bukirwa H, Staedke SG, Snow RW, Brooker S. Plasmodium infection and its risk factors in eastern Uganda. Malar J. 2010;9:2.

23. Nankabirwa J, Brooker SJ, Clarke SE, Fernando D, Gitonga CW, Schellenberg D, et al. Malaria in school-age children in Africa: an increasingly important challenge. Trop Med Int Health. 2014;19:1294–309.

24. Zeger de Beyl C, Kilian A, Brown A, Sy-Ar M, Selby RA, Randriamanantenasoa F, et al. Evaluation of community-based continuous distribution of long-lasting insecticide-treated nets in Toamasina II District, Madagascar. Malar J. 2017;16:327.

25. Kilian A, Woods Schnurr L, Matova T, Selby RA, Lokko K, Blaufuss S, et al. Evaluation of a continuous community-based ITN distribution pilot in Lainya County, South Sudan 2012–2013. Malar J. 2017;16:363.

26. Stuck L, Lutambi A, Chacky F, Schaettle P, Kramer K, Mandike R, et al. Can school-based distribution be used to maintain coverage of long-lasting insecticide-treated bed nets: evidence from a large scale programme in southern Tanzania? Health Policy Plan. 2017;32:980–9.

27. Smithuis FM, Kyaw MK, Phe UO, van der Broek I, Katterman N, Rogers C, et al. The effect of insecticide-treated bed nets on the incidence and prevalence of malaria in children in an area of unstable seasonal transmission in western Myanmar. Malar J. 2013;12:363.

28. Pinchoff J, Hamapumbu H, Kobayashi T, Simubali L, Stevenson JC, Norris DE, et al. Factors associated with sustained use of long-lasting insecticide-treated nets following a reduction in malaria transmission in Southern Zambia. Am J Trop Med Hyg. 2015;93:954–60.

29. Thwing J, Hochberg N, Eng JV, Issifi S, James Eliades M, Minkoulou E, et al. Insecticide-treated net ownership and usage in niger after a nationwide integrated campaign. Trop Med Int Health. 2008;13:827–34.

30. Mabaso ML, Sharp B, Lengeler C. Historical review of malarial control in southern African with emphasis on the use of indoor residual house-spraying. Trop Med Int Health. 2004;9:846–56.

19

Inter-sectoral approaches for the prevention and control of malaria among the mobile and migrant populations

Cho Naing[1,2*†] , Maxine A. Whittaker[2†] and Marcel Tanner[3†]

Abstract

Background: Malaria cases among mobile and migrant populations (MMPs) represent a large and important reservoir for transmission, if undetected or untreated. The objectives of this review were to identify which intersectoral actions have been taken and how they are applied to interventions targeted at the MMPs and also to assess the effect of interventions targeted to these special groups of population.

Results: A total of 36 studies met the inclusion criteria for this review. Numerous stakeholders were identified as involved in the intersectoral actions to defeat malaria amongst MMPs. Almost all studies discussed the involvement of Ministry of Health/Public Health (MOH/MOPH). The most frequently assessed intervention among the studies that were included was the coverage and utilization of insecticide-treated nets as personal protective measures (40.5%), followed by the intervention of early diagnoses and treatment of malaria (33.3%), the surveillance and response activities (13.9%) and the behaviour change communication (8.3%). There is a dearth of information on how these stakeholders shared roles and responsibilities for implementation, and about the channels of communication between-and-within the partners and with the MOH/MOPH. Despite limited details in the studies, the intermediate outcomes showed some evidence that the intersectoral collaborations contributed to improvement in knowledge about malaria, initiation and promotion of bed nets utilization, increased access to diagnosis and treatment in a surveillance context and contributed towards a reduction in malaria transmission. Overall, a high proportion of the targeted MMPs was equipped with correct knowledge about malaria transmission (70%, 95% CI 57–83%). Interventions targeting the use of bed nets utilization were two times more likely to reduce malaria incidence amongst the targeted MMPs (summary OR 2.01, 95% CI 1.43–2.6) than the non-users. The various intersectoral actions were often more vertically organized and not fully integrated in a systemic way within a given country or sub-national administrative setting.

Conclusion: Findings suggest that interventions supported by the multiple stakeholders had a significant impact on the reduction of malaria transmission amongst the targeted MMPs. Well-designed studies from different countries are recommended to robustly assess the role of intersectoral interventions targeted to MMPs and their impact on the reduction of transmission.

Keywords: Malaria, Mobile, Migrants, Intersectoral, Interventions, Review

*Correspondence: cho3699@gmail.com
†Cho Naing, Maxine A. Whittaker and Marcel Tanner contributed equally to this work
[1] Institute for Research, Development and Innovation (IRDI), International Medical University, Kuala Lumpur, Malaysia
Full list of author information is available at the end of the article

Background

The ultimate goal of the Global Technical Malaria Strategy 2016–2030 is to eliminate malaria from at least 35 countries by 2030 [1, 2]. In 2016, 91 countries reported on the indigenous malaria cases. Among these, 15 countries carried 80% of the global malaria burden [3]. In some of the pre-elimination countries, malaria is now limited to remote, forested areas, and often malaria cases are largely found in mobile and migrant populations (MMPs) [4]. The link between malaria transmission and human population movement (HPM) has been acknowledged many years ago [5]. Historically, it has been noted that the failure to consider HPM has been one factor contributing to the failure of malaria eradication campaigns in the 1950s and the 1960s [6–9].

As transmission declines due to concerted efforts of malaria control, it often becomes increasingly focal [10] or found as pockets of transmission [11]. Control programmes should target the remaining parasite reservoirs, deploying resources with increasing granularity [10] to populations who are at high risk of malaria transmission. This often includes MMPs. Numerous studies have reported that MMPs face many obstacles in accessing equitable essential healthcare services due to their living and working conditions, education level, gender, illegal migration status, language and cultural barriers, anti-migrant sentiments and lack of migrant-inclusive health policies, among others [12–14]. In the context of achieving and sustaining malaria elimination, there is a need to have health services that are used by MMPs and this requires specific service-delivery because they move into and through multiple localities that may have different malaria transmission levels and risks [13].

Efforts should be directed towards implementation of integrated interventions through multilateral partnerships across health and non-health sectors [12]. However, there are limited and mixed evidences about the success of intersectoral malaria-focussed activities and HPM. For instance, some studies reported there was no clear linkages between the health sectors and other sectoral ministries [14], while other studies showed reduction of malaria incidence through intersectoral activities [15]. Additionally, descriptions of successful intersectoral approaches to malaria in general, and in particular for MMPs are limited. Intersectoral interventions (activities/actions) for malaria in this review refers to the inclusion of several sectors in addition to the health sector when designing and implementing public policies to improve quality of life [16] for MMPs.

The current study address the research question: What sectors are addressing and implementing intervention(s) targeted towards malaria control of the MMPs?

The objectives were to:

- Identify what intersectoral actions have been taken and how they are applied to intervention(s) targeted at the MMPs,
- Establish which intervention(s) targeted to these special group of populations is/are effective and
- Identify the knowledge gaps and lessons learned about the interventions focused upon MMPs.

This systematic review was commissioned by the WHO/TDR (2017/721367-0).

Methods

The current review was carried out, following the Preferred Reporting Items for Systematic Reviews and Meta-Analyses (PRISMA) guideline [17] (Additional file 1). A conceptual framework for intersectoral activities addressing malaria and HPM is provided (Fig. 1). The framework identified three main domains that can contribute to the consequences of malaria interventions targeted towards the HPM. The domains included are the antecedents, the health problems and the key actors. The first domain, the antecedents which were considered in the present review include mobile population, migrants and IDPs. In general, these vulnerable populations have encountered multiple health problems. However, the focus of this study is primarily on malaria. The key factors that are involved in the implementation of interventions are also described. The two inter-linked factors are then identified as the sectors and the interventions involved where multiple sectors are involved. The sectors involved are broadly categorized as MOH, other ministries/non-health sectors (e.g., labour/social welfare department, immigrations departments, agriculture departments), agencies, non-governmental organizations (NGOs), community and so forth. The interventions where these sectors are involved are classified as (i) surveillance and response, (ii) test and treat, (iii) vector control and (iv) PPE/HE, in accordance with the global malaria control strategy. All these three domains are sequentially linked which contribute to the consequences of interventions implemented by the sectors, which are targeted to the HPM. The consequences are broadly identified as success (achieved the programme target), failure (unmet targets) or gap between the expectations and actual achievements of the sectors involved.

Study search

The relevant studies were searched in the health-related databases, such as PubMed, Medline, Embase, ProQuest, Global Health, and Google Scholar. Keywords used in the search included: malaria, *Plasmodium falciparum*, *Plasmodium vivax*, migrants, migration, hard-to-reach, marginalised, multisectoral, intersectoral, stakeholders with

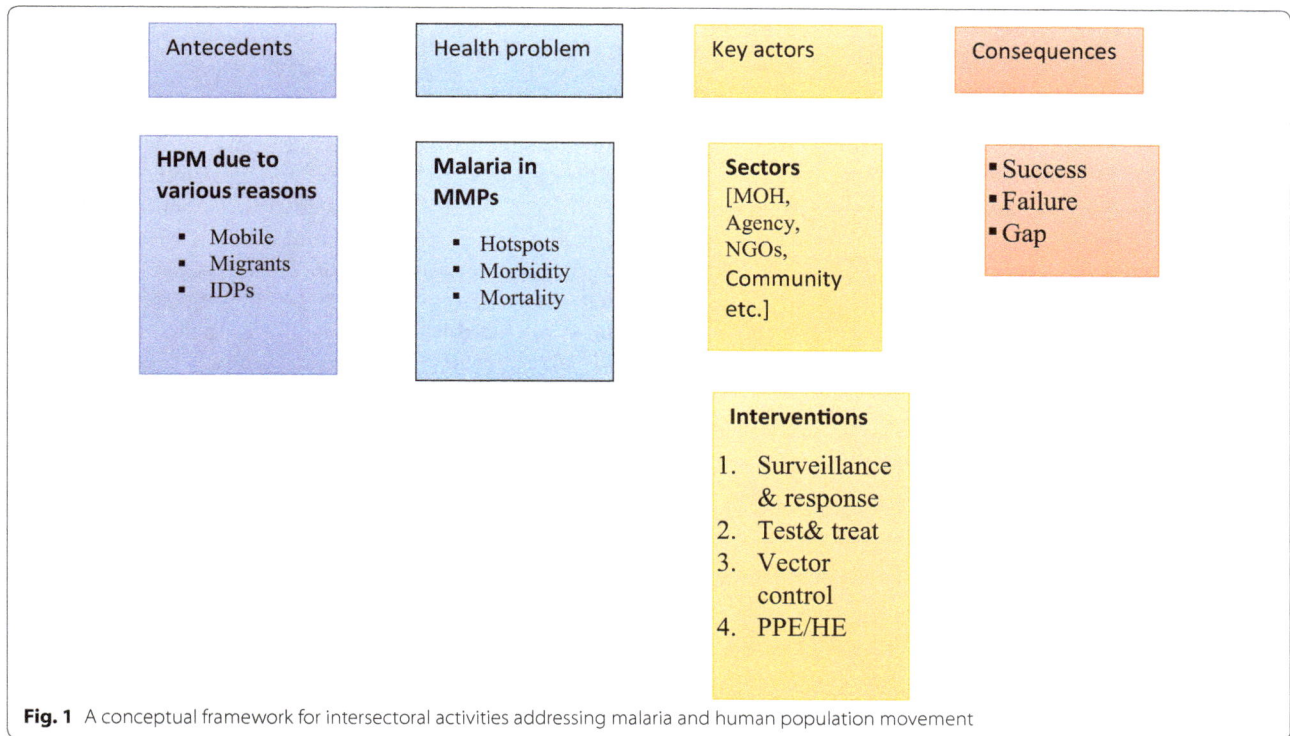

Fig. 1 A conceptual framework for intersectoral activities addressing malaria and human population movement

the use of Boolean operator, truncating and proximity operators, as appropriate. The search was extended to the WHO websites for Roll Back Malaria Partnership to end malaria (RBM) documents, the international agency websites including International Organization for Migration (IOM), United Nations High Commission for Refugees (UNHCR), United Nations Children's Fund (UNICEF) and the international NGOs websites including Population Services International (PSI).

Study selection

The selection criteria for the current review are provided as population, concepts and context in the PCC format [18].

Population (P)

Studies with participants having malaria and categorized as MMP, were included regardless of age, gender and their legal status. As theories and definitions of migration are diverse [11] and migration is not a definitive risk for malaria [19], the MMP in this review is defined in the context of malaria, rather than general definition of MMP. In the present study MMPs are defined as *"individuals who move to and/or from the endemic/studied areas for a certain period of time and live and/or work at a certain distance from forest and/or forest-like settings"* [20]. This can include internally displaced persons (IDPs)

(4), defined as individuals who have been forced to leave their homes or places of habitual residence, in particular, as a result of or in order to avoid the effects of armed conflict, situations of generalized violence, violations of human rights, or natural or man-made disasters, and who have not crossed an international border [21]. The present study classified the collective movement of all MMPs including IDPs as human population movement (HPM) [22].

Concepts (C)

All interventions targeting to the prevention or control of malaria were included. The interventions were summarized into five categories; (i) surveillance and response to surveillance, (ii) test and treat, (iii) health education/promotion, (iv) personal prevention and (v) vector control.

Contents (C)

Published and unpublished epidemiologic studies were considered, assessing interventions for malaria control, case studies (publications that describe implementation of interventions), position papers (publications that focus on policy) as well as a relevant narrative review (publication that include the description of actual or proposed interventions) with a focus on intersectoral collaboration for malaria control among MMPs. The following outcomes of intersectoral interventions targeted at MMPs were considered.

Interventions that

- Benefited participants (levels of knowledge, attitudes and practices of malaria control),
- Demonstrated positive behaviour changes with significant reduction in malaria incidence,
- Had increased detection of asymptomatic malaria cases,
- Demonstrated intersectoral coordination (qualitatively or quantitatively).

The search was limited to publications in English language between 1978 and 2017, regardless of the study location. An initial search was performed in February 2017, and repeated in July 2017 and May 2018 to update the study search. Articles that were primarily concerned with other issues rather than intersectoral collaboration to address malaria amongst MMPs were excluded.

Data extraction

Several steps were involved in data extraction in the present review. First, two investigators individually screened the titles and abstracts, and then selected full-text articles, according to the selection criteria. The two investigators independently extracted information from each included study using a data extraction form prepared for the review. The data extraction form had been pre-tested by the investigators on a sample of papers to check its utility, comprehensiveness and ease of use. Any discrepancy was resolved by consensus. Information collected were: first author and publication year, methods (design, year of data collection), location (country of study, setting), participants (sample size, characteristics), intersectoral action (sectors involved), interventions, outcomes, mechanisms for intersectoral action. For studies with qualitative information, the two investigators independently reviewed each article for a second time and then, coded for the major/prominent themes such as lessons learned for 'success' and/or 'challenges' encountered.

Data synthesis

Details of the included studies were combined as a narrative review by the domain of outcomes. If there were a minimum of three studies reporting the outcomes in similar ways, a meta-analysis of outcome data was performed. For qualitative information, the results from each theme were summarized in a tabular format. No judgment was made on the methodological quality of the included studies, as many of these were cross-sectional descriptive surveys, surveillance reports or retrospective chart/record reviews. Instead, the analyses were stratified by interventions identified.

Results

Figure 2 shows the four-phase PRISMA flow chart of the study selection process. The initial search yielded 174 citations. After the title and abstract screening, a total of 53 studies were considered and a final of 36 studies met our inclusion criteria [15, 20, 22–55]. A list of seventeen excluded studies along with the main reasons for exclusion is provided in Additional file 2. Table 1 provides the characteristics of the included studies. Of these studies, the vast majority of studies were cross-sectional descriptive surveys (78%, 28/36), four were case studies, two were reviews, and one study each was randomized trial and evaluation report.

Figure 3 shows the geographic distribution of the studies included. The key characteristics of the included studies are provided in Table 1. Eleven studies (30.5%) were from Myanmar [20, 25, 26, 35–37, 39, 48, 51, 54, 55], four studies (11.1%) from Cambodia [22, 40, 43, 52], three studies from French Guiana [45, 46, 48] and two studies each from China [15, 50], Thailand [23, 27], Sri Lanka [28, 32] and Uganda [24, 33]. The remaining ten single studies were done in Columbia [43], Congo [44], Ethiopia [41], Lao [52], Malaysia [38], Namibia [34], Pakistan [31], Sierra Leone [29], Suriname [30] and South America [47].

Stakeholders involved

The list of stakeholders in the intersectoral actions for malaria control among MMPs is presented in Additional file 3. A variety of stakeholders, such as MOH/MOPH, other government ministries, bilateral cooperation initiatives, private sectors, international and local NGOs, and faith-based organizations, were identified for intersectoral actions to defeat malaria amongst MMPs. Almost all studies discussed the involvement of MOH/MOPH, except two studies from Myanmar in which international NGOs (INGO) and faith-based organizations appeared to be the key actors [25, 26]. The other ministries involved were the Ministry of Mines and Energy in Columbia [42] and the Ministry of Education in French Guiana [46]. Bilateral cooperation activities such as the Trans-Kunene Malaria Initiative (TKMI) between the ministries of Namibia and Angola and 'SOSEK MALINDO' between the ministries of Malaysia and Indonesia were also identified. However, there is dearth of information on how these stakeholders shared roles and responsibilities for implementation, the channels of communication between-and-within the partners and with the MOH/MOPH. However, all but one study [15] provided clear information on the stakeholders, the type of services provision and duration of their stay in different places.

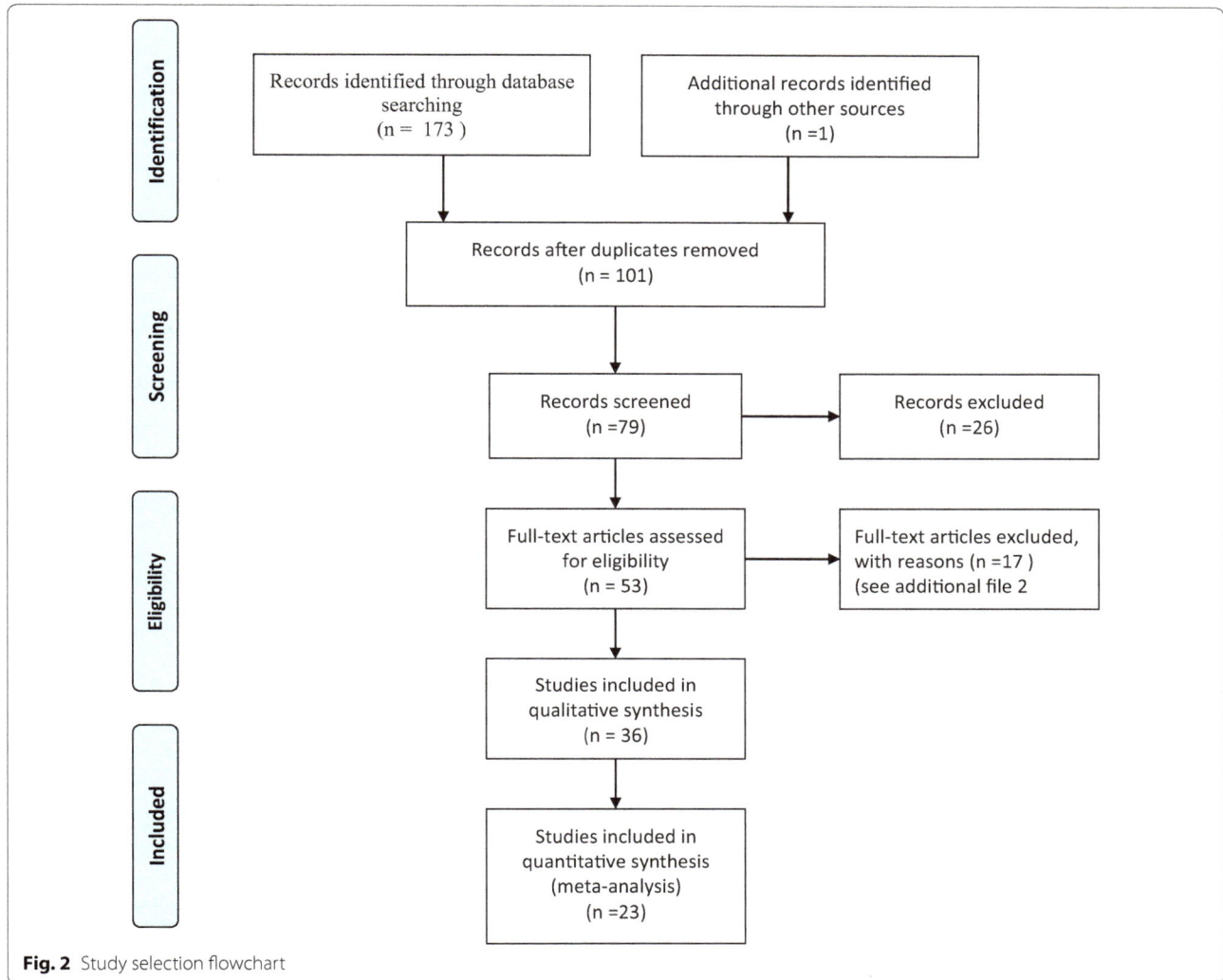

Fig. 2 Study selection flowchart

The interventions that the stakeholders involved/supported are presented in Additional file 4. Of these 36 studies included, the most frequently assessed intervention was the coverage and utilization of insecticide-treated nets (ITNs)/long-lasting insecticide-treated nets (LLINs) as personal protective measures (PPM) (40.5%), followed by the intervention of early diagnosis and treatment of malaria (33.3%), the surveillance and response activities (13.9%) and the behaviour change communication (BCC) (8.3%).

Lessons learned

Table 2 presents the summary of lessons learned on the intersectoral involvement for malaria control/elimination amongst MMPs. Almost all studies described the success factors for the intervention activities (e.g. ITNs), but there is limited description on which a particular agency/sector was involved and how they collaborated with each other in malaria control/elimination activities. Only three studies explicitly provided details on factors contributing towards the success of intersectoral involvement at the community level for MMPs. These were noted as: "*strengthened partnership and established the collaboration, coordination and cooperation channels among stakeholders*" [50, p. 8], "*prompt establishment of health care clinics, resource mobilization by international agencies and NGOs in response to the disaster*" [15, p. 7] and "*receipt of a steady source of detailed, accurate, government and NGO-sponsored information*" [53, p. 7]. Similarly there was limited discussion on the challenges encountered. Only 2 studies explicitly described "*The need to improve mechanisms of communication among multiple partners*" [36, p. 9] and "*the assurance of long-term, sustainable funding*" [28, p. 11].

Table 1 Characteristics of the included studies

No	Study[a] [reference no.]	Year of publication	Study design	Country	Targeted population
1	Soe et al. [55]	2017	Cross-sectional survey	Myanmar	Internal migrants
2	Phyo Than et al. [54]	2017	Cross-sectional survey	Myanmar	Migrant workers
3	Ly et al. [53]	2017	Cross-sectional survey using RDS[b]	Cambodia	Mobile and migrant population
4	Kounnavong et al. [52]	2017	Review	Lao	In-out migrations and military personnel
5	Crawshaw et al. [51]	2017	Cluster randomised trial	Myanmar	Migrant rubber tappers
6	Zhang et al. [50]	2016	Case study	China	Fever cases in the border areas
7	Vezenegho et al. [49]	2016	Survey	French Guiana	Forest workers
8	Nyunt et al. [48]	2016	Mixed method (qualitative and quantitative)	Myanmar	Local health volunteers for migrants
9	Krisher et al. [47]	2016	Case study	South America	Cross-border migrants
10	Douine et al. [46]	2016	Prospective, multicentre	French Guiana	Illegal gold miners
11	de Santi et al. [45]	2016	Cross-sectional survey	French Guiana	Illegal gold miners
12	Charchuk et al. [44]	2016	Cross-sectional survey	Congo	Internally displaced persons
13	Canavati et al. [43]	2016	Mixed method (qualitative and quantitative)	Cambodia	Seasonal workers
14	Castellanos et al. [42]	2016	Retrospective chart review	Columbia	Illegal gold miners
15	Schicker et al. [41]	2015	Cross-sectional survey (venue based survey)	Ethiopia	Migrant workers
16	Peeters et al. [40]	2015	Cross-sectional survey	Cambodia	Migrants
17	Nyunt et al. [39]	2015	Cross-sectional survey	Myanmar	Mobile population
18	MOH, Malaysia et al. [38]	2015	Case study	Malaysia (Sabah)	Migrants
19	Hlaing et al. [37]	2015	Cross-sectional survey	Myanmar	Internal migrants
20	Wai et al. [36]	2014	Cross-sectional survey	Myanmar	Migrant workers
21	Nyunt et al. [35]	2014	Cross-sectional survey	Myanmar	Migrant workers
22	Gueye et al. [34]	2014	Case study with mixed method	Namibia	Population in the border areas
23	Obol et al. [33]	2013	Cross-sectional survey	Uganda	Internally displaced persons
24	Kirkby et al. [32]	2013	Cross-sectional survey	Sri Lanka	People in a post-conflict setting
25	Qayum et al. [31]	2012	Cross-sectional survey	Pakistan	Internally displaced persons
26	Hiwat et al. [30]	2012	Case study	Suriname	Post-conflict district
27	Burns et al. [29]	2012	Randomized trial	Sierra Leone	Refugees
28	Abeyasinghe et al. [28]	2012	Case study	Sri Lanka	People in a conflict setting
29	Wangroongsarb et al. [27]	2011	Cross-sectional survey using RDS[b]	Thailand	Migrant workers
30	Mullany et al. [26]	2010	Pre-post comparison[c]	Myanmar	Mon state
31	Lee et al. [25]	2009	Evaluation report	Myanmar	Internally displaced persons
32	Kolaczinski et al. [24]	2006	Cross-sectional survey	Uganda	Internally displaced persons
33	Carrara et al. [23]	2006	Cross-sectional survey (before, during and after interventions)	Thailand	IDP
34	Guyant et al. [22]	2015	Review	Cambodia	Mobile and migrant population
35	IOM et al. [20]	2012	Review	Myanmar	Internal MMPs
36	Zhou et al. [15]	2016	Surveillance	China	Internally displaced persons

[a] First author of the study; [b] RDS: respondent-driven sampling (i.e. a sampling method based on snowball approach); [c] Seem as a before-after design

The outcome of interventions

A subset of eight studies from six countries was identified, that provided details on the proportion of MMPs with the correct knowledge about malaria as a mosquito borne disease [27, 31, 32, 37, 39, 41, 43, 53]. Overall, a pooled estimate was 70% (95% CI 57–83%), indicating a high proportion of the targeted MMPs had correct knowledge about malaria transmission (Fig. 4). There was a substantial variation within study heterogeneity, and the estimates varied from a low level 48% (95% CI 44–52%) in Ethiopia [41] to sufficient level of knowledge in Cambodia (93%, 95% CI 92–95%) [53]. Gaps were obvious even within the same country. For instance, 58% of MMPs located in the Myanmar Artemisinin Resistance

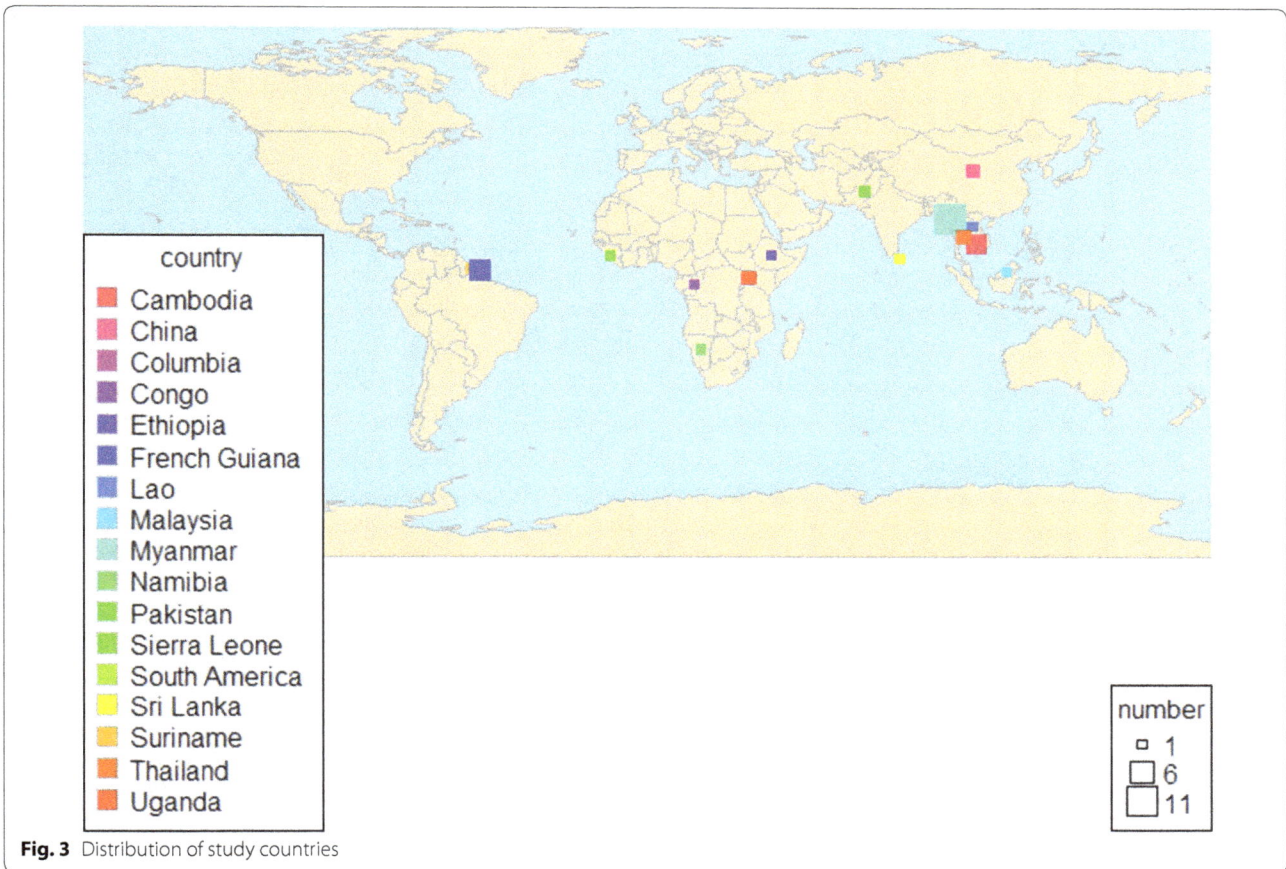

Fig. 3 Distribution of study countries

Containment (MARC) zone in Bago region alone [37] and 82% of MMPs located in the MARC zone in Kayin State, Mon State, Bago region and Tanintharyi region of Myanmar [39] had correct knowledge about malaria transmission. This implied that there might be variations in modes of delivery of health education (HE) messages.

Estimates of net ownership (including insecticide-treated clothing, ITC) amongst MMPs were available across fourteen studies from nine countries. Overall, a pooled estimate was 44% (95% CI 35–52%), indicating less than half of the targeted MMPs used ITNs. A subgroup of five studies conducted in Myanmar [35, 37, 39, 51, 54] also showed similar results (47%, 95% CI 28–66%) (Fig. 5). There was substantial heterogeneity (I^2 99.9%), indicating between-country and within-country variation. For instance, net utilization rate was relatively higher in studies from Pakistan (75%) [31] and Ethiopia (74%) [41], but was observed to have lower estimates in a study from Congo (16%) [44]. Qualitative studies reinforced that community acceptance of ITNs was a major factor in utilisation and vice versa. An example from Myanmar was *"I don't know that is ITN. I don't like it because it is too rough in texture with big pits. It looks like the nets used for animals such as buffalos and cows in my native town. Some of villagers use it to catch up fish"* [35 p. 5].

Interestingly, the paradoxical phenomenon of a high proportion of MMPs with knowledge about malaria transmission, but with a low proportion of net utilization was found in a study from Cambodia [53], and vice versa in a study from Ethiopia [41]. This implied that there was a gap between knowledge acquisition and the actual practice among these MMPs. Overall, a pooled analysis of four studies [31, 35, 37, 51] showed that a high proportion of participants were willing to buy ITNs/LLINs/ITCs (71%, 95% CI 53–89%) (Fig. 6). Variation in the willingness to purchase as supported by substantial heterogeneity (99.3%) may be linked to the level of understanding of and belief in the benefits of using ITNs [33]. Interestingly, one study in Myanmar reported the gap between willingness to buy ITNs/LLINs and affordability (88.5% vs. 60.2%) [36].

Among the studies that measured an outcome of malaria case reduction, five studies (with six datasets) provided data with comparable reporting methods [15, 23, 29, 41, 55] with either a comparison before and after

Table 2 Description of lessons learned from the intersectoral involvement for malaria control targeted to the mobile and migrant populations

Study, year	Country	Lessons learned (success)
Zhang, 2016 [50]	China	Strengthened the partnership and established the collaboration, coordination and cooperation channels among stakeholders. Health Poverty Action (HPA) is an example model
Zhou, 2016 [15]	China	Prompt establishment of health care clinics, resource mobilization by international agencies and NGOs in response to the disaster
Ly, 2017 [53]	Cambodia	Received a steady source of detailed, accurate, government and NGO-sponsored information
Zhou, 2016; [15] Carrara, 2006 [43]	China; Thailand	Significantly reduced incidence with effective management
Obol, 2015 [33]	Uganda	In all IDP camps, health care services and ITNs distribution etc. were solely provided by the emergency relief organisations and the UN
Lee, 2008 [25]	Myanmar	Feasibility of delivering effective disease control interventions in an area of active conflict through the trained volunteers
Kirkbya, 2012 [32]	Sri Lanka	Malaria is taught during grade 6 of the school curriculum, i.e. at the beginning of secondary school education
Nyunt, 2014 [35]	Myanmar	Free distribution was found as one of the major factors causing utilization of ITNs in migrant workers
Canavati, 2016 [43]	Cambodia	Targeted community was satisfied with the mobile malaria workers' services
Lessons learned (challenges)		
Wai, 2014 [36]	Myanmar	Need to improve mechanisms of communication among multiple partners
Wai, 2014 [36]	Myanmar	Need collaborative work between health department and administrators to inform and motivate the regular use of LLINs
Abeyasinghe, 2012 [28]	Sri Lanka	The assurance of long-term, sustainable funding
Ly, 2017 [53]; Wai, 2014 [36]; Wangroongsarb, 2011 [27]; Peeters, 2015 [40]	Cambodia; Myanmar; Thailand	Limited the effectiveness of health education message/IEC due to limited literary or language barrier in multilingual ethnic groups
Ly, 2017 [53]	Cambodia	~ 10% of participants treated for malaria did not have a confirmed diagnosis
Ly, 2017 [53]; Obol, 2013 [33]; Charchuk, 2016 [44]	Cambodia; Uganda;	Low net utilization rates
Zhou, 2016 [15]	China	Interventions exclusively to IDP camps, excluding local surrounding villages
Gueye, 2014 [34]	Namibia	Not appropriate timing of the spray season; Late payment of temporary spray men may have resulted in decreased morale and lower quality of IRS
Zhou, 2016 [15]; Wai, 2014 [36]; Wangroongsarb, 2011 [27]	China; Myanmar; Thailand	Lack of convenient access to health care facilities/limited access to formal health facility/health message; Transportation constraints to access health care facility
Wai, 2014 [36]	Myanmar	A gap in willingness to buy ITNs/LLINs and affordability
Canavati, 2016 [43]		Short stay of mobile malaria workers; Low utilization of mobile malaria workers
Carrara, 2006 [23]	Thailand	2-day artesunate regimen given, not a standard 3-day regimen
MOH, Malaysia, 2015 [38]	Malaysia	Undocumented migrant workers are a challenging group to access/trace for the malaria elimination intervention
Qayum, 2012 [31]	Pakistan	Limited distribution of ITNs; No worn out bed nets were replaced; some were not in a useable state

Table 2 (continued)

Study, year	Country	Lessons learned (success)
Lee, 2009 [25]	Myanmar	Exceeded the capacity to train volunteers or to monitor and evaluate their work; Inadequate training of volunteers and a lack of strong guidelines for recruiting villagers
Lee, 2009 [25]	Myanmar	Community health workers reluctance to delegate additional responsibilities to the volunteers
Lee, 2009 [25]	Myanmar	Recruitment, training and supervision of volunteers became more time consuming for clinic staff
Lee, 2009 [25]	Myanmar	Over-treatment of test-result negative patients by volunteers
Nyunt, 2014 [35]	Myanmar	Unpleasant insecticide smell of the nets

IDP internally displaced people, *IRS* indoor residual spraying, *ITN* insecticide treated bed net/material, *LLIN* long lasting insecticide treated bed net/material, *NGO* non-governmental organization

interventions or between intervention and no-intervention. An intervention for utilization of ITNs/LLINs was two times more likely to reduce malaria incidence amongst the targeted MMPs (summary OR 2.01, 95% CI 1.43–2.6) (Fig. 7). Amongst MMPs in China-Myanmar border areas, those who reported the habit of (always) sleeping under a bed net at night were likely to have a threefold reduction in malaria incidence compared to those who did not reported this behaviour (OR 3.2, 95% CI 2.9–3.7) [15]. Only one study on the Myanmar-Thailand borders provided data on outcome of early detection and treatment. It showed a 12% increase in malaria cases in the non-intervention groups compared to those MMPs under intervention (OR 1.12, 95% CI 1.09–1.16) [23].

The current findings showed that if BCC is integrated within an intervention, rather than stand-alone, people would initiate and sustain the desired behaviours (e.g. sleeping under LLINs). For instance, the Nyunt study in Myanmar used an integrated BCC approach of HE supporting bed net distribution [39] and the outcome was a high proportion of MMPs with adequate knowledge, whereas the Hlaing study in the same country was implemented using stand-alone HE approach [37].

There were several studies on the surveillance and response approach, but they combined data on MMPs and non-MMPs or did not clearly identify intersectoral actions there. Although they were not included in the current review, a common finding in these studies was the high levels of asymptomatic malaria. The detection of asymptomatic malaria was through active case detection (ACD) and reactive case detection (RCD) activities among MMPs. One of the included studies was conducted in the illegal gold mining population of French Guiana. It showed that RDTs and microscopy (used for surveillance) did not identify all the people who had malaria parasites [46]. Compared to PCR, the RDT sensitivity was very low (16%, 95% CI 9.9–27.7%)

as was microscopy (18%, 95% CI 11.6–27.1%). However, specificity was very high with RDT (99.1%, 95% CI 97.3–99.7%) or with microscopy (100%, 95% CI 98.8–100%). This would mean that 84% and 82% of humans carrying malaria parasites would have been missed by using only microscopy or only RDT, respectively. Several stakeholders, such as MOH, regional health agencies, the French Army Health Department, the Ministry of Foreign Affairs, the Home Affairs Ministry, the Overseas Territories Ministry, PAHO/WHO and the Global Fund, supported the interventions targeted to these high risk population in French Guiana [49]. There were very limited descriptions of the roles and responsibilities of communication channels between the stakeholders and with public sectors of the host country that can helped others adopt or adapt these approaches.

Discussion

The present review summarizes thirty-six studies across seventeen countries. This is the first systematic review which assessed intersectoral collaboration for malaria control targeted to MMPs in pre-elimination or elimination phases. *"Intersectoral action is a strategy used to deal with complex policy problems that cannot be solved by a single country, region, government, department, or sector. Intersectoral action has been brought to bear on specific determinants of health, diseases, populations (e.g. indigenous peoples, children), geographic communities, health behaviours, and risk factors"* [56, p. 7].

The major observations in this review are

- Malaria is a health problem amongst MMPs, including mining communities, who had limited access to formal healthcare facilities and low utilization of PPMs such as ITNs;

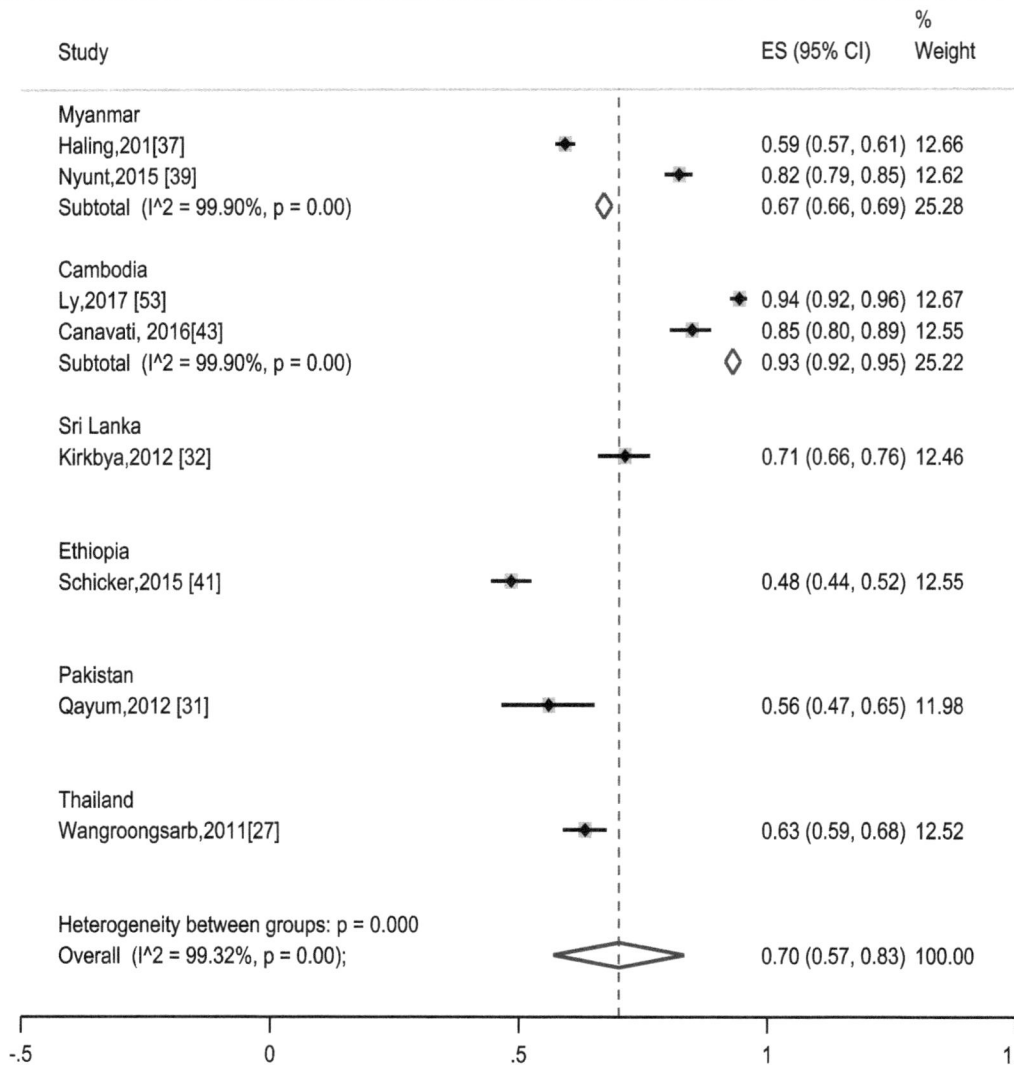

Fig. 4 Proportion of the mobile and migrant populations who correctly know malaria as a mosquito-borne disease. Effect size (ES) indicates proportion. Each included study is represented by squares at the estimated point of effect. The horizontal lines through the square illustrate the length of the confidence interval (CI). The longer the lines, the wider the CI, the less reliable the study results. A subtotal or the overall combined result is represented by a diamond with its centre indicating the pooled point estimate, while its width representing the CI for the pooled data. The wider the width of the diamond, the less reliable the pooled results

- Multiple stakeholders including public sectors, local and international agencies, NGOs, private sectors, employers of concern had been supporting the various interventions for malaria control/elimination targeted to these high risk populations;
- Although limited details were provided in the studies, the intermediate outcomes showed some evidence that the intersectoral collaborations contributed to the improvement in knowledge about malaria. This also initiated and promoted bed net utilization; increased access to diagnosis and treatment interven-

tions and contributed towards a reduction in malaria incidence.

The need for more detailed description of partnerships
Intersectoral collaboration to address health problems was described 50 years ago in the Alma Ata Declaration of 1978 [56]. The current review identified several agencies who played various roles such as suppliers of materials, provider of services or research collaborators through intersectoral approaches who targeted

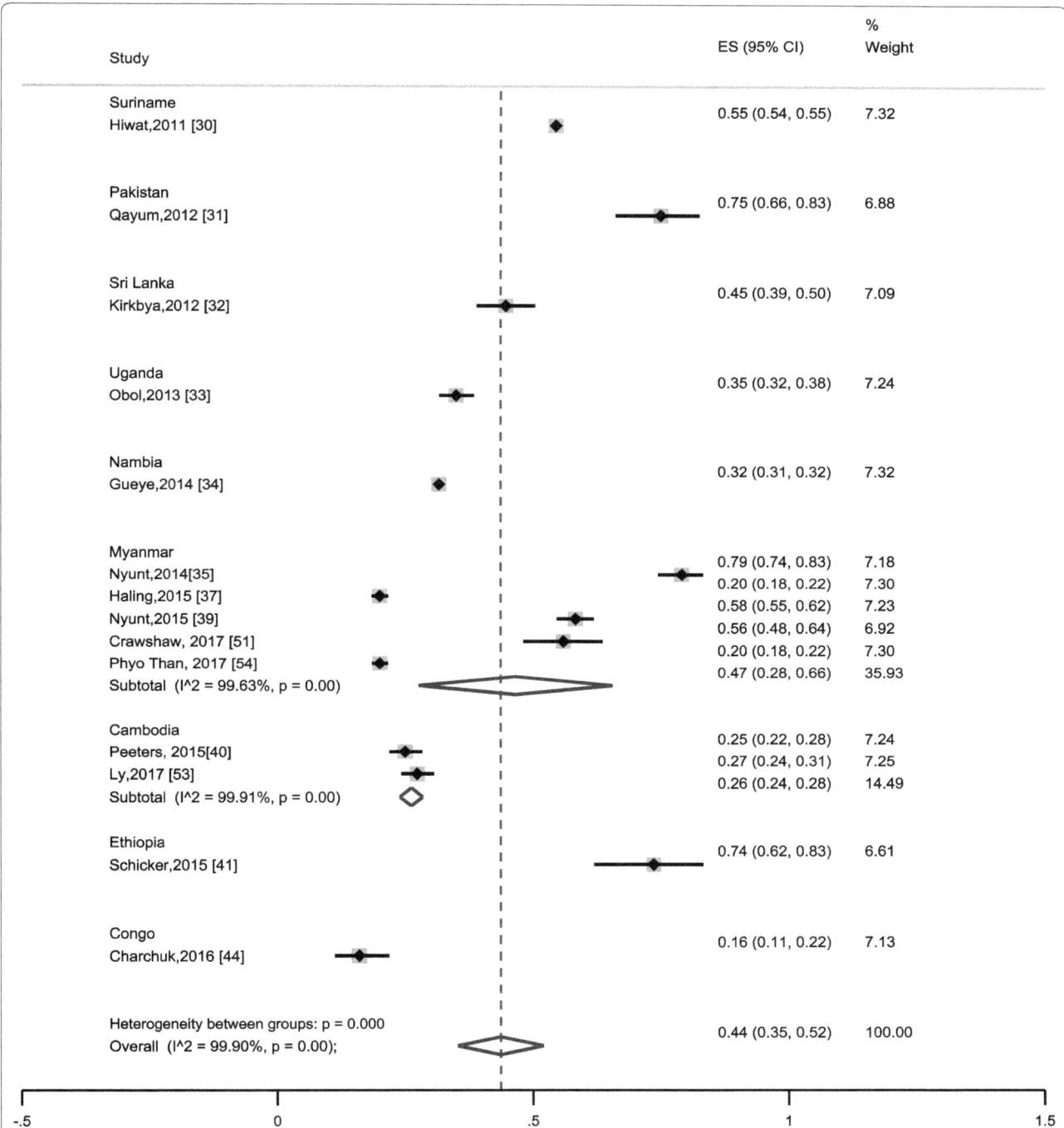

Fig. 5 Proportion of nets ownership among the mobile and migrant populations. Effect size (ES) indicates proportion. Each included study is represented by squares at the estimated point of effect. The horizontal lines through the square illustrate the length of the confidence interval (CI). The longer the lines, the wider the CI, the less reliable the study results. A subtotal or the overall combined result is represented by a diamond with its centre indicating the pooled point estimate while its width representing the CI for the pooled data. The wider the width of the diamond, the less reliable the pooled results

the MMPs. However, there was inadequate description and limited robust analysis of the contribution of these intersectoral actions made towards achieving the

targeted malaria control outcome. This was because these studies were designed to address their specific objectives, rather than to undertake a robust

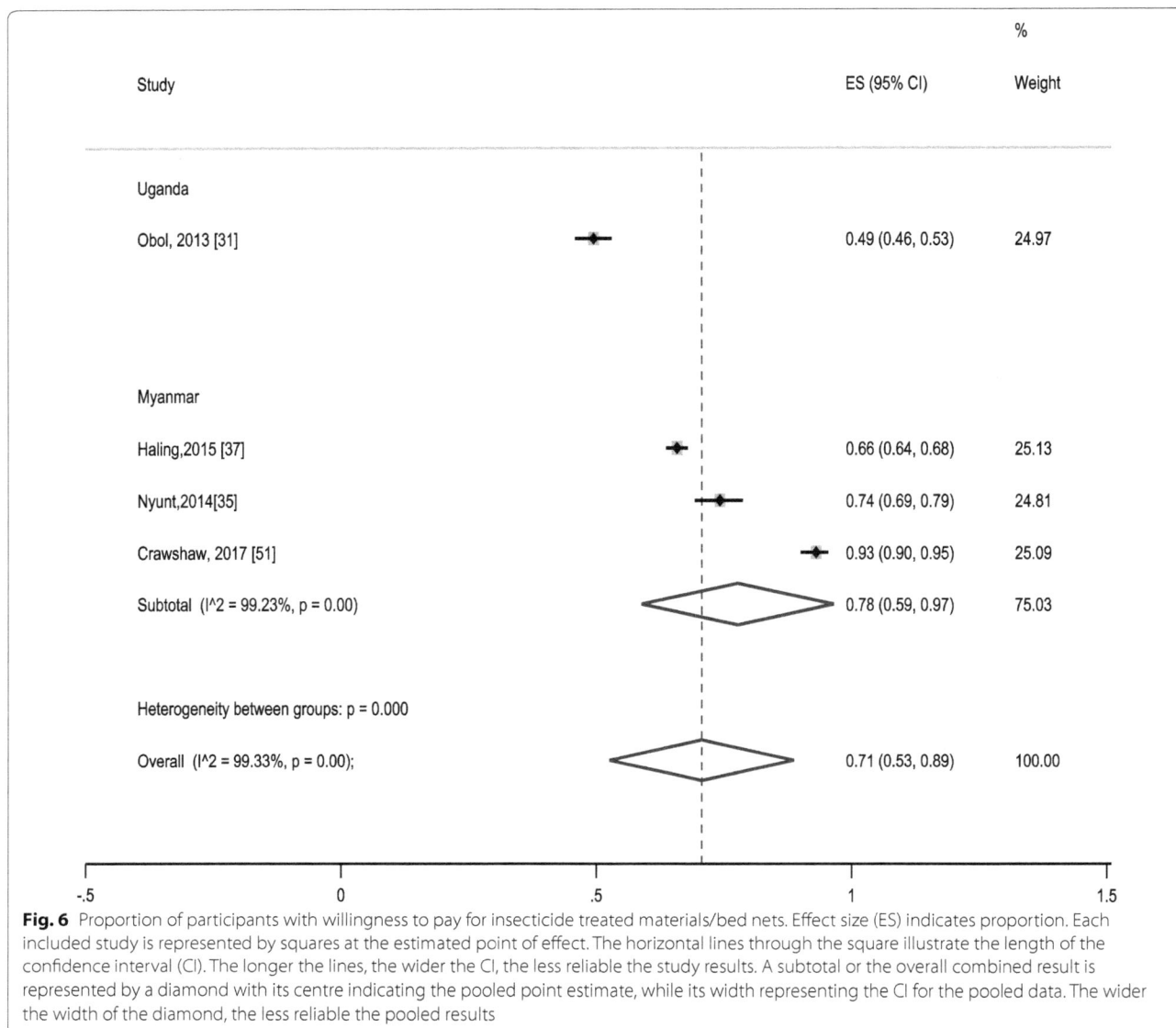

Fig. 6 Proportion of participants with willingness to pay for insecticide treated materials/bed nets. Effect size (ES) indicates proportion. Each included study is represented by squares at the estimated point of effect. The horizontal lines through the square illustrate the length of the confidence interval (CI). The longer the lines, the wider the CI, the less reliable the study results. A subtotal or the overall combined result is represented by a diamond with its centre indicating the pooled point estimate, while its width representing the CI for the pooled data. The wider the width of the diamond, the less reliable the pooled results

assessment of the intersectoral collaboration. Future studies are needed which are designed to assess the role of intersectoral interventions targeted to MMPs.

Although there was paucity of data, evidence was found that interventions targeted towards malaria in IDP camps/amongst MMPs could reduce malaria incidence/prevalence significantly in comparison to the surrounding villages or those villages without an intervention. Moreover, studies included in this review had highlighted the important role of intersectoral actions. An example from a study in Uganda was... *"In all IDP camps, health care services and ITN distribution etc. were solely provided by the emergency relief*

organisations and the UN was [33 p. 963]. In fact, the intersectoral collaboration is required *"because of the wide range of interests involved, additional effort and negotiation to reach a shared understanding of goals, approaches, respective roles, and accountability for outcomes"* [57].

It seemed that conditions in illegal mining camps in French Guiana showed less success against their desired outcomes that in other MMPs settings. A reason for this might be related to multiple factors including the complexities involved in accessing these populations, and because investing in "illegal" miners' health was not sanctioned or funded [46].

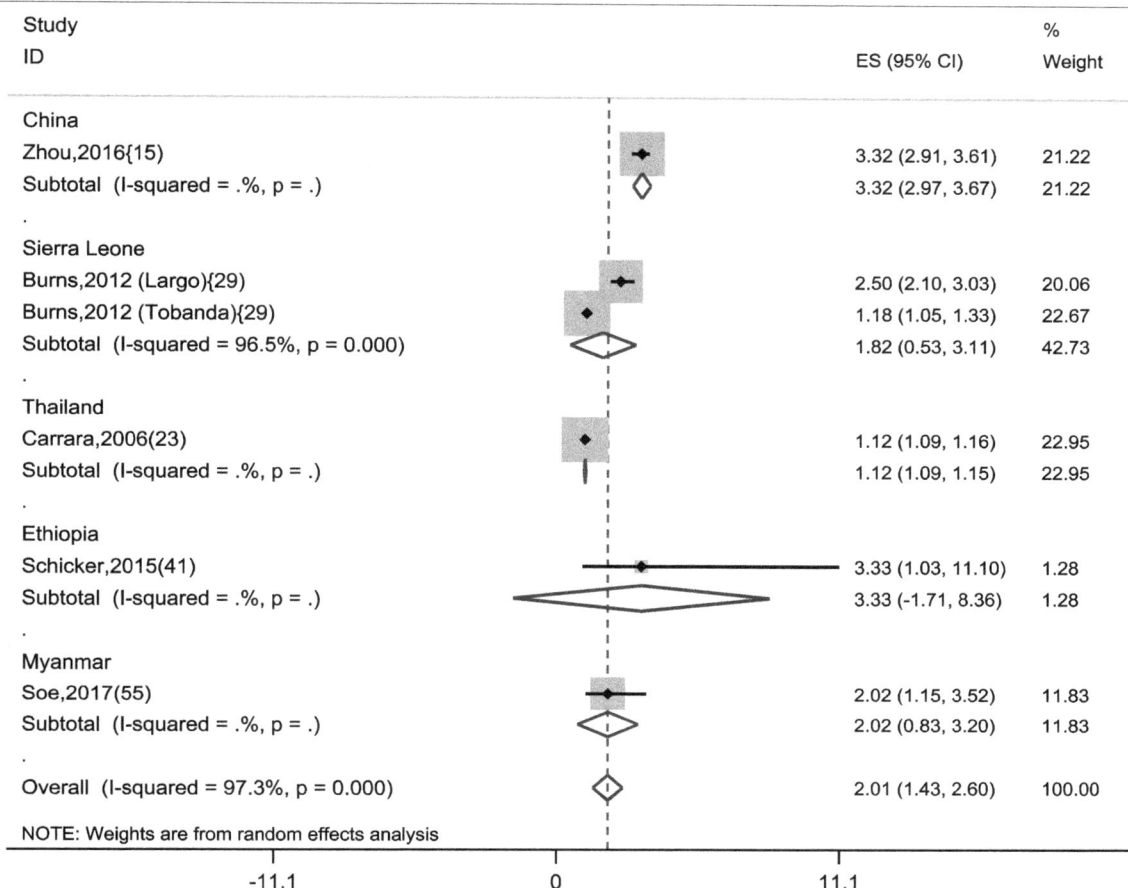

Fig. 7 Cases reduction related to the interventions compared to no-interventions for the mobile and migrant populations. Effect size (ES) indicates odds ratio and its 95% confidence interval (CI). Each included study is represented by squares at the estimated point of effect. The horizontal lines through the square illustrate the length of the CI. The longer the lines, the wider the CI, the less reliable the study results. A subtotal or the overall combined result is represented by a diamond with its centre indicating the pooled point estimate while its width representing the CI for the pooled data. The wider the width of the diamond, the less reliable the pooled results

Better segmentation of behaviour change communication is of immense value

MMPs were often targeted by interventions as a homogenous group, but in reality they have varying health beliefs, patterns of health behaviour and utilization of health services [18]. The current analysis confirmed this assertion by revealing the geographical variations in the level of knowledge about malaria transmission or net utilization. This difference was possibly related to type of interventions for MMPs. For instance, BCC is a term often used to describe any communication strategy with individuals or communities to promote positive behaviours appropriate to their settings.

The proportion of people equipped with knowledge about malaria transmission through the bite of (infective female) mosquitoes was higher, but the net utilization rates (ITNs/LLINs) were still at inadequate levels for personal protection. This implied that there was a gap between the knowledge and the actual practice amongst these populations. These discrepancies suggested a range of areas for investigation and improved interventions. For example, it needs well-designed BCC coupled with improved accessibility to, and affordability of, the means of protection in order to support people to convert their knowledge and supportive attitudes into malaria control practice. Moreover, other aspects of a supportive environment such as community and health services support, innovative methods of newer or modified means of protection and treatment that is acceptable, affordable and convenient for the population [36] must be included in an intervention.

In addition, factors linked to the social determinants of health such as income and education are often the strongest predictors of bed net use [51, 58]. An analysis of these factors was beyond the scope of this review but would be useful to undertake in future studies.

Broadening access to all beyond the MMPs

Interventions identified for the current review seemed to be designed by the partners/agencies/donors to specifically serve the IDP camps/MMPS, and excluded neighbouring villages. In the elimination phase, all instances of detected parasitaemia (including gametocytaemia only) are considered as 'malaria case' as they might lead to onward transmission, regardless of the presence or absence of clinical symptoms [59]. Hence, it is crucial to expand malaria intervention strategies in IDP camps to local surrounding villages in the border area [22]. The malaria control strategy in the critical period of pre/elimination phase in the areas of MMPs should be an *"all inclusive"* approach, by expanding services to those non-MMPs who share the same tyrannies of poor access to health services and programmes. However, there might be limitations in the 'agency' mission, funding and approvals that will not support this broadening of the target populations. Finding ways to scale up successful interventions utilized for MMPs to broader catchments may need different collaborations and should be studied.

Sustainability issues

An important issue related to the current findings was the sustainability of the agency/donor-dependent interventions. For instance, there was a gap between the willingness and ability of the populations to pay for ITNs [37], which would become the case should donor funding cease. This is of great concern as most of the MMPs within the border areas are poor and they have limited employment opportunities [58]. More detailed consideration of sustainability of malaria control interventions among various sub-populations of MMPs is required to achieve the targets of elimination and sustaining them in those populations and susceptible contiguous regions.

Study limitations

The findings of the intersectoral activities and the outcomes were exclusively based on research studies conducted in the IDP camps or areas where MMPs reside. It appears that the studies included in this review were not designed to study the outputs or outcomes from the processes for intersectoral approaches even when these approaches were the major platform for delivery of the intervention (e.g. ITN distribution or BCC activities). It is likely that countries have developed strategies for malaria control activities with MMPs through intersectoral actions that have not been published and are, therefore, not included in this review. Moreover, the reported findings could be geographically biased due to an unequal number of included studies and limited to generalizability towards MMPs/IDPs across countries.

Regarding the methodology, there was substantial heterogeneity among studies (I^2: 97.3%). The fact that I^2 value remained high in the meta-analysis implied that there might be factors inherent in the included studies; the individual characteristics of MMPs, migration patterns, level of malaria endemicity in their localities, the presence of co-infections/co-morbid conditions, and coverage of effective malaria interventions. Due to inadequate data, stratified analyses based on all these influencing factors were not possible. Future studies should consider these factors in their design.

Public health implications

Universal health coverage must be the goal for all people at risk of malaria including MMPs. Control of malaria and effective treatment was problematic since it was difficult for routine health sector activities, especially public sector, to locate, diagnose and treat infected people in these populations. Malaria programmes can adapt the methods of a wide-reaching "pre-surveillance assessment" process that has been done in the HIV programmes, as describe elsewhere [60]. Access to early diagnosis and effective treatment by promoting ACD and RCD and/or provision of innovative clinical treatment models such as mobile clinics are crucial for these populations. Moreover, the use of PPM and available healthcare services could be maximized through improved knowledge and supportive attitudes towards malaria control supported by effective BCC that were linked to improve provision of required "tools" for PPM.

It is important to segment health communications to address the specific language, cultural, gender specific, contextual and literacy needs in the MMPs. Well-developed and evidence-based IEC and BCC that are based on the needs, characteristics and culture of the MMPs including migrant workers are needed to increase knowledge of symptoms, prevention and control measures. In addition, sources and need for early diagnosis-based treatment and care and the risks associated with delays in treatment also need to be addressed. Community-based interventions and services through a network of village health workers and community volunteers to strengthen malaria prevention and control measures might be particularly useful for the MMPs who have limited access to health services [1, 27, 57].

Conclusions

The findings suggest that interventions supported by multiple stakeholders have a significant impact on reduction of malaria transmission in the targeted MMPs. It is important to realize that intersectoral action is a key strategy for various interventions targeted to those populations not usually reached by routine health services. A well-coordinated strengthened partnership of multiple stakeholders including employers of the targeted MMPs, public health sectors, other related ministries, private medical sectors and implementing NGOs is urgently needed to enhance the outcome of malaria control and elimination efforts targeting these often neglected and underserved populations. Well-designed studies from different countries to robustly assess the role of intersectoral interventions targeting the MMPs and the impact on the reduction of transmission are recommended.

Additional files

> **Additional file 1.** PRISMA checklist.
>
> **Additional file 2.** Excluded studies and the reasons for exclusion.
>
> **Additional file 3.** List of the stakeholders involved for malaria control among mobile and migrant populations.
>
> **Additional file 4.** Intersectoral involvement in the malaria intervention activities targeted to the mobile and migrant populations.

Abbreviations

ACD: active case detection; BCC: behaviour change communication; HE: health education; HPM: human population movement; HPA: Package of Health Poverty Action; IDP: internally displaced persons; IEC: information, education and communications; IOM: International organization for migration; ITC: insecticide treated clothing; ITN: insecticide treated nets; LLINs: long lasting insecticide treated nets; MARC: Myanmar Artemisinin Resistance Containment; MMP: mobile and migrant population; MOH: Ministry of Health; MOPH: Ministry of Public Health; NGO: non-governmental organizations; PCC: population, context, and contents; PPM: personal protective measures; PRISMA: Preferred Reporting Items for Systematic Reviews and Meta-Analyses; PSI: Population Services International; RBM: Roll Back Malaria; RCD: reactive case detection; RDT: rapid diagnostic test; TKMI: Trans-Kunene Malaria Initiative; UNDP: United Nations Development Programme; UNHCR: United Nations High Commission for Refugees; UNICEF: United Nations Children's Fund; WHO: World Health Organization.

Authors' contributions

Conceptualized: MT; Designed: MAW, CN; Data extracted: CN; Analysed: MT, MAW, CN; Interpreted: CN, MAW; CN: Drafted the manuscript together with MAW: MT: Added additional information. All authors read and approved the final manuscript.

Author details

[1] Institute for Research, Development and Innovation (IRDI), International Medical University, Kuala Lumpur, Malaysia. [2] Division of Tropical Health and Medicine, James Cook University, Townsville, QLD, Australia. [3] Swiss Tropical and Public Health Institute, Basel, Switzerland.

Acknowledgements

The authors are grateful to the UNICEF/UNDP/World Bank/WHO-the Special Programme for Research and Training in Tropical Diseases (TDR) for giving an opportunity to conduct this systematic review. The view expressed are solely those of the authors. We also thank the editors and anonymous reviewers for the comments provided and valuable input to improve the quality of manuscript. We thank our institutions for allowing us to perform this study and for providing us technical and administrative support. CN thanks Professor Joon Wah Mak for technical advice, Dr. Norah Htet Htet for assisting in the development of a conceptual framework and Dr Dinesh Kumar for additional input.

Competing interests

MAW and MT declare that they have no competing interests. CN is a recipient of a grant from the WHO/TDR (2017/721367-0).

Funding

WHO/TDR (2017/721367-0). The funders had no role in study design, data collection/analyses and manuscript preparation.

References

1. WHO. Global technical strategy and targets for malaria 2016–2030. Geneva: World Health Organization; 2015. http://www.who.int/malaria/areas/global_technical_strategy/en/. Accessed 12 May 2018.
2. WHO. Eliminating malaria. Geneva: World Health Organization; 2016. http://www.who.int/malaria/publications/atoz/eliminating-malaria/en/. Accessed 12 May 2018.
3. WHO. World malaria report 2017. Geneva: World Health Organization; 2017.
4. WHO. Mobile and migrant populations and malaria information systems. New Delhi, Geneva: SERO, World Health Organization; 2015.
5. Prothero RM. Disease and mobility: a neglected factor in epidemiology. Int J Epidemiol. 1977;6:259–67.
6. Bruce-Chwatt LJ. Malaria zoonosis in relation to malaria eradication. Trop Geogr Med. 1968;20:50–87.
7. Martens P, Hall L. Malaria on the move: human population movement and malaria transmission. Emerg Infect Dis. 2000;6:103–9.
8. Hay SI, Guerra CA, Tatem AJ, Noor AM, Snow RW. The global distribution and population at risk of malaria: past, present, and future. Lancet Infect Dis. 2004;4:327–36.
9. Cohen JM, Smith DL, Cotter C, Ward A, Yamey G, Sabot OJ, et al. Malaria resurgence: a systematic review and assessment of its causes. Malar J. 2012;11:122.
10. Sturrock HJW, Novotny JM, Kunene S, Dlamini S, Zulu Z, Cohen JM, et al. Reactive case detection for malaria elimination: real-life experience from an ongoing program in Swaziland. PLoS ONE. 2013;8:e63830.
11. Zimmerman C, Kiss L, Hossain M. Migration and health: a framework for 21st century policy-making. PLoS Med. 2011;8:e1001034.
12. IOM (International Organization for Migration). A global report on population mobility and malaria: moving towards elimination with migration in mind. 2013. https://www.iom.int/.../REPORT-14Aug2013-v3-FINAL-IOM-Global-Report-Populati. Accessed 1 March 2018.
13. Smith C, Whittaker M. Beyond mobile populations: a critical review of the literature on malaria and population mobility and suggestions for future directions. Malar J. 2014;13:307.
14. Mlozi MRS, Rumisha SF, Mlacha T, Bwana VM, Shayo EH, Mayala BK, et al. Challenges and opportunities for implementing an intersectoral approach in malaria control in Tanzania. Tanzania J Health Res. 2015;17:1–16.

15. Zhou G, Lo E, Zhong D, Wang X, Wang Y, Malla S, et al. Impact of interventions on malaria in internally displaced persons along the China–Myanmar border: 2011–2014. Malar J. 2016;15:471.
16. WHO. Intersectoral Action for Health (ISA). Geneva: World Health Organization; 2011 http://www.who.int/kobe_centre/interventions/intersectorial_action/ISA/en/ Accessed 6 February 2018.
17. Liberati A, Altman DG, Tetzlaff J, Mulrow C, Gotzsche PC, Ioannidis JP, et al. The PRISMA statement for reporting systematic reviews and meta-analyses of studies that evaluate healthcare interventions: explanation and elaboration. BMJ. 2009;339:b2700.
18. Institute The Joanna Briggs. Joanna Briggs Institute Reviewers' Manual: 2015 edition/Supplement. The Joanna Briggs Institute.: The University of Adelaide; 2017.
19. Ward M, Motus D, Mosca A. A global report on population mobility and malaria: Moving towards elimination with migration in mind. Geneva: International Organization for Migration; 2013.
20. IOM (International Organization for Migration). Malaria on the Move: Mapping of population migration and malaria in South-Eastern Region of Myanmar. 2012. https://reliefweb.int/report/myanmar/malaria-move-mapping-population-migration-and-malaria-south-eastern-region-myanmar. Accessed 6 February 2018.
21. UNHCR. Internally Displaced People. 2010. http://www.unhcr.org/en-my/internally-displaced-people.html. Accessed 6 February 2017. Accessed 9 March 2018.
22. Guyant P, Canavati SE, Chea N, Ly P, Whittaker MA, Roca-Feltrer A, et al. Malaria and the mobile and migrant population in Cambodia: a population movement framework to inform strategies for malaria control and elimination. Malar J. 2015;14:252.
23. Carrara VI, Sirilak S, Thonglairuam J, Rojanawatsirivet C, Proux S, Gilbos V, et al. Deployment of early diagnosis and mefloquineartesunate treatment of falciparum malaria in Thailand: The Tak Malaria Initiative. PLoS Med. 2006;3:e183.
24. Kolaczinski JH, Ojok N, Opwonya J, Meek S, Collins A. Adherence of community caretakers of children to pre-packaged antimalarial medicines (HOMAPAK®) among internally displaced people in Gulu district, Uganda. Malar J. 2006;5:40.
25. Lee TJ, Mullany LC, Richards AK, Kuiper HK, Maung C, Beyrer C. Mortality rates in conflict zones in Karen, Karenni, and Mon states in eastern Burma. Trop Med Int Health. 2006;11:119–27.
26. Mullany LC, Lee TJ, Yone L, Lee CI, Teela KC, Paw P, et al. Impact of community-based maternal health workers on coverage of essential maternal health interventions among internally displaced communities in eastern Burma: the MOM project. PLoS Med. 2010;7:e1000317.
27. Wangroongsarb P, Satimai W, Khamsiriwatchara A, Thwing J, Eliades JM, Kaewkungwal J, et al. Respondent-driven sampling on the Thailand-Cambodia border. II. Knowledge, perception, practice and treatment-seeking behavior of migrants in malaria endemic zones. Malar J. 2011;10:117.
28. Abeyasinghe RR, Galappaththy GNL, Gueye CS, Kahn JG, Feachem RG. Malaria control and elimination in Sri Lanka: documenting progress and success factors in a conflict setting. PLoS ONE. 2012;7:e43162.
29. Burns M, Rowland M, N'guessan R, Carneiro I, Beeche A, Ruiz SS, et al. Insecticide-treated plastic sheeting for emergency malaria prevention and shelter among displaced populations: an observational cohort study in a refugee setting in Sierra Leone. Am J Trop Med Hyg. 2012;87:242–50.
30. Hiwat H, Hardjopawiro LS, Takken W, Villegas L. Novel strategies lead to pre-elimination of malaria in previously high-risk areas in Suriname, South America. Malar J. 2012;11:10.
31. Qayum M, Zahur H, Ahmad N, Ilyas M, Khan A, Khan S. SPHERE-based assessment of knowledge and preventive measures related to malaria among the displaced population of Jalozai, Pakistan. J Pak Med Assoc. 2012;62:344–6.
32. Kirkby K, Galappaththy GN, Kurinczuk JJ, Rajapakse S, Fernando SD. Knowledge, attitudes and practices relevant to malaria elimination amongst resettled populations in a post-conflict district of northern Sri Lanka. Trans R Soc Trop Med Hyg. 2013;107:110–8.
33. Obol JH, Ononge S, Orach CG. Utilisation of insecticide treated nets among pregnant women in Gulu: a post conflict district in northern Uganda. Afr Health Sci. 2013;13:962–9.
34. Gueye CS, Gerigk M, Newby G, Lourenco C, Uusiku P, Liu J. Namibia's path toward malaria elimination: a case study of malaria strategies and costs along the northern border. BMC Public Health. 2014;14:1190.
35. Nyunt MH, Aye KM, Kyaw MP, Kyaw TT, Hlaing T, Oo K, et al. Challenges in universal coverage and utilization of insecticide-treated bed nets in migrant plantation workers in Myanmar. Malar J. 2014;13:211.
36. Wai KT, Kyaw MP, Oo T, Zaw P, Nyunt MH, Thida M, et al. Spatial distribution, work patterns, and perception towards malaria interventions among temporary mobile/migrant workers in artemisinin resistance containment zone. BMC Public Health. 2014;14:463.
37. Hlaing T, Wai KT, Oo T, Sint N, Min T, Myar S, et al. Mobility dynamics of migrant workers and their socio-behavioral parameters related to malaria in Tier II, artemisinin resistance containment zone, Myanmar. BMC Public Health. 2015;15:886.
38. MOH Malaysia, WHO, UCSF. Eliminating malaria: case-study 8. Progress towards elimination in Malaysia. Geneva: World Health Organization; 2015.
39. Nyunt MH, Aye KM, Kyaw MP, Wai KT, Oo T, Than A, et al. Evaluation of the behaviour change communication and community mobilization activities in Myanmar artemisinin resistance containment zones. Malar J. 2015;14:522.
40. Peeters GK, Gryseels C, Dierickx S, Bannister-Tyrrell M, Trienekens S, Uk S, et al. Characterizing types of human mobility to inform differential and targeted malaria elimination strategies in Northeast Cambodia. Sci Rep. 2015;5:16837.
41. Schicker RS, Hiruy N, Melak B, Gelaye W, Bezabih B, Stephenson R, et al. A venue-based survey of malaria, anemia and mobility patterns among migrant farm workers in Amhara Region, Ethiopia. PLoS One. 2015;10:e0143829.
42. Castellanos A, Chaparro-Narvaez P, Morales-Plaza CD, Alzate A, Padilla J, Arevalo M, et al. Malaria in gold-mining areas in Colombia. Mem Inst Oswaldo Cruz. 2016;111:59–66.
43. Canavati SE, Quintero CE, Lawford HL, Yok S, Lek D, Richards JS, et al. High mobility, low access thwarts interventions among seasonal workers in the Greater Mekong Sub-region: lessons from the malaria containment project. Malar J. 2016;15:434.
44. Charchuk R, Paul MK, Claude KM, Houston S, Hawkes MT. Burden of malaria is higher among children in an internal displacement camp compared to a neighbouring village in the Democratic Republic of the Congo. Malar J. 2016;15:431.
45. de Santi VP, Djossou F, Barthes N, Bogreau H, Hyvert G, Nguyen C, et al. Malaria hyperendemicity and risk for artemisinin resistance among illegal gold miners, French Guiana. Emerg Infect Dis. 2016;22:903–6.
46. Douine M, Musset L, Corlin F, Pelleau S, Pasquier J, Mutricy L, et al. Prevalence of *Plasmodium* spp. in illegal gold miners in French Guiana in 2015: a hidden but critical malaria reservoir. Malar J. 2016;15:315.
47. Krisher LK, Krisher J, Ambuludi M, Arichabala A, Beltrán-Ayala E, Navarrete P, et al. Successful malaria elimination in the Ecuador–Peru border region: epidemiology and lessons learned. Malar J. 2016;15:573.
48. Nyunt MH, Aye KM, Kyaw KT, Han SS, Aye TT, Wai KT, et al. Challenges encountered by local health volunteers in early diagnosis and prompt treatment of malaria in Myanmar artemisinin resistance containment zones. Malar J. 2016;15:308.
49. Vezenegho SB, Adde A, de Pommier Santi V, Issaly J, Carinci R, Gaborit P, et al. High malaria transmission in a forested malaria focus in French Guiana: How can exophagic *Anopheles darlingi* thwart vector control and prevention measures? Mem Inst Oswaldo Cruz. 2016;111:561–9.
50. Zhang J, Dong JQ, Li JY, Zhang Y, Tian Y-H, Sun X-Y, et al. Effectiveness and impact of the cross-border healthcare model as implemented by non-governmental organizations: case study of the malaria control programs by health poverty action on the China–Myanmar border. Infect Dis Poverty. 2016;5:80.
51. Crawshaw AF, Maung TM, Shafique M, Sint N, Nicholas S, Li MS, et al. Acceptability of insecticide-treated clothing for malaria prevention among migrant rubber tappers in Myanmar: a cluster-randomized non-inferiority crossover trial. Malar J. 2017;16:92.
52. Kounnavong S, Gopinath D, Hongvanthong B, Khamkong C, Sichanthongthip O. Malaria elimination in Lao PDR: the challenges associated with population mobility. Infect Dis Poverty. 2017;6:81.
53. Ly P, Thwing J, McGinn C. The use of respondent-driven sampling to assess malaria knowledge, treatment-seeking behaviours and preventive practices among mobile and migrant populations in a setting of artemisinin resistance in Western Cambodia. Malar J. 2017;16:378.

54. Phyo Than W, Oo T, Wai KT, Thi A, Owiti P, Kumar B, et al. Knowledge, access and utilization of bed-nets among stable and seasonal migrants in an artemisinin resistance containment area of Myanmar. Infect Dis Poverty. 2017;6:138.

55. Soe HZ, Thi A, Aye NN. Socioeconomic and behavioural determinants of malaria among the migrants in gold mining, rubber and oil palm plantation areas in Myanmar. Infect Dis Poverty. 2017;6:142.

56. WHO. ALMA-ATA Primary Health care. Geneva: World Health Organization; 1978. p. 1978.

57. Public Health Agency of Canada (PHAC)-WHO. Crossing sectors- experiences in intersectoral action, public policy and health. 2008.

58. Moore SJ, Min X, Hill N, Jones C, Zaixing Z, Cameron MM. Border malaria in China: knowledge and use of personal protection by minority populations and implications for malaria control: a questionnaire-based survey. BMC Public Health. 2008;8:344.

59. WHO. Disease surveillance for malaria elimination: an operational manual. Geneva: World Health Organization; 2012.

60. Jacobson JO, Cueto C, Smith JL, Hwang J, Gosling R, Bennett A. Surveillance and response for high-risk populations: what can malaria elimination programmes learn from the experience of HIV? Malar J. 2017;16:33.

Permissions

List of Contributors

Ellen Bruske and Matthias Frank
Institute of Tropical Medicine, University of Tuebingen, Wilhelmstr. 27, 72074 Tuebingen, Germany

Thomas D. Otto
Malaria Programme, Wellcome Trust Sanger Institute, Hinxton CB10 1SA, UK
Present Address: Centre of Immunobiology,Institute of Infection, Immunity & Inflammation, College of Medical, Veterinary and Life Sciences, University of Glasgow, Glasgow, UK

Oléfongo Dagnogo and Joseph Allico Djaman
UFR Biosciences, Félix Houphouët-Boigny University, BP V 34, Abidjan 01, Côte d'Ivoire
Institut Pasteur of Côte d'Ivoire, 01 BP 490, Abidjan 01, Côte d'Ivoire

Aristide Berenger Ako, David N'golo Coulibaly and André Offianan Touré
Institut Pasteur of Côte d'Ivoire, 01 BP 490, Abidjan 01, Côte d'Ivoire

Lacinan Ouattara
Department of Food Science and Technology, Nangui Abrogoua University, 02 BP 801, Abidjan 02, Côte d'Ivoire

Noel Dougba Dago
UFR Sciences Biologiques, Péléforo Gon Coulibaly University, BP1328 Korhogo, Côte d'Ivoire

Angel Dillip
Ifakara Health Institute, Dar-es-Salaam, Tanzania

Zawadi M. Mboma and Lena M. Lorenz
Ifakara Health Institute, Dar-es-Salaam, Tanzania
London School of Hygiene and Tropical Medicine, London, UK

Karen Kramer
National Malaria Control Programme, Dar-es-Salaam, Tanzania
Swiss Tropical and Public Health Institute, Basel,Switzerland
University of Basel, Petersplatz 1, 4003 Basel, Switzerland

Hannah Koenker
PMI VectorWorks, Johns Hopkins Center for Communication Programs, Baltimore, MD, USA

George Greer
U.S. President's Malaria Initiative, U.S. Agency for International Development, Dar es Salaam, Tanzania

Gerardo Rojo-Marcos
Hospital Universitario Príncipe de Asturias, Ctra de Meco s/n, 28805 Alcalá de Henares, Madrid, Spain

José Miguel Rubio-Muñoz
Instituto de Salud Carlos III, Majadahonda, Madrid, Spain

Andrea Angheben
Ospedale Sacro Cuore - Don Calabria, Negrar, Verona, Italy

García-Rodríguez
Hospital General Universitario de Valencia, Valencia, Spain

Israel Molina-Romero
11 Hospital Vall D´Hebron-Drassanes, Barcelona, Spain

Rogelio López-Vélez
Hospital Universitario Ramón y Cajal, Madrid, Spain

Esteban Martin-Echevarría
Hospital Universitario de Guadalajara, Guadalajara, Spain

Matilde Elía-López
Complejo Hospitalario de Navarra, Pamplona, Navarra, Spain

José Llovo-Taboada
Complejo Hospitalario Universitario de Santiago de Compostela, A Coruña, Spain

Fiona Macintyre, Hanu Ramachandruni, Jeremy N. Burrows, Anna Thomas, Jörg J. Möhrle, Stephan Duparc, Rob Hooft van Huijsduijnen, Winston E. Gutteridge, Timothy N. C. Wells and Wiweka Kaszubska
Medicines for Malaria Venture, Route de Pré Bois 20, 1215 Geneva, Switzerland

René Holm
Drug Product Development, Janssen R&D, Johnson & Johnson, Turnhoutseweg 30, 2340 Beerse, Belgium
Department of Science and Environment, Roskilde University, 4000 Roskilde, Denmark

Brian Greenwood
Faculty of Infectious and Tropical Diseases, London School of Hygiene and Tropical Medicine, London, UK

Nicholas J. White
Faculty of Tropical Medicine, Mahidol University, Bangkok, Thailand
Centre for Tropical Medicine and Global Health, Nuffield Department of Medicine, University of Oxford, Oxford, UK

Madhavinadha Prasad Kona, Raghavendra Kamaraju, Rajendra Mohan Bhatt, Nutan Nanda, Mehul Kumar Chourasia, Dipak Kumar Swain, Shrity Suman, Sreehari and Uragayala
ICMR-National Institute of Malaria Research, Sector-8, Dwarka, New Delhi 110077, India

Martin James Donnelly
Liverpool School of Tropical Medicine, Liverpool, UK

Immo Kleinschmidt
Department of Infectious Disease Epidemiology, London School of Hygiene and Tropical Medicine, London, UK

Veena Pandey
Department of Biotechnology, Kumaun University, Nainital, India

Kyaw Thu Hein, Thae Maung Maung and Kyaw Ko Ko Htet
Department of Medical Research, Ministry of Health and Sports, Yangon, Myanmar

Hemant Deepak Shewade and Jaya Prasad Tripathy
International Union Against Tuberculosis and Lung Disease (The Union), South-East Asia Office, New Delhi, India
International Union Against Tuberculosis and Lung Disease (The Union), Paris, France

Swai Mon Oo
Population Services International, Yangon, Myanmar

Zaw Lin
Vector Borne Disease Control Program, Ministry of Health and Sports, Nay Pyi Taw, Myanmar

Aung Thi
National Malaria ControlProgram, Ministry of Health and Sports, Nay Pyi Taw, Myanmar

Oleg Mediannikov
Aix Marseille Univ, IRD, AP-HM, MEPHI, IHU-Méditerranée Infection, Marseille, France

El Hadji Amadou Niang
Aix Marseille Univ, IRD, AP-HM, MEPHI, IHU-Méditerranée Infection, Marseille, France
Laboratoire d'Ecologie Vectorielle et Parasitaire, Faculté des Sciences et Techniques, Université Cheikh Anta Diop, Dakar, Senegal
VITROME,Campus International, UCAD-IRD, Dakar, Senegal

Hubert Bassene
VITROME,Campus International, UCAD-IRD, Dakar, Senegal
Aix Marseille Univ, IRD, AP-HM, SSA, VITROME, IHU-Méditerranée Infection, Marseille, France

Florence Fenollar
Aix Marseille Univ, IRD, AP-HM, SSA, VITROME, IHU-Méditerranée Infection, Marseille, France

Patrick Makoundou and Mylène Weill
Institut des Sciences de l'Evolution (ISEM), CNRS-Université de Montpellier-IRD-EPHE, Montpellier, France

Richard Eastman, Carleen Klumpp-Thomas, Crystal McKnight and Craig Thomas
National Center for Advancing Translational Sciences, National Institutes of Health, Bethesda, MD, USA

Kimberly F. Breglio
National Center for Advancing Translational Sciences, National Institutes of Health, Bethesda, MD, USA
Nuffield Department of Medicine, University of Oxford, Oxford, UK

Rajarshi Guha
National Center for Advancing Translational Sciences, National Institutes of Health, Bethesda, MD, USA.
Vertex Pharmaceuticals, Boston, MA, USA

Roberto Amato
Wellcome Sanger Institute, Wellcome Genome Campus, Hinxton, Cambridge, UK

Pharath Lim, Juliana M. Sa, Sundar Ganesan and Rick M. Fairhurst
National Institute of Allergy and Infectious Diseases, National Institutes of Health, Bethesda, MD, USA

David W. Dorward
Rocky Mountain Laboratories, National Institute of Allergy and Infectious Diseases, National Institutes of Health, Bethesda, MD, USA

David Roberts
Radcliffe Department of Medicine, Medical Sciences Division, University of Oxford, Oxford, UK

Anna Katharina Simon
Kennedy Institute of Rheumatology and Medical Research Council Human Immunology Unit, Weatherall Institute of Molecular Medicine, University of Oxford, Oxford, UK

Martin C. Akogbeto
Centre de Recherche entomologique de Cotonou (CREC), Cotonou, Benin

Albert S. Salako, Idelphonse Ahogni and Casimir Kpanou
Centre de Recherche entomologique de Cotonou (CREC), Cotonou, Benin
Faculté des Sciences et Techniques de l'Université d'Abomey-Calavi, Abomey-Calavi, Benin

Roseric Azondekon
Centre de Recherche entomologique de Cotonou (CREC), Cotonou, Benin
University of Wisconsin Milwaukee, Milwaukee, WI, USA

André A. Sominahouin
Centre de Recherche entomologique de Cotonou (CREC), Cotonou, Benin
Faculté des Sciences Humaines et Sociales de l'Université d'Abomey-Calavi, Abomey-Calavi, Benin

Arthur Sovi
PMI VectorLink Project, Abt Associates, Bamako, Mali

Filémon Tokponnon
Programme Nationale de Lutte contre le Paludisme, Cotonou, Benin

Virgile Gnanguenon
PMI VectorLink Project, Abt Associates, Bujumbura, Burundi

Fortuné Dagnon
US President's Malaria Initiative, US Agency for International Development, Cotonou, Benin

Laurent Iyikirenga
PMI VectorLink Project, Abt Associates, Cotonou, Benin

Luis L. Fonseca and Eberhard O. Voit
The Wallace H. Coulter Department of Biomedical Engineering, Georgia Institute of Technology and Emory University, Atlanta, GA 30332-2000, USA
Malaria Host–Pathogen Interaction Center, Emory Vaccine Center, Yerkes National Primate Research Center, Emory University, Atlanta, GA 30322, USA

The MaHPIC Consortium
Malaria Host–Pathogen Interaction Center, Emory Vaccine Center, Yerkes National Primate Research Center, Emory University, Atlanta, GA 30322, USA

Chester J. Joyner, Celia L. Saney, Alberto Moreno and Mary R. Galinski
Malaria Host–Pathogen Interaction Center, Emory Vaccine Center, Yerkes National Primate Research Center, Emory University, Atlanta, GA 30322, USA
Division of Infectious Diseases, Department of Medicine, Emory University, Atlanta, GA 30322, USA

John W. Barnwell
Malaria Host–Pathogen Interaction Center, Emory Vaccine Center, Yerkes National Primate Research Center, Emory University, Atlanta, GA 30322, USA

Malaria Branch, Division of Parasitic Diseases and Malaria, Centers for Disease Control and Prevention, Atlanta, GA 30322,USA

Endalew Zemene and Abebaw Tiruneh
School of Medical Laboratory Sciences, Faculty of Health Sciences, Jimma University, Jimma, Ethiopia

Delenasaw Yewhalaw
School of Medical Laboratory Sciences, Faculty of Health Sciences, Jimma University, Jimma, Ethiopia
Tropical and Infectious Diseases Research Centre, Jimma University, Jimma, Ethiopia

Cristian Koepfli, Ming-Chieh Lee and Guiyun Yan
Program in Public Health, College of Health Sciences, University of California at Irvine, Irvine, CA 92697, USA

Asnakew K. Yeshiwondim
PATH/MACEPA, Addis Ababa, Ethiopia

Dinberu Seyoum
Department of Statistics, College of Natural Sciences,Jimma University, Jimma, Ethiopia

Welbeck A. Oumbouke, Alphonsine A. Koffi and Raphael N'Guessan
Department of Disease Control, London School of Hygiene and Tropical Medicine, London, UK
Institut Pierre Richet (IPR)/Institut National de Santé Publique (INSP), Bouaké, Côte d'Ivoire

Innocent Z. Tia
Institut Pierre Richet (IPR)/Institut National de Santé Publique (INSP), Bouaké, Côte d'Ivoire

Antoine M. G. Barreaux, Eleanore D. Sternberg and Matthew B. Thomas
Department of Entomology, Center for Infectious Disease Dynamics, The Pennsylvania State University, University Park, PA 16802, USA

Halfan S. Ngowo
Environmental Health and Ecological Sciences Department, Ifakara Health Institute, Kiko Avenue, Mikocheni, Dar es Salaam, United Republic of Tanzania

Irene R. Moshi
Environmental Health and Ecological Sciences Department, Ifakara Health Institute, Kiko Avenue, Mikocheni, , Dar es Salaam, United Republic of Tanzania

School of Public Health, Faculty of Health Sciences, University of the Witwatersrand, Parktown, Johannesburg, South Africa

Ladislaus L. Mnyone
Environmental Health and Ecological Sciences Department, Ifakara Health Institute, Kiko Avenue, Mikocheni, , Dar es Salaam, United Republic of Tanzania
School of Public Health, Faculty of Health Sciences, University of the Witwatersrand, Parktown, Johannesburg, South Africa
Sokoine University of Agriculture, Pest Management Centre, , Morogoro, Tanzania

Fredros O. Okumu
Environmental Health and Ecological Sciences Department, Ifakara Health Institute, Kiko Avenue, Mikocheni, , Dar es Salaam, United Republic of Tanzania
School of Public Health, Faculty of Health Sciences, University of the Witwatersrand, Parktown, Johannesburg, South Africa
Institut de Recherche en Sciences de la Santé, Bobo-Dioulasso, Burkina Faso
Institute of Biodiversity, Animal Health and Comparative Medicine, University of Glasgow, Glasgow G12 8QQ, UK

Yeromin P. Mlacha
Environmental Health and Ecological Sciences Department, Ifakara Health Institute, Kiko Avenue, Mikocheni, Dar es Salaam, United Republic of Tanzania
Swiss Tropical and Public Health Institute (Swiss TPH), Basel, Switzerland
University of Basel, Basel, Switzerland
Sokoine University of Agriculture, Pest Management Centre, , Morogoro, Tanzania

Lenore Manderson
School of Public Health, Faculty of Health Sciences, University of the Witwatersrand, Parktown, Johannesburg, South Africa

Kanako Komaki-Yasuda
Department of Tropical Medicine and Malaria, Research Institute, National Center for Global Health and Medicine, Tokyo 162-8655, Japan

Jeanne Perpétue Vincent
Department of Tropical Medicine and Malaria, Research Institute, National Center for Global Health and Medicine, Tokyo 162-8655, Japan
Graduate School of Comprehensive Human Sciences, University of Tsukuba, Ibaraki 305-8575, Japan

Shigeyuki Kano
Department of Tropical Medicine and Malaria, Research Institute, National Center for Global Health and Medicine, Tokyo 162-8655, Japan.
Graduate School of Comprehensive Human Sciences, University of Tsukuba, Ibaraki 305-8575, Japan.
SATREPS Project for Parasitic Diseases, Vientiane, Lao People's Democratic Republic

Satoru Kawai
Department of Tropical Medicine and Parasitology, Dokkyo Medical University, Tochigi 321-0293, Japan.
SATREPS Project for Parasitic Diseases, Vientiane, Lao People's Democratic Republic

Moritoshi Iwagami
Department of Tropical Medicine and Malaria, Research Institute, National Center for Global Health and Medicine, Tokyo 162-8655, Japan
SATREPS Project for Parasitic Diseases, Vientiane, Lao People's Democratic Republic

Amy Lynd, Ambrose Oruni, Arjen E. van't Hof, John C. Morgan, Dimitra Pipini, Kevin A. O'Kines, Martin J. Donnelly and David Weetman
Liverpool School of Tropical Medicine, Liverpool, UK

Leon Bwazumo Naego
Avenue de l'infirmerie, Quartier Yola Bokonzo, Gemena, Sud Ubangi, Democratic Republic of Congo

Thierry L. Bobanga
University of Kinshasa, Kinshasa, Democratic Republic of Congo

Bolanle Olapeju, Matthew Lynch, Angela Acosta, Sean Blaufuss, Eric Filemyr, Hunter Harig, April Monroe, Richmond Ato Selby and Hannah Koenker
PMI VectorWorks Project, Johns Hopkins Center for Communication Programs, School of Public Health, 111 Marketplace, Baltimore, MD 21202, USA

Ifta Choiriyyah
Department of Population, Family and Reproductive Health, Johns Hopkins University Bloomberg School of Public Health, Baltimore, USA

Albert Kilian
PMI Vector- Works Project, Tropical Health LLP, Montagut, Spain

Cho Naing
Institute for Research, Development and Innovation (IRDI), International Medical University, Kuala Lumpur, Malaysia
Division of Tropical Health and Medicine, James Cook University, Townsville, QLD, Australia

Maxine A. Whittaker
Division of Tropical Health and Medicine, James Cook University, Townsville, QLD, Australia.

Marcel Tanner
Swiss Tropical and Public Health Institute, Basel, Switzerland

Index

www.ingramcontent.com/pod-product-compliance
Lightning Source LLC
Chambersburg PA
CBHW061300190326
41458CB00011B/3725